Hand and Upper Extremity Rehabilitation

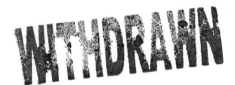

THIRD EDITION

Hand and Upper Extremity Rehabilitation

A PRACTICAL GUIDE

Editors

Susan L. Burke, OTR/L, CHT, MBA
Regional Director, Hand and Upper
 Extremity Program
Department of Hand Therapy
Curtis National Hand Center
Union Memorial Hospital
Baltimore, Maryland

James P. Higgins, MD
Attending Hand Surgeon
Curtis National Hand Center
Union Memorial Hospital
Baltimore, Maryland

Michael A. McClinton, MD
Attending Hand Surgeon
Curtis National Hand Center
Union Memorial Hospital
Baltimore, Maryland

Rebecca J. Saunders, PT, CHT
Senior Hand Therapist and Upper
 Extremity Physical Therapist
Department of Hand Therapy
Curtis National Hand Center
Union Memorial Hospital
Baltimore, Maryland

Lauren Valdata, PT, CHT
Senior Hand Therapist and Upper
 Extremity Physical Therapist
Department of Hand Therapy
Curtis National Hand Center
Union Memorial Hospital
Baltimore, Maryland

Illustrator **Joyce Lavery**

Photographer **Mark Swisher**

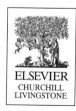

ELSEVIER
CHURCHILL
LIVINGSTONE

ELSEVIER
CHURCHILL
LIVINGSTONE

11830 Westline Industrial Drive
St. Louis, Missouri 63146

HAND AND UPPER EXTREMITY REHABILITATION
Copyright © 2006, 1998, 1993 by Elsevier Inc.

NOTICE

ISBN-13: 978-0-443-06663-4
ISBN-10: 0-443-06663-9

Acquisitions Editor: Kathy Falk
Publishing Services Manager: Patricia Tannian
Project Manager: Kristine Feeherty
Designer: Amy Buxton

Printed in the United States of America

Last digit is the print number: 9 8 7 6 5 4 3

To the founders of Union Memorial Hospital's Raymond M. Curtis Hand Center:
Raymond M. Curtis, MD
E.F. Shaw Wilgis, MD
Gaylord L. Clark, MD
Frederik C. Hansen, Jr., MD
Rodney W. Schlegel, PT, ECS, and
Janice Maynard, OTR,
and to all of the hand and upper extremity patients past, present, and future

Contributors

Lauren Adelsberger, OTR/L, CHT
Occupational Therapist
Curtis National Hand Center
Union Memorial Hospital
Baltimore, Maryland

Bonnie J. Aiello, PT, CHT
Physical Therapist
Regional Rehab at Pasadena
Pasadena, Maryland

Mallory S. Anthony, RPT, MMSc, CHT
Formerly with Curtis National
  Hand Center
Union Memorial Hospital
Baltimore, Maryland

Romina P. Astifidis, MS, PT, CHT
Clinic Manager and Physical
  Therapist
Curtis National Hand Center at
  Lutherville
Lutherville, Maryland
Regional Rehabilitation at National
  Rehabilitation Hospital
Baltimore, Maryland

Tara Barasch, MOT, OTR/L
Occupational Therapist
Curtis National Hand Center at
  Lutherville
Lutherville, Maryland

Judith Bell-Krotoski, OTR, CHT, FAOTA
Captain, USPHS (Ret.)
Private Teaching and Consulting
Hand Therapy Research;
Former Chief Hand and OT/
  Clinical Research Therapist
USPHS National Hansen's
  Disease Programs
Baton Rouge, Louisiana

Nicole E. Bickhart, OTR/L, CHT
Staff Hand Therapist
Outpatient Rehabilitation
NRH Regional Rehab at
  Pasadena
Pasadena, Maryland

Arlynne Pack Brown, PT, MPH
Formerly with Curtis National
  Hand Center
Union Memorial Hospital
Baltimore, Maryland

Ronald Burgess, MD
Clinical Associate Professor of
  Orthopedic Surgery
University of Kentucky
Lexington, Kentucky
Clincical Associate Professor of
  Orthopaedic Surgery
University of Cincinnati
Cincinnati, Ohio

Gregory K. Davis, MPT, CHT
Senior Staff Therapist
Hand & Orthopedic Physical
 Therapy Associates
Levittown, Pennsylvania

Heather DeLaney, DPT, OCS
Clinic Director
Physiotherapy Associates
Baltimore, Maryland

Lauren M. DeTullio, MS, OTR/L
Hand Therapist, Occupational
 Therapist
Hand Therapy Department
The Philadelphia Hand Center, P.C.
King of Prussia, Pennsylvania

**Frank DiGiovannantonio,
OTR, CHT**
Chief Operating Officer
Rehabilitation Centers of Southern
 Maryland
Waldorf, Maryland

Dale Eckhaus, OTR/L, CHT
Senior Hand Therapist
Curtis National Hand Center
Union Memorial Hospital
Baltimore, Maryland

Anne Edmonds, PT, CHT
Physical Therapist
Physiotherapy Associates
Clarksville, Maryland

Juan Martin Favetto, MD
Clinical Instructor
Division of Hand Surgery
University of Louisville School of
 Medicine
Louisville, Kentucky
President of Medical Staff
St. Joseph East Hospital
Lexington, Kentucky

Mary Formby, OTR, CHT
Clinical Specialist
Curtis National Hand Center
Union Memorial Hospital
Baltimore, Maryland

**Gregory A. Hritcko, MS, OTR/L,
CHT**
Director
Hand Therapy of Greater
 Binghamton
Johnson City, New York

Robert C. Kahlert, OTR/L, CHT
Industrial Rehabilitation Clinical
 Specialist
Curtis Work Rehabilitation Services
Union Memorial Hospital
Baltimore, Maryland

**Donna M. Keegan, M.Ed, CRC,
CVE**
Program Coordinator
Curtis Work Rehabilitation
 Services
Curtis National Hand Center
Union Memorial Hospital
Baltimore, Maryland

Brenda A. Kelly, PT, CHT
Senior Physical Therapist
Department of Rehabilitation
 Therapies
University of Iowa Hospitals and
 Clinics
Iowa City, Iowa

**Michele A. Klein, OTR/L,
CHT**
Senior Hand Therapist
Curtis National Hand Center
Union Memorial Hospital
Baltimore, Maryland

Barbra J. Koczan, MPT, CHT
Physical Therapist
Outpatient Hand Rehab
Curtis National Hand Center at
 Lutherville
Lutherville, Maryland

**Beth Farrell Kozera, OTR,
CHT**
Director of Hand Therapy
Rehabilitation Division
Orthopaedic Specialty Center
Owings Mills, Maryland

Scott H. Kozin, MD
Associate Professor
Department of Orthopaedic Surgery
Temple University;
Attending Hand Surgeon
Shriners Hospital for Children
Philadelphia, Pennsylvania

Paige E. Kurtz, MS, OTR/L, CHT
Senior Hand Therapist
HealthSouth Rehabilitation Center
Melbourne, Florida

Rebecca N. Larson, OTR/L
Occupational Therapist
Outpatient Hand Therapy
Tracy Caulkins Physiotherapy
  Center
Lebanon, Tennessee

Georgiann F. Laseter, OTR, FAOTA, CHT
Hand Rehabilitation Services
Dallas, Texas

Jason Leadbetter, PT
Clinical Coordinator, Physical
  Therapist
Union Memorial Sports Medicine
  at Stadium Place
Baltimore, Maryland

Ann Leman-Domenici, LCSW-C
Clinical Social Worker
Hand Therapy
Curtis National Hand Center
Union Memorial Hospital
Baltimore, Maryland

Linda Luca, OTR/L, CHT
Senior Hand Therapist
Curtis National Hand Center
Union Memorial Hospital
Baltimore, Maryland

Cheryl S. Lutz, MS, OTR/L
Upper Extremity Team Leader
Shriners Hospital for Children
Philadelphia, Pennsylvania

Gary M. Lynch, MS, PT, ATC, CSCS
Owner
Gary M. Lynch Physical
  Therapy
Forest Hill, Maryland

William McKay, OTR/L, CHT
Lead Hand Therapist
Montgomery Orthopaedics
Kensington, Maryland

Shelby Moore, PTA
Physical Therapist Assistant
Outpatient Hand Therapy
Curtis National Hand Center at
  Lutherville
Lutherville, Maryland

Mary Schuler Murphy, OTR/L, CHT
Clinical Specialist
Curtis National Hand Center
Union Memorial Hospital
Baltimore, Maryland

William L. O'Neill, Jr, MD
Clinical Instructor
Division of Hand Surgery
University of Louisville School of
  Medicine
Louisville, Kentucky
Chief of Plastic Surgery
Saint Joseph Healthcare
Lexington, Kentucy

Greg Pitts, MS, OTR/L, CHT
Clinical Director, Rehab
Kentucky Hand and Physical
  Therapy
Lexington, Kentucky

Rebecca J. Saunders, PT, CHT
Senior Hand Therapist and Upper
  Extremity Physical Therapist
Department of Hand Therapy
Curtis National Hand Center
Union Memorial Hospital
Baltimore, Maryland

Jane Imle Schmidt, PT, CHT
Hand Therapy Coordinator
Central Maryland Rehabilitation
  Center
Columbia, Maryland

Terri M. Skirven, OTR/L, CHT
Director
Hand Therapy
The Philadelphia Hand Center, P.C.
King of Prussia, Pennsylvania

Corie Sullivan, OTR/L, CHT
Occupational Therapist
Outpatient Network
NRH Regional Rehab
Baltimore, Maryland

Lorie Theisen, OTR/L, CHT
Clinic Manager
Regional Rehab at Pasadena
Pasadena, Maryland

Stephen C. Umansky, MD
Attending Hand Surgeon
Section of Orthopedics and Sports
  Medicine
Lexington Clinic
Lexington, Kentucky

Lauren Valdata, PT, CHT
Senior Hand Therapist and Upper
  Extremity Physical Therapist
Department of Hand Therapy
Curtis National Hand Center
Union Memorial Hospital
Baltimore, Maryland

Tracy Videon, MPT, ATC
Union Memorial Sports Medicine
  Center at Bel Air
Bel Air, Maryland

J. Martin Walsh, OTR/L, CHT
Adjunct Instructor
Hand Therapy Certification
  Program
Samuel Merritt College
Oakland, California
Hand Occupational Therapist
Outpatient Occupational Therapy
  Department
Sutter Roseville Medical Center
Roseville, California

Mark T. Walsh, PT, MS, CHT, ATC
Instructor
Programs in Rehabilitation Sciences
Drexel University
Philadelphia, Pennsylvania
Co-owner and President
Hand & Orthopedic Physical
  Therapy Associates
Levittown, Pennsylvania

Linda Coll Ware, OTR, CHT
Occupational Therapist
Rehabilitation Department
Johns Hopkins Bayview Medical
  Center
Baltimore, Maryland

Jason A. Willoughby, OTR/L, CHT
Managing Partner
Kentucky Hand and Physical
  Therapy, PLLC
Lexington, Kentucky

Barbara Wilson, ORT/L, CHT
Senior Occupational Therapist
Curtis National Hand Center
Union Memorial Hospital
Baltimore, Maryland

Foreword

Throughout my career, I have been fortunate to witness the growth of hand care from scattered pockets of expertise across the country to nearly uniform availability of quality surgery and therapy. During that same interval, I have also witnessed the growth of Union Memorial Hospital's leadership in providing and teaching quality care for diseased and injured hands. And now I see further growth of a work that is already classic—*Hand and Upper Extremity Rehabilitation: A Practical Guide*.

The growth in these three areas is not unrelated or coincidental. At the end of World War II, Dr. Raymond M. Curtis caught a zeal for perfection in hand care from the founding members of the American Society for Surgery of the Hand. He settled in Baltimore and quietly developed his expertise. More important, he shared his passion with all who would listen. I met Dr. Curtis when I was a junior orthopedic surgery resident in the 1970s. While we residents ate our lunch in the doctors' dining room at Children's Hospital, Dr. Curtis would mark up paper placemats with anatomical sketches and explain to us the details of the morning's surgical procedures. Practically hoarse, he would suddenly look at his watch, realize that it was time to return to the operating room, take a quick sip of tea, and head back to work, his lunch untouched. His passion was infectious. Testimony of it today is the eminence of the Curtis National Hand Center at Union Memorial Hospital, the understated elegance of quality care and teaching represented in *Hand and Upper Extremity Rehabilitation: A Practical Guide*, and the book's daily use worldwide.

Readers unfamiliar with the first (1993) and second (1998) editions of *Hand Rehabilitation: A Practical Guide* will quickly come to value the succinct melding of everyday useful advice from surgeons and therapists. This should come as no surprise because Dr. Curtis gathered general, orthopedic, and plastic surgeons as well as physical and occupational therapists around him to share every expertise available. We visual learners also value greatly the frequent inclusion of photographs and line drawings. Those readers who have worn out copies of the first two editions should unhesitatingly take the third edition to heart as well. New chapters include more shoulder topics, which are entirely related to the global "hand," and more wrist topics, which reflect the flurry of current research on this, the body's most compact, complex linkage of joints. Evidence-based practice of hand therapy also makes its debut, a valuable addition that would undoubtedly bring a twinkle to Dr. Curtis's eye, for he was originally from Missouri, the "Show Me State." And in a broader sense, that is exactly what *Hand and Upper Extremity Rehabilitation: A Practical Guide* does.

Everyone holding this book, by only a few degrees of separation at most, benefits from Dr. Curtis's passion for perfection in hand care and hand care education. Read the book. Share the passion.

Roy A. Meals, MD
Clinical Professor of Orthopaedic Surgery
UCLA School of Medicine
Los Angeles, California

Preface

Hand and Upper Extremity Rehabilitation: A Practical Guide provides therapists with a quick-reference overview and treatment guidelines for conditions commonly seen in a hand therapy clinic. This third edition retains the structure of the previous editions but has been thoroughly updated with new chapters, outcomes data to guide patient expectations from therapy, and updated text and references throughout. The contributors to this edition come from within the Curtis National Hand Center at Union Memorial Hospital and their affiliates and from leading hand therapists across the country.

This text is intended for both the new and experienced therapist when treating a patient with a given diagnosis. The outline format with numerous illustrations and photographs provides a thorough but efficient guide for the therapist and treatment recommendations. The book can be studied as a text or consulted in preparation for a clinical session.

This edition also offers a chapter on research in hand therapy with a focus on internet resources as more outcomes information becomes available. We believe the coming years will bring new insights in treatment of patients with hand injury or dysfunction. Hand therapists can have an important role in research efforts to improve treatment.

As in the previous editions, we hope the third edition provides a valuable resource for quality care of hand and upper extremity patients.

Susan L. Burke
James P. Higgins
Michael A. McClinton
Rebecca J. Saunders
Lauren Valdata

Acknowledgments

We thank Dr. Richard Hinton of Orthopaedics Sports Medicine and Drs. Keith Segalman, Michael Murphy, Raymond Wittstadt, and E.F. Shaw Wilgis of the Curtis National Hand Center, Union Memorial Hospital, for their medical review of the chapters in this book. Dr. Gaylord Clark, one of the original hand surgeons at the Curtis National Hand Center and an editor of the first two editions, contributed invaluable expertise and enthusiasm in the early stages of planning for the third edition. We also want to thank Thomas J. Graham, MD, Chief of the Curtis National Hand Center, for his support of this project.

We thank our photographer, Mark Swisher, for his expert assistance in providing the many new photographs needed for the third edition. We also thank the photographer from the second edition, Peter Andrews, and Joyce Lavery for all new illustrations in the third edition.

We thank Kathy Falk, Robin Sutter, and the editorial staff at Elsevier for their expertise and guidance throughout the revision process. We also received support, guidance, and project management from the medical editors in Orthopaedics and Hand Surgery at Union Memorial Hospital, Lyn Camire and Anne Mattson. In addition, we would like to acknowledge the Curtis National Hand Center staff for their assistance throughout this project.

Above all, we thank the many hand therapists who contributed their time and expertise to this edition and the previous editions of this text.

Contents

PART **ONE**

Wound Management, 1

1. **Wound Care,** Heather DeLaney   3

2. **Skin Grafts and Flaps,** Linda Coll Ware and Mallory Anthony   17

3. **Burns,** Linda Coll Ware   29

4. **Scar Management,** Tara Barasch   39

PART **TWO**

Nerve Injuries and Compression, 51

5. **Sensibility Testing,** Judith Bell-Krotoski   53

6. **Median Nerve Compression,** Bonnie J. Aiello   87

7. **Ulnar Nerve Compression,** Nicole E. Bickhart   97

8. **Radial Nerve Compression,** Greg Pitts and Stephen C. Umansky   109

9. **Thoracic Outlet Syndrome,** Mallory S. Anthony   121

10. **Nerve Repair,** Linda Luca   139

11. **Desensitization and Reeducation,** Rebecca N. Larson   151

12. **Tendon Transfers for Median Nerve Palsy,** Michele A. Klein   165

13. **Tendon Transfers for Ulnar Nerve Palsy,** Michele A. Klein   175

14. **Tendon Transfers for Radial Nerve Palsy,** Arlynne Pack Brown   187

15. **Brachial Plexus Injuries,** Mark T. Walsh and Gregory K. Davis   195

16. **Complex Regional Pain Syndrome,** Romina P. Astifidis   215

PART **THREE**

Tendon Injuries, 225

17. Flexor Tendon Repair, Mary Formby   227

18. Flexor Tendon Reconstruction, Barbara Wilson   245

19. Flexor Tenolysis, Barbara Wilson   261

20. Management of Extensor Tendon Repairs, Rebecca J. Saunders   271

21. Extensor Tendon Imbalance: Mallet Finger, Swan-Neck Deformity, Boutonniere Deformity, Jason A. Willoughby, Juan Martin Favetto, and William L. O'Neill, Jr   293

22. Extensor Tendon Tenolysis, Rebecca J. Saunders   311

23. Complex Extensor Reconstruction, Rebecca J. Saunders 319

PART **FOUR**

Shoulder, 327

24. Shoulder Tendonitis, Mary Schuler Murphy   329

25. Rotator Cuff Repairs, Mary Schuler Murphy   345

26. Glenohumeral Instability, Gary M. Lynch   359

27. Humeral Fractures, Mary Schuler Murphy   369

28. Shoulder Arthroplasty, Anne Edmonds   389

PART **FIVE**

Elbow, 397

29. Epicondylitis, Jason Leadbetter   399

30. Elbow Fractures and Dislocations, Jane Imle Schmidt   409

31. Elbow Arthroscopy, Frank DiGiovannantonio   423

32. Elbow Arthroplasty, Anne Edmonds   431

PART **SIX**

Wrist and Distal Radial Ulnar Joint, 439

33. Wrist and Hand Tendinopathies, Romina P. Astifidis   441

34. Wrist Arthroscopy, William McKay   453

35. Carpal Fractures and Instabilities, Terri M. Skirven and Lauren M. DeTullio   461

36. Triangular Fibrocartilage Injuries, Greg Pitts and Ronald Burgess   475

37. External and Internal Fixation of Unstable Distal Radius Fractures, Georgiann F. Laseter   489

38. Ulnar Head Resection, Frank DiGiovannantonio   507

39. Proximal Row Carpectomy, Corie Sullivan   517

40. Wrist Arthroplasty, Brenda A. Kelly   523

41. Wrist Arthrodesis, Beth Farrell Kozera   529

PART SEVEN

Hand, 537

42. Dupuytren's Disease, Dale Eckhaus   539

43. Ligament Injuries of the Hand, Barbra J. Koczan and Shelby Moore   547

44. Digital Fracture Rehabilitation, Gregory A. Hritcko   561

45. Replantation, J. Martin Walsh   581

46. Digital Amputation and Ray Resection, Linda Coll Ware   597

47. Metacarpal and Proximal Interphalangeal Joint Capsulectomy,
Rebecca J. Saunders   605

48. Thumb Carpometacarpal Joint Arthroplasty,
Rebecca J. Saunders   617

49. Metacarpophalangeal Joint Arthroplasty, Lorie Theisen   625

50. Proximal and Distal Interphalangeal Joint Arthroplasty,
Lorie Theisen   633

51. Small Joint Arthrodesis of the Hand, Lauren Adelsberger   641

PART EIGHT

Special Topics, 647

52. Conservative Management of Arthritis, Paige E. Kurtz   649

53. Congenital Differences in the Hand and Upper Extremity,
Cheryl S. Lutz and Scott H. Kozin   659

54. Therapeutic Management of the Performing Artist,
Lauren Valdata   689

55. Special Considerations and Common Injuries of Athletes,
Tracy Videon   707

56. Management of Upper Extremity Amputations, Lorie Theisen   715

57. Social Work Services, Ann Leman-Domenici   721

58. Industrial Rehabilitation Services, Donna M. Keegan and
Robert C. Kahlert   727

59. Evidence-Based Practice in Hand and Upper Extremity
Therapy, Heather DeLaney   739

Index, 745

PART **ONE**

Wound Management

Wound Care

1

Heather DeLaney

Therapists and physicians involved with the treatment of hand injuries know that even a small wound can be detrimental to hand function. Hand structures are made up of dense connective tissue, and essential to normal hand function is the ability of these strong connective tissue structures to glide in relation to one another. The formation of scar tissue after injury can significantly impede gliding and thus decrease function. A thorough understanding of wound management throughout all phases of wound healing is important in developing a comprehensive treatment program.

During the initial phases of wound healing, the focus is on preservation of function through prevention of edema, to reduce subsequent fibrosis, and maintenance of gliding surfaces. Wound closure is facilitated based on knowledge of wound healing and effective dressing techniques.

During the final phases of wound healing—the scar maturation phase—the therapist's role is to apply controlled stress to the scar, thereby increasing gliding potential and allowing the most functional outcome.

The following guideline suggests evaluation and wound care techniques that should help the clinician expedite wound closure, minimize scar formation, and achieve optimum functional results.

DEFINITION

A **wound** is a disruption of the anatomic or functional continuity of tissue.
I. Elective or surgical wound: a wound that has been "designed, executed, and repaired...under ideal, controlled, and aseptic circumstances"[1]; in general, these wounds heal rapidly
II. Traumatic open wound
   A. Tidy: Clean laceration, minimal tissue damage, and minimal contamination
   B. Untidy: Significant amount of tissue damage with uncertain viability of underlying structures; may have a higher degree of contamination
   C. Infected wound: presently infected

SURGICAL PURPOSE

I. To achieve rapid healing of soft tissue, to minimize scar formation, and to allow for the maximum function of the underlying anatomic components (e.g., tendon, nerve, blood vessels, bone). Soft tissue coverage may be required if deeper vital structures are exposed.
   A. Split-thickness skin grafts (STSG) (epidermis and part of dermis) or full-thickness (FTSG) (epidermis and underlying dermis): replace skin in areas where adequate subcutaneous tissues remain to protect underlying structures and vascularize the graft.
   B. Flap coverage is necessary if the wound bed has exposed vital structures or if the bed has either a poor chance or no chance of providing vascularization for a graft.
   C. Vacuum-assisted closure (VAC) may be used by the physician to accelerate debridement and promote healing by applying controlled levels of negative pressure. The negative pressure is thought to remove excess interstitial fluid, decrease local edema, and promote increased blood flow to the area.[2]

TREATMENT GOAL

I. Promote wound closure as quickly as possible with minimal scar formation.
II. Restore active range of motion (AROM) and passive range of motion (PROM) in the involved area, through scar management, splinting, stretching, and range of motion (ROM) exercises.
III. Maintain full ROM of all uninvolved joints of the upper extremity.
IV. Increase strength and promote return of upper extremity function to optimum level.
V. Reduce chances for hypertrophic scar formation.

INDICATIONS/PRECAUTIONS FOR THERAPY

I. Indications[1]
   A. Presence of a yellow or black wound
   B. A red wound in need of protection from adverse mechanical influences
   C. Loss of ROM and function during scar maturation phase
II. Precautions
   A. Infection
   B. Damage to deep vital structures
   C. Extreme pain
   D. Severe edema

THERAPY

Understanding Wound Physiology

Wound healing occurs in an overlapping sequence of events (Fig. 1-1; Box 1-1).

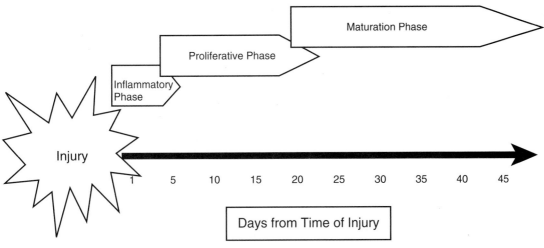

FIG. 1-1 Wound healing timeline.

I.   Inflammatory phase (injury to 6 days)
   A. Vasoconstriction: mediated by norepinephrine to slow blood loss
      in the affected area[3]
   B. Vasodilation: Noninjured vessels in the area vasodilate in
      response to chemicals released by injured tissues.[3]
   C. Clot formation: temporarily occludes the vessels to slow or stop
      bleeding

BOX 1-1 Wound Healing Phase Timetable

  I. Epithelialization (begins within a few hours after wounding)
    A. Regeneration of epithelial layer through four stages: mobilization, migration, proliferation, and differentiation of epithelial cells
    B. Covers exposed dermis
    C. May be complete in 6 to 48 hours after suturing (longer in wound healing by secondary intention)
  II. Inflammatory (substrate or lag phase: from wounding to 3 to 5 days)
    A. Vascular response (5 to 10 minutes of vasoconstriction followed by vasodilation)
    B. Phagocytosis (neutrophils and macrophages rid wound of bacteria and foreign debris)
 III. Fibroplasia (latent phase: days 4 to 5 to days 14 to 28)
    A. Fibroblasts enter wound and begin synthesizing collagen (scar tissue).
    B. Tensile strength increases with deposition of collagen.
    C. Angiogenesis (neovascularization): capillary budding begins, to form new blood vessels
    D. Formation of granulation tissue (new collagen and new capillaries, red in appearance)
 IV. Scar maturation or remodeling (days 14 to 28 up to several years)
    A. Strength increases through gradual intramolecular and intermolecular cross-linking of collagen molecules.
    B. Changes occur in form, bulk, and architecture of collagen (i.e., ongoing collagen synthesis versus lysis cycle; more organized orientation of collagen fibers with applied stress).
    C. Appearance of scar changes from red and raised to more pale and flat as maturation occurs.
  V. Contraction (days 4 to 5 up to day 21)
    A. Movement of wound margins toward center of wound defect
    B. Myofibroblasts (modified fibroblasts) are thought to be responsible for wound contraction.

          D. Phagocytosis: Macrophages produce collagenase and proteoglycan-degrading enzymes to facilitate debridement.

  II.   Proliferative phase (6 to 21 days): formation of granulation tissue

          A. Epithelialization: regeneration of the epithelial layer through four stages: mobilization, migration, proliferation, and differentiation of epithelial cells

          B. Fibroplasia/collagen production: Fibroblasts begin collagen synthesis, forming a thin, weak-structured, unorganized framework.[3]

          C. Wound contracture: regulated by myofibroblasts

          D. Neovascularization: development of new blood supply as a result of angiogenesis

          E. Immobilization may be required at this stage due to tenuous tensile strength of the collagen framework and fragility of the thin-walled capillaries.[3]

 III. Maturation phase (21 days to 2 years)

          A. Collagen synthesis/lysis balance: The balanced process of remodeling can last 12 to 24 months.[3]

          B. Collagen fiber orientation: affected by application of stress during wound healing

Wound Evaluation

   I.   Patient history

          A. Age

          B. Occupation and avocational interests

          C. Alcohol, tobacco, or caffeine use

          D. Metabolic status: Underlying disease affecting circulation (e.g., diabetes, vascular disorders)

          E. Nutritional status

          F. Medications (i.e., steroids, anticoagulants)

          G. Psychological/intelligence factors that could improve wound healing.

  II.   Wound history

          A. Mechanism of injury

          B. Time interval between injury and onset of treatment

             1. Acute: Acute inflammatory stage lasts no longer than 2 weeks.[3]

             2. Chronic: greater than 4 weeks in the inflammatory stage; can lead to loss of function because there is ultimately more scar tissue and adhesion formation.[1]

 III. Subjective evaluation

          A. Pain description

          B. Changes in sensation

  IV. Objective evaluation

          A. Observation/inspection[1]

             1. Wound hydration

                a. Desiccation

                b. Maceration

             2. Inflammatory reaction

                a. Pain

  b. Swelling
   (1) Redness and edema extending well beyond the wound boundaries may indicate cellulitis
  c. Redness
   (1) Lymphangitis: streaking redness
  d. Temperature
3. Drainage
  a. Amount: none, scant, minimal, moderate, or high
  b. Color
  c. Odor: presence or absence of foul odor
  d. Consistency
   (1) Transudate: clear and watery
   (2) Exudate: thick and yellowish
   (3) Pus: thicker and yellow-brown
4. Adjacent tissues
  a. Trophic skin changes: may indicate complex regional pain syndrome development
  b. Skin color
   (1) Redness: inflammation present
   (2) Blueness: cyanotic; venous obstruction
   (3) Pallor: arterial obstruction
  c. Hematoma/seroma: collection of blood and/or serum, usually clotted.
  d. Bleb: a blood- or serum-filled blister
5. Type of closure
  a. Primary: Immediate wound closure (e.g., tidy wound)
   (1) Closure: sutures, staples, Steri-Strips, graft or flap
   (2) Fixation: K-wire, pull-out wire, external fixator
   (3) VAC closure: used in large wounds; often used in severe Dupuytren's disease to reduce wound tension during the postoperative period
  b. Delayed primary: Wound is left open after injury because the degree of bacterial contamination or the extent of vascular impairment is in doubt. Usually left open 4 to 5 days, then closed with minimal risk of infection.
  c. Secondary intention: Wound closes through natural biological processes of epithelialization, inflammation, fibroplasia, scar maturation, and contraction. Commonly used for heavily contaminated wounds and for superficial wounds with extensive tissue loss.
6. Clinical measurements
  a. Wound configuration
  b. Location of wound
  c. Length and width dimensions
  d. Wound depth
  e. Presence of tunneling
  f. Color: universal classification system for open wounds
   (1) Red: definite border, granulation tissue present, with apparent revascularization (Fig. 1-2)

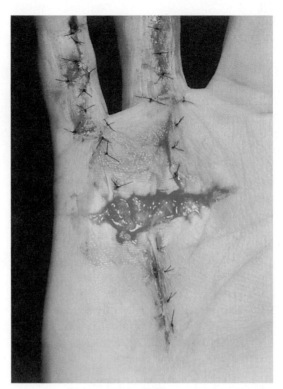

FIG. **1-2** A red wound in a Dupuytren's fasciectomy 3 days after surgery. The wound in the palm is beefy red, without infection, with epithelial, endothelial myofibroblast, and fibroblast cellular activity taking place. Note that the digital wounds are already epithelized. (From Mackin EJ, Callahan AD, Skirven TM, et al. [eds]: Hunter-Mackin-Callahan Rehabilitation of the Hand and Upper Extremity. 5th Ed. Vol. 1. Mosby, St. Louis, 2002.)

    (2) Yellow: creamy ivory to a canary yellow; draining, purulent, and characterized by slough that is liquid or semi-liquid; contains pus, yellow fibrous debris, or viscous surface exudates (Fig. 1-3)

    (3) Black: dark-brown to gray-black; covered with eschar or thick necrotic tissue (Fig. 1-4)

7. Edema measures
   a. Circumferential: referenced to bony landmarks
   b. Volumetric: with the use of a volumeter, which measures the amount of displaced water as a measure of mass of the extremity

8. Other measures
   a. If a flap or graft has been used, check for color, viability, swelling, tightness of suture line, and so on.
   b. ROM measures as appropriate
   c. Sensibility testing as indicated

Wound Management

Wound management contributes to the healing process by protecting the wound fluids, preventing/managing infection, controlling mechanical influences, and influencing the collagen maturation process.[1]

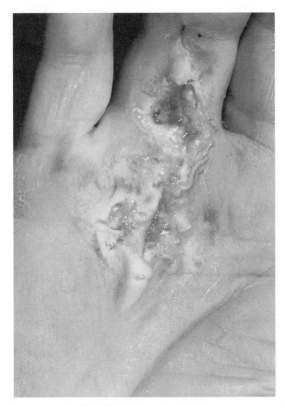

FIG. **1-3** A yellow wound infected with *Pseudomonas* in a postsurgical Dupuytren's fasciectomy closed by primary intention with subsequent dehiscence. Although some of the green color is from skin pencil, the wound is yellow-green with a distinctive odor. Cellular activity is dominated by the macrophage, which is stimulated by bacteria and inflammation. (From Evans RB: Hand Clin 7:409-432, 1991.)

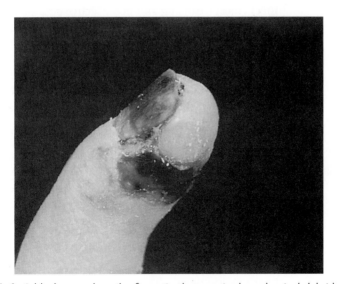

FIG. **1-4** A black wound on the fingertip that required mechanical debridement in therapy after whirlpool. The macrophages are working to clean the area of bacteria and debris. The fibroblasts and endothelial cells will begin to synthesize collagen and new vessels as the debris is removed. (From Mackin EJ, Callahan AD, Skirven TM, et al. [eds]: Hunter-Mackin-Callahan Rehabilitation of the Hand and Upper Extremity. 5th Ed. Vol. 1. Mosby, St. Louis, 2002.)

I. Protecting the wound environment: The goal is to maintain home-
    ostasis in order to create an environment for granulation formation
    and angiogenesis.
    A. Wound cleansing
        1. Purpose: To remove unattached cellular debris from the
           wound bed
        2. Indications
            a. Yellow and sloughing wound
            b. Edematous and glassy wound
            c. Highly contaminated wound
        3. Types of cleansing[1]
            a. Normal sterile saline
            b. Other agents: typically cytotoxic to healing tissues, thus
               delaying healing; therefore, should be used only on
               necrotic tissues, and discontinued in the presence of gran-
               ulation tissue
                (1) Povidone-iodine solution (0.001%): indicated for treat-
                    ment *Staphylococcus aureus,* although less effective in
                    exudating wounds; toxic to skin and mucous membranes
                (2) Sodium hypochlorite (0.25% to 0.50%): controls wound
                    sepsis but is cytotoxic to fibroblasts; it is less toxic in
                    the form of chloramine-T (Chlorazene).
                (3) Dakin solution (0.45% to 0.5% sodium hypochlorite
                    and 0.4% boric acid): indicated for streptococci, staphy-
                    lococci, and pyocyaneus microorganism. Local skin irri-
                    tation may occur when full-strength solution is applied.
                (4) Acetic acid solution: Although acetic acid is effective in
                    killing *Pseudomonas aeruginosa,* it has been found that
                    it does not significantly enhance the healing process.
                (5) Hydrogen peroxide: Foaming action is often used for
                    mechanical cleansing and nonselective debridement.
                    Should not be used on healthy granulation tissue or
                    closed/tunneling wounds. Must be flushed with
                    normal sterile saline after use.
                (6) Topical antibiotics (Neosporin, Silvadene, Furacin):
                    Studies done in animal populations have not provided
                    conclusive evidence on the benefits or detriments of
                    topical antibiotics.
    B. Debridement
        1. Purpose: remove necrotic and devitalized tissue
        2. Indications:
            a. Rid wound of necrotic tissue to facilitate the proliferative
               phase
            b. Prevent infection
            c. Correct abnormal wound repair
        3. Types
            a. Selective: removes only necrotic tissue
                (1) Sharp debridement: the use of scalpel, scissors, and
                    forceps to remove devitalized tissue easily from the
                    wound with no bleeding
                (2) Enzymatic debridement: the use of topical enzymes
                    formulated to break down specific necrotic tissues

(a) Fibrinolytic and proteolytic enzymes: used on the top portions of necrotic wounds

(b) Collagenases: break down undenatured collagen that is often responsible for anchoring stubborn necrotic tissue to wound surface

(3) Autolytic debridement: The most selective form of debridement, because it relies on the normal activity of white blood cells to phagocytize necrotic issue. Debridement occurs when natural enzymes sequestered under a synthetic dressing promote the action of macrophages. It is contraindicated for infected wounds, prolonged use (greater than 2 weeks), or premature removal of dressings before the phagocytic action has occurred.

a. Nonselective

(1) Wet-to-dry dressings

(a) Limit to wounds with a high percentage of necrotic tissue because of the acute trauma they cause to healthy granulation tissue.

(b) Should not be used if they cause bleeding or pain or on exposed tendons

b. Topical agents: as discussed earlier, should be used for the purpose of cleansing and bacteria control

c. Surgical debridement: An outpatient procedure requiring anesthesia; typically sacrifices some viable tissue in exchange for rapid results.

d. Forceful irrigations: effective to remove superficial, nonattached cellular debris; can deliver cleansing agents and clean malodorous wounds

e. Hydrotherapy: debride loosely adherent necrotic tissue, soak off adherent dressings, and cleanse a wound of dirt, foreign contaminants, and toxic residue

C. Dressings

1. Gauze

a. Frequent changes can cause necrosis of healing tissues by removal of important exudates

b. Permeable to bacteria

c. Fibers may become embedded, causing inflammation and delayed healing.

2. Calcium alginate: Fibers turn into biocompatible gel to provide a moist environment for autolytic debridement.

3. Semipermeable films: balance wound hydration with normal to no exudates without macerating the periwound (Fig. 1-5)

4. Semipermeable foams: able to absorb moderate to high amounts of exudates, typically without macerating the periwound.

5. Impermeable hydrocolloids: provide an anaerobic wound environment because they are impermeable to water, bacteria, and oxygen or other gases

6. Semipermeable hydrogel: able to conform to the wound while absorbing only small amounts of exudates; allows exudates to pass through to the secondary dressing

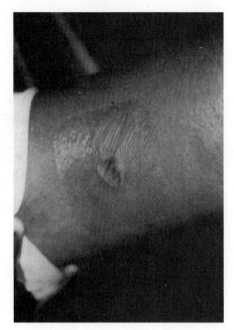

FIG. **1-5** Semipermeable dressing.

II. Minimizing mechanical influence
 A. Edema
  1. Elevation
  2. Controlled motion
  3. Bulky dressing
 B. Hematoma
  1. Increases fibrosis and scar formation; serves as a culture
   medium for bacteria, increasing the risk for infection
 C. Wound site tension
  1. Associated problems
   a. May reduce the rate of repair
   b. Compromises tensile strength
   c. Increases the final width of the scar
  2. Management
   a. Wound tape
   b. Pressure dressings
   c. Splinting
III. Influencing the collagen maturation process
 A. Initiated from first day of treatment
  1. Infection prevention
  2. Avoid exaggerated inflammatory state
  3. Maintain moist wound environment
 B. Adhesion control
  1. Controlled motion with respect to tensile strength
 C. Cutaneous scars
  1. Pressure garments
  2. Elastomer molds
  3. Silicone gel sheeting

D. Hypertrophic scars
   1. Found in areas of high tension and movement
   2. Use topical silicone gel sheeting
   3. Paper tape

COMPLICATIONS

I. Infections
II. Wound dehiscence/loss of graft or flap
III. Abnormal scar formation
   A. Hypertrophic
   B. Keloid

EVALUATION TIMELINE

Wound status and type of dressing should be assessed at every treatment, during initial and discharge evaluations, and each time a progress evaluation is indicated for the patient, until the wound is healed. After wound closure, description of scar and resulting limitations of motion, strength, and function should be noted.

TABLE **1-1** Wound Healing Process: Characteristics of Various Dressing Choices

Characteristic	Calcium Alginate Dressings	Semipermeable Films	Semipermeable Foams	Hydrogels	Hydrocolloids
Commercial brands	Sorbsan Kaltostat Curasorb	OpSite Tegaderm Polyskin II	Allevyn NU-DERM Flexzan	Vigilon NU-GEL Elasto-Gel	DuoDERM Comfeel Tegasorb
Absorption	Good	Fair	Good/Excellent	Poor/Fair	Good
Autolytic debridement	Minimal to maximal	Minimal	Minimal to moderate	Minimal to maximal	Minimal to moderate
Use on infected wounds	Yes	No	No	No	No
Type of wound	Wet	Superficial	Yellow	Superficial	Yellow
Maintains moisture	Yes	Yes	Yes	Yes	Yes
Conformity	Good	Good	Poor on irregular surfaces	Excellent	Poor on irregular surfaces
Irritate with removal	No	Minimal	Minimal to none	No	Minimal
Permeability to oxygen	Good	Good	Good	Good	No
Permeable to bacteria, urine, etc.	Yes	Yes	No	Yes	No
Maintains wound temperature	Yes	No	Yes	Cools	Yes
Allows visual monitoring	No	Yes	No	Yes	No
Pain at site	Decreases	Decreases	Decreases	Decreases	Decreases

Data from McCulloch JM, Kloth LC, Feedar JA: Wound Healing: Alternatives in Management. 2nd Ed. FA Davis, Philadelphia, 1995.

OUTCOMES

Table 1-1 summarizes the characteristics of various wound dressings.

REFERENCES

1. McCulloch JM, Kloth LC, Feedar JA: Wound Healing: Alternatives in Management. 2nd Ed. FA Davis, Philadelphia, 1995
2. Information available at: http://www.worldwidewounds.com/2001/may/Thomas/Vacuum-Assisted-Closure.html (accessed March 21, 2005)
3. Evans RB, McAuliffe JA: Wound classification and management. In Mackin EJ, Callahan AD, Skirven TM, et al. (eds): Hunter-Mackin-Callahan Rehabilitation of the Hand and Upper Extremity. 5th Ed. Mosby, St. Louis, 2002, p. 311

SUGGESTED READINGS

Alvarez O, Rozint J, Wiseman D: Moist environment for healing: matching the dressing to the wound. Wounds 1:35, 1989

Arem AJ, Madden JW: Effects of stress on healing wounds: I. Intermittent non-cyclical tension. J Surg Res 20:93, 1976

Ahn ST, Monafo WW, Mustoe TA: Topical silicone gel: a new treatment for hypertrophic scars. Surgery 106:781, 1989

Brennan SS, Foster ME, Leaper DJ: Antiseptic toxicity in wounds healing by secondary intention. J Hosp Infect 8:263, 1986

Bruster J, Pullium G: Gradient pressure. Am J Occup Ther 37:485, 1983

Bryant W: Clinical Symposia: Wound Healing. CIBA Pharmaceutical Co., Summit, NJ, 1977

Burkhalter WE: Wound classification and management. In Hunter JM, Schneider LH, Mackin EJ, et al. (eds): Rehabilitation of the Hand: Surgery and Therapy. 3rd Ed. Mosby, St. Louis, 1990, p. 167

Carrico T, Merhof A, Cohen I: Biology of wound healing. Surg Clin North Am 64:721, 1984

Clark JA, Cheng JC, Leung KS, et al.: Mechanical characterization of human postburn hypertrophic skin during pressure therapy. J Biomech 20:397, 1987

Cohen K: Can collagen metabolism be controlled: theoretical considerations. J Trauma 25:410, 1985

Cohn GH: Hyperbaric oxygen therapy: promoting healing in difficult cases. Postgrad Med Oxygen Ther 79:89, 1986

Davies D: Scars, hypertrophic scars, and keloids. Br Med J Clin Res 290:1056, 1985

Donnell M: Pros and cons of wound care techniques for the upper extremity: practice forum. J Hand Ther 3:128, 1991

Silastic Gel Sheeting [monograph]. Dow Corning Wright, Arlington, TN, 1989

Groves AR: The problem with scars. Burns 13:S15, 1987

Henning JP, Roskam Y, Van Gemert MJ: Treatment of keloids and hypertrophic scars with an argon laser. Lasers Surg Med 6:72, 1986

Hunt TK (ed): Wound Healing and Wound Infection: Theory and Surgical Practice. Appleton-Century-Crofts, East Norwalk, CT, 1980

Hunt TK, Dunphy J: Fundamentals of Wound Management. Appleton-Century-Crofts, East Norwalk, CT, 1979

Hunt TK, Hussain Z: Wound microenvironment. In Cohen IK, Diegelman RF, Lindblad WJ (eds): Wound Healing: Biochemical and Clinical Aspects. WB Saunders, Philadelphia, 1992, p. 274

Hunt TK, Lavan FB: Enhancement of wound healing by growth factors. N Engl J Med 321:111, 1989

Jensen LL, Parshley PF: Postburn scar contractures: histology and effects of pressure treatment. J Burn Care Rehabil 5:119, 1984

Johnson CL: Physical therapists as scar modifiers. Phys Ther 64:1381, 1984

Johnson CL: Wound healing and scar formation. Top Acute Care Trauma Rehabil 1:1, 1987

Kanzler MH, Gorsulowsky DC, Swanson NA: Basic mechanisms in the healing cutaneous wound. J Dermatol Surg Oncol 12:1156, 1986

Kloth LC, Feedar JA: Acceleration of wound healing with high voltage, monophasic, pulsed current. Phys Ther 68:503, 1988

Lawrence JC: The aetiology of scars. Burns 13:S3, 1987

Linares HA, Kischer CA, Dobrkovsky M, et al.: On the origin of the hypertrophic scar.
    J Trauma 13:70, 1973

Madden JW: Wound healing: the biological basis of hand surgery. In Hunter JM, Schneider
    LH, Mackin EJ, et al. (eds): Rehabilitation of the Hand: Surgery and Therapy. 3rd Ed.
    Mosby, St. Louis, 1990, p. 181

Malick MH, Carr JA: Flexible elastomer molds in burn scar control. Am J Occup Ther
    34:603, 1980

Martin GR, Peacock EE: Current perspectives in wound healing. In Cohen IK, Diegleman
    RF, Lindblad WJ (eds): Wound Healing: Biochemical and Clinical Aspects. WB Saunders,
    Philadelphia, 1992

McAuliffe JA, Seltzer DG: HIV disease: basic science and treatment implications.
    In Hunter JM, Mackin EJ, Callahan AD (eds): Rehabilitation of the Hand: Surgery
    and Therapy. 4th Ed. Mosby, St. Louis, 1995, p. 261

Michlovitz SL: Thermal Agents in Rehabilitation. 2nd Ed. FA Davis, Philadelphia, 1990

Nathan R, Taras JS: Common infections in the hand. In Hunter JM, Mackin EJ, Callahan
    AD (eds): Rehabilitation of the Hand: Surgery and Therapy. 4th Ed. Mosby, St. Louis,
    1995, p. 251

Nicolai JP, Bronkhorst FB, Smale CE: A protocol for the treatment of hypertrophic scars and
    keloids. Aesthetic Plast Surg 11:29, 1987

Noe JM: Dressing the acutely injured hand. In Wolfort FG (ed): Acute Hand Injuries:
    A Multispecialty Approach. Little, Brown, Boston, 1980, p. 241

Noe JM, Keller M: Can stitches get wet? Plast Reconstr Surg 81:82, 1988

Peacock EE: Wound Repair. 3rd Ed. WB Saunders, Philadelphia, 1984

Peacock EE, Madden JW, Trier WC: Biologic basis for the treatment of keloids and hypertrophic
    scars. South Med J 63:755, 1970

Perkins K, Davey RB, Wallis K: Current materials and techniques used in a burn scar
    management programme. Burns 13:406, 1987

Pollack SV: Wound healing: a review. J Dermatol Surg Oncol 5:389, 1979

Quinn KJ: Silicone gel in scar treatment. Burns 13:S33, 1987

Quinn KJ, Evans JH, Courtney JM, et al: Non-pressure treatment of hypertrophic scars.
    Burns 12:102, 1985

Reid W: Hypertrophic scarring and pressure therapy. Burns 13:S29, 1987

Rodeheaver G, Bellamy W, Kody M, et al: Bactericidal activity and toxicity of iodine-containing
    solutions in wounds. Arch Surg 117:181, 1982

Rose MP, Deitch EA: The clinical use of a tubular compression bandage, Tubigrip, for
    burn-scar therapy: a critical analysis. Burns 12:58, 1985

Ross R: Wound healing. Sci Am 220:40, 1969

Rudolph R: Wide spread scars, hypertrophic scars, and keloids. Clin Plast Surg 14:253, 1987

Smith KL: Wound care for the hand patient. In Hunter JM, Schneider LH, Mackin EJ, et al.
    (eds): Rehabilitation of the Hand: Surgery and Therapy. 3rd Ed. Mosby, St. Louis, 1990,
    p. 172

Smith KL: Wound care for the hand patient. In Hunter JM, Mackin EJ, Callahan AD (eds):
    Rehabilitation of the Hand: Surgery and Therapy. 4th Ed. Mosby, St. Louis, 1995, p. 232

Surveyer JA, Cloughtery DM: Burn scars: fighting the effects. Am J Nurs 83:746, 1983

Ware LC, Anthony MS: Burns and open wounds of the hand. In Home Study Course 95-2.
    Topic: The Wrist and Hand. Orthopaedic Section. APTA, Inc., Alexandria, VA, 1995, pp. 1-18

Weeks P, Wray C: Hand Management: A Biological Approach. Mosby, St. Louis, 1973

Wessling N, Ehleben CM, Chapman V, et al: Evidence that use of a silicone gel sheet
    increases range of motion over burn wound contractures. J Burn Care Rehabil 6:503,
    1985

Westaby S (ed): Wound Care. Mosby, St. Louis, 1986

Wheeland RG: The newer surgical dressings and wound healing. Dermatol Clin 5:393, 1987

Wiseman DM, et al: Wound dressings: design and use. In Cohen IK, Diegelman RF,
    Lindblad WJ (eds): Wound Healing: Biochemical and Clinical Aspects. WB Saunders,
    Philadelphia, 1992, p. 562

Skin Grafts and Flaps

2

Linda Coll Ware
Mallory Anthony

Wounds with significant tissue loss often require skin grafts or flaps for adequate wound closure. In the hand, replacement of soft tissue warrants special attention by the therapist to achieve maximum functional outcome. Dorsal skin is thinner, elastic, and loose enough not to restrict flexion; it must provide a barrier to cover tendons and joints.[1] Volar skin is thick and tough and has a system of fibrous septae to maintain its stability (to withstand pressure and friction caused by grasp and pinch); at the same time, it is loose and elastic enough to allow motion and to retain its function of sensibility.[1]

The immediate short-term goals for soft tissue replacement are (1) to produce primary healing, (2) to prevent infection, and (3) to preserve the viability of exposed underlying structures.[2] The long-term benefits of adequate skin replacement are (1) to provide a durable skin cover to withstand everyday use; (2) to provide sensation at key points in the hand; (3) to permit mobility of underlying structures, especially tendons; (4) to permit later reconstruction procedures to repair the deep structures, if necessary; and (5) to prevent the development of contractures.[2]

Skin grafts are used to replace skin in areas where adequate circulation is available and underlying structures are protected by adequate subcutaneous tissue[2] (Table 2-1). A split-thickness skin graft (STSG) usually is obtained from the thigh, buttock, or abdomen. Compared with full-thickness

TABLE 2-1 Characteristics of Skin Flaps and Grafts

Type of Soft Tissue Coverage	Vascularity/Take	Donor Site Closure
STSG	3 days	Secondary intention
FTSG	57 days	Primary intention
Free tissue transfer	Immediate	Primary closure or skin graft
Pedicled flaps	Approximately 3 wk	Primary closure or skin graft

STSG, Split-thickness skin graft; *FTSG,* full-thickness skin graft.

skin grafts (FTSG), these skin grafts (1) are more suitable on large and contaminated wounds, (2) take more readily, (3) are less prone to infection, and (4) offer a large supply of donor sites. One major disadvantage is its increased tendency to contract during healing. Meshing of an STSG is occasionally indicated on suboptimal wound beds, where the risk of infection and/or hematoma is great and meshing is necessary to allow drainage of exudate and/or blood.[2] Meshing may also be used in cases of donor site shortage (e.g., extensive burns), to allow expansion of the graft.[2]

An FTSG usually is obtained from the hypothenar eminence, the medial aspect of the arm, or the groin. These skin grafts (1) provide increased durability, (2) afford better protection, (3) establish better sensibility, (4) contain more epidermal appendages, (5) contract less than STSGs, (6) provide increased cosmesis and color match, and (7) are more suitable for small, clean wounds (Fig. 2-1).

Firm "take" of a skin graft requires good recipient bed vascularity, free from increased levels of bacteria and devitalized tissue. After application, a skin graft first survives by means of transudate from the wound (plasmatic circulation).[1] Later, the ingrowth of capillary buds into the skin graft from the wound bed provides the necessary vascularity. Optimal beds for skin grafts include muscle, fascia, and granulation tissue. Suboptimal beds include denuded bone or tendon.

Skin flaps are needed for soft tissue coverage if the recipient bed provides poor vascularity, if the wound is too large for primary or secondary wound healing, or if vital structures are exposed.[3] A skin flap consists of dermis and subcutaneous tissue elevated from its underlying bed.

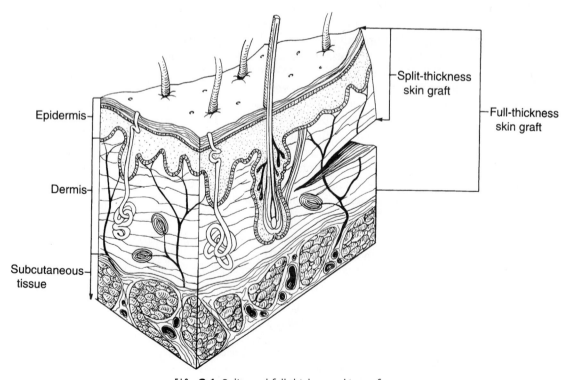

FIG. 2-1 Split- and full-thickness skin grafts.

It maintains vascularity through its base (pedicle). A flap can be classified as pedicle or free. A pedicle flap remains attached to the recipient site and may require later detachment. A free flap is transferred by dividing its vascular pedicle and resuturing the pedicle to recipient vessels in the recipient site.

A pedicle flap may be classified according to its vascular supply from the skin, which is present in four vascular layers. These layers are the subdermal, subcutaneous, fascial, and muscular layers, shown in Fig. 2-2. A flap that receives its blood supply from the subdermal layer is called a random flap.[3] The vascular supply of an axial flap comes from the subcutaneous, fascial, or muscular layer.[3]

Pedicle flaps, such as a groin flap, can provide sufficient tissue coverage in all but the most massive defects.[3] On the negative side, (1) the hand may be dependent during attachment, resulting in prolonged immobilization; (2) these flaps require a minimum of two operative procedures; (3) the blood supply on which the pedicle flap initially depends is cut at the time of detachment, making the flap dependent on peripheral vascularity

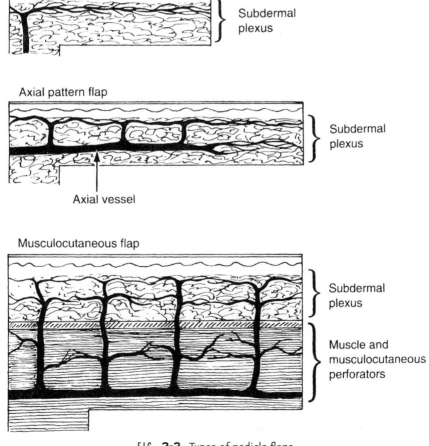

FIG. **2-2** Types of pedicle flaps.

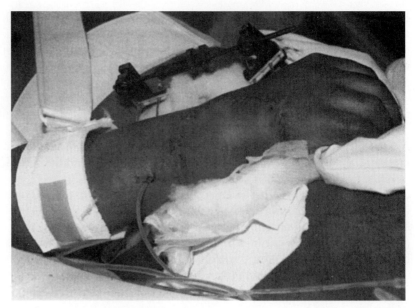

FIG. **2-3** Pedicle flap from groin for soft tissue defect. External fixator for treatment of distal forearm fracture.

(less dependable and robust); and (4) the flap may be avulsed by a very young or incompetent patient (Fig. 2-3).

The edges of all these skin flaps initially depend on nutrition by perfusion through microcirculation, before neovascularization (capillary budding) occurs and sufficient blood supply has grown across into the flap from the surrounding tissues. Approximately 3 weeks is required before healing is sufficient to allow pedicle division.

A free flap provides immediate vascularity. Vein grafts are sometimes necessary if the vascular pedicle is stretched at the repair site. Free flaps offer many advantages over the pedicle flap: (1) the recipient limb is mobile and free of prolonged attachment to the donor, permitting elevation and early mobilization; (2) free flaps frequently require only one operative procedure; (3) they bring their own blood supply, increasing the potential for healing, especially in a poorly vascularized and scarred bed; (4) they can be cut to fit the defect with precision (almost limitless choice of size and thickness)[4]; and (5) they can carry additional tissues (i.e., bone, tendon, nerves, and muscle).

Tissue expanders can be used for the expansion and growth of new skin needed for reconstruction. A tissue expander is a silicone balloon expander that is placed under the skin and then gradually filled with saline over time, causing the skin to stretch and grow. Tissue expansion works by stimulating the growth of new skin. It takes advantage of the skin's ability to stretch, similar to the stretching of a woman's abdomen during pregnancy.

Independent of the type of soft tissue coverage chosen for the patient, the goals are to promote wound healing, decrease edema, provide effective scar management, and help restore optimal range of motion (ROM) and function for these patients.

DEFINITIONS

I. **Graft:** a portion of tissue, such as skin, periosteum bone, or fascia, that is removed free and transferred to correct a defect in the body. A graft may consist of skin only (skin graft), or it may be a composite of tissues such as muscle and bone (composite graft).[5]

II. **Flap:** a portion of tissue that is partly removed from its place of origin to correct a defect in the body, as in pedicle flaps, or is completely severed from its origin, as in free flaps. A flap may consist of skin only (including its subdermal plexus of vessels), or it may be a composite of tissues such as skin, muscle, or bone (composite flap).[5] A flap contains its own vascular supply (Fig. 2-4).

III. Types of tissue transfers
  A. Free tissue transfers
    1. **STSG:** a free graft of skin that includes the epidermis and part of the dermis (may be meshed if moderate serous drainage is expected or if the recipient bed is suboptimal for vascularity)
    2. **FTSG:** a free graft of skin that includes the whole thickness of epidermis and dermis; contains dermal appendages and nerve endings, with the exception of subcutaneous sweat glands and some pacinian corpuscles
    3. **Free vascularized tissue transfer:** a composite flap with its vascular pedicle completely cut and transferred to the recipient site for immediate microvascular anastomoses (e.g., free groin flap, free latissimus flap)

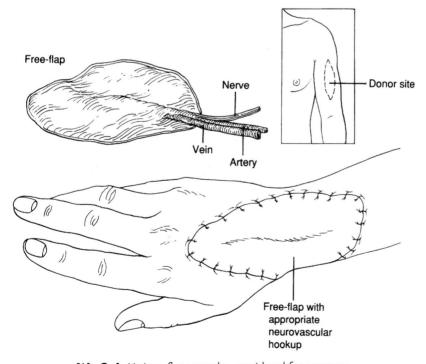

FIG. **2-4** Various flaps may be considered for coverage.

B. Pedicled flaps
1. **Random flaps:** designed to fit the recipient defect without attention to specific nutrient vessels in the pedicle.[5] There is no anatomically recognized arterial or venous system, and the flap receives its blood supply from the dermal-subdermal plexus (e.g., Z-plasty, V–Y advancement, rotation flap, transposition flap).
2. **Axial flaps:** designed so that the pedicle has within it identifiable, direct, cutaneous vascular elements[5]
   a. Cutaneous: axial flaps whose vessels supply skin alone and proceed directly to it (e.g., groin flap).
   b. Fasciocutaneous: axial flaps whose vessels first supply fascia (e.g., radial forearm flap).
   c. Myocutaneous or musculocutaneous: axial flaps whose vessels first supply muscle (e.g., latissimus dorsi flap).
   d. Island flap: axial flap whose pedicle has been reduced to the point that it consists only of nutrient blood vessels with or without nerves (e.g., neurovascular digital island flap).
IV. Location of grafts/flaps
   A. Local (from skin adjacent to the defect)—for example, transposition (Z-plasty), advancement (V–Y advancement), or rotation (fillet flap)
   B. Regional (from elsewhere on the limb)—for example, lateral arm flap, cross-finger flap, or thenar flap
   C. Distant (from other parts of the body)—for example, abdominal or groin flap

SURGICAL PURPOSE

To provide wound coverage of open areas to protect underlying structures. Each graft/flap type has a very specific reason for being used, and each has well-defined risk/benefit ratios.

TREATMENT GOALS

I. Provide adequate wound care and promote wound healing of graft, flap, and/or donor site.
II. Restore active range of motion (AROM) and passive range of motion (PROM) in affected areas underlying flaps/grafts.
III. Maintain full ROM of all uninvolved joints.
IV. Return to optimum level of function.

INDICATIONS FOR TISSUE COVERAGE

I. STFG and FTSG are used to replace skin in areas in which adequate subcutaneous tissues remain to protect underlying structures and adequate circulation is available
II. Flaps are indicated for wounds in which there is bone devoid of periosteum, tendon devoid of paratenon, or cartilage devoid of perichondrium; vital structures are exposed; or later reconstruction is planned.

PRECAUTIONS FOR THERAPY

I. Decreased graft/flap viability as observed by color change noted in postoperative evaluation
    A. Infection (cardinal signs: warmth, redness, pain, edema, and wound drainage)
    B. Mechanical problems: establishment of barrier between wound bed and graft (e.g., hematoma)
    C. Inadequate preparation of recipient bed
    D. Inadequate surgical technique
II. Damage and repair to deep vital structures
III. Extreme pain
IV. Severe edema

THERAPY

I. Preoperative management
    A. Provide sterile whirlpool, dressing changes, and debridement of recipient wound area, if indicated, in preparation for tissue coverage.
    B. Patient education to prepare patient for pedicle or free flap. This may include instruction in one-handed techniques and information regarding clothing (e.g., the type of clothing that will best accommodate the arm while it is attached to a groin flap).
    C. Maximize ROM and increase strength in muscle to be trans-ferred for planned functional muscle flap (nonemergency basis).
II. Postoperative evaluation
    A. Please refer to wound management evaluation, Chapter 1.
    B. Graft/flap viability assessment (general guidelines)[3]
       1. Observe color
          a. Random pattern flap
             (1) Pink: healthy
             (2) Pale with faint blue/gray tinge: inadequate arterial supply
             (3) Angry red first, then progressively purple red and purple blue: inadequate venous supply
          b. Axial pattern flap
             (1) Very pale pink: healthy
             (2) Waxy pallor (white tinged with yellow or brown): vascular compromise
          c. Free flaps
             (1) Pink: healthy
             (2) White or mottled appearance: arterial problems
             (3) Dusky blue: venous problems
       2. Observe refill after blanching by fingertip pressure or by running a blunt point across the flap.
          a. Slow refill (greater than 2 seconds) with pale flap: arterial insufficiency
          b. Rapid refill with bluish flap: venous insufficiency (e.g., kinking of pedicle)
       3. Temperature of flap
          a. Marked decrease in temperature between flap and tissue adjacent to flap may indicate impaired blood flow.
       4. Monitor pulsatile flow within the flap

III. Postoperative management of skin grafts[1,5,6]

A. Grafts are immobilized and protected 3 to 5 days for STSG and 5 to 7 days for FTSG.

1. Immobilization is accomplished by splinting in a protective position to decrease the risk of shear force.

B. Beginning 3 to 7 days postoperatively daily dressing changes with nonadherent gauze my be instituted. NOTE: Loss of a graft is usually the result of fluid accumulation under the graft (hematoma) or shear forces. Care must be taken during dressing changes not to rub the healing graft.

C. Once adherence of skin graft is evident (3 to 7 days), begin gentle ROM exercises (under supervision of therapist only). It may be desirable to conduct exercise without dressing in place to avoid a shearing force on the wound and to observe the skin graft.

D. Elevation to decrease edema

E. Once complete epithelialization is evident (10 to 14 days), begin gentle application of topical lubricant to healed areas. Graft sites are dry due to lack of secondary protective skin structures.

F. Beginning 2 weeks postoperatively, gentle massage, scar softening modalities, pressure garments, and compressive wraps may be used over a well-vascularized graft to decrease edema and begin scar management. Shearing forces must be avoided, and the treating physician should be consulted.

G. Splinting

1. Early/protective: to immobilize joints in functional position, eliminate tension on repaired structures, protect the healing graft, and prevent shearing forces.

2. Late (6 weeks): to apply stress to scar, increase ROM and prevent contracture formation.

H. Continue ROM exercises and advance aggressively to increase strength, endurance, and function.

I. Monitor return of sensation.

J. Patients must protect both donor and recipient sites against sun exposure for at least 6 months to 1 year.

IV. Postoperative management of flaps[5]

A. Pedicle (axial)

1. Left attached and immobilized 2 to 3 weeks (to allow new vascular ingrowth to the flap from the recipient bed); immobilized by dressing, tape, slings or splints

2. Use gauze pads in areas where maceration is a problem.

3. Coban and retrograde massage may be used to free digits, and thereby decrease edema, if no stress is placed on attachment.

4. Maintain ROM in uninvolved joints.

5. After flap detachment

a. Promote wound healing.

b. Decrease edema.

c. Regain full AROM/PROM in uninvolved joints.

d. Reestablish AROM/PROM in affected area.

e. Scar management to both recipient and donor sites.

B. Free tissue transfer[3,5]

1. Postoperatively protected with sterile dressing and splint

2. Vascular status is critical in the first few days postoperatively. (Patient is kept warm and should abstain from caffeine and nicotine. Make sure circumferential dressings are not too tight.)

3. Elevation, to heart level only, to decrease edema. Extensive elevation may impair arterial inflow. No compression wraps until 3 weeks postoperatively and with physician approval.

4. Wound care for donor and recipient sites. If wounds are dry and healing well, minimal dressing is required.

5. Monitor vascularity: observe color, temperature, and capillary refill time. A Doppler ultrasound study may be used to monitor vascular flow.

6. AROM to uninvolved joints.

7. 2 weeks postoperatively: Sutures and staples removed. AROM of involved joints if vascular status is stable and deeper structures are not involved.

8. 3 to 4 weeks postoperatively: gentle massage, scar-softening modalities, and compressive wraps if vascular status is stable.

9. 6 to 8 weeks postoperatively: splinting and passive ROM exercise as healing permits.

10. 8 weeks postoperatively: Patient can resume normal daily activities using the hand.

11. Continue ROM exercises and add activities to increase strength, endurance, and function.

12. Heavy and stressful activities allowed at 3 months.

13. Monitor return of sensation.

C. Functional muscle flap (free tissue transfer)[5]

1. Immobilized for 3 weeks in relaxed position. During this immobilization phase, once vascular stability is achieved (usually by 1 to 2 weeks), and with physician approval, PROM of uninvolved joints may be initiated.

2. Continue gentle PROM exercise until preoperative ROM is achieved.

3. As clinical signs of reinnervation are noted (4 to 7 months postoperatively), active-assisted range of motion (AAROM) exercises may be initiated.

4. Muscle stimulation, active exercise, and resistive exercise may be added as muscle strengthens.

V. Donor sites

A. Monitor donor site for development of hypertrophic scar.

B. Massage with topical lubricant and application of pressure may be initiated for scar management, as wound healing permits.

C. Be aware of loss of sensibility in donor site and educate patient, if a nerve has been taken for a transfer.

VI. Tissue expanders

A. Monitor for infection

B. Site may be painful after expansion, limiting motion in nearby joints.

POSTOPERATIVE COMPLICATIONS

I. Loss of graft/flap

A. Hematoma or seroma

    B. Infection
    C. Vascular compromise
      1. Kinking of pedicle attachment.
      2. Compression of arterial supply for free flap.
      3. Inadequate preparation of recipient bed.
II.   Extreme pain
III. Severe edema
IV. Excess scarring due to a long interval between injury and time of coverage

EVALUATION TIMELINE

I.   Graft/flap viability status should be assessed at initial evaluation, and during every treatment session, until the graft or flap is well taken.
II.   Joint motion affected by graft/flap should be assessed initially when graft/flap is stable and at least once a month thereafter.
III. Description of scar should be assessed, as well as sensory status, strength, and function during follow-up evaluations.

FUNCTIONAL OUTCOMES

It is unusual that an injury involves soft tissue only without associated injury of vital underlying structures. Refer to Chapters 3 and 23 for additional functional outcomes.

Hallock reported a series of 33 limbs requiring 16 local fascia flaps, 22 free flaps, 1 multistaged distant pedicle flap, and 1 local muscle flap. Conclusions drawn included the following: the shoulder girdle and axilla were reached by local trunk muscle or fascia flaps; the upper limb is conducive to coverage with specific local fascia flaps; and the distal upper extremity may be best served by a free flap.[7]

REFERENCES

1. Jones NF, Lister GD: Free skin and composite flaps. In Green DP (ed): Operative Hand Surgery. 4th Ed. Churchill Livingstone, New York, 1999, p. 1159
2. Smith PF: Skin loss and scar contractures. In Burke FD, McGrouther DA, Smith PJ (eds): Principles of Hand Surgery. Churchill Livingstone, New York, 1990, p. 31
3. Lister G, Pederson WC: Skin flaps. In Green DP (ed): Operative Hand Surgery. 4th Ed. Churchill Livingstone, New York, 1999, p. 1783
4. Chase RA: Skin and soft tissue. In Taras JS, Schneider LH. Atlas of Hand Surgery. Vol. 2. WB Saunders, Philadelphia, 2000
5. Levin LS, Moorman GJ, Heller L: Management of skin grafts and flaps. In Mackin EJ, Callahan AD, Skirven TM, et al. (eds): Rehabilitation of the Hand and Upper Extremity. 5th Ed. Mosby, St. Louis, 2002, p. 344
6. Simpson RL, Gartner MC: Management of burns of the upper extremity. In Mackin EJ, Callahan AD, Skirven TM, et al. (eds): Rehabilitation of the Hand and Upper Extremity. 5th Ed. Mosby, St. Louis, 2002, p. 1504
7. Hallock GG: The utility of both muscle and fascia flaps in severe upper extremity trauma. J Trauma. 53:61-65, 2002

SUGGESTED READINGS

Beasley RW: Hand Injuries. WB Saunders, Philadelphia, 1981
Brown PW: Open injuries of the hand. In Green DP (ed): Operative Hand Surgery. 4th Ed. Churchill Livingstone, New York, 1998, p. 1533

Browne EZ Jr: Complications of skin grafts and pedicle flaps. Hand Clin 2:353-359, 1986

Fisher JC: Skin grafting. In Georgiade GS, Reifkohl R, Levi LS (eds): Plastic Maxillofacial and Reconstructive Surgery. 3rd Ed. Baltimore, Williams & Wilkins, 1997

German G, Sherman R, Levin LS: Decision Making in Reconstructive Surgery: Upper Extremity. Springer, New York, 2000

Lister G: Injury. In The Hand: Diagnosis and Indications. 2nd Ed. Churchill Livingstone, New York, 1984, p. 1

Michon J: Complex hand injuries: surgical planning. In Tubiana R (ed): The Hand. Vol. 2. WB Saunders, Philadelphia, 1985, p. 196

Morrison WA, Gilbert A: Complications in microsurgery. In Tubiana R (ed): The Hand. Vol. 2. WB Saunders, Philadelphia, 1985, p. 145

Tsuge K, Kanaujia RR, Steichen JB: Comprehensive Atlas of Hand Surgery. Year Book Medical Publishers, Chicago, 1989

Ware LC, Anthony MS: Burns and open wounds of the hand. In Home Study Course 95-2. Topic: The Wrist and Hand. Orthopedic Section. APTA, Inc., Alexandria, VA, 1995, Chapter 2

Wolfort FG: Acute Hand Injuries: A Multispecialty Approach. Little, Brown, Boston, 1980

Burns 3

Linda Coll Ware

Hand burns are the most common of all thermal injuries.[1] Burns of the hand and upper extremity can result in severe functional limitation and esthetic deformity.[2] Normal skin serves several functions essential for life:

1. It guards against invasion of bacteria.
2. It regulates body temperature.
3. It prevents excess loss of body fluids.
4. It protects deeper structures from injury.
5. It protects against ultraviolet rays of the sun.
6. It protects nerve endings responsible for sensation.

When a burn injury has occurred and skin is lost, the body is vulnerable to infection, fluid loss, and injury to deeper structures.

Functional and cosmetic results after burn injuries are directly related to the severity of the burn and the body's ability to prevent infection and form satisfactory scars.[3] The severity of thermal injuries depends on the depth of skin destruction. Superficial partial-thickness burns involve destruction of the epidermis and possibly portions of the dermis; in deep partial-thickness burns, most of the dermal layers are destroyed. There is complete destruction of the epidermal and dermal layers in full-thickness burns.

Wound severity is sometimes unclear, and it is not always determined until several days after burn injury, because a burn "evolves" over several days. It is possible for a deep partial-thickness burn to convert into a full-thickness burn if left untreated. It is not surprising, therefore, that several treatment approaches have arisen in recent years: conservative treatment with topical antibiotics to permit spontaneous healing, early total excision and immediate grafting, delayed excision and grafting (later than 14 days), and sequential tangential excision and grafting.[3]

Therapeutic intervention of the burned upper extremity requires a therapist trained specifically in wound/graft care, splinting to prevent deformities and contractures, edema control, scar management, and pain control. Close monitoring of the patient's response to treatment (wound status, range of motion [ROM], skin integrity) is necessary to determine whether treatment methods are effective. As well, close communication with the surgeon is vital initially, postoperatively, and throughout the course of treatment. The following protocol serves as a guideline for treatment of thermal injuries to the hand and upper extremity.

DEFINITION

Burns are injuries to skin and underlying soft tissues caused by contact with dry heat (e.g., fire), moist heat (e.g., steam, hot liquid), chemicals, electricity, friction, or radiant energy.[4] The following is a discussion of thermal injuries according to the level of injury (Fig. 3-1).

I.   Partial-thickness burns[5]
   A. **Superficial partial-thickness:** first- or second-degree burn (i.e., destruction of epidermis and possibly portions of upper dermal layers). Appears red, bright pink, blistered, moist, and soft. Painful. No grafting is necessary for healing. Wound will heal by reepithelialization in 10 to 14 days, resulting in no restrictive scarring with full hand function.
   B. **Deep partial-thickness[5]:** deep second-degree burn. Destruction of epidermis and greater portion of dermal layer (hair follicles, sweat glands). Appears red or white, with the absence of blisters and sometimes a moderate thickness eschar.[1] Sensation and pain may be diminished. Potential conversion to full-thickness burn. Delayed healing taking 14 to 21 days and can result in poor-quality skin, risking hypertrophic scarring and contracture formation. Early resurfacing with better-quality skin must be considered.[1]

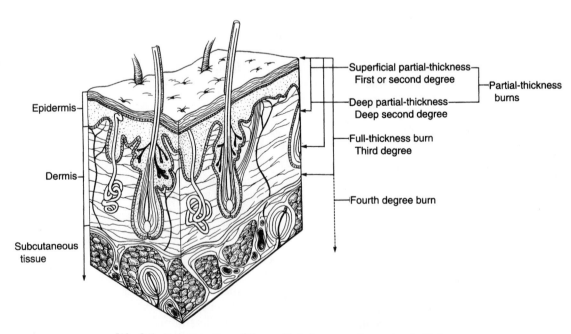

FIG. **3-1** Categorization of thermal injuries according to level of injury.

II. **Full-thickness burn**[1,5]: third-degree burn. Destruction of entire epidermis and dermal layers (hair follicles, nerve endings, sweat glands). Appears white or tan, waxy, dry, and leathery, with a thick, inelastic eschar. No pain or sensation. Requires skin graft resurfacing.

III. **Fourth-degree burn:** Deep soft tissue damage to fat, muscle, tendon, and bone. Appears charred. Electrical burns may show this level of destruction, with thrombosed blood vessels, destruction of nerves along pathway, fractures, and dislocations. Requires extensive surgical procedures and possibly amputations.

IV. Stages of burn recovery

    A. **Acute stage** refers to the time from initial injury until wound closure; estimated up to 2 weeks

    B. **Rehabilitation stage** is from wound closure to scar maturation; estimated 2 weeks to 2 years

    C. **Reconstructive stage** refers to the time during reconstructive surgery to correct contractures or scarring

TREATMENT AND SURGICAL PURPOSE

The goal of managing the burned upper extremity is to restore maximum function with stable esthetic soft tissue coverage at the earliest possible time. Skin grafting is frequently required to achieve this. Therapeutic exercise, proper positioning, and splinting are essential in preventing contracture formation and lost motion and preserving function.

TREATMENT GOALS FOR ACUTE BURN STAGE

    I. Promote wound closure.

    II. Protect exposed tendons and joints.

    III. Maximize functional recovery through prevention of the following

        A. Contractures

        B. Infection

        C. Muscle disuse atrophy

        D. Tendon adherence and rupture

        E. Capsular and ligament shortening

    IV. Decrease edema.

    V. Control pain.

    VI. Regain full ROM.

    VII. Minimize excess scar formation.

    VIII. Assist with psychological recovery.

    IX. Restore functional independence.

TREATMENT GOALS FOR REHABILITATION STAGE

    I. Maximize functional recovery through prevention of the following

        A. Contractures

        B. Muscle disuse atrophy

        C. Tendon adherence

        D. Capsular and ligament shortening

    II. Control pain.

    III. Regain full ROM.

    IV. Minimize excess scar formation.

    V. Restore functional independence.

    VI. Increase strength and endurance.

TREATMENT GOALS FOR RECONSTRUCTION STAGE

I.   Correct positioning and protection to promote healing of reconstructive procedure.
II. Regain full ROM.
III. Minimize excess scar formation.
IV. Restore functional independence.
V.   Increase strength and endurance.
VI. Return to work.

INDICATIONS FOR SURGERY

I.   Tangential excision/grafting: indicated for deep partial-thickness burns
II. Full-thickness excision: indicated for full-thickness burns
III. Circumferential thermal burn may require an escharotomy
IV. Electrical burn: may require fasciotomy[3]
V.   Burn scars requiring contracture release or resurfacing: FTSGs, flaps, tissue expanders, and skin substitutes

POSTOPERATIVE INDICATIONS/PRECAUTIONS FOR THERAPY

I.   Contraindications/precautions for the acute burn stage
     A. Overstretching and vigorous exercise (especially the proximal interphalangeal [PIP] joint)
     B. Occlusive dressing (interferes with evaluation of perfusion)[3]
     C. Splinting straps may apply pressure that interferes with circulation. Gauze wraps should be used.
     D. Pressure may increase severity of burn.[6]
     E. Discontinue ROM or use protective ROM to exposed joints or tendons.[6]
     F. Discontinue ROM or pain-free ROM only if patient complains of deep joint pain due to possible heterotrophic ossification.[6]
     G. Cellulitis[7]
II. Precautions during the rehabilitation and reconstructive stage
     A. Patient should use sun block or avoid strong sunlight.
     B. Patient will be less able to tolerate cold weather and will require gloves to remain warm.
     C. New skin will blister easily and break open.

POSTOPERATIVE THERAPY FOR THE ACUTE BURN STAGE

I.   See graft care guidelines for specific management.
II. See wound care guidelines for specifics on management of wounds.
III. Superficial partial-thickness burns
     A. First 48 hours: keep hand elevated.[3,6] Gently cleanse the wound. Jets from whirlpool will be too painful. See physician regarding debridement approach. Dress with nonadherent dressing. Begin gentle active range of motion (AROM) and passive range of motion (PROM) to pain tolerance. Splinting is not required. Patient should be moving hand, fingers, and wrist.
     B. Two days to healing of wounds: Encourage independence in activities of daily living (ADL); full mobility.

IV. Deep partial-thickness burns if not grafted
  A. Up to 72 hours after surgery: Keep hand elevated to decrease edema.[3,6] Irrigate wound with saline. Remove debris. Dress with nonadherent dressing. Pain control. Begin gentle AROM. AROM exercise should be performed every hour.[1] Splinting is required only if patient is unable to complete exercises.
  B. Hook and fist exercises may be initiated as long as tendons and joints are not exposed.
  C. Dorsal hand burns are splinted in intrinsic-plus position; that is, wrist in 20 degrees to 30 degrees extension; finger metacarpophalangeal (MCP) joints in 70 degrees flexion; interphalangeal (IP) joints in full extension; thumb positioned halfway between radial and palmar abduction, with MCP flexed 10 degrees and IP fully extended[1,3,7] (Fig. 3-2).
  D. Palmar burns only are splinted with wrist in 30 degrees of extension and fingers in extension with thumb abducted and extended.[3]
  E. Once edema has decreased, splint only at night, if needed. Begin PROM to tolerance. Encourage use of hand for light activities.
  F. Once wound has healed: begin gradual strengthening as tolerated.
V. Full-thickness burn: excision and grafting of deep partial-thickness burn
  A. Preoperatively splint as described earlier. Protected AROM exercises to prevent tendon rupture.
    1. Wrist and MCP joints positioned in extension, with PIP and distal interphalangeal (DIP) joints in flexion.
    2. PIP and DIP joints positioned in extension, with the MCP joints flexed.
  B. Immediately postoperative: Hand is elevated. Splint as described previously.
  C. 3 to 5 days postoperatively: First dressing change.[3] Reintroduction of motion depends on graft adherence. Motion should not be started on grafts that appear macerated or discolored or if excess bleeding is present. Begin AROM when dressings are off to observe the graft. Continue splinting at night and between exercises.

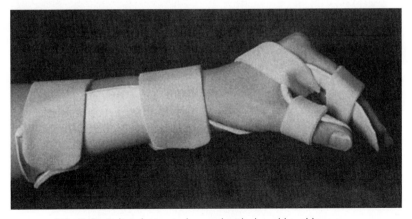

FIG. **3-2** Splint design to be used with dorsal hand burns.

D. 5 to 7 days postoperatively: Daily dressing changes. Continue AROM exercises. Begin active-assisted range of motion (AAROM) and PROM. Encourage light ADL.[3] Splint only at night.

E. After 7 days: Discontinue splinting time during the day unless patient begins to develop deformities, but continue night splinting. Encourage use of hand for all self-care activities.

F. Various skin substitutes have become commercially available, including cultured epithelial autografts, AlloDerm, and Integra. Consult with the physician and manufacturer for therapy guidelines.

POSTOPERATIVE THERAPY FOR THE REHABILITATION STAGE

I. Scar massage and retrograde massage can be initiated once tissue is adherent, even if small open areas exist.

II. Begin early application of pressure to minimize scar formation: elastomer and silicone gel sheeting (Fig. 3-3) (watch for maceration), Coban or Ace wraps, Tubigrip bandages, or Isotoner gloves can be used as early forms of pressure therapy.

III. Custom burn garments should be ordered once the burn wound is almost healed and there are only a few open areas no larger than a quarter[8]; garments are applied when higher shear forces can be tolerated[9] (Fig. 3-4). Elastomer inserts or silicone gel sheeting may be worn under custom compression garments.[6]

IV. Prolonged stretch to scar contractures. Low load over a long period can be achieved through splinting, serial casting, exercises (pulleys), and positioning.

V. Begin strengthening and occupational training.

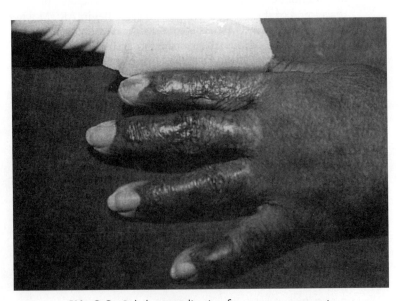

FIG. 3-3 Gel sheet application for scar management.

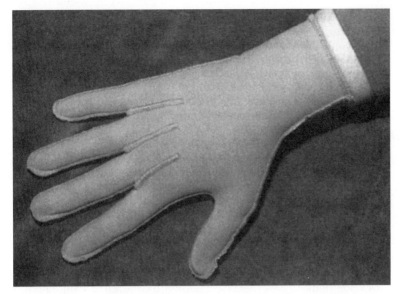

FIG. 3-4 Compressive garments are used to minimize hypertrophic scarring.

Keep in mind that contractures sometimes do not develop until 3 to 4 weeks postoperatively. Scar tissue remains active for 6 months to 2 years. Patients should continue to see their therapists for scar management and splinting to prevent contracture formation.

POSTOPERATIVE THERAPY FOR THE RECONSTRUCTIVE STAGE

   I.   Immobilization immediately after surgery. Length of immobilization depends on type of coverage used (i.e., FTSG or flap). Consult physician.

  II. Begin ROM with physician approval and night splinting

 III. Pressure therapy

 IV. Strengthening

  V. Return to work

POSTOPERATIVE COMPLICATIONS

   I.   Infection

  II. Blisters from shear force

 III. Contractures: may require surgical reconstruction (see Chapter 2)

     A. Boutonniere deformity (most common)[10]

       1. Treated with a finger gutter splint to position PIP joint in extension for 6 to 8 weeks

       2. Treated with serial casting over dressings keeping PIP joint extended for 6 to 8 weeks, with the cast being changed daily if needed to change dressing

       3. Treated with K-wire fixation for 3 weeks, followed by splinting

     B. Web space contractures, especially the thumb and index finger web space

       1. Treated with splinting and elastomer

   C. Swan neck deformity
    1. Treated with splinting
 IV. Heterotrophic ossification (more common in the elbow)
  V. Pain
 VI. Vascular insufficiency with chronic edema
 VII. Psychological issues: posttraumatic stress syndrome

EVALUATION TIMELINE

  I. Wound evaluation with careful attention to exposed tendons or joints: acute stage
  II. ROM: all stages. Notify physician of joint contractures. Early reconstructive surgery may be indicated.
 III. Sensation: all stages
 IV. Scar assessment: rehabilitation and reconstruction stages
  V. Strengthening: rehabilitation and reconstruction stages
 VI. Fine motor skills: rehabilitation and reconstruction stages
 VII. Developmental assessments/screening in children: rehabilitation and reconstruction stages

FUNCTIONAL OUTCOMES

Research on functional restoration of the burned upper extremity has shown encouraging results. The deepest burns requiring grafts show the most dysfunction in ROM, grip strength, and coordination.

Sheridan and coworkers,[9] over a 10-year period, treated 659 patients with 1047 acutely burned hands. They reported normal function in 97% of those with superficial injuries and 81% of those with deep dermal and full thickness injuries requiring surgery. Only 9% included injuries involving the extensor mechanism, joint capsule, or bone. Ninety percent were able to independently perform activities of daily living.

Barillo and colleagues[11] reported on 82 burned hands, 64 of which required grafting. Total active motion averaged 220.6 degrees at discharge and 229.9 degrees at 3 months after injury. Mean hand grip strength was 60.8 pounds at discharge and 66.0 pounds at 3 months after injury.

von Heimburg and associates[12] assessed sensation in patients with deep partial-thickness hand burns who underwent debridement and grafting with STSG. Assessments were performed at 2 weeks and at 1, 3, 6, and 12 months after grafting. Light touch and sharp/dull discrimination were found to be intact. Two-point discrimination varied with each patient. Tactile gnosis and stereognosis were good in all burned hands.

REFERENCES

1. Helm PA: Burn rehabilitation: dimensions of the problem. Clinic Plast Surg 19:551-560, 1992
2. Howell JW: Management of the acutely burned hand. In Richard RL, Staley MJ (ed): Burn Care and Rehabilitation: Principles and Practice. FA Davis, Philadelphia, 1994
3. Achauer BM: The burned hand. In Green DP (ed): Operative Hand Surgery. 4th Ed. Churchill Livingstone, New York, 1999, p. 2045
4. Simpson RL, Gartner MC: Management of burns of the upper extremity. In Mackin EJ, Callahan AD, Skirven TM, et al. (eds): Rehabilitation of the Hand and Upper Extremity. 5th Ed. Mosby, St. Louis, 2002, p. 1475

5. Barret JP, Herndon DN (ed): Color Atlas of Burn Care. WB Saunders, New York, 2001
6. Serghiou MA, et al.: Comprehensive rehabilitation of the burn patient. In Herndon DN (ed): Total Burn Care. 2nd Ed. WB Saunders, New York, 2002, p. 563
7. Ware LC, Anthony MS: Orthopaedic Physical Therapy: Burns and Open Wounds of the Hand. Home Study Course 95-2. Orthopaedic Section. American Physical Therapy Association, LaCrosse, WI, 1995
8. Richard RL, Staley MJ: Burn Care and Rehabilitation: Principles and Practice. FA Davis, Philadelphia, 1994
9. Sheridan RL, Hurley J, Smith MA, et al.: The acutely burned hand: management and outcome based on a ten-year experience with 1047 acute hand burns. J Trauma 38:406-411, 1995
10. deLinde GG, Knothe B: Therapist's management of the burned hand. In Mackin EJ, Callahan AD, Skirven TM, et al. (eds): Rehabilitation of the Hand and Upper Extremity. 5th Ed. Mosby, St. Louis, 2002, p. 1492
11. Barillo DJ, Harvey KD, Hobbs CL, et al.: Prospective outcome analysis of a protocol for surgical and rehabilitative management of burns to the hand. Plast Reconstr Surg 100:1442-1451, 1997
12. von Heimburg D, Bahm J, Sporkmann C, et al.: The burned hand: a computer-assisted study of late function of 67 burned and operated hands [German]. Unfallchirurg 105:606-611, 2002

SUGGESTED READINGS

Belliappa PP, McCabe SJ: The burned hand. Hand Clin 9:313-324, 1993
Clarke HM, Wittpenn GP, McLeod AM, et al.: Acute management of pediatric hand burns. Hand Clin 6:221-232, 1990
Frist W, Ackroyd F, Burke J, et al.: Long-term functional results of selective treatment of hand burns. Am J Surg 149:516, 1985
Fisher SV, Helm PA: Comprehensive Rehabilitation of Burns. Williams & Wilkins, Baltimore, 1982
Harrison DH, Parkhouse N: Experience with upper extremity burns: the Mount Vernon experience. Hand Clin 9:11-209, 1990
Herndon D (ed): Total Burn Care. 2nd Ed. WB Saunders, New York, 2002
Kealy GP, Jensen KT: Aggressive approach to physical therapy management of the burned hand. Phys Ther 68:683, 1988
Levine NS, Buchanan T: The care of burned upper extremities. Clin Plast Surg 13:107-113, 1986
Malick M, Carr J: Manual on Management of the Burned Patient. Harmanville Rehabilitation Center, Pittsburgh, 1982
Robson MC, Smith DJ, Vanderzee AJ: Making the burned hand functional. Clin Plast Surg 19:663-671, 1992
Sykes PJ: Severe burns of the hand: a practical guide to their management [review article]. J Hand Surg Br 16:6, 1991
Tredget E: Management of the acutely burned upper extremity. Hand Clin 16:187-202, 2000

Scar Management

4

Tara Barasch

The formation of scar is a normal physiological process that occurs during healing of wounds after accidental tissue disruption or surgery. Excessive scar tissue can interfere with regaining full range of motion (ROM), thereby limiting a patient's functional use of the affected extremity. In addition, an unfavorable scar can be emotionally and socially devastating. Many factors determine scar formation, including a person's age,[1] genetic make-up,[2] health status,[3] wound tension,[4] wound hydration,[5] surgical method used,[1] severity of wound, location of wound,[3] and whether the wound is closed by primary intention or by secondary intention and injection.

There are three main phases of wound healing: the inflammatory phase, fibroplasia, and scar maturation. The **inflammatory phase** occurs after tissue injury and lasts for approximately 5 days. The main objective of this phase is to clear the wound of debris.[3] The next phase of wound healing is **fibroplasia**, which occurs between the third and fifth day and lasts from 2 to 6 weeks. Fibroblasts begin synthesizing collagen, resulting in a scar that is raised and red. Viewed under a microscope, the collagen fibers are oriented in a random configuration, as opposed to a linear fashion as in normal collagen tissue (Fig. 4-1). This is caused by an imbalance between the rate of collagen deposition and that of collagen destruction, which can last up to 4 months. At 3 weeks, wounds gain 20% of final tensile strength; they will reach only 70% of preinjury skin tensile strength once fully matured.[2] The last phase of wound healing is the **scar maturation** or remodeling phase, which begins between the second and third weeks and lasts approximately 1 to 2 years.[6] The rate of collagen synthesis and lysis becomes balanced during this phase, resulting in a paler, softer, and flatter scar.[3] It is during this phase that scar can be greatly influenced to promote tissue gliding and thus increase function. If not managed properly, scars can become problematic, resulting in contracture, adhesion formation, or an abnormal formation. The following guideline will assist the hand therapist in managing scar during the wound healing process after injury, primary surgery, or scar revision surgery. Influencing the factors responsible for morphological change in scar tissue is an important aspect in the restoration of the patient's normal hand function.

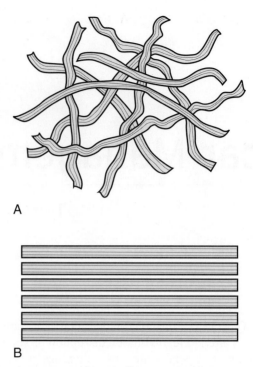

FIG. **4-1 A,** Random pattern of new collagen tissue. **B,** Linear pattern resembling normal collagen tissue.

DEFINITION

    I. **Scar management:** the use of various techniques to remodel/realign the collagen fibers of tissue to promote tissue excursion and improve cosmetic appearance. Initiated after suture removal.

    II. **Hypertrophic scar:** raised, red, itchy scar overgrowth that is confined within the margin of the wound or incision and typically manifests within the first 3 months after injury or surgery. Usually responds to therapy and will flatten eventually within 1 to 2 years.[7,8]

    III. **Keloid scar:** raised, red, and itchy scar overgrowth that extends beyond the margin of the original wound; noted after the first several months up to several years after injury. Often does not respond to therapy and remains elevated. Also, has a high rate of recurrence after revision surgery.[7,8]

TREATMENT PURPOSE

To promote wound or incision closure with minimal scar tissue adhesion, maximal tissue gliding, and acceptable appearance.

TREATMENT GOALS

    I. Restore normal functional use of the involved upper extremity.
    II. Promote tissue gliding to allow ROM.
    III. Improve the appearance of the scar.
    IV. Resolve pain, pruritus (itchiness), and hypersensitivity.
    V. Prevent/treat present or impending joint contracture.

NONOPERATIVE INDICATIONS/PRECAUTIONS FOR THERAPY

I.   Indications
     A. Normal scar: to prevent hypertrophic and/or keloid scar formation
     B. Abnormal scar (hypertrophic or keloid): to flatten and soften
II. Precautions
     A. Infection: a prolonged inflammatory phase may result in infection, leading to increased collagen production.[2,9]
     B. Delayed wound closure: occurs if necrotic tissue is not removed, thus inhibiting the edges of the wound from re-epethializing; this causes an increased risk in the formation of abnormal scar.[2]
     C. Edema: may increase fibroblast production by sustaining an environment susceptible to infection. Also may decrease motion and lead to permanent joint contracture.
     D. Wound tension: Overly aggressive splinting and exercise may increase wound site tension, which in turn delays healing of wound, increases scar width, increases likelihood of necrosis, and decreases tensile strength of wound.[9]
     E. Hypersensitivity: see Chapter 11 on desensitization techniques if present.
     F. Lack of sensation: Use caution in the application of modalities.
     G. Pain: progress treatment gently as tolerated by patient.
     H. Sun exposure: immature scars are prone to burning, which can result in permanent darkening of the healing scar. Sun exposure should be avoided for at least 1 year.
     I. Early aggressive scar massage/therapy: Because the strength of the wound is still very weak during the end of the inflammatory phase and the beginning of the fibroplasia phase, there is great risk of causing an inflammatory response.[10] In addition, vigorous treatment can cause blisters[7] and increase the possibility of hypertrophic scar by increasing fibroblast activity.[11]
     J. Skin maceration: This occurs secondary to continued wear of pressure garments or gel sheets. Instruct patient in frequent skin checks and proper hygiene with the wearing of splints, compression garments, and gel sheets.

NONOPERATIVE THERAPY

I.   Scar evaluation
     A. Location: Note whether scar crosses joints or tendons; risk of contracture is high at these sites.[12]
     B. Type: normal, hypertrophic, keloid (note if widespread).
     C. Pliability: Note whether scars are immature (thick, rigid, and elevated) or mature (flattened, softened, and pale) and whether fibrous bands (frequently seen in burn wounds) are present.[13]
     D. Size: Note width, length, thickness, and height.
     E. Color[3]
        1. Vascularization: Immature scars are red or purplish in color, raised, and blanch to touch; mature scars no longer blanch and are flattened, pale, and closer to patient's normal skin color.
        2. Pigmentation: Hyperpigmentation can indicate problematic scars; hypopigmentation indicates a flat, mature scar.

F. Sensibility: Note hypersensitivity or abnormal sensation.

G. Temperature: Compare against adjacent normal tissue. A warmer scar may indicate a hypertrophic scar, because they contain more cellular activity than mature scars do.[3]

H. Subjective: The patient's perception of the scar can be measured by using a rating scale (Fig. 4-2).[3] Variables assessed include pain, color, size, and itchiness.

II.   Scar management

A. Medical intervention: administered by physician

1. Intralesional corticosteroid injection: flattens scar by decreasing protein synthesis. An example is triamcinolone acetonide.[8,14]

2. Lidocaine patch: decreases itchiness[15] and pain.[16]

3. Interferon injection: inhibits collagen synthesis. Examples used include α-, β-, and γ-interferon.[14,17]

4. Cryosurgery: flattens scar tissue through necrosis. Liquid nitrogen is most commonly used.[14]

5. Laser surgery: reduces erythema, flattens scar, and improves scar texture by causing tissue damage. The flashlamp-pumped pulsed-dye laser (PDL) is the most common type.[14]

6. Antihistamines: reduces pruritus, decreases inflammation, and decreases collagen synthesis.[18] An example is diphenhydramine (Benadryl).

7. Verapamil (calcium channel blocker) injection or topical cream: induces collagen destruction and decreased collagen production.[18]

8. Radiation: destroys the collagen-producing fibroblasts after scar revision surgery.[8,11,14,18]

9. Digit Widget[19]: worn according to doctor's discretion. Promotes contracted tissue to grow.

B. Therapeutic intervention

1. Silicone gel sheets (Fig. 4-3, A), hydrogel sheets,[11,18] digital gel caps (Fig. 4-3, B), Silastic molds (Fig. 4-4): increase skin hydration, resulting in decreased capillary activity, collagen deposition, and hyperemia. The outcome is usually a softer, flatter scar.* Gel caps also assist in edema reduction in the digits. Suggested wearing schedule is during sleep and occasionally during the waking hours totaling at least 12 hours.[17] Limit daytime use, especially over joints, to allow full motion. Gel sheets and putty molds can be secured with compressive garments such as an elastic sleeve (Tubigrip) or self-adherent elastic wrap (Coban), which may also aid in further scar remodeling (see discussion of compressive garments).

2. Compressive garments[12,21]: Isotoner glove (Fig. 4-5), Tubigrip, or Coban wrapping can be used to provide pressure; this results in decreased blood flow and oxygenation of tissue, thereby decreasing collagen production and increasing collagen degradation. Pressure also facilitates realignment of collagen bundles to produce a flatter scar. The recommended amount of compression pressure is 24 mm Hg.[11]

*References 5, 8, 9, 13, 14, 20.

Name _____   Date _____

Scar Self-rating Scale

*The following questions relate to your scar **over the past week.***

PRESENCE OF SYMPTOMS

Over the past week, has your scar been . . .

	Itchy	Hard	Painful
	Tight	Red	Height of scar has increased

CONCERN FOR EACH SYMPTOM

Rate how much each symptom has bothered you over the past week while performing your usual activities, by choosing the number that best describes the amount of bother you have on a scale of 0 to 10. A zero (0) means the symptom did not bother you at all, and a ten (10) means you were extremeiy bothered by the symptom.

Please rate how bothersome the symptom has been:

Itchy
0 1 2 3 4 5 6 7 8 9 10
No bother   Extremely bothered

Hard
0 1 2 3 4 5 6 7 8 9 10
No bother   Extremely bothered

Tight
0 1 2 3 4 5 6 7 8 9 10
No bother   Extremely bothered

Red
0 1 2 3 4 5 6 7 8 9 10
No bother   Extremely bothered

Painful
0 1 2 3 4 5 6 7 8 9 10
No bother   Extremely bothered

Increased height of scar
0 1 2 3 4 5 6 7 8 9 10
No bother   Extremely bothered

PAIN
Rate the average amount of pain in your scar over the past week, by choosing the number that best describes your pain on a scale of 0 to 10. A zero (0) means you did not have any pain, and a ten (10) means you had the worst pain you have ever experienced or you could not do the activity because of pain.

Please rate your pain:
At rest
0 1 2 3 4 5 6 7 8 9 10
No pain   Worst ever

When doing a task holding an object
in your hand
0 1 2 3 4 5 6 7 8 9 10
No pain   Worst ever

COLOR
Rate the color of your scar over the past week, by choosing the number from the scale below that best describes the color of your scar for the majority of the time.

Please rate the color of your scar:
0 Normal   1 Pink   2 Red   3 Purple

COMPLIANCE
Rate the compliance of your scar over the past week, by choosing the number from the scale below that best describes the skin texture.

0	Normal, feels like the skin on the rest of your hand
1	Minimal resistance to pressure
2	Moderate resistance to pressure
3	Firm, inflexible, not easily moved, resistant to pressure
4	Tums white when stretched
5	Is tight when stretched, permanent shortening of scar, producing deformity, distortion, contracture

Thank you for taking the time to answer these questions.

FIG. 4-2   Surgical scar self-rating scale. (From McOwan CG, Mac Dermid JC, Wilton J: J Hand Ther 14(2): 77-85, 2001.)

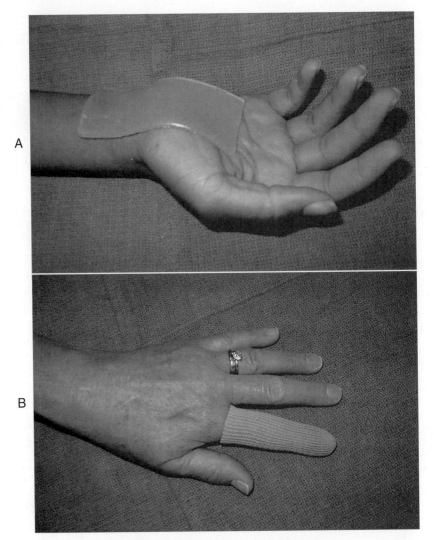

FIG. **4-3** **A,** Gel sheet. **B,** Gel cap.

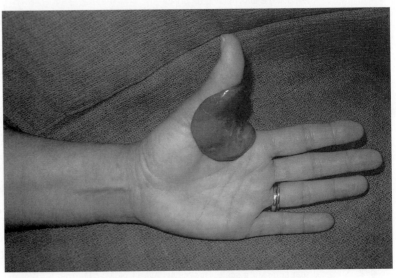

FIG. **4-4** Elastomer mold.

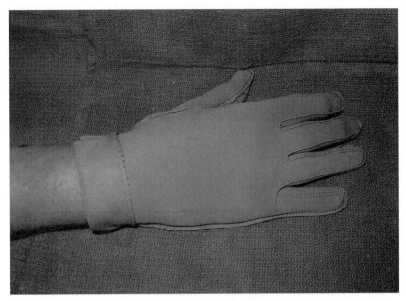

FIG. **4-5** Isotoner glove.

Compressive garments can also be used to secure gel sheets and Silastic molds. Instruct patient to avoid seam lines in hand by wearing glove inside out.

3. Scar massage: After wound closes, begin massage of the scar with lotion several times per day. Use enough pressure to blanch scar. Massage helps to break up collagen fibers, resulting in a softer, flatter, and paler scar.[7] Massage also decreases tissue stiffness and promotes tissue mobility,[21] thus preventing scar contracture.[22]

4. Active/passive range of motion (AROM/PROM): facilitates tissue gliding and increased scar tissue length to prevent scar adhesion and contracture.[23]

5. Stress application: Low-load, prolonged stretch produces permanent elongation of soft tissue.[23]
   a. Static progressive splints[11]: worn for 30- to 45-minute sessions at least three times a day. Patient may also wear during sleep if tolerated.
   b. Joint Active System (JAS)[24]: worn 30 minutes in direction of stretch three times per day.
   c. Serial casting[11]: Apply cast every 3 to 4 days with serial stretch until desired result is achieved. Patient performs AROM/PROM and strengthening exercises between casts.

6. Modalities
   a. Superficial heat: softens soft tissue and increases tissue extensibility. Examples include moist heat packs, paraffin wax, and fluidotherapy.
   b. Deep heat: Thermal ultrasound[11,22] increases collagen extensibility when combined with stretch to increase ROM. Continue applying stretch for 5 to 10 minutes afterward, while tissue is cooling, for optimal results.[25]
   c. Functional electrical stimulation (FES): promotes tendon gliding through scar tissue.

    d. Iontophoresis: helps to reduce excessive scar formation.
     (1) Saline[21]: 2% concentration; negative polarity
     (2) Iodine[25]: 5% to 10% concentration; negative polarity
   7. Topical creams
    a. Mederma (over the counter): helps to smooth, soften, and improve the appearance of scars.[18]
    b. Hydrocortisone: decreases itchiness.
   8. Paper tape: prevents stretching of scar and therefore prevents hypertrophic scarring. Apply tape after wound closure along incision line longitudinally.[9]
   9. Natural ointments (topical vitamins A and E): decrease collagen production as well as inflammation.[5,14]
  C. Functional
   1. Encourage and engage patient in purposeful tasks to restore functional use in
    a. Activities of daily living (ADLs)
    b. Work/productive tasks
    c. Leisure activities
   2. Protect scar as needed: discourage rubbing and scratching.
  D. Surgical intervention
   1. Revision/excision: see later discussion.
   2. Skin grafting, flaps: provide wound coverage if there is significant tissue loss (see Chapter 2).

NONOPERATIVE COMPLICATIONS

 I. Infection
 II. Abnormal scar formation
  A. Hypertrophic
  B. Keloid
 III. Joint contracture
 IV. Tissue adhesion
 V. Decreased function
 VI. Undesirable appearance

NONOPERATIVE OUTCOMES

The use of silicone gel sheeting has been proven to be effective in preventing and improving abnormal scars. Ahn and colleagues[26] found that silicone gel sheeting inhibits hypertrophic scar formation when worn for 2 months for at least 12 hours per day. A 2002 study conducted by Mustoe and co-workers[17] demonstrated gel sheeting as an effective means of preventing hypertrophic scars and keloids as well. In 1995, Katz[20] showed a 55% improvement in chronic hypertrophic or keloid scars with the use of silicone gel sheeting for 2 months. In addition, the effectiveness of gel sheeting in the softening of scar tissue and in reducing pruritus has been documented.[8]

INDICATIONS/PRECAUTIONS FOR SCAR REVISION SURGERY

 I. Indications
  A. Limited motion (joint contracture unresolved with conservative treatment)
  B. Functional loss

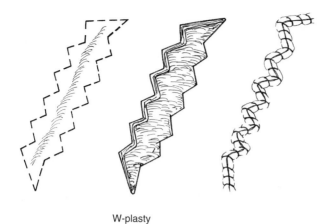

W-plasty

FIG. 4-6 In scar revision surgery, the scar is excised by the W-plasty closure procedure.

     C. Disfigurement

     D. In rare cases, hypertrophic or keloid scars that do not respond to therapy

  II. Precautions: same as nonoperative precautions

SURGICAL DEFINITION

Scar revision/excision: surgical procedure performed 3 to 6 months after the scar maturation phase to improve function and appearance and to correct disfigurement or contracture. The scar is excised and sutured by the W-plasty (Fig. 4-6), Z-plasty (Fig. 4-7), or geometric broken-line closure procedure.

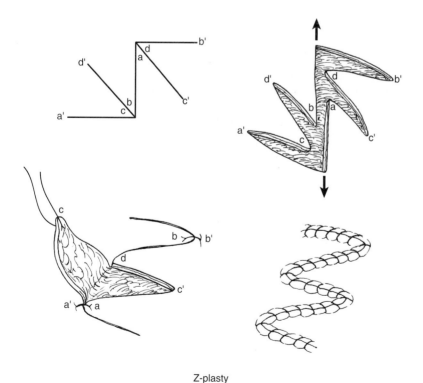

Z-plasty

FIG. 4-7 Z-plasty closure procedure.

Not only do these techniques prevent wound tension, thereby minimizing the recurrence of an abnormal scar growth, but they also camouflage the scar as a jagged line, diffused light making it much less noticeable.[2]

SURGICAL PURPOSE

I.   Improve appearance of scar
II. Improve function
III. Correct disfigurement or contracture

SURGICAL GOALS[27]

I.   To flatten scar
II. To similarly match color and texture of adjacent skin
III. To align incision with relaxed skin tension lines
IV. To elongate scar and break up longitudinal line of scar by using a nonlinear surgical technique

POSTOPERATIVE THERAPY

Scar evaluation and management are the same as for nonoperative therapy; however, immediate therapy is very important postoperatively for optimal results in preventing recurrence of abnormal scar.

POSTOPERATIVE COMPLICATIONS

Complications are the same as for nonoperative therapy; however, the recurrence of an abnormal scar is an additional unwanted complication after scar revision surgery.

EVALUATION TIMELINE

Scar management begins after suture removal or wound closure. Continue scar management for 6 to 12 months. Re-evaluate periodically to monitor both subjective and objective change.

POSTOPERATIVE OUTCOMES

Scar revision surgery alone results in a 45% to 100% recurrence rate[11] of hypertrophic or keloid scar. Combining revision surgery with therapy and medication can improve these statistics significantly. For instance, combining with corticosteroid injections results in a recurrence rate of less than 50%.[11] Moreover, in a 1998 study by Su and colleagues,[11] the combination of surgery, therapy (gel sheets and pressure), and radiation treatment decreased the rate to less than 10%.

REFERENCES

1. Koopman C: Cutaneous wound healing: an overview. Otolaryngol Clin North Am 28: 835-845, 1995
2. Moran ML: Scar revision. Otolaryngol Clin North Am 34:767-780, 2001
3. McOwan CG, MacDermid JC, Wilton J: Outcome measures for evaluation of scar: a literature review. J Hand Ther 14:77-85, 2001

4. Atiyeh BS, Ioannovich J, Al-Amm CA, et al.: Improving scar quality: a prospective clinical study. Aesthetic Plast Surg 26:470-476, 2002

5. Chang CWD, Ries WR: Nonoperative techniques for scar management and revision. Facial Plast Surg 17:283-287, 2001

6. Madden JW: Wound healing: the biological basis of hand surgery. Clin Plast Surg 3:181-186, 1976

7. Edwards J: Scar management. Nurs Stand 17(52):39-42, 2003

8. Alster TS, Tanzi EL: Hypertrophic scars and keloids. Am J Clin Dermatol 4:235-243, 2003

9. Evans RB, McAuliffe JA: Wound classification and management. In Mackin EJ, Callahan AD, Skirven TM, et al. (eds): Hunter-Mackin-Callahan Rehabilitation of the Hand and Upper Extremity. 5th Ed. Mosby, St. Louis, 2002, pp. 325-326

10. Poochareon VN, Berman B: New therapies for the management of keloids. J Craniofac Surg 14:654-657, 2003

11. Su CW, Alizadeh K, Boddie A, et al.: The problem scar. Clin Plast Surg 25:451-465, 1998

12. Puzey G: The use of pressure garments on hypertrophic scars. J Tissue Viability 12:11-15, 2001

13. deLinde LG, Knothe B: Therapist's management of the burned hand. In Mackin EJ, Callahan AD, Skirven TM, et al. (eds): Hunter-Mackin-Callahan Rehabilitation of the Hand and Upper Extremity. 5th Ed. Mosby, St. Louis, 2002, pp. 1492-1523

14. Tsao SS, Dover JS, Arndt KA, et al.: Scar management: keloid, hypertrophic, atrophic, and acne scars. Semin Cutan Med Surg 21:46-75, 2002

15. McClinton MA: Personal communication, March 25, 2005

16. Galer BS, Jensen MP, Ma T, et al.: The lidocaine patch 5% effectively treats all neuropathic pain qualities: results of a randomized, double-blind, vehicle-controlled, 3-week efficacy study with use of the neuropathic pain scale. Clin J Pain 18:297-301, 2002

17. Mustoe TA, Cooter RD, Gold MH, et al.: International clinical recommendations on scar management. Plast Reconstr Surg 110:560-571, 2002

18. Roseborough IE, Grevious MA, Lee RC: Prevention and treatment of excessive dermal scarring. J Natl Med Assoc 96:108-116, 2004

19. Agee JM: Reversing PIP joint contractures: applicability of the Digit Widget external fixation system. Hand Biomechanics Lab 1-10, 2002

20. Katz BE: Silicone gel sheeting in scar therapy. Therapeutics for the Clinician 56:65-67, 1995

21. Micholovitz SL: Ultrasound and selected physical agent modalities in upper extremity rehabilitation. In Mackin EJ, Callahan AD, Skirven TM, et al. (eds): Hunter-Mackin-Callahan Rehabilitation of the Hand and Upper Extremity. 5th Ed. Mosby, St. Louis, 2002, p. 1758

22. Demling RH, SeSanti L: Scar management strategies in wound care. Rehab Manag 14:26-30, 2001

23. Pettengill KMS: Therapist's management of the complex injury. In Mackin EJ, Callahan AD, Skirven TM, et al. (eds): Hunter-Mackin-Callahan Rehabilitation of the Hand and Upper Extremity. 5th Ed. Mosby, St. Louis, 2002, pp. 1415-1418

24. Bonutti PM, Windau JE, Ables BA, et al.: Static progressive stretch to reestablish elbow range of motion. Clin Orthop (303):128-134, 1994

25. Cameron MH: Physical agents in rehabilitation: from research to practice. WB Saunders, Philadelphia, 1999, pp. 280-282, 402-405

26. Ahn ST, Monafo WW, Mustoe TA: Topical silicone gel for the prevention and treatment of hypertrophic scar. Arch Surg 126:499-504, 1991

27. Horswell BB: Scar modification: techniques for revision and camouflage. Atlas Oral Maxillofac Surg Clin North Am 6:55-72, 1998

SUGGESTED READINGS

Bayat A, McGrouther DA, Ferguson MW: Skin scarring. BMJ 326:88-92, 2003

Cohen IK, Diegelmann, RE, Lindblad WJ: Wound healing: biomechanical and clinical aspects. WB Saunders, Philadelphia, 1992

Donnelly C, Wilton J: The effects of massage to scars on AROM movement and skin mobility. Br J Hand Ther 7:5-11, 2002

Hardy MA: The biology of scar formation. Phys Ther 69:1014-1024, 1989

Har-Shai Y, Amar M, Sabo E: Intralesional cryotherapy for enhancing the involution of hypertrophic scars and keloids. Plast Reconstr Surg 111:1841-1852, 2003

Lupton JR, Alster TS: Laser scar revision. Dermatol Clin 20:55-65, 2002

O'Kane S: Wound remodeling and scarring. J Wound Care 11:296-299, 2002
Paper S: The management of scars. J Wound Care 2:354-360, 1993
Schweinfurth JM: Future management of scarring. Facial Plast Surg 17:279-282, 2001
Sherris D, Larrabee W, Murakami C: Management of scar contractures, hypertrophic scars, and keloids. Otolaryngol Clin North Am 28:1057-1062, 1995

PART **TWO**

Nerve Injuries and Compression

Sensibility Testing 5

Judith Bell-Krotoski

Today, it is possible to repair peripheral nerves and maintain or regain degrees of peripheral nerve function with varying success. Advances in the understanding of disease, injury, and neurophysiology offer new knowledge on how nerves are damaged and how they repair themselves. Documentation of the direction of change in peripheral nerve function—improvement, *status quo*, or worsening—requires clear and exacting measurement of nerve status. Sensitive, repeatable and valid testing can document the results of treatment with evidence, substantiate the value of therapy in patient recovery, and help identify the most successful treatments and treatment outcomes. A clear test of physical nerve status is critical in patient evaluation for direct correlations with treatment intervention. One must first determine the physical status of the nerve, rather than how the patient is adapting to degrees of loss in function. Secondarily, understanding is needed of an impaired or recovering patient's ability to adapt and retrain abnormal sensory processes. Recent studies have demonstrated the plasticity of the brain in response to amputation and injury and offer renewed hope that reeducation does influence physiologic recovery.[1]

It stands to reason that test instruments that are relied upon for meaningful clinical information should be as objective and as repeatable in test stimuli as possible. *Testing of sensibility can be subjective if it relies on the response of the patient to determine intact or impaired neural processes.* The challenge in testing should not be used as an excuse to use unrepeatable and unreliable tests for measurement. On the contrary, it becomes even more important to use measurements that are as exacting and repeatable as possible to unmask and reveal the specific physiological status and changes in neural status, which can be directly correlated with treatment.

DEFINITIONS

I. **Epicritic sensation:** Sufficient degrees of sensibility present to provide useful touch recognition—may be two-point discrimination or touch-pressure threshold detection that is protective level or above.[2]

II. **Hypersensitivity:** Change in sensitivity of the end-organ receptors in the skin after injury; often associated with areas of *diminuted* threshold detection to light touch that are hyperirritable and increased in pain sensitivity.

III. **Innervation density:** As used in sensibility measurement, the density (number) of end-organ receptors in a cutaneous area, often reduced in number after nerve repair and regeneration, even after optimal recovery of the nerve; associated with two-point discrimination testing.

IV. **Mechanoreceptors:** Neural end organs in the skin that respond to deformation or stretch.

V. **Provocative tests:** Tests that can elicit signs and symptoms of peripheral nerve involvement—used for early recognition of developing problems in patients with a good history of nerve involvement who have nerves that still score "within normal limits" to standard tests.

VI. **Referred touch:** Missed reference of point or area detection, most often found after nerve repair and regeneration—tends to improve with maturation of the nerve and use of the hand.

VII. **Reeducation:** Retraining of neural events occurring at the end organs, and patient recognition/discrimination of neural events; actually begins immediately after injury but is believed to be most responsive to therapeutic programmed instruction after sufficient neural return has occurred to allow useful discrimination of touch recognition.

VIII. **Sensation:** The acceptance and activation of impulses in the afferent nerve fibers of the nervous system.[3]

IX. **Sensibility:** The conscious appreciation and interpretation of the stimulus that produced sensation.[3]

   A. **Graphesthesia:** The ability to detect symbols drawn on the fingertips as evidence of light touch recognition and discrimination.

   B. **Texture discrimination:** The ability to recognize small differences in texture as evidence of touch recognition and discrimination.

   C. **Stereognosis:** The ability to discriminate between similarly sized and shaped objects (central nervous system [CNS] recognition).

   D. **Protective sensation:** Sufficient degree of sensibility to avoid burns and other injury from external pressure, heat, or sharp objects.

   E. **Loss of protective sensation:** Degree of impairment or loss in protective function of the terminal nerve fibers and sensory end organs that places a patient in danger of burns and other injury (from unrecognized external pressure or during use of an extremity with a slowed or absent response to temperature and pain).[4]

X. **Touch-pressure threshold detection level:** Increasing or decreasing levels of light-touch to deep-pressure mechanoreceptor response that correlate in general with a hierarchy of sensibility capacity (levels of functional detection, recognition, and discrimination).

XI. **Tactile gnosis:** Touch knowledge; use of sensibility and CNS knowledge of neural events occurring at the terminal nerve fibers and end organs that Moberg[5] described as object recognition.

TREATMENT PURPOSE

Sensibility evaluation is intended to examine the peripheral nerve system, which is composed of motor, sensory, and sympathetic nerve fibers. Three major nerve branches innervate the hand and upper extremity: the ulnar, median, and radial branches. The motor nerve fibers terminate in the muscles that they respectively innervate, and the sensory nerve fibers terminate in the skin. Other fibers terminate in the blood vessels and hair follicles.[6] All sensibility evaluation is performed with the peripheral nerves and their normal variations in mind.

Data from patient sensibility evaluations overall contain both quantitative and qualitative elements that help provide insight and information regarding the degree of impairment and function of the patient. The examiner needs to focus testing and evaluation time on "minimal critical measures" that can be obtained accurately and consistently and provide the most reliable information for treatment consideration and monitoring of peripheral nerve status.

GOALS

I. The initial goal in sensibility evaluation is to identify correctly the physical status of the peripheral nerves (i.e., determine the degree of nerve function or impairment).[7-9]
    A. Clinical evaluation consists of a good history and examination of the integrity of the peripheral nerves, including sensory, motor, and sudomotor function.
    B. Quantitative evaluation primarily consists of measurements of neural mechanoreceptor end organs in the skin that can reveal and quantify the status of the nerves. Initial evaluation allows the establishment of a baseline in status for subsequent measurements. Other tests may need to be added to determine specific diagnoses.
    C. Subsequent repeat testing determines the character and direction of change in nerve status.
II. The second goal in sensibility evaluation is measurement of patient use and adaptation. Adaptation does require CNS cortical reasoning and includes skills of the patient, which can vary from patient to patient. Patient use of an extremity with impaired sensibility can vary depending on CNS function, extent of nerve injury, and whether muscle function is also involved.

INDICATIONS AND PRECAUTIONS

I. Indications
    A. Nerve compressions, repetitive use syndromes, and so on
        1. The establishment of a baseline and subsequent testing enables treatment considerations in early stages and allows early recognition of "acute episodes."
        2. As measured with commonly used tests, neural change in physiological function can be measured as change in light-touch perception, and later, with progression, as changes in temperature, deep pressure, or pain; it can progress to a point at which all of epicritic touch that is protective is lost, except for some deep pressure and pain response, before total loss of all neural function occurs.[2,4]

   3. Early detection of developing problems allows treatment
      intervention at a point before nerve impairment has become
      irreversible and there is a loss of protective sensation.
B. Nerve repairs, grafts, replantations, and so on
   1. Measurements are best made before nerves are repaired, if
      possible, to allow documentation of differences on subsequent
      examinations and to clearly detect early neural return.
   2. The rate of axonal regeneration is typically 1 to 5 mm/day or
      1 inch/month, but some repairs return faster and others
      more slowly.
   3. In general, a nerve graft is expected to return more slowly and to
      a lesser degree than a simple nerve repair. The quality of return
      is somewhat dependent on the length the nerve has to regrow,
      with shorter distances sometimes showing better return.
   4. Referred touch is a common phenomenon after nerve repair
      and is most extreme when the nerve is first regenerating.
   5. As a repaired nerve regenerates, nerve axons may not always
      reinnervate the same fascicles, and sensory fibers may be
      cross-innervated with other sensory fibers and motor fibers.
   6. Localization of touch tends to normalize as the hand is used
      and the new nerve matures.
   7. Point and area localization usually improve with reeducation,
      but touch-pressure threshold detection does not.
   8. Regenerating nerves usually produce spontaneous
      sensations, which are sometimes painful and uncomfortable
      "electrical," pin-prick, moving touch, itching, buzzing,
      tickling, or hot and cold sensations.
   9. Patients need to be told to expect spontaneous sensations
      before or soon after the repair, so that they know what to
      anticipate, and that such signals from the injured nerve are a
      good sign indicating that the nerve is alive and repairing.
   10. If patients are informed that abnormal sensations are to be
       expected only after they have complained about them, they
       often believe that the treating staff personnel are just trying
       to make them feel better. The difference in attitude can be
       dramatic.
   11. In general, spontaneous aberrant sensations normalize as
       the nerve matures, but they often take 1 year or longer to
       disappear.
   12. Unwanted spontaneous sensations can remain a problem in
       some patients for years, particularly in replanted hands.
   13. The possibility that some patients will react adversely to these
       sensations in replanted hands should be considered in
       decisions of whether to reattach a hand or part. Some patients
       have actually requested that their replanted hand be removed.
C. Underlying neuropathic disease causing ischemia and dysfunction
   1. Some patients have underlying neuropathic disease and
      dysfunction as a basis of their abnormality in sensibility.
   2. Patients with neuropathic disease often have a stocking glove
      pattern to their sensory loss.
   3. Patients with diabetes often have a dying-back pattern of the
      peripheral nerves related to ischemia.

4. Patients with underlying neuropathic disease can be tested with the same measures used for patients with repetitive use, compression, and entrapment syndromes or lacerations.

5. Patients with CNS disorders may have normal neural potential for sensibility but abnormal central recognition; they require other forms of testing.

II. Precautions

A. All peripheral nerve testing needs to be done in a quiet area where the patient can be relaxed and free of distraction.

B. Measurements and test instruments should be kept as consistent as possible between and across patients, with critical measures established on all patients and other tests added as indicated for individual patients and specific patient conditions.

C. Specific questions need to be asked regarding which conditions make the symptoms worse, and which help, because these give clues to the cause of the problems.

D. Time elapsed is particularly important in nerve compression and entrapment syndromes; long-standing unchanging impairment is less likely to improve with treatment.

E. In repaired nerves, the time before repair, the condition of the repaired nerve, and postoperative tension and positioning are important to record.

F. Pain or hypersensitivity can be an inhibiting factor to any patient measurement. The area, type, and degree of pain are important to record.

G. The American Society for Surgery of the Hand (ASSH) and the International Federation of Societies for Surgery of the Hand (IFSSH) have developed an Impairment Classification that addresses pain: Sensory Deficits and/or Pain Interference from Peripheral Nerve Disorders (IFSSH, 2004) (Appendix 5-1).

THERAPY (EVALUATION)

I. Provocative tests

A. When a patient with nerve compression or entrapment syndrome scores "within normal limits" on testing, or there is a good history of nerve symptoms returning after suture, provocative tests are sometimes helpful.

B. Before there are measurable sensory changes, signs and symptoms can sometimes be elicited and measured, which, when combined with a good history, can indicate nerve return or the need for treatment at a point before changes are otherwise quantifiable.

C. The peripheral nerves in patients with nerve entrapment or compression are examined for points of tenderness or discomfort at typical sites of entrapment, and the results are recorded as part of the physical examination.[10]

D. A positive Phalen's test can elicit signs of median nerve compression at the wrist (Fig. 5-1).

E. Elbow flexion with traction placed on the ulnar nerve can elicit signs and symptoms of nerve compression at the elbow (Fig. 5-2).

F. Forearm pronation with wrist flexion can elicit symptoms of radial sensory nerve compression (Fig. 5-3).
G. If a patient who tests "within normal limits" states that his or her symptoms become worse after a particular activity, it is sometimes helpful to test the patient before and after that activity. Some patients have symptoms during or after periods of stress but have results that are "within normal limits" after a

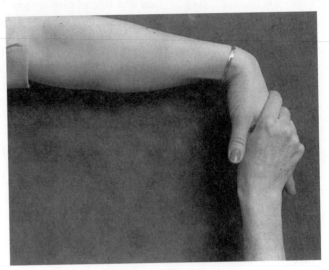

FIG. **5-1** Phalen's test.

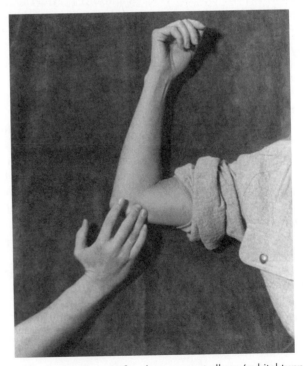

FIG. **5-2** Provocative test for ulnar nerve at elbow (cubital tunnel).

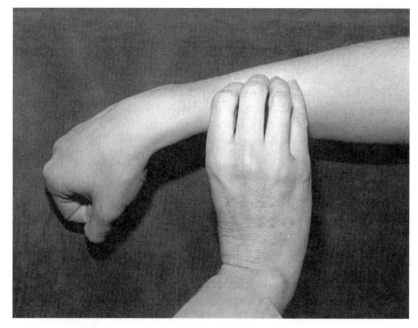

FIG. **5-3** Provocative test for radial sensory nerve compression.

period of rest. When they report for evaluation, they are
frequently taking off from their normal work, have perhaps slept
later, and may have had a leisurely morning before testing.

H. A positive Tinel's sign distal to the point of nerve suture is the
earliest sign that a repaired nerve is returning, although it is not
a quantifiable test.[11] Tapping over the nerve 4 to 6 weeks after
injury can elicit shocking and shooting sensations distal to the
site of suture and signal regrowth of a nerve.

II. Sympathetic nerve status

A. The condition and appearance of the hand being evaluated should
be examined, with particular attention given to areas of vasomotor
change, sweating change, and absence of "gooseflesh" response
(excluding palm).

B. Dryness or hardening of skin can correspond with areas of
sensory diminution. Areas of callus sometimes correspond with
areas of sensory diminution (e.g., a patient squeezes harder in
using the fingers to obtain previous sensory feedback levels).
Any suspect areas are recorded and examined closely during
sensibility testing.

C. A fingertip-wrinkling test can demonstrate areas of denervation
at the fingertips in children with early lacerations of ulnar or
median nerves (not accurate after a period of potential nerve
return).[12] The patient's fingertips are soaked in water at
approximately 40° C for 30 minutes, and "wrinkling" or
shriveling is observed to occur, or not, in fingertips that
correspond to the nerves in question.

III. Nerve conduction velocity

A. Sensory and motor nerve conduction testing should be done for
patients with entrapment or compression if it is available and
can be done with careful technique.

B. Although nerve conduction testing is relatively objective, in that it does not require the subjective response of the patient for measurement, this examination also varies with the skill of the examiner, interpretation of results, quality of the instrument, time of day, temperature of the room, and other variables.

C. Given correct instrument calibration, procedure, and interpretation, the test can produce invaluable information regarding the physical nerve status, anatomical level of involvement, and specific nerves involved.

D. If indicated, electroneuromyographers usually recommend examining both extremities of the patient, including ulnar, median, and radial branches, from the neck down.

E. Many peripheral nerve problems are bilateral, and "double crush" involvement (more than one level of slowing) or multiple nerve involvement is possible.

F. Nerve conduction velocity studies do not directly correlate with what a patient can or cannot detect at the end organs (i.e., the potential ability of the patient to "feel").[13-15] There is a loose correlation, for example, if sensory nerve conduction is greatly slowed; and there usually is a diminution in measurement of touch-pressure threshold detection, and often in innervation density testing, but it is not a direct correlation. One test measures the speed at which the nerve conducts, and the others measure the potential of the sensory end organs to respond to a signal.

G. It is not expected that a direct correlation will be found between speed of nerve conduction and end-organ function, because these are different measurements. Tested independently, but considered together, the tests give added insight into nerve status and specific nerve involvement. For instance, it is possible to have an absent nerve conduction response, leading an examiner to believe that the nerve being measured is unresponsive and no longer treatable, yet, in some cases, residual response may be present on deep pressure detection threshold testing, leading one to consider that the nerve still is alive and potentially recoverable (i.e., treatable).

IV. Muscle testing

A. Brief muscle testing should be performed along with sensibility testing to provide more information on the character and status of the peripheral nerves, and on the intrinsic versus extrinsic muscle balance of the fingers and thumb.

B. Testing of one or two muscles for each nerve is essential (consistent on Hand Screen) but others may be added in testing as indicated.

C. Usually muscle testing is done as a prelude to sensibility testing, and it has the effect of also relaxing the patient and making the testing situation more comfortable due to direct interchange and contact between patient and therapist.

D. It is important to also consider the muscles in doing sensibility testing, because the peripheral nerves include both motor and sensory fibers.

E. Sensory fibers are usually affected first in compression syndromes, and sensory rather than motor impairment is usually the first to recover after laceration.

F. Muscle abnormality in any of the three major nerves that innervate the upper extremity can signal which sensory areas to check or measure more closely.

G. The ASSH and the IFSSH have developed an Impairment Classification that addresses muscle testing: Motor Strength and Loss of Range of Motion (IFSSH, 2004) (Appendix 5-2).

V. Monofilament testing for touch-pressure detection threshold level

A. Test instrument

1. The Semmes-Weinstein Monofilament Test, developed specifically for measuring touch-pressure threshold detection levels, is increasingly gaining recognition and use worldwide.[16]

2. The diameter and length of the monofilament predicts its force of application. If the length is 68 mm from where it leaves the rod, and the diameter is correct, the monofilament will apply an intended force of application within a small range.[17]

3. Measurement of touch-pressure threshold detection levels provides a clear understanding of the area and degree of return to the repaired nerve or nerves (Fig. 5-4).

4. The Original Long Set of 20 monofilaments was not arranged in a predetermined size progression based on specific numerical intervals of application force; rather, it was arranged according to available diameters that produce increasing force. Therefore, not all of the monofilaments in the long kit are needed for most testing. They have been identified and grouped according to the descriptive "levels of function" found, compared with patient functional discrimination tests. The test most often used has been shortened to those five or six monofilaments

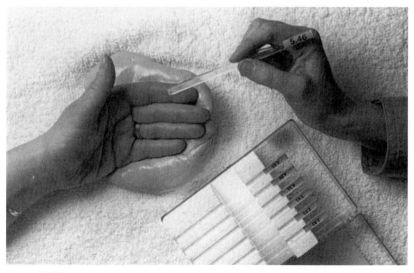

FIG. **5-4** Use of Semmes-Weinstein monofilaments.

that are most useful in predicting changes in levels of function.[2,4,18,19]

5. Reporting of the source, type, and calibration of test used is critical to any studies and publications regarding the monofilament test.

6. Although this is an exact test when used correctly, all monofilament tests are dependent on technique and instrument calibration for validity.[20]

B. Test protocol

1. Questions considered during evaluation:

a. *Is a nerve normal or not (within normal limits)?* Patient populations may be screened for those with impairment in nerve status, using the monofilament most consistent with "normal thresholds." This shortens the time needed for testing patients, because, if the result is normal, there is usually no need to proceed with more detailed testing. Exceptions occur if nerve conduction tests are abnormal or if the patient history indicates that a patient deserves to be retested or monitored closely.

b. *If a nerve is abnormal, how abnormal is it (degree of diminution in physiological nerve function)?* Does the patient have only slight or severe diminution, or even loss? If only mild diminution is present, the patient may need only to be followed and retested periodically. If the abnormality is moderate to severe, it is only a matter of time before the nerve impairment becomes permanent, if it is not already permanent. If the injury is recent, the patient with nerve impairment at least deserves consideration of whether there is potential for recovery with treatment intervention. Subsequent tests can demonstrate changes in status.

c. *What is the direction of the "change in status" with subsequent tests and treatment (improved,* status quo, *or worsened)?* Nerves do not usually cease to function at a single point in time unless there is severe compression or laceration. Most nerve involvements caused by disease or repetitive injury show areas of mild diminution long before they show more severe involvement, and then progress to loss of nerve function. In contrast, a nerve that has lost function will usually show only deep pressure recognition and response to heavier monofilaments until there is more return and recognition of lighter-force monofilaments. But these patterns are not absolute, and in patients with compression it is often found that an injured nerve attempts to recover but has continued episodes of diminution and incomplete recovery. A nerve that has been demonstrating good return after laceration and repair may become entangled in scar tissue at some point and cease improving or become worse. Only sequential measurement can reveal the exact status and direction of change in status, if any.

d. *What is the quality of neural status and function?* What is the level of tactile discrimination compared with other sensibility tests of graphesthesia, texture discrimination, stereognosis, temperature, and pain?

e. *What other tests are needed?* For the overall picture of patient status and possibilities of treatment intervention, results of testing are often used in the context of triangulation of findings; that is, they are used, as a minimum, with additional tests of nerve conduction as well as qualitative assessments of patient history and functional use.

2. Procedure for Hand Screen or mapping

a. For comparisons with normative data to be valid, the test protocol used should be the same as that used to establish the normative data. Normative data for the Semmes-Weinstein type monofilaments are available.[8,9,21,22]

b. Monofilament testing is now included in the Impairment Classification Guidelines created and endorsed by both the ASSH and IFSSH and used by the American Medical Association (AMA). These recommend a standard protocol and grading (IFSSH, 2004) (Appendix 5-3): "Testing begins with the lightest filaments for screening normal areas. If these filaments are detected, it is not necessary to use heavier filaments. If they are not detected, progressively heavier filaments are used until a filament is recognized, or the patient does not respond to any filament. As the patient closes the eyes, the monofilament is applied perpendicular to the body surface, and pressure is increased until the monofilament bends. The filaments are applied at least three times to an unresponsive site. This is done to ensure delivery of the desired threshold force, as the light filaments can sometimes be applied at an angle and result in too light a force. One response out of three is considered a correct response. Testing begins by establishing an area that tests within normal limits, to allow the patient to become familiar with the procedure, and the examiner to establish a normal sensibility area for reference. This area can be revisited frequently, to ascertain that what the subject cannot detect in the test site, cannot also be detected in the normal control site."

3. Additional procedure detail

a. The patient is shown examples of the touch of the monofilament and asked to respond with a "yes" when it is detected.

b. The subject closes the eyes and turns the head, or the line of vision is occluded with a screen (e.g., file folder). The subject is not blindfolded, because this can be distracting and introduces hygiene considerations.

c. A *site of reference* can be established on the distal volar forearm or higher up the extremity, even on the face or back, if necessary.

d. The site of reference is marked and returned to frequently if there is no response to an area tested, to ensure a differential—that a monofilament not responded to at a test site is responded to in the reference site. This eliminates uncertainty.

e. For accuracy, each monofilament is applied in a smooth application of about 1.5 seconds, held for 1.5 seconds, and removed in 1.5 seconds.

f. The filament should not be "bounced" against the skin, unless the examiner is intending to deliver a slightly heavier force of application (e.g., checking to see whether the subject might respond if the monofilament were slightly heavier).

g. The filament should not be jerked away or lifted quickly, because this can produce a burst of stimulus to the end organs in the skin.

h. Establishing a rhythm in application helps the subject anticipate the timing of stimulation. At any time, the rhythm may be interrupted to ensure that the patient is responding to the stimulus and not just saying "yes." If the patient continues to say "yes" when not being touched, this can be pointed out to the patient, which almost always creates the focus needed.

i. The 2.83 monofilament is tested first, because if the result is "normal" there is no need to proceed with heavier monofilaments and the test is over in a short time.

j. Once areas that are "normal" are quickly eliminated, progressively heavier monofilaments are used to fill in areas in which there is not response, until detection levels are identified or it is established there is no response to any monofilament. Hand Screen monitoring sites (Fig. 5-5) are tested first, usually from distal to proximal, but the examiner randomly moves around to test these and any other sites added to avoid the subject's anticipation of the next site to be tested (to eliminate a potential source of a false-positive result).

k. At any time, the sequence and timing of application may be interrupted to ensure that the patient is actually responding to the stimulus and not just giving a "yes" response.

l. Mapping in addition to the Hand Screen simply requires more test sites sufficient in area and number to map out the desired area, in contrast to areas of response that are "within normal limits." A full mapping is most often done on initial testing, with a follow-up Hand Screen.

m. The lightest monofilaments (up to 5.07 in the long kit of 20) are applied in three applications. The patient usually responds to the first monofilament within three applications, and this is important to ensure that the correct force of these very fine monofilaments has been delivered. (This procedure is identical to that used in normative studies for the monofilaments.)

n. Examiners do not have to be concerned about summation of touch, because there is no summation of touch for

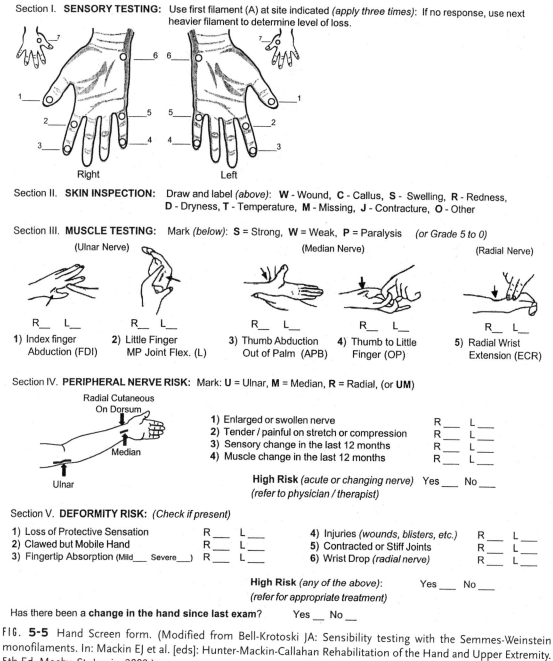

Section I. **SENSORY TESTING:** Use first filament (A) at site indicated *(apply three times)*: If no response, use next heavier filament to determine level of loss.

Right   Left

Section II. **SKIN INSPECTION:** Draw and label *(above)*: **W** - Wound, **C** - Callus, **S** - Swelling, **R** - Redness, **D** - Dryness, **T** - Temperature, **M** - Missing, **J** - Contracture, **O** - Other

Section III. **MUSCLE TESTING:** Mark *(below)*: **S** = Strong, **W** = Weak, **P** = Paralysis   *(or Grade 5 to 0)*

(Ulnar Nerve)   (Median Nerve)   (Radial Nerve)

R__ L__   R__ L__   R__ L__   R__ L__   R__ L__

1) Index finger   2) Little Finger   3) Thumb Abduction   4) Thumb to Little   5) Radial Wrist
   Abduction (FDI)   MP Joint Flex. (L)   Out of Palm (APB)   Finger (OP)   Extension (ECR)

Section IV. **PERIPHERAL NERVE RISK:** Mark: **U** = Ulnar, **M** = Median, **R** = Radial, (or **UM**)

Radial Cutaneous
On Dorsum

Median

Ulnar

1) Enlarged or swollen nerve   R ___ L ___
2) Tender / painful on stretch or compression   R ___ L ___
3) Sensory change in the last 12 months   R ___ L ___
4) Muscle change in the last 12 months   R ___ L ___

High Risk *(acute or changing nerve)* Yes ___ No ___
(refer to physician / therapist)

Section V. **DEFORMITY RISK:** *(Check if present)*

1) Loss of Protective Sensation   R ___ L ___   4) Injuries *(wounds, blisters, etc.)*   R ___ L ___
2) Clawed but Mobile Hand   R ___ L ___   5) Contracted or Stiff Joints   R ___ L ___
3) Fingertip Absorption (Mild___ Severe___) R ___ L ___ 6) Wrist Drop *(radial nerve)*   R ___ L ___

High Risk *(any of the above)*:   Yes ___ No ___
(refer for appropriate treatment)

Has there been a **change in the hand since last exam**?   Yes ___ No ___

FIG. 5-5 Hand Screen form. (Modified from Bell-Krotoski JA: Sensibility testing with the Semmes-Weinstein monofilaments. In: Mackin EJ et al. [eds]: Hunter-Mackin-Callahan Rehabilitation of the Hand and Upper Extremity. 5th Ed. Mosby, St. Louis, 2002.)

touch recognition (as there can be for temperature or pain). It is not possible to change the detection level by continued stimulation or retraining, and this is one reason the monofilament test is a good test (i.e., there is no learning curve).[23] Where in doubt, it is best to retest sites to establish the correct level of detection, rather than report a false-negative finding.

     o. For the Hand Screen, because a limited number of sites are tested, each site is revisited at least three times if the patient does not respond.

     p. The level of monofilament identified by number is recorded on a form, and color-coded at the site tested, or filled in to make a map. The same form may be used to record localization testing information, areas of two-point discrimination tested, and results from inspection of the hand (e.g., callus, dryness, wounds), and all other sensibility tests performed, on one report.

     q. See Appendix 5-3 for Semmes-Weinstein Monofilaments Interpretation and Relationship to Function, and Scale of Interpretation of Monofilaments.

4. Hand Screen (see Fig. 5-5)

     a. The minimum monofilaments for an examination can be used at test sites specific to each nerve (ulnar, median, and radial) to maximize information on specific nerves and normal or abnormal level of detection.

     b. A Hand Screen Form with other information important in peripheral nerve monitoring and recording of monofilaments detected at each data point on a hand drawing is the simplest record and documentation.

     c. The critical Minikit monofilaments include the "cutoff" detection level for normal men and women (2.83 marking number), and "cutoff" filaments for each functional detection level (3.61, 4.31, 4.56, and 6.65 marking numbers).

     d. Time required is often reduced to 10 minutes for the Hand Screen.

     e. The data points (test sites) may be numerically coded for direct comparisons in relation to treatment.

     f. The data points lend well to graphs of patient peripheral nerve function with comparison of treatment results over time.

     g. When examiners use the same data points, data collected in the same test protocols may be compared between patients and across patient populations for information on similarities of findings and differences among treatment programs and clinics.

     h. Lighter monofilaments, found in the 20-monofilament set, are sometimes added to the Hand Screen when testing for earliest detection of compression syndromes (in subjects with a good history but score "within normal limits").[24]

     i. A few heavier monofilaments are sometimes added for monitoring earliest return after nerve suture (the 5.56 monofilament, approximately 10 g, is most commonly added).

     j. The Hand Screen data points for each nerve may be compared consistently, regardless of the number of additional data sites used, in a Hand Screen, a full hand mapping, or a full upper extremity mapping of threshold response.

k. The Hand Screen test and Form are in general domain for use and may be copied.

l. Scoring the Hand Screen:

(1) Each monofilament is given a weighted grade for detection level—normal, 5 points; diminished light touch, 4 points; diminished protective sensation, 3 points; loss of protective sensation, 2 points; residual deep pressure sensation, 1 point; and untestable, 0 points—at each site, then totaled for a numerical score for each nerve and also overall.

(2) Muscle testing is included to monitor muscles specific to each peripheral nerve. Each muscle is given a weighted grade (5 to 0 points, respectively) for normal, good, fair, poor, trace, and absent results, and totaled for a numerical score for each nerve and overall.

(3) Other information is consistently included on the Hand Screen Form regarding the skin condition and presence of trophic changes or callus, tenderness or pain over nerves when palpated, and the relative quiescence or acuteness of peripheral nerve symptoms.

(4) A Disability Classification indicator (based on the World Health Organization Disability Classification of 1984) is also included, and scoring is explained on the form.

6. Known errors in use of the monofilaments:

a. Bouncing the filaments against the skin (increases force of application).

b. Using a point-localization test to change the results (confuses results and mapping).

c. Applying the lightest monofilaments only once (lighter than 5.07 marking number).

d. Asking for two "yes" responses out of three trials (should be one out of three, as in normative studies).

e. Bending the monofilament until it forms a "C" curve.

f. Cutting off a monofilament to increase its force of application.

g. Testing with a more-than-slightly bent monofilament.

h. Accepting a monofilament application that slid across a finger or other skin area.

i. Applying a monofilament in less than 1.5 seconds (increases force of application).

j. Not establishing an area of reference on the patient as being "within normal limits."

k. Testing the patient in a noisy area.

l. Testing the patient in extremes of temperature (can change calibration).

V. Point or area localization of touch

A. Localization of touch is often abnormal after nerve suture and should be assessed separately as another test.

B. Patterns of return of localization vary from the patterns of touch-pressure detection threshold, and the two should not be tested together, or one test changed because of the other, as has been done in some test protocols for the monofilaments.

C. Point or area localization can be quickly and easily assessed in areas of abnormality that have been determined by touch-pressure threshold testing.

D. Testing is done by the examiner's touching (with a small dowel or probe) a spot distal to a nerve suture for the patient to identify and point to with an identical probe in the subject's other hand.

E. The centimeters of distance and the direction from the point stimulated that are indicated by the patient comprise the measurement of amount of referral.

F. Multiple stimulations usually show multiple distances and directions, and these can be indicated on a form (Hand Screen) by arrows.

G. The subject's vision is occluded during testing.

H. The results in centimeters of distance measured with a small ruler are noted.

I. Improvement is recognized in reduced distances of referral on subsequent testing.

J. Referred touch tends to normalize (become closer to within 1 cm) as a nerve regrows and returns, from proximal to distal, with proximal areas showing improvement before distal ones do.

VI. Two-point discrimination for innervation density

A. Test instrument

1. The two-point discrimination test has been the most frequently and most widely used of the sensibility tests.

2. Moberg, who first popularized the test, has maintained that the standard two-point discrimination test is the most useful test in determining "tactile gnosis."

3. Dellon named the original test the "static" two-point discrimination test and introduced a "moving" two-point discrimination test for earlier detection in patients with axonal return after nerve repair.

4. Both "static" and "moving" two-point discrimination tests are most accurate at the fingertips, with a wider spread between points of detection more proximally on the hand and upper extremity and on other areas of the body.[25,26]

5. The Disk-Criminator (Post Office Box 16392, Baltimore, MD 21210) has advantages over other two-point discrimination instruments in that it has graduated, preset, standard millimeter distance tips for testing, and the weight of each disc is relatively light.

6. If the weight of the instrument is used in an attempt to control the force of application, the application force of the instrument is more controlled than when there is no limit to force applied.[27]

7. The test is still subject to wide variation in application force and vibration of the examiner's hand, as well as variations from examiner to examiner.

8. Pressure should not be added in addition to the weight of the instrument in testing.

9. The weight of the instrument cannot be used as a control in various positions in which gravity is reduced and the examiner is left to simulate the weight of the instrument.

10. Test/retest studies can be found in the literature for two-point discrimination that report repeatable testing.[28-30]

11. Sometimes two-point discrimination values can be normal when there is diminution to touch-pressure at the level of diminished protection. In controlled neural compression in normal subjects, it was demonstrated that two-point discrimination values remain normal long after nerve conduction, monofilament, and vibration testing detect changes. In addition, after release of compression, two-point discrimination is the last test to return to normal values.[14]

12. Many investigators now agree that the two-point discrimination test is not sensitive enough for early detection in patients with nerve compression, and that decreased two-point discrimination is a late finding.[31]

13. Lundborg and colleagues reported that "two-point discrimination may never return to normal or measurable levels after repair of major nerve trunks in adults, even in cases where there is good recovery of perception of touch/pressure, useful dexterity, good grip strength and no pain or discomfort."[32]

B. Test protocol

1. General considerations

a. Because the fingertips are the distalmost points of innervation for the ulnar and median nerves, the status of these nerves can often be assessed at the fingertips, and the test is most frequently used at the fingertips (Fig. 5-6).

b. The test can be quickly performed for comparison in sites of abnormality identified by touch-pressure threshold testing.

c. Some examiners start with the smallest distance and others with the greatest distance between the probes.

2. The Impairment Classification created and endorsed by the ASSH and IFSSH and used by the AMA, recommends a standard protocol and grading for two-point discrimination testing (see Appendix 5-1):

a. "During the test, the patient's hand should be fully supported and the vision occluded. Testing is started distally and proceeds proximally. Because light-touch discrimination is being tested, the pressure applied should be very light (10 to 15 g) and must not produce a point of blanching or skin indentation. The most common error is to apply too much pressure which will completely change the results because more pressure will bring more receptors into the field of stimulation and cause more skin deformation.[33,34] The two points are applied in a longitudinal orientation and must make contact exactly at the same time to avoid recognition factors related to time-dynamics rather than spatial orientation.[1] A series of one or two-point touches is applied randomly at an interval of no less than 3 to 5 seconds and the subject immediately

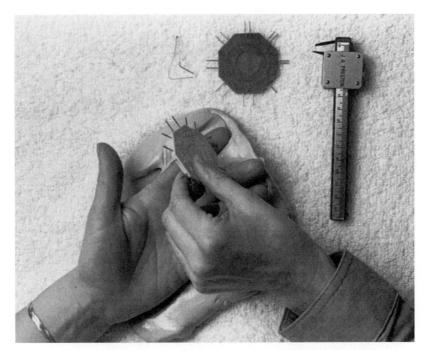

FIG. 5-6 Devices that may be used to assess two-point discrimination.

indicates whether one or two points are felt. At least two out of three responses must be accurate for scoring.[8] The distance between the caliper tips is set first at 5 mm and progressively increased until the required accurate responses are elicited, at which time the distance is recorded."

b. A classification that recognizes this important functional differentiation was suggested by Gelberman and associates[35] and by Fess,[36] and was adopted by the ASSH for interpretation of two-point discrimination scores: normal, less than 6 mm; fair, 6 to 10 mm; poor, 11 to 15 mm; protective, one point perceived; and anesthetic, no point perceived.

3. Grading
   a. Most examiners agree that detection of less than 6 mm of distance is normal in the fingertip pulp.[8,37-39]
   b. Moberg maintained that recognition of distances of 6 to 15 mm is required for tactile gnosis, and that greater than 15 mm represents a useless finger.[5,40]
   c. For standard grading, the protocol and classification of the ASSH is recommended: normal, less than 6 mm; fair, 6 to 10 mm; poor, 11 to 15 mm (ASSH, 1983).[36]

4. Known errors in use of two-point instruments
   a. Using different techniques or instruments for measuring the same patients or groups.
   b. Using blanching as a control for force of application (blanching occurs with different force in different fingers and skin areas).[20]

      c. Applying increased force of application in addition to the weight of the instrument.

      d. Bouncing an instrument against the skin (increases force).

      e. Assuming that the application force of a hand-held instrument is less than 2 to 4 g (unless force is controlled).

      f. Assuming that the application force of a hand-held instrument is repeatable within a small gram range or standard deviation (unless force is controlled).

VII. Moving two-point discrimination

    A. Dellon realized the limitation in conventional two-point discrimination testing for detection of early nerve return and was searching for a more sensitive test when he introduced the moving two-point discrimination test.

    B. The instrument and technique are the same as for the conventional test, except that the instrument is drawn along the length of the finger proximally to distally, with prongs side by side.

    C. Patients with returning peripheral nerves will detect a "moving" two-point stimulus before a "static" conventional one, providing a positive response earlier in nerve recovery.

    D. Several authors report a good correlation between moving two-point tests and object identification.[41-43]

    E. The moving two-point-discrimination test[37,44] is advocated by Dellon as useful in the evaluation of recovering nerve function because a patient can detect response to this stimulus before response to a "static" (nonmoving) two-point stimulus.

VIII. Vibration detection

    A. Vibration testing with tuning forks has been a frequently used test among neurologists, and it was earlier advocated by Dellon for recognition of returning nerve function.

    B. Vibration testing is limited in its usefulness for providing specific test information in patients with nerve compression or nerve repairs by its lack of suitably controlled instruments.

    C. Tuning forks are so uncontrolled that they will only be mentioned here.

    D. The largest criticism of tuning forks for testing of vibration, in addition to their hand-held application, is that their actual vibration and frequency in cycles per second are masked by the large-amplitude signals produced when they are applied to the patient's skin.[20]

    E. The tuning forks were designed to produce a frequency stimulus for measuring hearing; they were not designed to slap against the skin at varying amplitudes for measuring sensibility.

    F. Detection of the vibration of tuning forks, at either 30 or 256 Hz, can still be accomplished by some patients who have a known partial nerve loss, possibly by bone conduction and overflow of stimulation to other areas.

    G. Vibration as produced by tuning forks for sensory reeducation after nerve repair may be useful and may have a role in sensory reeducation, as do any other tools that can stimulate returning axons and excite sensory end organs.

    H. Dellon advocated that the perception of a 30-Hz tuning fork distal to the site of nerve suture is a helpful early sign of nerve return and usually can be detected before a 256-Hz tuning fork.

    I. Dellon[37] also suggested that perception of a 256-Hz tuning fork to indicate enough sensory return for formal reeducation techniques can be effective, and many examiners use this test as a useful guideline in reeducation of patients.

IX. Computerized sensibility tests

    A. Dyck and associates[7,45] used computer-controlled test stimuli in experimental studies to evaluate touch-pressure, vibration, and thermal cutaneous sensation.

    B. An automated tactile tester (ATT) was designed by Horch and Tuckett for light-touch, vibration, two-point discrimination, and thermal sensations.[46]

    C. Lundborg and coworkers[47] reported good results with computerized vibration instruments that are force controlled, specific and sensitive, but not generally available in the United States.

    D. Gelberman and Szabo used experimental computerized instruments for vibration that are available in the United States, but they reportedly have not been satisfied that instrument designs are yet sufficiently controlled and repeatable to be used for reliable clinical testing.[14,24] Experimental research is expensive, but it is hoped that highly controlled computerized vibration tests will become more available and may play a larger role in future clinical testing of sensibility.

    E. Another computerized instrument designed primarily for two-point discrimination testing is the NK Hand Assessment. Nebojsa Kovacevic invented the NK Hand Assessment computerized two-point discrimination test and believed that the ability of the platform to hold and deliver the instrument probes and to adjust these to a specific distance from the site to be tested were important factors for a repeatable control of force of application.[26]

    F. Dellon purchased the rights to the NK instrument, adapted the equipment to his specifications, and now sells it as the Pressure Sensitive Device (PSSD). (See Appendix 5-4 for sample quantitative testing results and a PSSD Quantitative Testing Form.) The PSSD has improved control on force of application for one-point and two-point testing over the hand-held tests with no or limited control. The stimulus device reportedly has a damping mechanism in its design for reducing vibration of the examiner's hand, but it is still hand-held in application to the patient being tested. Computerized instruments are intended to apply controlled force or pressure.[26,42,45-49]

OUTCOMES

I. Outcome studies are needed to help substantiate the critical elements that should be measured in practice.[50]

II. All of the tests have in common detection of thresholds for normal patients, all identify change in sensibility, and the results are often clearer in testing when these results are considered together. (See Appendix 5-5 for a Sensory Testing Relative Guide.)

III. Today clinical tests have been further developed through an evolution in understanding of neurophysiology and technology, but many need improved instrument control before their results can be relied upon in clinical testing.

IV. The examiner of sensibility has to have one foot in understanding the intent and development of tests, as well as their strengths and weaknesses, and one foot in the future, remaining open to newer knowledge and tests.

REFERENCES

1. Lundborg G, Rosen BG: The Two-Point Discrimination Test: Time for a Reappraisal? Department of Hand Surgery, Malm University Hospital, Malm, Sweden. In Press.
2. Werner JL, Omer GE: Evaluating cutaneous pressure sensation of the hand. Am J Occup Ther 24:347, 1970
3. Omer GE Jr: Sensation and sensibility in the upper extremity. Clin Orthop 104:30-36, 1974
4. Von Prince K, Butler B: Measuring sensory function of the hand in peripheral nerve injuries. J Occup Ther 21:385-396, 1967
5. Moberg E: Objective methods for determining the functional value of sensibility in the hand. J Bone Joint Surg Br 40:454-476, 1958
6. Mountcastle VB: Medical Physiology. 14th Ed. Mosby, St. Louis, 1980, pp. 348-390
7. Dyck PJ, Obrian PC, Bushek W, et al.: Clinical versus quantitative evaluation of cutaneous sensation. Arch Neurol 33:651-656, 1979
8. Omer GE, Bell-Krotoski J: Sensibility testing. In: Omer GE, Spinner M, Van Beek MA (eds): Management of Peripheral Nerve Problems. WB Saunders, Philadelphia, 1998, pp. 3,11-28
9. Bell-Krotoski J, Fess EE, Figarola JH, et al.: Threshold detection and Semmes-Weinstein monofilaments. J Hand Ther 8:155, 1995
10. Eversmann WW: Compression and entrapment neuropathies of the upper extremity. J Hand Surg Am 8:759, 1983
11. Tinel J: The "tingling" sign in peripheral nerve lesions. In Spinner M (ed): Injuries to the Major Branches of Peripheral Nerves of the Forearm. 2nd Ed. WB Saunders, Philadelphia, 1978, pp. 8-11
12. O'Riain S: New and simple test of nerve function in the hand. BMJ 3:615-616, 1973
13. Almquist E, Ecg-Olofsson O: Sensory nerve-conduction velocity and two-point discrimination in sutured nerves. J Bone Joint Surg Am 52:791-796, 1970
14. Gelberman RH, Szabo RM, Williamson RV, et al.: Sensibility testing in peripheral nerve compression syndromes: an experimental study in humans. J Bone Joint Surg Am 65:632-638, 1983
15. Breger DE: Correlating Weinstein-Semmes monofilament mapping with sensory nerve conduction parameters in Hansen's disease patients: an update. J Hand Ther I:33-37, 1987
16. Weinstein S: Reminiscences on the history and development of the Semmes-Weinstein monofilaments. Presented at the Conference on Biomechanics of Deformity and Treatment of the Insensitive Hand, Gillis W. Long Hansen's Disease Center, Carville, LA, May 4-6, 1992
17. Bell-Krotoski J, Tomancik E: The repeatability of testing with the Semmes-Weinstein monofilaments. J Hand Surg Am 12:155, 1987
18. Bell JA: Light touch–deep pressure measurement with the Semmes-Weinstein monofilaments. In: Hunter JM, Schneider LH, Mackin EJ, Bell JA (eds): Rehabilitation of the Hand. Mosby, St. Louis, 1978
19. Bell-Krotoski JA: Light touch–deep pressure testing using Semmes-Weinstein monofilaments. In: Hunter JM, Schneider LH, Mackin EJ, Callahan AD (eds): Rehabilitation of the Hand: Surgery and Therapy. 3rd Ed. Mosby, St. Louis, 1990, p. 585

20. Bell-Krotoski JA, Buford WL Jr: The force/time relationship of clinically used sensory testing instrument. J Hand Ther 10:297-309, 1997; 1:76, 1988

21. Semmes J, Weinstein S: Somatosensory Changes After Penetrating Brain Wounds in Man. Harvard University Press, Cambridge, MA, 1960

22. Weinstein S: Tactile sensitivity of the phalanges. Percept Mot Skills 14:351-354, 1962

23. Robert LaMotte, PhD: Personal communication, 1979.

24. Szabo RM, Gelberman RH, Dimick MP: Sensibility testing in patients with carpal tunnel syndrome. J Bone Joint Surg Am 66:60, 1984

25. Weinstein S: Intensive and extensive aspects of tactile sensitivity as a function of body part, sex, and laterality. In Kenshalo DR (ed): The Skin Senses. Charles C Thomas, Springfield, EL, 193-218, 1968

26. Bell-Krotoski JA: Advances in sensibility evaluation. Hand Clin 7:527, 1991

27. Louis DS, Greene TL, Jacobson KE, et al.: Evaluation of normal values for stationary and moving two-point discrimination in the hand. J Hand Surg Am 9:552-555, 1984

28. Dellon AL, MacKinnon SE, Crosby PM: Reliability of two-point discrimination measurements. J Hand Surg Am 12:693-696, 1987

29. MacKinnon SE, Dellon AL: Two-point discrimination tester. J Hand Surg Am 10: 906-907, 1985

30. Novak CB, MacKinnon SE, Williams JI, et al.: Establishment of reliability in the evaluation of hand sensibility. J Plast Reconstr Surg 92:311-322, 1993

31. Katz JN, Simmons BP: Clinical practice. Carpal tunnel syndrome. N Engl J Med 346:1807-1812, 2002

32. Lundborg G, Rosen B, Dahlin LB, et al.: Tubular repair of the median or ulnar nerve in the human forearm: a 5-year follow-up. J Hand Surg Br 29:100-107, 2004

33. Moberg E: Two-point discrimination test: a valuable part of hand surgical rehabilitation in tetraplegia. Scand J Rehabil Med 22:127-134, 1990

34. Moberg E: Reconstructive hand surgery in tetraplegia, stroke and cerebral palsy: some basic concepts in physiology and neurology. J Hand Surg Am 1:29-34, 1976

35. Gelberman R, Urbaniak J, Bright D, et al.: Digital sensibility following replantation. J Hand Surg Am 3: 313-319, 1978

36. Fess EE: Documentation: essential elements of an upper extremity assessment battery. In Mackin EJ, Callahan AD, Skirven TM, et al. (eds): Hunter-Mackin-Callahan Rehabilitation of the Hand and Upper Extremity. 5th Ed. Mosby, St. Louis, 2001, pp. 263-283

37. Dellon AL: Evaluation of Sensibility and Re-education of Sensation in the Hand. Williams & Wilkins, Baltimore, MD, 1981

38. Gellis M, Pool R: Two-point discrimination distances in the normal hand and forearm: application to various methods of fingertip reconstruction. Plast Reconstr Surg 59:57-63, 1977

39. Moberg E: Methods for examining sensibility in the hand. In: Flynn JE (ed): Hand Surgery. Williams & Wilkins, Baltimore, MD, 435-439, 1966

40. Moberg E: Aspects of sensation in reconstructive surgery of the upper extremity. J Bone Joint Surg Am 46:817-825, 1964

41. Chassard M, Pham E, Comtet JJ: Two-point discrimination tests versus functional sensory recovery in both median and ulnar nerve complete transections. J Hand Surg Br 18:790-796, 1993

42. Dellon ES, Keller KM, Moratz V, et al.: Validation of cutaneous pressure threshold measurements for the evaluation of hand function. Ann Plast Surg 38:485-492, 1997

43. Novak C, MacKinnon S, Kelly L: Correlation of two-point discrimination and hand function following median nerve injury. Ann Plast Surg 31:495-498, 1993

44. Dellon AL: The moving two-point discrimination test: clinical evaluation of the quickly adapting fiber receptor system. J Hand Surg Am 3:474-481, 1978

45. Dyck PJ, Zimmerman IR, Obrien PC, et al.: Introduction of automated systems to evaluate touch-pressure, vibration, and thermal cutaneous sensation in man. Ann Neurol 4:502-510, 1978

46. Horch K, Hardy M, Jimenez S, et al.: An automated tactile tester for evaluation of cutaneous sensibility. J Hand Surg Am 17:829, 1992

47. Lundborg G, Gelberman R, Minteer-Convery M, et al.: Median nerve decompression in the carpal tunnel: functional response to experimentally induced controlled pressure. J Hand Surg Am 7:252-259, 1982

48. Dellon AL: A numerical grading scale for peripheral nerve function. J Hand Ther 6:152, 1993

49. Tassler PL, Dellon AL: Correlation of measurements of pressure perception using the pressure-specified sensory device with electrodiagnostic testing. J Occup Environ Med 37:862-866, 1995
50. Bindra RR, Dias JJ, Heras-Palau C, et al.: Assessing outcome after hand surgery: the current state. J Hand Surg Br 28:289-294, 2003

SUGGESTED READINGS

Bell-Krotoski JA: Sensibility testing: state of the art. In: Hunter JM, Mackin EJ, Callahan AD, et al. (eds): Rehabilitation of the Hand: Surgery and Therapy. 4th Ed. Mosby, St. Louis, 1995, p. 109

Bell-Krotoski JA: Correlating sensory morphology and tests of sensibility with function. In: Hunter JM, Schneider LH, Mackin EJ (eds): Tendon and Nerve Surgery in the Hand: A Third Decade. Mosby, St. Louis, 1997, pp. 49-62

Bell-Krotoski J, Weinstein S, Weinstein C: Testing sensibility, including touch-pressure, two-point discrimination, point localization, and vibration. J Hand Ther 6:114, 1993

Buford WL: Clinical assessment, objectivity, and the obiquitous laws of instrumentation. J Hand Ther 8:149-154, 1995

Darian-Smith I, Kenins P: Innervation density of mechanoreceptors supplying glabrous skin of the monkey's index finger. J Physiol 309:147-155, 1980

Dellon AL: Sensibility testing. In Gelberman RH (ed): Operative Nerve Repair and Reconstruction. Lippincott-Raven, Philadelphia, 1991, p. 135

Dellon AL: Management of peripheral nerve problems in the upper and lower extremity using quantitative sensory testing. Hand Clin 15:697-715, 1999

Dellon AL, Kallman CH: Evaluation of functional sensation in the hand. J Hand Surg Am 8:865-870, 1983

Duteille F, Petry D, Poure L, et al.: A comparative clinical and electromyographic study of median and ulnar nerve injuries at the wrist in children and adults. J Hand Surg Br 26:58-60, 2001

Gibson JJ: Observations on active touch. Psychol Rev 69:477-491, 1962

Gordon G: Active Touch. Pergamon Press, Elmsford, NY, 1978

Greenspan JD, Lamotte RH: Cutaneous mechanoreceptors of the hand: experimental studies and their implications for clinical testing of tactile sensation. J Hand Ther 6:75, 1993

Johansson RS, Vallbo AB: Tactile sensibility in the human hand: relative and absolute densities of four types of mechanoreceptive units in glabrous skin. J Physiol 286: 283-300, 1979

Johnson KO, Hsiao SS: Neural mechanisms of tactual form and texture perception. Ann Rev Neurosci 15:227-250, 1992

Kets CM, Van Leerdam ME, Van Brakel WH, et al.: Reference values for touch sensibility thresholds in healthy Nepalese volunteers. Leprosy Rev 67:28-38, 1996

Kenshalo DR: The Skin Senses. Plenum Press, New York, 1968, pp. 195-218

LaMotte RH, Srinivasan MA: Tactile discrimination of shape: response of slowly adapting mechanoreceptive afferents to a step stroked across the monkey fingerpad. J Neurosci 7:1655-1671, 1987

Lundborg G, Lie-Stenstrom AK, Sollerman C, et al.: Digital vibrogram: a new diagnostic tool for sensory testing in compression neuropathy. J Hand Surg Am 11:693-699, 1986

MacDermid JC, Kramer JF, Roth JH: Decision making in detecting abnormal Semmes-Weinstein monofilament thresholds in carpal tunnel syndrome. J Hand Ther 7:158-162, 1994

MacKinnon SE, Dellon AL: Diagnosis of nerve injury. In: MacKinnon SE, Dellon AL (eds): Surgery of the Peripheral Nerve. Thieme Medical Publishers, New York, 1988, p. 65

MacKinnon SE, Dellon AL: Sensory rehabilitation after nerve injury. In: MacKinnon SE, Dellon AL (eds): Surgery of the Peripheral Nerve. Thieme Medical Publishers, New York, 1988, p. 521

Ochs S: A brief history of nerve repair and regeneration. In: Jewett DL, McCarroll HR Jr: Nerve Repair and Regeneration, Mosby, St. Louis, 1980, p. 5

Omer GE, Spinner M, Van Beek MA (eds): Management of peripheral nerve problems. WB Saunders, Philadelphia, 1998, p. 556

Phillips JR, Johnson KO: Tactile spatial resolution: II. Neural representation of bars, edges, and gratings in monkey primary afferents. J Neurophysiol 46:1192-1203, 1981

Rosen B: Recovery of sensory and motor function after nerve repair: rationale for evaluation. J Hand Ther 9: 315-327, 1996

Rosen B, Lundborg G: A new model instrument for outcome after nerve repair. Hand Clin 19:463-470, 2003

Rozental TD, Beredjiklian PK, Guyette TM, et al: Intra- and interobserver reliability of sensibility testing in asymptomatic individuals. Ann Plast Surg 44:605-609, 2000

Vanderhooft E: Functional outcomes of nerve grafts for the upper and lower extremities. Hand Clin 16:93-104, 2000

Waylett-Rendall J: From the periphery to the somatosensory cortex: a global view of nerves and their function. J Hand Ther 6:71, 1993

Waylett-Rendall J: Sensibility evaluation and rehabilitation. Orthop Clin North Am 9:43-56, 1988

Waylett-Rendall J: Sequence of sensory recovery: a retrospective study. J Hand Ther 2:245, 1989

Werner G, Mountcastle VB: Neural activity in mechanoreceptive cutaneous afferents: stimulus response relations, Weber functions and information transmission. J Neurophysiol 28:359-397, 1965

World Health Organization: Sixth Report of the WHO Expert Committee on Leprosy. Technical Report Series No. 768. WHO, Geneva, Switzerland, 1988

APPENDIX **5-1**

American Society for Surgery of the Hand (ASSH) and International Federation of Hand Surgeons (IFSSH) Impairment Classification Recommendations (Sensory and Pain)

5.3D IMPAIRMENT DETERMINATION PRINCIPLES

Impairments of sensory function resulting from peripheral nerve disorders are determined by multiplying the percentage of severity of loss of sensibility level and/or associated pain interference by the assigned upper extremity impairment value for maximum sensory deficit of the structure involved. The classification of severity grades is shown in Part A in the following table and the impairment determination procedure in Part B. The impairment determination method of sensory/motor deficits is further detailed in Section 5.2. Clinical judgment is applied to select an appropriate percentage of severity from the range listed for each severity grade; the maximum value is not applied automatically. Note that this table is not to be used for rating pain that is not related to documented nerve injury or disease, nor for pain in the distribution of a nerve that has not been injured, except in diagnosed cases of reflex sympathetic dystrophy (CRPS I).

Upper extremity impairment due to sensory deficits and/or associated pain interference resulting from peripheral nerve disorders: Grade of severity classification (a) and impairment determination procedure (b). Interpretation of Part A: Classification corresponds to the following:

Grade 4: Diminished light touch, with good (<6 mm) to fair (6-10 mm) two-point discrimination, localization of sensory stimuli, and good protective sensibility. Abnormal sensations or pain, if present, are minimal and forgotten during activity.

Grade 3: Diminished light touch and two-point discrimination. There may be mislocalization of sensory stimuli with some abnormal or increased irritability sensations, or pain that interferes with activities. Protective sensibility is normal.

Grade 2: Decreased protective sensibility, which is defined as a conscious appreciation of pain, temperature, or pressure before tissue damage results from the stimulus. The hand function is diminished. There may be mislocalization and overresponsiveness (hyperesthesia or paresthesia, hyperpathia, or allodynia) to sensory stimuli that results in decreased manipulative skills and grip function and complaints of hand weakness. It is possible to have a gross appreciation of two-point discrimination (11-15 mm) at this level.

Sensory Deficits and/or Pain Interference from Peripheral Nerve Disorders

A. CLASSIFICATION

Grade	Sensibility Level and/or Associated Pain Interference	Sensory Deficit %
5	No loss of sensibility, abnormal sensation, or associated pain interference	0
4	Distorted superficial tactile sensibility (diminished light touch and good to fair two-point discrimination) with or without minimal abnormal sensations, or associated pain interference which is forgotten during activity	5-25
3	Distorted superficial tactile sensibility (diminished light touch and two-point discrimination) with normal protective sensibility and some abnormal sensations, or slight associated pain which interferes with some activities	30-50
2	Decreased superficial cutaneous pain and tactile sensibility (diminished protective sensibility) with abnormal sensations, or moderate associated pain interference which may prevent some activities	60-80
1	Absent superficial pain and tactile sensibility (absent protective sensibility) with some retained deep cutaneous pain and deep pressure sensibility, and abnormal sensations, or severe associated pain interference which prevents most activity	90-95
0	Absent sensibility, abnormal sensations, or severe associated pain interference which prevents all activity	100

B. IMPAIRMENT DETERMINATION PROCEDURE

I   Localize area of involvement: cutaneous innervation, or dermatomes.

II   Identify nerve structure(s) involved: origins and functions of peripheral nerves of upper extremity, cutaneous innervation, dermatomes, brachial plexus.

III   Grade severity of sensory deficit or pain according to above classification (a).

IV   Locate maximum upper extremity impairment value for sensory deficit or pain of each nerve structure involved: spinal nerves, brachial plexus, and major peripheral nerves.

V   *Multiply* percent of severity of sensory deficit by maximum upper extremity impairment value to obtain upper extremity impairment for each nerve structure involved.

B derived from Kline DG, Hudson AR: Operative Results for Major Nerve Injuries, Entrapments, and Tumors. WB Saunders, Philadelphia, 1995, p. 89; Moberg E: Sensibility in reconstructive limb surgery. In Fredericks S, Brody GS (eds): Symposium on the Neurologic Aspects of Plastic Surgery. CV Mosby, St. Louis, 1978, pp. 30-35; Omer GE Jr, Bell-Krotoski J: Evaluation of clinical results following peripheral nerve suture. In Omer GE Jr, Spinner M, Van Beek AL (eds): Management of Peripheral Nerve Problems. 2nd ed. WB Saunders, Philadelphia, 1998, pp. 340-349; Seddon HJ: Surgical Disorders of the Peripheral Nerves. 2nd ed. Churchill Livingstone, Edinburgh, Scotland, 1975; Swanson AB: Surg Clin North Am 44:925-940, 1964; and Swanson AB, de Groot Swanson G: Evaluation of permanent impairment in the hand and upper extremity. In Doege TC (ed): Guides to the Evaluation of Permanent Impairment. 4th ed. American Medical Association, Chicago, 1993.

Grade 1: No protective sensibility. Individuals have little use of the hand, cannot manipulate objects outside their line of vision, and have a tendency to injure themselves easily. However, they can feel a pinprick and have deep-pressure sensibility, and they are not totally asensory. Pain and/or overresponse can be severe.

Grade 0: Asensory hand with severe pain, overreactive responses, and no functional use.

APPENDIX **5-2**

American Society For Surgery of the Hand (ASSH) and International Federation of Hand Surgeons (IFSSH) Impairment Classification Guidelines: Sensory Deficits and/or Pain Interference from Peripheral Nerve Disorders (IFSSH, 2004) (Muscle)

5.4 MOTOR FUNCTION IMPAIRMENT EVALUATION

Precise anatomic knowledge is prerequisite to properly select the muscle function tests that correlate to the specific nerve structure(s) involved. Maneuvers for individual muscle testing are well described in the literature. Some muscles display a dual or variable pattern of nerve supply and require special consideration. Individuals with long-standing nerve injury or those who have lost function of individual muscles, for example, after a free flap transfer, usually recruit adjacent muscles to replace lost functions. Such movements may lead to false interpretation of standard muscle function tests.

Upper extremity impairment due to motor strength and range of motion deficits resulting from peripheral nerve disorders based on individual muscle grading: Grade of severity classification (a) and impairment determination procedure (b).

Motor Deficits

A. CLASSIFICATION

Grade	Motor Strength and Loss of Range of Motion	Motor Deficit %
5	Complete active range of motion against gravity with full resistance	0
4	Complete active range of motion against gravity with some resistance	5-25
3	Complete active range of motion against gravity only, without resistance	30-50
2	Complete active range of motion with gravity eliminated	60-80
1	Evidence of slight contractility; no joint movement	90-95
0	No evidence of contractility	100

B. IMPAIRMENT DETERMINATION PROCEDURE

1   Identify the key muscles for the motion involved, such as flexion, extension, etc.
2   Identify nerve structure(s) involved: origins and functions of peripheral nerves of upper extremity, motor innervation, brachial plexus.
3   Grade severity of motor deficit of individual muscles according to above classification (a).
4   Locate maximum upper extremity impairment value for motor deficit of each nerve structure involved: spinal nerves, brachial plexus, major peripheral nerves.
5   *Multiply* percent of severity of motor deficit by maximum upper extremity impairment value to obtain upper extremity impairment for each nerve structure involved.

B adapted from Lovett RW. From Omer GE Jr, Bell-Krotoski J: Evaluation of clinical results following peripheral nerve suture. In Omer GE Jr, Spinner M, Van Beek AL (eds): Management of Peripheral Nerve Problems. 2nd ed. WB Saunders, Philadelphia, 1998, p. 341; Seddon HJ: Surgical Disorders of the Peripheral Nerves. 2nd ed. Churchill Livingstone, Edinburgh, Scotland, 1975; and Swanson AB, de Groot Swanson G: Evaluation of permanent impairment in the hand and upper extremity. In Doege TC (ed.): Guides to the Evaluation of Permanent Impairment. 4th ed. American Medical Association, Chicago, 1993.

Techniques to examine muscle power are based on the use of gravity and resistance. The Lovett method, originally proposed in 1917, is most commonly used. Manual grading of muscle strength is based on the ability of a normal muscle unit to contract and move a bone-joint lever arm through its full active range of motion with full resistance. Palpation of the muscle-tendon unit helps evaluate muscle contractility.[25]

APPENDIX **5-3**

Semmes-Weinstein Monofilaments Interpretation and Relationship to Function*

A. INTERPRETATION AND RELATIONSHIP TO FUNCTION

The interpretation of monofilament force levels was based on the review I made of 150 cases and 200 tests of patients with peripheral nerve problems at the Philadelphia Hand Center, Ltd., Philadelphia, from 1976 to 1978. Subsequent discussion of the data with von Prince and experience in use of the interpretation in patients with peripheral nerve problems over the last 15 years has continued to support the relationship of force thresholds to functional sensibility. Comparisons were made between the Semmes-Weinstein monofilaments and other tests of sensibility routinely given to patients as a test battery.

Normal touch is a recognition of light touch, and therefore deep pressure, that is within normal limits. This level is the most significant of all levels because it allows the examiner to distinguish between areas of normal sensibility and areas of sensory diminution.

Diminished light touch is diminished recognition of light touch. If a patient has diminished light touch, provided that his motor status and cognitive abilities are in play, he has fair use of his hand, his graphesthesia and stereognosis are both close to normal and adaptable, he has good temperature appreciation, he definitely has good protective sensation, he most often will have fair to good two-point discrimination, and he may not even realize he has had a sensory loss.

Diminished protective sensation is just that. If a patient has diminished protective sensation, he will have diminished use of his hands, he will have difficulty manipulating some objects, he will have a tendency to drop some objects, and he may complain of weakness of his hand, but he will have an appreciation of the pain and temperature that should help keep him from injury, and he will have some manipulative skill. Sensory reeducation can begin at this level. It is possible for a patient to have a gross appreciation of two-point discrimination at this level (7 to 10 mm).

Loss of protective sensation is again what it says. If a patient has loss of protective sensation he will have little use of his hand, he will have a diminished, if not absent, temperature appreciation, he will not be able to manipulate objects outside his line of vision, he will have a tendency to injure

*From Bell-Krotoski JA: Sensibility testing: state of the art. In Hunter JM, Mackin EJ, Callahan AD, et al. (eds): Rehabilitation of the Hand: Surgery and Therapy. 4th Ed. Mosby, St. Louis, 1995, p. 109.

himself easily, and it may even be dangerous for him to be around machinery. He will, however, be able to feel a pinprick and have deep pressure sensation, which does not make him totally asensory. Instructions on protective care are helpful to prevent injury.

If a patient is *untestable*, he may or may not feel a pinprick but will have no other discrimination of levels of feeling. If a patient feels a pinprick in an area otherwise untestable, it is important to note this during the mapping. Instructions on protective care of the hand are mandatory at this level to prevent the normally occurring problems associated with the asensory hand.

Force of Semmes-Weinstein monofilaments relative to "Levels of Function." All 20 available monofilaments are shown, the Minikit monofilaments used in a shortened version of the test and Hand Screen are in bold. The monofilaments can be used for testing and mapping anywhere on the body, except for the contact areas of the foot, which requires a 3.61 monofilament for normal.

B. Scale of Interpretation of Monofilaments

Color	Functional Level	Filament Markings	Calculated Force (g)
Green	Normal	1.65-**2.83**	0.0045-0.068
Blue	Diminished light touch	3.22-**3.61**	0.166-0.408
Purple	Diminished protective sensation	3.84-**4.31**	0.697-2.06
Red	Loss of protective sensation	**4.56**	3.63-447
	Loss of protective sensation/Residual deep pressure	**6.65**	
Red-lined	Untestable	>6.65	>447

Force data from Semmes J, Weinstein S: Somatosensory Changes After Penetrating Brain Wounds in Man. Harvard University Press, Cambridge, MA, 1960. Minikit monofilaments are in bold. Descriptive levels are based on other scales of interpretation and collapse of data from 200 patient tests.

APPENDIX 5-4

Quantitative Sensory Testing

A. QUANTITATIVE SENSORY TESTING (EXAMPLE)

Pressure Sensory One/Two-Point Device

Location	1-PT Static (GM/SQMM)	2-PT Static (GM/SQMM)	Distance (mm)	1-PT Moving (GM/SQMM)	2-PT Moving (GM/SQMM)	Distance (mm)
Left						
Index	40.0	30.2	10.1	36.0	49.8	10.1
Little	1.0	2.5	5.5	1.0	0.7	5.5
Thenar palm	39.3	37.2	22.0	57.0	25.5	22.0
Right						
Index	53.6			85.5	76.8	13.5
Little	1.4	2.9	6.0	0.9	2.2	6.2
Thenar palm	73.5	76.3	25.0	60.8	60.6	25.0

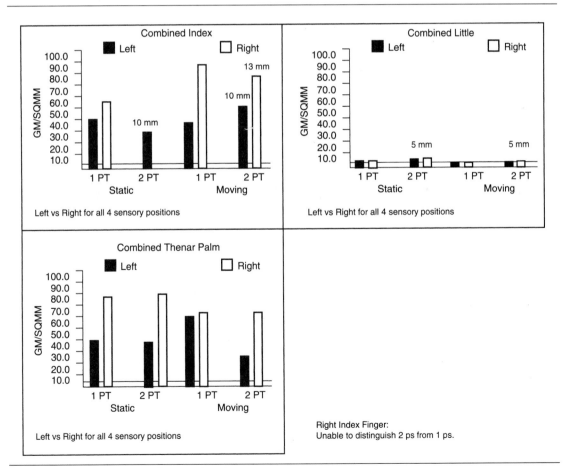

Right Index Finger:
Unable to distinguish 2 ps from 1 ps.

GM/SQMM, Grams per square millimeter; *PT*, point.
Courtesy Lee Dellon, MD, Baltimore, Md.

B. PRESSURE SENSITIVE DEVICE: QUANTITATIVE TESTING FORM

Pressure Sensory One/Two-Point Device

Location	1-PT static (GM/SQMM)	2-PT static (GM/SQMM)	Distance (mm)	1-PT moving (GM/SQMM)	2-PT moving (GM/SQMM)	Distance (mm)
Left						
Index						
Little						
Thenar palm						
Right						
Index						
Little						
Thenar palm						

APPENDIX **5-5**

Sensory Testing (Relative Guideline)

Touch/Pressure Threshold (Monofilaments)	Functional Level	Innervation Density (Two-Point)	Vibration	Other Tests
Normal touch (2.36-2.83)	Normal level of function	*Moving two-point 2-3 mm (good) *Static two-point 2-5 mm (good)	†Computerized vibration tests	—
Diminished light touch (3.22-3.61)	Good use of hand, close to normal graphesthesia and tactile discrimination	Moving two-point 4-6 mm (fair) Static two-point 7-10 mm (fair)	—	Moberg Object Pick-up (Dellon Modification)
Diminished protective sensation (3.84-4.31)	Fair use of hand, difficulty manipulating some objects, tendency to drop some objects, may complain of weakness	Static two-point 11-15 mm (poor)	‡256-Hz tuning fork	—
Loss of protective sensation (4.56-6.56)	Markedly decreased or absent stereognosis, slowed response to hot or sharp objects	—	—	Abnormal temperature and pain recognition; protective care techniques important to prevent injury
(Loss of protective) Deep pressure 6.65	Absent stereognosis and poor response to hot or sharp objects, but residual deep pressure sensation	—	‡30-Hz tuning fork	Minimal to absent temperature and pain recognition; protective care techniques important to prevent injury
Untestable no response to 6.65	Nonfunctional sensibility	—	—	May still detect pin prick, and proprioception

*Varies according to instrument and force of application.
†Depends on control and accuracy of the test for high and low frequency; most use fixed frequency and variable amplitude.
‡Tuning forks are a gross indicator, not specific measurement; highly variable in force of application that can mask intended frequency.

Median Nerve Compression

6

Bonnie J. Aiello

The proximal median nerve may be impinged in several areas down the length of the forearm (Box 6-1). The patient may experience pain in the volar surface of the distal arm or proximal forearm with increased activity. The patient may have decreased sensibility of the radial three and one-half digits but a negative Phalen's test.

The anterior interosseus nerve, a branch of the median nerve as it passes deep to the pronator teres, may cause nonspecific pain in the proximal forearm that increases with activity, but no sensory problems. Patients have weakness of flexor digitorum profundus of the index and middle fingers, the flexor pollicis longus, and the pronator quadratus.

In the carpal tunnel, the nerve is impinged beneath the transverse carpal ligament. Patients present with decreased sensation in the radial three and one-half digits, thenar clumsiness, and weakness in the lumbricals of the index and middle fingers. They may have a positive Phalen's test (Fig. 6-2) and a positive Berger's test.[1]

BOX 6-1 Sites for Median Nerve Impingement

1. Ligament of Struthers in the distal third of the humerus beneath the supracondylar process.
2. Lacertus fibrosis at the elbow joint if the median nerve is superficial to the flexor muscle mass, thereby exposing it to compression with supination and pronation.
3. In between heads of the pronator muscle; usually caused by hypertrophy of the muscle mass or by the aponeurotic fascia on the deep surface of the head of the pronator teres muscle (Fig. 6-1).
4. At the arch of flexor digitorum superficialis (FDS) as the median nerve passes deep to it.

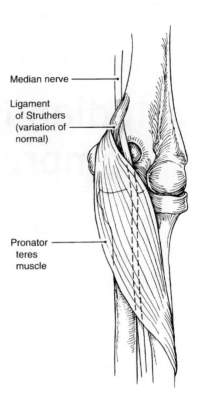

FIG. **6-1** Anatomy of pronator syndrome.

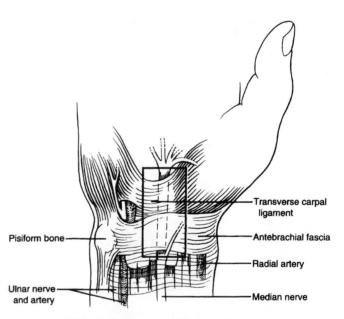

FIG. **6-2** Anatomy of the carpal tunnel.

DEFINITION

Impingement of the median nerve in the proximal forearm, under the pronator teres, at the anterior interosseus level or carpal tunnel. Median nerve compression is a common cumulative trauma.

Pathologic Anatomy and Staging of Compression

In **early compression**, the epineural blood flow is impaired, causing decreased axonal transport. Morphologic changes are absent.[2] The patient complains of intermittent symptoms, tests positive only for provocative tests, and can be found to be hypersensitive to 256 cps.[3] These patients do the best with conservative therapeutic management.[3]

In **moderate compression**, persistent interference of intraneural microcirculation is present along with epineural and intrafascicular edema.[2] Intraneural fibrosis may be present; however, wallerian degeneration has not taken place. There is decreased vibratory sensation, positive findings on provocative tests, and thenar weakness; the patient complains of abnormal sensation.

In **severe compression**, long-standing epineural edema may be followed by endoneural edema and fibrosis.[2] There may be loss of fibers. Electromyography (EMG) shows denervation potentials in the muscles supplied by the median nerve. Persistent sensory changes, abnormal static two-point discrimination greater than 4 mm, and thenar atrophy are present.[3]

These pathologic, histologic, and clinical findings determine which path of treatment to follow.

TREATMENT AND SURGICAL PURPOSE

To reduce compressive forces on the median nerve in the carpal tunnel. Nonoperative methods rely on decreasing demands on the hand and wrist to reduce inflammation of the flexor tendon synovium. This is usually accomplished by work modification, wrist splinting, and antiinflammatory medications. Surgery is directed at enlarging the carpal tunnel by releasing the transverse carpal ligament, which allows more space for the median nerve.

The median nerve can be compressed in the proximal forearm, resulting in pronator syndrome or anterior interosseous nerve compression. Surgery for these compression syndromes involves an antecubital incision with division of the structures (e.g., bicipital aponeurosis, superficial head of the pronator teres, origin of the superficialis muscle) and release of the anterior interosseous nerve branch if needed.

TREATMENT GOALS

   I.   Decrease pain and paresthesias
  II.   Increase or maintain muscle strength
 III.   Maintain function of the hand
 IV.   Education

NONOPERATIVE INDICATIONS/PRECAUTIONS FOR THERAPY

I. Indications
   A. Intermittent paresthesias or pain, clumsiness
   B. Positive provocative tests
   C. Hypersensitive to 256 cps[3]
II. Precautions
   A. Decreased tunnel size (e.g., prior fracture)
   B. Increased tunnel contents (e.g., cysts)
   C. Neuropathic conditions
   D. Inflammatory conditions
   E. Fluid balance problems
   F. Congenital problems[4]

NONOPERATIVE THERAPY

I. Proximal compression
   A. Long arm splint in 90 degrees of elbow flexion and neutral wrist position for 3 to 4 weeks followed by night wear for about the same amount of time
   B. Nonsteroidal antiinflammatory drugs (NSAIDs)
   C. Phonophoresis[5]
   D. Iontophoresis[5]
   E. Cryotherapy
   F. Allow elbow and wrist active range of motion (AROM) to maintain it during the day
   G. Tendon and nerve gliding[6-8]
   H. Ergonomic assessment and recommendations
   I. Strengthening of affected muscles (Table 6-1)
II. Distal compression
   A. Wrist splint 3 to 4 weeks in neutral position followed by night wear for approximately the same amount of time[3,5,9-14] (Fig. 6-3). The splint may include the metacarpal phalangeal joints in neutral position if the lumbricals are well developed.[1]

TABLE 6-1 Muscle Innervations

Nerve	Muscles Innervated
Median nerve	Pronator teres
	Flexor carpi radialis
	Flexor digitorum superficialis
Anterior interosseus nerve	Flexor digitorum profundus to the index and middle fingers
	Flexor pollicis longus
	Pronator quadratus
Terminal median nerve	Abductor pollicis
	Opponens pollicis
	Lumbricals to the index and middle fingers

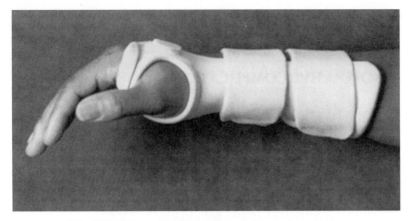

FIG. **6-3**   Wrist splint for use in carpal tunnel syndrome.

    B. Phonophoresis[5]
    C. Iontophoresis[5]
    D. Cryotherapy[5]
    E. NSAIDs[11,13,15]
    F. Tendon and nerve glides[6-8]
    G. Ergonomic assessment and recommendations
    H. Strengthening for affected muscles (see Table 6-1)
    I. Patients who are not candidates for carpal tunnel release but
       have severe compression require sensory precautions and may
       use a carpometacarpal joint splint to hold the thumb in useful
       opposition.
    J. Carpal bone mobilization[16]

NONOPERATIVE COMPLICATIONS

    I.   Persistent pain, paresthesias
   II.   Progression of thenar atrophy
 III.   Progression of nerve damage
 IV.   Decreased function

OPERATIVE INDICATIONS/PRECAUTIONS
FOR THERAPY

   I. Indications
       A. Failed conservative treatment
       B. Moderate to severe compression—evidenced by weakness in
          abduction and/or diminished sensation
  II. Precautions
       A. Decreased size of tunnel (e.g., prior fracture)
       B. Increased contents in tunnel (e.g., cysts)
       C. Neuropathic conditions
       D. Inflammatory conditions
       E. Fluid balance problems
       F. Congenital problems[4]

POSTOPERATIVE THERAPY

I. Pronator syndrome
  A. Postoperative immobilization
    1. Day 3 to 5: bulky dressing. Allow full AROM to the digits. Elbow and wrist AROM flexion and extension are limited only by the patient's complaints and the dressing. Gradually increase activity as the patient's symptoms permit.[17]
                              OR
    2. Elbow 90 degrees for 5 to 10 days, then motion exercise as tolerated.[12,17]
  B. Scar management
  C. Ergonomic assessment and recommendations
  D. Strengthening of all affected muscles
  E. Nerve and tendon gliding[6-8]
II. Anterior interosseus
  A. Bulky dressing supporting the elbow and wrist. Allow full digital AROM and wrist flexion and extension. Strengthening at 7 to 10 days postoperatively unless the pronator was elevated.[17]
  B. If the pronator teres was elevated, splint supporting the elbow and the wrist should be held between 45 degrees and full pronation for 2 to 3 weeks. Digit AROM should begin immediately. AROM of the elbow and wrist should begin in week 3 and strengthening at 3 to 4 weeks.[17]
  C. Scar management
  D. Ergonomic assessment and recommendations
  E. Strengthening for all affected muscles
  F. Nerve and tendon gliding[6-8]
III. Carpal tunnel release
  A. Days 1 to 14
    1. Patient's wrist immobilized in neutral. AROM all digits. Nerve and tendon gliding.
  B. Day 15
    1. Suture removal
    2. Wrist AROM
    3. Continue AROM to all digits
    4. Desensitization if needed
    5. Scar management started
  C. Day 21: Strengthening of affected muscles
  D. Day 28
    1. Sensory evaluation and retraining
    2. Work hardening may begin
    3. Ergonomic assessment and recommendations

POSTOPERATIVE COMPLICATIONS

I. Infection, dehiscence
II. Neuroma
III. Continued pain, numbness
IV. Hypersensitive scar
V. Reflex sympathetic dystrophy (RSD)
VI. Incomplete release

EVALUATION TIMELINE

I. Initial or preoperative visit
   A. Sensory evaluation
   B. AROM
   C. Manual muscle test (MMT)
II. For nonoperative therapy: Repeat above tests monthly.
III. Postoperative therapy
   A. First postoperative visit
      1. AROM
      2. Wound evaluation
   B. 3 weeks postoperative: MMT
   C. 4 weeks postoperative
      1. Sensory evaluation repeated monthly

OUTCOMES

I. Nonoperative: The outcome depends on the length and severity of compression and the ability to modify the activity and the time spent doing the activity.[1]
II. Postoperative: The outcome depends on the symptom duration and severity, the incision length, scar tenderness, pillar pain, patient motivation, insurance coverage, and specific work requirements.[1] Consider job requirements, sensory and strength deficits, and pain.
   A. For light or sedentary work, return is between 2 and 4 weeks. For work requiring much repetition or heavy activity, the recuperation period is longer.[1]
   B. Return to work also can be broken down by incision type[1-3]
      1. Limited palmar excision: 21 days
      2. Endoscopic carpal tunnel release: 25 to 28 days
   C. Grip and pinch strengths return to preoperative levels by 2 to 3 months, with maximal improvement by 10 months.[18,19]
   D. Two-point discrimination may remain abnormal after 2 years in half of the patients.[20]
   E. Compression symptoms may reoccur in 1.7% to 3.1% of patients.[21,22]

REFERENCES

1. Evans RB: Therapist's management of carpal tunnel syndrome. In Mackin EJ, Callahan AD, Skirven TM et al. (eds): Hunter-Mackin-Callahan Rehabilitation of the Hand and Upper Extremity. 5th Ed. Mosby, St. Louis, 2002
2. Gelberman R, Szabo RM, Williamson RV: Sensibility testing in peripheral nerve compression syndromes. J Bone Joint Surg 65A:632, 1983
3. Dellon AL, MacKinnon SE: Surgery of the Peripheral Nerve. Thieme Medical Publishers, New York, 1988
4. Szabo RM: Carpal tunnel syndrome. In Szabo RM (ed): Nerve Compression Syndromes: Diagnosis and Treatment. Slack, Thorofare, NJ, 1989
5. Griffin JE: Physical Agents for Physical Therapists. 2nd Ed. Charles C Thomas, Springfield, MO, 1982
6. Rozmaryn LM, Dovelle S, Rothman ER, et al.: Nerve and tendon gliding exercises and the conservative management of carpal tunnel syndrome. J Hand Ther 11:171-179, 1998
7. Akalin E, El O, Peker O, et al.: Treatment of carpal tunnel syndrome with nerve and tendon gliding exercises. Am J Phys Med Rehab 81:108-113, 2002

8. Butler DS: Mobilisation of the Nervous System. Churchill Livingstone, Melbourne, 1991
9. Carragee E, Hentz V: Repetitive trauma and nerve compression. Orthop Clin North Am 19:157, 1988
10. Phalen G: Clinical evaluation of 398 hands. Clin Orthop 83:29, 1972
11. Spinner R, Bachman JW, Adadio PC: The many faces of carpal tunnel syndrome. Mayo Clin Proc 64:829, 1989
12. Green D: Operative Hand Surgery. 2nd Ed. Churchill Livingstone, New York, 1988
13. Greenspan J: Carpal tunnel syndrome: a common but treatable cause of pain. Postgrad Med 84:34, 1988
14. Weiss ND, Gordon L, Bloom T, et al.: Position of the wrist associated with the lowest carpal tunnel pressures: implications for splint design. J Bone Joint Surg 77A: 1695-1699, 1995
15. Calliet R: Hand Pain and Impairment. 3rd Ed. FA Davis, Philadelphia, 1982
16. Tal Akabi A, Rushton A: An investigation to compare the effectiveness of carpal bone mobilisation and neurodynamic mobilisation as methods of RX for CTS. Man Ther 5:214-222, 2000
17. Eversman WW: Proximal median nerve compression. Hand Clin 8:307, 1992
18. Katz JN, Fossel KK, Simmons BP, et al.: Symptoms, functional status, and neuromuscular impairment following carpal tunnel release. J Hand Surg 20A:549, 1995
19. Leach WJ, Esler C, Scott TD: Grip strength following carpal tunnel decompression. J Hand Surg 17A:1003, 1992
20. Hayes EP, Carney K, Wolf J, et al.: Carpal tunnel syndrome. In Mackin EJ (ed): Rehabilitation of the Hand and Upper Extremity. Part VIII: Compression Neuropathies. Elsevier, St. Louis, 2002
21. Langloh NH, Linscheid RL: Reccurrent and unrelieved carpal tunnel syndrome. Clin Orthop 83:41, 1972
22. Cobb TK, Amadio PC: Reoperation for carpal tunnel syndrome. Hand Clin 12:313, 1996

SUGGESTED READINGS

Daniels L, Worthingham C: Muscle Testing. 4th Ed. WB Saunders, Philadelphia, 1986

Dellon AL: Functional sensation and its re-education. Clin Plast Surg 11:95, 1984

DiBenedetto M, Mitz M: New criteria for sensory nerve conduction especially useful in diagnosis of carpal tunnel syndrome. Arch Phys Med Rehabil 67:586, 1986

Elias JM: Treatment of carpal tunnel syndrome with vitamin B6. South Med J 80:882, 1987

Gainor BJ: Modified exposure for pronator syndrome decompression: a preliminary experience. Orthopedics 16:1329, 1993

Gelberman R, Aronson D, Weisman MH: Carpal tunnel syndrome. J Bone Joint Surg 62A:1181, 1980

Gelberman R, Rydevik B, Pess G, et al.: Carpal tunnel syndrome: a scientific basis for clinical care. Orthop Clin North Am 19:115, 1988

Golding R, Selverajah K: Clinical tests for carpal tunnel syndrome: an evaluation. Br J Rheumatol 25:388, 1986

Higgins JP, Graham TJ: Carpal tunnel release via limited palmar incision. Hand Clin 18:219-230, 2002

Mackin EJ, Callahan AD, Skirven TM, et al.: Hunter-Mackin-Callahan Rehabilitation of the Hand and Upper Extremity. 5th Ed. Mosby, St. Louis, 2002

Kaplan SJ, Glickel SZ, Eaton RG: Predictive factors in the nonsurgical treatment of carpal tunnel syndrome. J Hand Surg 15B:106, 1990

Kelly CP, Pulisetti D, Jamieson AM: Early experience with endoscopic carpal tunnel release. J Hand Surg 19B:18, 1994

Kulick MI, Gordillo G, Javidi T, et al.: Long-term analysis of patients having surgical treatment for carpal tunnel syndrome. J Hand Surg 11A:59, 1986

Lamb DW: The Practice of Hand Surgery. 2nd Ed. Blackwell Scientific, Boston, 1989

Lister GD, Bledsole RB, Klein H: The radial tunnel syndrome. J Hand Surg 4:52, 1979

Litchmeen HM, Triedman MH, Silver CM, et al.: The carpal tunnel syndrome (a clinical and electrodiagnostic study). Int Surg 50:269, 1968

Lucketti R, Schoenhuber R, Landi A: Assessment of sensory nerve conduction in carpal tunnel syndrome before, during, and after operating. J Hand Surg 13B:386, 1988

Lundborg G, Stanstrom AK, Sollerman C, et al.: Digital vibrogram: a new diagnostic tool for sensory testing in compression neuropathy. J Hand Surg 11A:693, 1986

Masear VR, Hayes JM, Hyde AG: An industrial cause of carpal tunnel syndrome. J Hand
   Surg 11A:222, 1986

Mesgarzadeh M, Schenk CD, Bonakdarpour A: Carpal tunnel: MR imaging, part I: normal
   anatomy. Musculoskel Radiol 171:743, 1989

Mesgarzadeh M, Schenk CD, Bonakdarpour A, et al.: Carpal tunnel: MR imaging,
   part II: normal anatomy. Musculoskel Radiol 171:749, 1989

Murphy RX, Jennings JF, Wukich DK: Major neurovascular complications of endoscopic
   carpal tunnel release. J Hand Surg 19A:114, 1994

Nathan P, Kenistan R: CTS and its relation to general physical condition. Hand Clin
   9:253, 1993

Nelson R, Currier D: Clinical Electrotherapy. Appleton & Lange, East Norwalk, CT, 1987

Omer G: Median nerve compression at the wrist. Hand Clin 8:317, 1992

Phalen G: The carpal tunnel syndrome. J Bone Joint Surg 48A:211, 1966

Rehak DC: Protonator syndrome. Clin Sports Med 20:531-540, 2001

Robbins H: Anatomical study of the median nerve in the carpal tunnel and etiologies of the
   carpal tunnel syndrome. J Bone Joint Surg 45A:953, 1963

Rotman MB, Donovan JP: Practical anatomy of the carpal tunnel. Hand Clin 18:219-230,
   2002

Spinner M: Injuries to the Major Branches of Peripheral Nerves in the Forearm.
   WB Saunders, Philadelphia, 1978

Sunderland S: Nerve and Nerve Injuries. 2nd Ed. Churchill Livingstone, New York, 1978

Waylett-Rendall J: Sensibility evaluation and rehabilitation peripheral nerve problems.
   Orthop Clin North Am 19:43, 1988

Wild E, Geberich SG, Hunt K, et al.: Analysis of wrist injuries in workers engaged in
   repetitive tasks. AAOHN J 35:356, 1987

Ulnar Nerve Compression

7

Nicole E. Bickhart

The ulnar nerve may be compressed at any point in its course from the axilla to the hand. Certain anatomic constraints make it particularly vulnerable to compression at the wrist and elbow.[1] The elbow is the most common site for ulnar nerve compression. The boundaries for compression begin 10 cm proximal to the elbow and end about 5 cm distal to the joint. The literature suggests more than five potential sites of compression, including the ligament of Struthers, the medial intermuscular septum, the medial epicondyle, the cubital tunnel, and the deep flexor pronator aponeurosis.[1,2]

The **cubital tunnel** is a bony canal formed by the ulnar collateral ligament, the trochlea, and the medial epicondylar groove and is roofed by the triangular arcuate ligament. The ulnar nerve that runs through this bony tunnel is responsible for sensation in the fifth and ulnar half of the fourth digit and supplies the ulnar intrinsics, flexor digitorum profundus fourth and fifth, and flexor carpi ulnaris[3] (Fig. 7-1).

Any irritation to the nerve at that level can cause severe pain, dysesthesias, deformity, and dysfunction of grip and pinch strength. Fine motor coordination is also affected. "Claw hand," or metacarpophalangeal (MCP) hyperextension with concurrent inability to fully extend the proximal interphalangeal (PIP) and distal interphalangeal (DIP) joints in the ring and little fingers, may also occur with severe compression.

Conservative treatment consists of patient education to limit activities and positions that provoke symptoms, appropriate splinting for rest and reduction of neural tension, and antiinflammatory modalities to decrease swelling in the closed-space tunnel.

Surgically, the nerve is decompressed, or moved under skin or muscle out of the compressed space. Rehabilitation is directed according to the structure disrupted to regain range of motion (ROM) and restore neural mobility.

Guyon's canal is the bony canal formed by the volar carpal ligament, the hook of the hamate, and the hamate. Both the ulnar nerve and the ulnar artery run through this tunnel and can be affected by a space-maintaining lesion or a decrease in the actual tunnel area (Fig. 7-2).

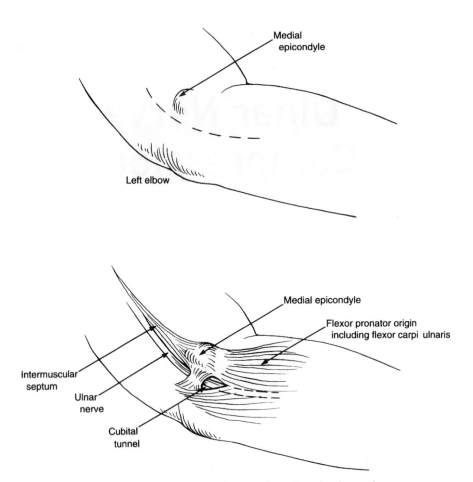

FIG. 7-1 Anatomy of the ulnar nerve in the cubital tunnel.

Motor and sensory deficits are present for all ulnar nerve–innervated areas distal to the canal. They may be distinguished from cubital tunnel deficits by the absence of any dorsal sensory branch symptoms. Compression may be caused by blunt trauma,[3] an occult tumorous condition[4,5] (e.g., lipoma, ganglion cyst), or a fracture of the hamate, ring, or little finger metacarpal bones.[3]

This deficit must be managed postsurgically, after the space-maintaining lesion or fracture has been alleviated, with splinting, muscle strengthening, and sensory reeducation.

DEFINITION

Cubital tunnel syndrome may be defined as compression of the nerve at the elbow as it passes through the area of the cubital tunnel. The pathophysiology is linked not only to compression but also to traction, friction, and nerve elongation. Cubital tunnel pressure has been found to be six times higher with the positions of elbow flexion, wrist extension, and shoulder abduction.[6,7] Other causative factors include recurrent subluxation, dislocations, rheumatoid arthritis, excessive elbow valgus, bony spurs, synovial cysts, and trauma.

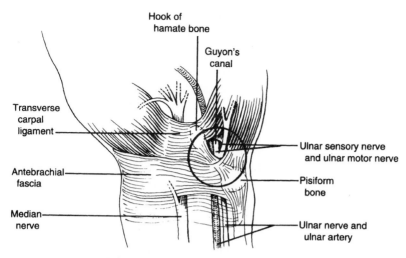

Hook of
hamate bone

Guyon's
canal

Transverse
carpal
ligament

Ulnar sensory nerve
and ulnar motor nerve

Antebrachial
fascia

Pisiform
bone

Median
nerve

Ulnar nerve and
ulnar artery

FIG. **7-2** Ulnar nerve in Guyon's canal.

Compression of the nerve in Guyon's canal may be defined as compression of the nerve at the wrist as it passes through Guyon's canal. Guyon's canal is divided into three anatomic zones. Zone 1 is at the wrist and proximal to the canal with both motor and sensory deficits. Zone 2 is at the exit of the canal and involves only the deep motor branch. Zone 3 is also at the exit of the canal but involves only the sensory branch.[8]

SURGICAL PURPOSE

I.   Cubital tunnel: to release compression of the ulnar nerve at the medial epicondyle of the elbow (see Fig. 7-1). Surgical methods have a spectrum from simple ligament release, to subcutaneous or submuscular transposition of the ulnar nerve, to medial epicondylectomy. All of these techniques are designed to remove the compressive forces from the nerve.

II. Guyon's canal: to release pressure on the ulnar nerve as it passes from the wrist into the palm by dividing the supporting fibro-osseous ligaments or removing space-occupying lesions from the channel. Surgery also may correct fractures of the hook of the hamate or reconstruct thrombosis of the ulnar artery.

TREATMENT GOALS

I.   Decrease painful paresthesias and hypersensitivity.
II.   Increase muscle strength to return to full use.
III. Prevent deformity.
IV.   Prevent recurrence with education, behavior modification, and ergonomic intervention to modify unavoidable deficits in activities of daily living (ADL) and for postural correction.
V.   Maintain and educate about protective and functional sensation.
VI.   Increase ROM and restore soft tissue mobility.
VII. Protect soft tissue repairs and manage scar.

NONOPERATIVE INDICATIONS/PRECAUTIONS

I. Indications: Intervention is based on stages of compression severity. Mild stages are generally treated conservatively. If conservative treatment fails and/or if the patient presents with moderate to severe compression symptoms, surgery is indicated.[9] Stages of compression severity are as follows.

   A. Mild: intermittent paresthesias, increased vibratory perception, complaints of clumsiness or loss of coordination, positive elbow flexion test, positive Tinel's sign

   B. Moderate: intermittent paresthesias, decreased vibratory perception, measurable grip and pinch weakness, positive Tinel's sign, positive elbow flexion test, finger crossing may be abnormal

   C. Severe: persistent paresthesias, decreased vibratory perception, abnormal two-point discrimination, measurable pinch and grip weakness. Muscle atrophy is present; claw deformity may be present. Clawing may be more pronounced with Guyon's canal compression where ulnar intrinsics are weak and flexor digitorum profundus is strong. Wartenberg's sign is positive when the fifth digit rests abducted from the fourth digit due to interosseous weakness. A Froment sign is positive when attempts to lateral pinch result in excessive thumb interphalangeal (IP) joint flexion. Positive Tinel's sign, positive elbow flexion test, finger crossing usually abnormal, electrodiagnostic testing usually positive for moderate or severe compression. Paresthesias that radiate down the medial forearm to the ulnar 1.5 digits and compression at the elbow may be differentiated from compression at Guyon's canal by the presence of dorsal sensory branch symptoms in the proximal compressions.

II. Precautions

   A. Diabetes

   B. Alcohol abuse–associated peripheral neuropathy

   C. Other peripheral neuropathic disease

III. Nonsurgical precautions

   A. Pain caused by immobilization

   B. Persistent pain, numbness, deformity

NONOPERATIVE TREATMENT (MILD DEGREE OF COMPRESSION)

I. Cubital tunnel syndrome: A thorough understanding of the anatomy and pathophysiology of nerve compression as it relates to the upper quarter is needed to guide clinical decision-making. Double and multiple crush syndromes, thoracic outlet syndrome, and various tendon disorders can coexist with cubital tunnel syndrome, leading to a complex clinical presentation.[10]

The extremity is immobilized with the elbow flexed 30 to 45 degrees[1,2,6,11,17] in either an anterior or posterior splint. The wrist can also be included, to rest the flexor carpi ulnaris muscle (Fig. 7-3). The splint is typically used for 3 months at night, but it can be used full-time for persistent symptoms.[12] The addition of a steroid injection has not been found to be of benefit in the treatment of cubital tunnel syndrome.[13] An elbow pad or Heelbo is

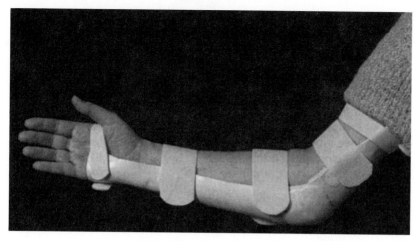

FIG. **7-3** Long arm splint.

used during the day to limit pressure over the cubital tunnel; it can be reversed to cover the antecubital fossa at night, to limit elbow flexion in lieu of a rigid splint. Symptomatic pain relief may be used with caution at insensate or hypersensitive areas. ROM is maintained. Imbalances in ROM, muscle tendon length, and strength are addressed. Positional education is stressed to avoid external nerve compression (e.g., leaning on the elbow, excessive elbow flexion) as well as overhead activity and use of vibratory tools. Postural education is also helpful for patients with proximal nerve symptoms, including the use of soft rolls at night to maintain a neutral spine position. Nerve gliding techniques can be performed as part of an overall plan to improve soft tissue mobility; however, treatment should proceed cautiously, because overmobilization can cause an exacerbation of symptoms.[12]

NONOPERATIVE COMPLICATIONS

I.   Pain caused by immobilization
II. Persistent pain, numbness, deformity

SURGICAL TREATMENT (MODERATE TO SEVERE COMPRESSION)

I.   Decompression: The aponeurosis is divided. The procedure only minimally disturbs the nerve, so no postoperative immobilization period is required.[11] A soft dressing is used postoperatively and active range of motion (AROM) is encouraged.
II. Anterior transposition: The ulnar nerve is moved anteriorly beneath a skin flap (subcutaneous transposition) or beneath the flexor muscle mass parallel to the median nerve (submuscular transposition).
     A. Subcutaneous transposition: Splint elbow in 45 degrees flexion, with forearm in neutral rotation and wrist in neutral for 2 weeks. Gentle AROM is then started. Progress to resisted exercise at 4 weeks.

    B. Submuscular transposition: Splint elbow in 45 degrees flexion, with forearm in neutral rotation and wrist in neutral for up to 3 weeks. At 1 to 2 weeks, start elbow flexion only, with wrist supported. At week 2, remove sling and begin gradual elbow extension exercises. At week 5, begin strengthening exercises.

III. Medial epicondylectomy: The medial epicondyle and distal part of the supracondylar ridge are resected. Bulky soft dressing is applied immediately, and AROM may start in 2 to 7 days. At week 2, begin passive range of motion (PROM). Progress to resisted ROM as tolerated.

POSTOPERATIVE INDICATIONS/PRECAUTIONS FOR THERAPY

    I. Cubital tunnel
        A. Indications
            1. Moderate to severe compression
            2. Failed conservative treatment
        B. Precautions
            1. Diabetes
            2. Alcohol abuse–associated peripheral neuropathy
            3. Other peripheral neuropathic disease

   II. Guyon's canal
        A. Indications: Confirmed presence of a neuropathy in the region of the wrist (especially if it is progressive); that is, the presence of combined or isolated motor or sensory neuropathy with no dorsal sensory branch symptoms.[1]
        B. Precautions
            1. Nonunited fractures
            2. Malignant conditions
            3. Alcohol abuse
            4. Diabetes
            5. Other neurologic disease

POSTOPERATIVE THERAPY

Cubital Tunnel

A thorough understanding of the surgical procedure and what soft tissue structures have been reconstructed is critical before postoperative rehabilitation is initiated. For instance, the flexor pronator origin may be partially or fully detached, thus requiring immobilization for soft tissue healing. Other surgeons do not advocate protecting the muscle origin and begin AROM at all the joints.

    I. Pain relief may be obtained via appropriate modalities.
   II. Scar management may be started as soon as wounds are healed.
 III. Splint to prevent deformity as indicated.
 IV. Assess sensory status.
  V. Postural and positional education
 VI. ROM of uninvolved joints is encouraged (i.e., shoulder and digit ROM).
VII. Specific treatment
    A. Decompression

1. Week 1
   a. Use of soft dressing and initiation of AROM
   b. Sensory assessment
   c. Wound care and edema control
   d. Exercise to promote gliding of the ulnar nerve to prevent scarring of the nerve to the surgical bed[14]
2. Week 2: As ROM progresses, initiate gentle strengthening exercises.
B. Submuscular transposition: Check with physician regarding protection of the flexor-pronator origin. If no protection is needed, then rehab is similar to that of the subcutaneous transposition.
   1. Week 1
      a. Splint in 45 degrees of flexion, with slight forearm pronation and wrist in neutral for 8 days to 3 weeks to protect the flexor pronator muscle origin.
      b. Sensory assessment
      c. Wound care and edema control
   2. Week 2: AROM of elbow, 30 degrees to full flexion with wrist and forearm supported in neutral.
   3. Week 3: AROM of elbow extension and flexion, wrist motion to patient's comfort.
   4. Week 4: PROM
   5. Week 5: resisted ROM
C. Subcutaneous transposition
   1. Week 1
      a. Splint in 45 degrees elbow flexion for up to 2 weeks. Gentle AROM is started at all joints. Progress to resistive exercises at 4 weeks.
      b. Sensory assessment
      c. Wound care and edema control
   2. Week 2: Discontinue splint; progress AROM.
   3. Week 3: PROM
   4. Week 4: resisted ROM
D. Medial epicondylectomy
   1. Week 1
      a. Bulky dressing
      b. Sensory assessment
      c. Wound care
      d. AROM
   2. Week 2: PROM
   3. Week 4: resisted ROM

Guyon's Canal

I. Because causes of compression of the ulnar nerve are varied, the cause must be addressed before rehabilitation of the nerve injury (e.g., proper splintage or fixation for appropriate fractures or removal of any space-maintaining mass). If a repetitive trauma is suspected (i.e., occupational- or sports/hobby-related injury), the patient is advised to rest the hand and avoid pressure at the hypothenar eminence.[8] A wrist immobilization splint may be used.
   A. Pain relief may be obtained via appropriate modalities.

B. Scar management
C. After protective splinting for cause of compression (3 days for ganglion tumor removal, 4 weeks for fracture), claw deformity may be addressed with an MCP block splint.
D. Sensory reeducation
E. Patient education about decreased sensitivity must be addressed immediately.
F. Strengthening may be started at 4 to 6 weeks for fracture (if healed), or after AROM is noted at ulnar innervated muscles.

POSTOPERATIVE COMPLICATIONS

I.   Cubital tunnel
     A. Laceration of the medial antebrachial cutaneous nerve
     B. Pain caused by immobilization
     C. Persistent flexion contractures
     D. Muscle rupture
     E. Infection
     F. Persistent pain, numbness, deformity
     G. Hypersensitive scar, heavy raised scar
     H. Incomplete decompression
     I. Postoperative nerve and or triceps tendon subluxation
II. Guyon's canal
     A. Painful paresthesias and persistent dysesthesias
     B. Decreased muscle strength atrophy
     C. Persistent numbness

EVALUATION TIMELINE

I.   Cubital tunnel
     A. Initial
        1. Pain
        2. Sensation and peripheral nerve screening
        3. Wound (for surgical patients)
        4. ROM (as directed by surgical repair)
     B. Monthly
        1. Sensory
        2. Manual muscle test (MMT)
        3. Pain
        4. ADL
     C. Specific surgical procedure
        1. Decompression
           a. 1 week: ROM
           b. 4 weeks: MMT, sensory, pain
        2. Submuscular
           a. Week 2: AROM, flexion with wrist and forearm supported
           b. Week 3: AROM, extension with wrist as tolerated by patient
           c. Week 4: PROM, sensory
           d. Week 5: MMT

    3. Subcutaneous
      a. 2 weeks: AROM
      b. 3 weeks: PROM
      c. 4 weeks: MMT, sensory
    4. Epicondylectomy
      a. 1 week: AROM
      b. 2 weeks: PROM
      c. 4 weeks: MMT, sensory
      d. Repeat monthly

II.   Guyon's canal
    A. Initial
      1. Sensory
      2. Pain
      3. ROM
      4. Manual muscle test (MMT)
    B. Biweekly
      1. ROM
    C. Monthly
      1. MMT
      2. Sensory

OUTCOMES

Ulnar nerve entrapment is the second most common nerve entrapment to the upper extremity.[14] The treatment for ulnar nerve compression is documented extensively throughout the literature with many different surgical techniques and outcomes. Dellon[15] provided general guidelines. He reported excellent results in 50% of patients with mild neuropathy treated nonsurgically and 90% excellent results in those treated with surgery regardless of the procedure. He also reported that nonoperative treatment and decompression surgery were mostly unsuccessful in treating moderate neuropathies; however, epicondylectomy provided excellent results in 50% of cases. Most literature describes resumption of full activities by 3 to 4 months after surgery; however, specific studies have shown an expedited return to work (RTW) or ADL and reduction of flexion contractures after early mobilization with therapy. Nathan and colleagues[14] reported that simple decompression combined with a program of early physical therapy resulted in good or excellent long-term relief in 89% of cases and an average RTW interval of 20 work days. Serdage[16] compared early versus delayed mobilization in cubital tunnel release and epicondylectomy procedures and found that the early mobilization group had an average RTW of 1 to 4 months, whereas the delayed mobilization group had an average RTW of 2 to 8 months. A significant reduction in the incidence of elbow flexion contractures was also reported with early mobilization.

REFERENCES

1. Khoo D, Carmichael SW, Spinner R: Ulnar nerve anatomy and compression. Orthop Clin North Am 27:317-328, 1996
2. Posner MA: Compressive ulnar neuropathies at the elbow: I. Etiology and diagnosis. J Am Acad Orthop Surg 6:282-288, 1998
3. Heuthoff S: Medial epicondylectomy for the treatment of ulnar nerve compression at the elbow. J Hand Surg Am 15:22-29, 1990

4. Eversmann WW Jr: Entrapment and compression neuropathies. In Green DP (ed): Operative Hand Surgery. 2nd Ed. Churchill Livingstone, New York, 1988, p. 1452

5. Silver M, Gelberman R, Gellman H: Carpal tunnel syndrome: associated abnormalities in ulnar nerve function and the effect of carpal tunnel release in these abnormalities. J Hand Surg Am 10:710, 1985

6. Gelberman RH, Yamaguchic K, Hollstien SB, et al.: Changes in interstitial pressure and cross-sectional area of the cubital tunnel and of the ulnar nerve with flexion of the elbow: an experimental study in human cadavera. J Bone Joint Surg Am 23:992-997, 1998

7. Wright TW, Glowczewskie F, Cowin D, et al.: Ulnar nerve excursion and strain at the elbow and wrist associated with upper extremity motion. J Hand Surg Am 26:655-662, 2001

8. Moneim MS: Ulnar nerve compression at the wrist: ulnar tunnel syndrome. Hand Clin 8:337-343, 1992

9. Dellon AL: Patient evaluation and management considerations in nerve compression. Hand Clin 8:229-239, 1992

10. Mackinnon SE: Double and multiple "crush" syndromes: double and multiple entrapment neuropathies. Hand Clin 8:369-390, 1992

11. Posner MA: Compressive ulnar neuropathies at the elbow: II. Treatment. J Am Acad Orthop Surg 6:289-297, 1998

12. Blackmore SM: Therapist's management of ulnar neuropathy at the elbow. In Hunter JM, Mackin EJ, Callahan AD (eds): Rehabilitation of the Hand: Surgery and Therapy. 4th Ed. Vol. 1. Mosby, St. Louis, 1995

13. Hong CZ, Long HA, Kanamedala RV, et al.: Splinting and local steroid injection for the treatment of ulnar neuropathy at the elbow: clinical and electrophysiological evaluation. Arch Phys Med Rehabil 77:573-577, 1996

14. Nathan PA, Kenniston RC, Meadows KD: Outcome study of ulnar nerve compression at the elbow treated with simple decompression and an early programme of physical therapy. J Hand Surg Br 20:628-637, 1995

15. Dellon AL: Review of treatment results for ulnar nerve entrapment at the elbow. J Hand Surg Am 14:688-700, 1989

16. Serdage H: Cubital tunnel release and medial epicondylectomy: effect of timing of mobilization. J Hand Surg Am 22:863-866, 1997

17. Bozentka DJ: Cubital tunnel pathophysiology. Clin Orthop Relat Res 351:90-94, 1998

SUGGESTED READINGS

Adelaar RS: The treatment of the cubital tunnel syndrome. J Hand Surg Am 9:90, 1984

Amako M, Nemoto K, Kawaguchi M, et al.: Comparison between partial and minimal medial epicondylectomy combined with decompression for the treatment of cubital tunnel syndrome. J Hand Surg Am 25:1043-1050, 2000

Amirjani N, Thompson S, Satkunam L, et al.: The impact of ulnar nerve compression at the elbow on the hand function of heavy manual workers. Neurorehabil Neural Repair 12:118-123, 2003

Arle JE, Zager EL: Surgical treatment of common entrapment neuropathies in the upper limbs. Muscle Nerve 23:1160-1174, 2000

Baker C: Evaluation, treatment and rehabilitation involving a submuscular transposition of the ulnar nerve at the elbow. Athletic Training 23:10, 1988

Beroit BG: Neurolysis combined with the application of a Silastic envelope for ulnar nerve entrapment at the elbow. Neurosurgery 20:594, 1987

Bowers WH: The distal radioulnar joint. In Green DP (ed): Operative Hand Surgery. 2nd Ed. Churchill Livingstone, New York, 1988, p. 973

Butler D: Mobilization of the nervous system. Churchill Livingstone, Edinburgh, 1991

Clark C: Cubital tunnel syndrome. JAMA 241:801, 1979

Craven P, Green DP: Cubital tunnel syndrome treatment by medial epicondylectomy. J Bone Joint Surg Am 62:986, 1980

Dellon AL: Review of treatment results for ulnar nerve entrapment at the elbow. J Hand Surg Am 14:688, 1989

Dellon AL, Hament W, Gittelshon A: Nonoperative management of cubital tunnel syndrome. Neurology 43:1673, 1993

Dellon A, MacKinnon S: Surgery of the Peripheral Nerve. Theme Medical Publisher, New York, 1988

Dellon A, MacKinnon S: Surgery of the peripheral nerve. Theme Medical Publishing, New York, 1988, p. 197

Dellon AL: Operative technique for submuscular transposition of the ulnar nerve. Contemp Orthop 16:17, 1988

Dimond ML, Lister GD: Cubital tunnel syndrome treated by long-arm splintage [abstract]. J Hand Surg Am 10:430, 1985

Eaton RG: Anterior transposition of the ulnar nerve using a non-compressing fasciodermal sling. J Bone Joint Surg Am 62:820, 1980

Folberg CR, Weiss AP, Akelman E: Cubital tunnel syndrome—part II: treatment. Orthop Rev 23:233, 1994

Foster RJ: Factors related to the outcome of surgically managed compressive ulnar neuropathy at the elbow level. J Hand Surg 6:181, 1981

Hicks D, Toby EB: Ulnar nerve strains at the elbow: the effect of in situ decompression and medial epicondylectomy. J Hand Surg 27:1026-1031, 2002

Idler RS: General principles of patient evaluation and nonoperative management of cubital tunnel syndrome. Hand Clin 12:397-403, 1996

Kleinman WM: Cubital tunnel syndrome: anterior transposition as a logical approach to complete nerve decompression. J Hand Surg Am 24:886-897, 1999

Kurvers H, Verhaar J: The results of operative treatment of medial epicondylitis. J Bone Joint Surg Am 77:1374-1379, 1995

Leffert RD: Anterior submuscular transposition of the ulnar nerve by the Learmonth technique. J Hand Surg Am 7:147, 1982

Lowe JB 3rd, Novak DB, Mackinnon SE: Current approach to cubital tunnel syndrome. Neurosurg Clin North Am 12:267-284, 2001

Manske PR, Johnson RJ, Pruitt DL, et al.: Ulnar nerve decompression at the cubital tunnel. Clin Orthop 274:231, 1992

Matev B: Cubital tunnel syndrome. Hand Surg 8:127, 2003

Moneim MS: Ulnar nerve compression at the wrist. Hand Clin 8:337, 1992

O'Rourke PJ, Quinlan W: Fracture dislocation of the 5th metacarpal resulting in compression of the deep branch of the ulnar nerve. J Hand Surg Br 18:190, 1993

Oswald TA: Anatomic considerations in evaluation of the proximal ulnar nerve. Phys Med Rehabil Clin North Am 9:777-794, 1998

Rayan GM: Proximal ulnar nerve compression. Hand Clin 8:2:325, 1992

Rengachary S, Arjunan K: Compression of the ulnar nerve in Guyon's canal by a soft tissue giant cell tumor. Neurosurgery 8:400, 1980

Thurman RT, Jindal P, Wolff TW: Ulnar nerve compression in Guyon's canal caused by calcinosis in scleroderma. J Hand Surg Am 16:739, 1991

Varitimidis SE, Riano F, Sotereanos DG: Recalcitrant post-surgical neuropathy of the ulnar nerve at the elbow: treatment with autogenous saphenous vein wrapping. J Reconstr Microsurg 16:273-277, 2000

Zahrawi F: Acute compression ulnar neuropathy at Guyon's canal resulting from lipoma. J Hand Surg Am 9:238, 1984

Radial Nerve Compression

8

Greg Pitts and Stephen C. Umansky

The radial nerve consists of fibers from the fifth through the eighth cervical roots in the majority of cases. It arises from the posterior cord of the brachial plexus. It exits the triangular space bounded by the teres major superiorly, the humerus and lateral head of the triceps laterally, and the long head of the triceps medially. At that point it supplies the triceps with innervation. From there, it courses along the posterior humerus in the spiral groove, giving off the posterior antebrachial cutaneous nerve, and pierces the lateral intermuscular septum to enter the anterior compartment of the arm. It then crosses the elbow anterior to the axis of rotation, only to course posteriorly again to the extensor compartment of the forearm, where it innervates the brachioradialis and extensor carpi radialis longus (ECRL). It then branches into the superficial radial nerve and the posterior interosseous nerve (PIN), which dives deep to the supinator to innervate it as well as the extensor carpi radialis brevis (ECRB), extensor digitorum, extensor digiti minimi, abductor pollicis longus (APL), extensor pollicis brevis (EPB), extensor pollicis longus, and extensor indicis proprius. The terminal branch of the PIN is a sensory nerve that supplies the dorsal capsule of the wrist joint. The superficial radial nerve supplies a small motor branch to the ECRB, then exits the deep fascia in the anterior compartment under brachioradialis, only to traverse posterior yet again to supply sensation to the dorsal aspect of the thumb, index, middle, and one half of the ring finger (Fig. 8-1).[1-3]

It is perhaps this tortuous course through the upper extremity that brings about the multiple compressive syndromes of the radial nerve. The four most described syndromes are radial nerve palsy at the spiral groove (Saturday night palsy), PIN syndrome, radial tunnel syndrome, and Wartenberg's syndrome. These produce a spectrum of compressive phenomena from mild paresthesias to dysfunction of all radially innervated muscles. Without appropriate treatment, severe disability may result.

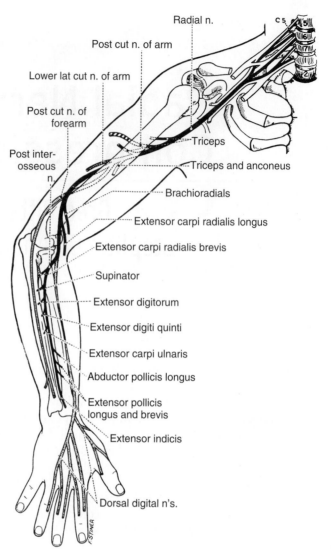

FIG. **8-1** The course and distribution of the radial nerve. (From Haymaker W, Woodhall B: Peripheral nerve injuries: principles of diagnosis. WB Saunders, Philadelphia, 1953.)

RADIAL NERVE PALSY

Definition

Radial nerve palsy in the spiral groove that is not caused by acute trauma (fractured humerus) is typically brought on by external compression. The classic scenario is falling into a deep or intoxicated sleep with compression on the posterior humerus by the arm of a chair. It produces a combined sensory and motor syndrome (hypesthesia to the dorsum of the forearm and hand, along with weak wrist extensors, digital extensors, and thumb extension). This syndrome is often referred to as Saturday night palsy.

Other mechanisms of compression consist of fractures of the humerus or blunt trauma to the upper arm.

Nonoperative Therapy

Initial management is aimed at keeping joints supple and preventing contracture. This is accomplished with a forearm-based dynamic extensor outrigger splint. The splint is designed and applied to allow the patient to conduct a natural grasp reflex. This enables the patient to pursue neuro-motor control rehabilitation while performing self-care activities of daily living (ADLs) with independence. The splint helps prevent adaptive shortening of the digital and wrist flexors while protecting the extensor mechanism from elongation.

Evaluation and Treatment Guidelines for Radial Nerve Palsy

I.   A custom forearm-based dynamic extensor outrigger is fabricated on the first day of treatment (Fig. 8-2).
     A. The selection of splint type is based on the following considerations
        1. Manual muscle test (MMT) evaluation of the ECRB of less than 3/5 (volar-based splint)
        2. Chronic problems with adaptive shorting of flexor compartment (flexor carpi radialis [FCR], flexor digitorum superficialis [FDS], flexor digitorum profundus [FDP]) and joint contractures of digits and wrist (volar-based splint)
        3. A large forearm muscle mass that inhibits flexor tenodesis with a dorsal approach splint (volar-based splint)
        4. For all others, use a dorsal-based dynamic extensor outrigger.
II. A custom forearm-based wrist gauntlet splint with the wrist at 30 to 45 degrees of extension is fabricated within the first week for night use to rest the hand from the dynamic outrigger.
     A. The gauntlet splint becomes the main splint once the evaluation yields an MMT score of ECRB 4/5 and extensor digitorum communis (EDC) 3+/5 (Fig. 8-3).
     B. The wrist splint is discontinued if MMT ECRB is 4+/5.

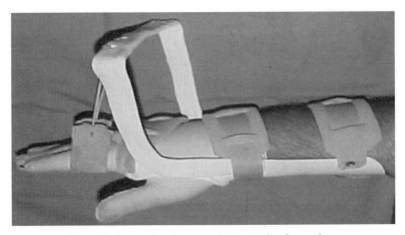

FIG. 8-2 Dynamic extensor outrigger with edema glove.

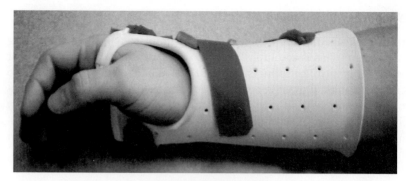

FIG. 8-3 Wrist gauntlet.

III. Functional
    A. Functional ADL training for the wrist and digit extensors is started in active therapy.
    B. The patient conducts active and passive range of motion (AROM/PROM) exercises to facilitate neuromotor control, diminish extrinsic flexor tightness and intrinsic tightness, and restore muscle balance.[4,5]
    C. If digital extensors return to 4/5, progress the rehabilitation process with strength and endurance training.
    D. Start gradual exposure to overhead activities, torquing tasks, and torquing tasks with load.
        1. Isometric strengthening with grip and hold (work at 10% or less of maximum voluntary effort [MVE])
        2. Isotonic strengthening with putty (focus on complete excursion of FDP)
        3. Isotonic wrist flexion and extension with weight
    E. Once the patient is asymptomatic with isometric grasp and linear isotonic wrist flexion and extension, exposure to low-load repetitive grasping may be attempted.
    F. A work conditioning/hardening program can be initiated for injured workers at the 10- to 12-week point, to facilitate the return to work process, if the patient has functional grasp reflex with basic ADL tasks.
    G. A wrist splint allows an increase in the patient's exposure to a work program while still protecting the patient from injury.

Operative Indications

Although most of these injuries are demyelinating in nature, and signs of recovery are seen in approximately 6 weeks, functional return of a nerve that has undergone axonotmesis (interruption of the nerve fiber with continuity of the fibrous sheath) returns at a rate of 1 mm/day. At that rate, it may take 6 months to see recovery of the most proximally innervated muscles (brachioradialis and ECRL). Failure of recovery of radial nerve function is an operative indication.[6]

    Surgery may consist of direct repair or grafting of the radial nerve (almost exclusively in traumatic cases); or transfer of tendons to restore wrist extension, digital extension, and thumb interphalangeal joint extension; or a combination of repair and tendon transfer, typically for wrist extension (see Chapter 14).

POSTERIOR INTEROSSEOUS NERVE SYNDROME AND RADIAL TUNNEL SYNDROME

The radial nerve is susceptible to compression after the point at which it bifurcates into the superficial radial nerve and the PIN at the level of the supinator. This produces two clinically distinct syndromes with identical pathology.

Definitions

I.   **Posterior interosseous nerve (PIN) syndrome** is characterized by the insidious onset of weakness of wrist extension (leading to extension in radial deviation from ECRL), digital extension, and thumb interphalangeal joint extension.
II. **Radial tunnel syndrome** is characterized by tenderness over the radial nerve at the proximal or distal edge of the supinator. It may be increased by passive pronation or active supination.

   Either syndrome may be caused by a mass (lipoma, ganglion, radiocapitellar synovitis) compressing the radial nerve. Other anatomic sites of compression follow the mnemonic *FREAS*: *F*ibrous bands anterior to the radiocapitellar joint, *R*ecurrent radial artery branches (leash of Henry), fibrous origin of the *E*xtensor carpi radialis brevis, the *A*rcade of Frohse (proximal fascial origin of supinator), and the distal edge of the *S*upinator.[6,7]

Nonoperative Therapy for Posterior Interosseous Nerve Syndrome

I.   A custom forearm-based dynamic extensor outrigger is fabricated on the first day of treatment.
     A. The selection of splint type is based on the following considerations
        1. MMT evaluation of the EDC of less than 3/5 (volar-based splint)
        2. Chronic problems with adaptive shortening of flexor compartment (FCR, FDS, FDP) and joint contractures of digits and wrist (volar-based splint)
        3. A large forearm muscle mass that inhibits flexor tenodesis with a dorsal approach splint (volar-based splint)
II. Functional
     A. The therapist should attempt to diminish joint capsule problems. Grade I and II joint mobilization techniques may be necessary to prevent digit, wrist, and forearm dysfunction.
     B. The patient will focus on AROM/PROM exercises to diminish extrinsic flexor tightness and intrinsic tightness and restore muscle balance.
     C. Functional ADL training for the wrist and digit extensors is started in active therapy.
     D. If digital extensors return to 4/5, progress the rehabilitation process with strength and endurance training.

E. A work conditioning/hardening program can be initiated for injured workers once a functional grasp reflex with basic ADL tasks has been restored and grip strength is 70% to 80% of that on the nonaffected side.

Nonoperative Therapy for Radial Tunnel Syndrome

I.   Weeks 0 to 3
   A. The patient is placed in a wrist splint in 30 to 45 degrees of extension to enhance function by resting the extensor compartment.
   B. The patient is encouraged to wear the splint continually with all ADLs.
   C. The purpose of the splint is to diminish the pain reflex and to diminish pressure on the radial nerve by putting a slack in the ECRB.
   D. Patient education should focus on the following
      1. Avoidance of the following tasks
         a. Pronation/supination functional tasks
         b. Large reach envelopes with arms extended at shoulder level or overhead and wrists flexed while forearm is placed in pronation. (This reach creates an increase in neurotension and decreased efficiency of movement.)
      2. Energy conservation and joint protection techniques, to include use of both hands supinated while conducting ADLs, instrumental activities of daily living (IADLs), and work activities.
      3. Use appropriate balanced tools while in the work environment, and avoid high-force tasks with torque or with heavy pronation or supination. *NOTE: The patient should focus on avoidance of mechanical stress along the radial tunnel extensor wad area with the use of counterforce braces.
      4. Workers should be aware of the potential for compression of the radial nerve by the wrist gauntlet splint proximal strap.
II.   Weeks 3+
   A. Clinical treatment
      1. Moist heat to the volar and dorsal compartments
         a. Avoid direct heating of the arcade of Frohse
      2. Radial nerve glides
      3. Ulnar nerve glides
      4. Median nerve glides
      5. Tendon gliding
         a. Basic-4 hand postures
         b. Overhead fisting
   B. Modalities as indicated
   C. Patient education on risk factors
      1. Mechanical stress
      2. Large reach envelopes
      3. Vibration
      4. Lift with pronated forearm
      5. Supination with force
   D. *NOTE: All exercises are conducted below the pain threshold to avoid increasing a pain reflex.
   E. Gradual exposure to strengthening and functional tasks

1. Start gradual exposure to overhead activities, torquing tasks, and torquing tasks with load.
2. Isometric strengthening with grip and hold (work at 10% or less of MVE).
3. Isotonic strengthening with putty (focus on complete excursion of FDP).
4. Isotonic wrist flexion and extension with weight.
5. Once the patient is asymptomatic with isometric grasp and linear isotonic wrist flexion and extension, exposure to low-load repetitive grasping may be attempted.

Operative Indications and Technique

Operative decompression of the radial nerve is indicated after failure of nonoperative treatment to resolve the motor findings (PIN syndrome) or pain (radial tunnel syndrome).

In each case, the radial nerve is approached through either an anterior, posterior, or anterior brachioradialis splitting approach. The posterior approach affords the best exposure for the distal supinator and may be combined with an anterior approach proximally. The brachioradialis splitting approach may use a transverse incision. The dissection is carried to the level of the radial head and supinator muscle. Radiocapitellar osteophytes or synovitis, ganglia, and lipomata are identified at this point and excised. The radial recurrent vessels (identified as they traverse the surgical field deep to the superficial radial nerve and superficial to the PIN) are cauterized and divided. The ECRB fascial edge is released, exposing beneath it the supinator, which is identified by its transverse-running fibers. The proximal edge of the supinator is released to expose the radial nerve. The muscle fibers of the supinator do not usually need to be released. There is sometimes a tight distal fascial edge of supinator that needs to be released. This is not well visualized from the brachioradialis splitting incision.[7-9]

Postoperative Management for Radial Tunnel Syndrome

I. Days 5 to 7
   A. Postoperative dressings are removed, and a light compressive bandage is applied.
   B. Patient is checked for signs and symptoms of infection.
   C. The patient is provided with education on wound care.
   D. AROM exercises are initiated for the wrist, forearm, and elbow.
      1. These are to be conducted every hour for 5 to 10 minutes total exercise time.
      2. These exercises will include
         a. Radial nerve glides
         b. Ulnar nerve glides
         c. Median nerve glides
         d. Tendon gliding
            (1) Basic-4 hand postures
            (2) Overhead fisting
   E. Patients will find it helpful to have a wrist gauntlet splint fabricated to enhance function by resting the extensor compartment while not conducting exercises.

*NOTE: All exercises are conducted below pain threshold to avoid increasing pain.

      F. Sutures are removed and silicone and elastomer are applied.

      G. Scar massage can be initiated with the use of Dycem, or a padded vibrator can be used to diminish scar pain with direct application over scar.

II.   4 weeks postoperative

      A. Focus should be on restoration of full, pain-free neural glide before starting a strengthening program.

      B. Strengthening may be initiated with the following

         1. Gentle isotonic putty for grasp and pinch

         2. Patient is encouraged to conduct basic self-care ADL activities and IADL tasks such as cooking and preparing meals.

         3. The patient continues to avoid heavy lifting, push/pull activities, torquing tasks, pronation, supination, and yard work at this time.

III. 6 weeks postoperative

      A. Start isometric strengthening with a 10-pound gripper: hold 30 seconds, rest 1 minute, perform five times, twice per day.

         1. Progress program with 10-pound gripper to hold 1 minute, rest 1 minute, perform five times, twice per day.

      B. Start wrist flexion/extension strengthening exercises below pain threshold (once all extrinsic flexor and extensor tightness and muscle guarding are diminished).

      C. Continue all nerve gliding and tendon gliding and scar management therapies.

IV. 8 to 10 weeks postoperative

      A. Start gradual exposure to overhead activities, torquing tasks, and torquing tasks with load.

         1. Isometric strengthening with grip and hold (work at 10% or less of MVE)

         2. Isotonic strengthening with putty (focus on complete excursion of FDP)

         3. Isotonic wrist flexion and extension with weight

      B. Once the patient is asymptomatic with isometric grasp and linear isotonic wrist flexion and extension, exposure to low-load repetitive grasping may be attempted.

      C. If the patient is asymptomatic with repetitive grasping, then progress to the following tasks

         1. Overhead, pronation, supination, ulnar and radial deviation, and weight-bearing tasks

         2. The following sequence is recommended

            a. First introduce the torque motion patterns of ulnar and radial deviation, followed by pronation and supination.

            b. Next is torque motion with gradual increase in load.

            c. The final stage is torque motion with load and pace.

               *NOTE: This is critical for return-to-work issues.

      D. The patient is strongly encouraged to avoid vibratory tools (e.g., weed-eaters, lawnmowers, torque wrenches) in the rehabilitation process until 10 to 12 weeks after surgery.

      E. Patients are encouraged to conduct only those exercises that are within their pain-free motion, gradually regaining AROM.

   F. Neuromotor control tasks with the use of ADL activities at end-
      range are very helpful in restoring functional ROM.

Postoperative Complications

   I.   Failure to relieve pain or restore function
   II. Infection
   III. Nerve injury
   IV. Hematoma leading to nerve compression
   V.   Painful neuroma
   VI. Lateral antebrachial cutaneous nerve injury
   VII. Painful scar

WARTENBERG SYNDROME

Definition

Wartenberg's syndrome, or cheiralgia paresthetica, is compression of the
sensory branch of the radial nerve at the wrist. It is thought that the lesion
arises from the point at which the nerve exits the deep tissues between
brachioradialis and ECRL in the distal forearm. Tight watches, bracelets or
handcuffs may compress the nerve distal to this tether, causing paresthesias in the dorsal thumb, index, and/or middle fingers and hand. Pain is
usually referable to the superficial radial nerve between the brachioradialis
and ECRL. Antiinflammatory medications, thumb spica splinting, and
corticosteroid injections may also improve symptoms.[10]

Nonoperative Therapy

   I.   Treatment is based on the following considerations
        A. Numbness and tingling symptoms in the radial sensory nerve
           distribution increase with pronation, wrist flexion, elbow exten-
           sion, and shoulder abduction.
        B. Finkelstein's test increases numbness and tingling symptoms in
           the radial sensory nerve distribution.
        C. MMT evaluation of APL and EPB 5/5 with no pain.
        D. Chronic problems with muscle cocontraction and guarding of
           wrist flexors and extensors with ADL tasks.
   II. A forearm thumb spica splint is used to diminish neurotension on
        the radial sensory nerve (Fig. 8-4).
   III. Active treatment
        A. Radial nerve glides
        B. Joint mobilization (wrist, hand, and digits) to inhibit joint
           pain reflex
        C. Transcutaneous electrical nerve stimulation (TENS) unit radial
           sensory nerve distribution[11]
        D. The patient will conduct AROM/PROM exercises to facilitate
           neuromotor control and diminish extrinsic and intrinsic
           tightness and restore muscle balance.
   IV. Patient education on risk factors
   V.   Activities at home and work to avoid
        A. Large reach envelope with arms extended at shoulder level or
           overhead and wrists flexed with forearm placed in pronation.

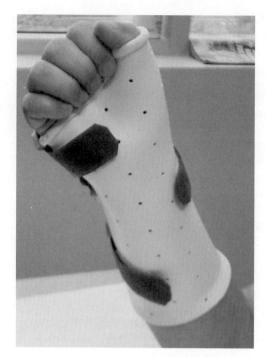

FIG. **8-4** Forearm-based thumb spica.

    (This reach creates an increase in neurotension and decreased efficiency of movement.)

    B. Vibration

    C. Pronation coupled with wrist extension

    D. Gloves and other equipment that place direct mechanical stress on the radial sensory nerve

    E. Use of personal articles that are offending factors (e.g., wristwatch, bracelet)

VI. A strengthening can be initiated once the patient has normalized AROM and has a reduced pain reflex.

    A. *NOTE: All tasks are conducted below a pain reflex.

Operative Indications/Technique

Operative decompression of the superficial radial nerve usually follows exhaustive nonoperative management that does not relieve the paresthesias and is rarely done. The fascia overlying the brachioradialis and ECRL is incised, and the nerve is carefully dissected. A partial excision of the tendon of brachioradialis is sometimes indicated.[10]

Postoperative Treatment

I. Days 5 to 7

    A. Postoperative dressings are removed, and a light compressive bandage is applied.

    B. The patient is checked for signs and symptoms of infection.

    C. The patient is provided with education on wound care.

    D. AROM exercises are initiated for the wrist, forearm, and elbow.
       1. These are to be conducted every hour for 5 to 10 minutes total exercise time.
       2. These exercises include the following:
         a. Radial nerve glides
         b. Ulnar nerve glides
         c. Median nerve glides
         d. Tendon gliding (see Chapter 19)
           (1) Basic-4 hand postures
           (2) Overhead fisting
    E. Patients will find it helpful to have a forearm thumb spica splint fabricated to enhance function by resting the decompressed radial sensory nerve while not conducting exercises (see Fig. 8-4).
    F. *NOTE: All exercises are conducted below the pain threshold, to avoid increasing pain.

Postoperative Complications

   I. Painful scar
  II. Nerve injury
 III. Failure to relieve symptoms
 IV. Infection

OUTCOMES

Triangular fibrocartilage complex injuries have many stages and severity indexes. Symptoms can go unnoticed for years and become symptomatic with trauma or competitive activity. A good outcome depends on communication between the surgeon and the therapist to fully understand the surgical techniques and map out a reasonable treatment program. To ensure proper compliance of the treatment program the patient should understand the injury, healing timelines of the surgery, and risk factors of ADL tasks. Education will help the patient have reasonable return-to-function expectations and should be completed before surgery.

Most studies demonstrate a good functional outcome with improved AROM and strength and a decrease in pain and strength within functional limits for ADL tasks.[12] However, a competitive level of activity is the most difficult type of function to regain. These types of activities include pronation/supination, ulnar and radial deviation, and overhead tasks. The hand therapist should progressively and safely expose these risk factors to the patient based on the stage of healing, the type of repair performed, and the type of movement patterns needed for gainful employment.

REFERENCES

1. Eaton CJ, Lister GD: Radial nerve compression. Hand Clin 8:345-357, 1992
2. Hollinshead HW: Anatomy for Surgeons: Back and Limbs. Lippincott Williams & Wilkins, Philadelphia, 1982
3. Netter FH: Atlas of Human Anatomy. CIBA-GEIGY, Summit, NJ, 1991
4. Hunter JM, Schneider LH, Mackin EJ, et al. (eds): Rehabilitation of the Hand and Upper Extremity. 5th Ed. Mosby, St. Louis, 2002
5. Morrey BF (ed.): The Elbow and Its Disorders. 3rd Ed. WB Saunders, St. Louis, 2002
6. Green DP: Radial nerve palsy. In Green DP, Hotchkiss RN, Pederson WP (eds): Green's Operative Hand Surgery. 4th Ed. Churchill Livingstone, New York, 1993

7. Lister GD, Belsole RB, Kleinert HE: The radial tunnel syndrome. J Hand Surg Am 4:52-59, 1979

8. Jebson Peter JL, Engber WD: Radial tunnel syndrome: long-term results of surgical decompression. J Hand Surg Am 22:889-896, 1997

9. Ritts GD, Wood MB, Lindscheid RL: Radial tunnel syndrome: a ten year surgical experience. Clin Orthop 219:201-205, 1987

10. Dellon AL, Mackinnon SE: Radial sensory nerve entrapment in the forearm. J Hand Surg 11A:199-205, 1986

11. Gersh M: Electrotherapy in Rehabilitation. 2nd Ed. FA Davis, Philadelphia, 2002

12. Palmer AK: The distal radial ulnar joint. Anatomy, biomechanics, and triangular fibrocartilage complex abnormalities. Hand Clin 3:31-40, 1987

SUGGESTED READINGS

American Society for Surgery of the Hand. The Hand: Primary Care of Common Problems. 2nd Ed. Churchill Livingstone, New York, 1990

Andrews JR, Wilk KE: The Athlete's Shoulder. Churchill Livingstone, New York, 1994

Beasley RW: Tendon transfers for radial nerve palsy. Orthop Clin North Am 1:439-445, 1970

Brand PW, Hollister A: Clinical Mechanics of the Hand. 3rd Ed. Mosby, St. Louis, 1990

Butler DS: The Sensitive Nervous System. Noigroup Publications, Adelaide, Australia, 2002

Cameron MH: Physical agents in rehabilitation: from research to practice. WB Saunders, St. Louis, 1999

Cannon NM (ed): Diagnosis and Treatment Manual for Physicians and Therapists. The Hand Rehabilitation Center, Indianapolis, IN, 2001

Chuinard RG, Boyes JH, Stark HH, et al: Tendon transfers for radial nerve palsy: use of the superficialis tendons for digital extension. J Hand Surg Am 3:560-570, 1978

Cooney WP, Linscheid RL, Dobyns JH (eds): The Wrist: Diagnosis and Operative Treatment. Mosby–Year Book, St. Louis, 1998

Fess EE, Philips CA, Gettle-Harmon K: Hand Splinting Principles and Methods. 3rd Ed. Mosby–Year Book, St. Louis, 2001

Green DP, Hotchkiss RN, Pederson WP (eds): Green's Operative Hand Surgery. 4th Ed. Churchill Livingstone, St. Louis, 1998

Hoppenfeld S, Hutton R: Physical Examination of the Spine and Extremities. Prentice-Hall, Saddle River, NJ, 1976

Kendall F, McCreary EK: Muscles: Testing and Function. 5th Ed. Lippincott Williams & Wilkins, Philadelphia, 1999

Magee DJ: Orthopedic Physical Assessment. 3rd Ed. WB Saunders, St. Louis, 1997

McCulloch JM, Kloth LD, Feedar JA (eds): Wound Healing: Alternatives in Management. 3rd Ed. FA Davis, Philadelphia, 2001

Michlovitz SL (ed.): Thermal Agents in Rehabilitation. 3rd Ed. FA Davis, Philadelphia, 1996

Nordin M, Frankel VH (eds): Basic Biomechanics of the Musculoskeletal System. 2nd Ed. Lippincott Williams & Wilkins, Philadelphia, 2001

Smith P: Lister's The Hand: Diagnosis and Indications. 4th Ed. WB Saunders, St. Louis, 2002

Stanley B, Tribuzi S: Concepts in Hand Rehabilitation. FA Davis, Philadelphia, 1992

Szabo RM: Entrapment and Compression Neuropathies. In Green DP, Hotchkiss RN, Pederson WP (eds): Green's Operative Hand Surgery. 4th Ed. Churchill Livingstone, New York, 1993

Tubiana R: Examination of the Hand and Wrist. 2nd Ed. Blackwell Science, Malden, MA, 1998

Thoracic Outlet Syndrome 9

Mallory S. Anthony

The thoracic outlet is the triangular channel through which the nerves and vessels of the arm leave the neck and thorax. The medial portion is bounded by the anterior scalene muscle anteriorly, the medial scalene muscle posteriorly, the clavicle superiorly, and the first rib inferiorly. As one moves laterally, the thoracic outlet boundaries include the coracoid, the pectoralis minor muscle, and its tendinous insertion into the coracoid and the deltopectoral fascia. The structures at risk of compression in this area are the subclavian artery, the subclavian vein, and the brachial plexus. The subclavian artery arches over the first rib, behind the anterior scalene muscle and in front of the medial scalene muscle. It then passes under the subclavius muscle and clavicle and enters the axilla beneath the pectoralis minor muscle. The subclavian vein follows the same course, except that it passes anteriorly rather than posteriorly to the anterior scalene muscle. The brachial plexus follows the route of the subclavian artery, but it lies a little more posteriorly and laterally.[1]

There are three potential spaces for compression of the brachial plexus and neurovascular structures[2] (Fig. 9-1). The first and most medial is the scalene triangle, bordered by the scalenus anterior and scalenus medius, and inferiorly by the first rib (see Fig. 9-1, *A*). The subclavian artery and brachial plexus travel within this triangle. Compression at this site would have no venous component, because the subclavian vein travels anteriorly to this space. The second space is the costoclavicular region, bordered superiorly by the clavicle and inferiorly by the first rib (see Fig. 9-1, *B*). The third potential space is the subcoracoid space, where the anterior deltopectoral fascia, the pectoralis minor, and the coracoid could all be sources of compression (see Fig. 9-1, *C*).

The causes of thoracic outlet syndrome (TOS) can be related to compressive neuropathy, postural abnormalities, or entrapment neuropathy.[2] Compression neuropathy can occur from anatomic causes such as muscle hypertrophy, adaptic shortening of surrounding fascia, or space-occupying lesions (e.g., cervical rib, bifid clavicle), all of which can decrease the sizes of potential spaces. Postural abnormalities, which frequently involve a forward head and rounded shoulders (e.g., tight scalenes and pectoralis minor

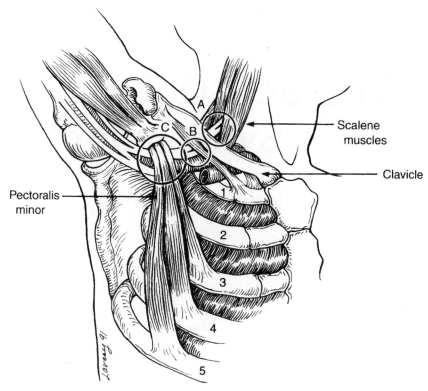

FIG. **9-1** Thoracic outlet anatomy with possible sites of compression. **A,** Scalene triangle; **B,** costoclavicular region; **C,** subcoracoid space.

muscle) can decrease the space of the scalene triangle and subcoracoid space, respectively, compressing the neurovascular structures. Patients with compression problems (anatomic or postural) usually have insidious onset of pain, no history of trauma, and often early signs of repetitive stress.[2] They frequently have predictable symptom distribution over the lower trunk (C8 to T1), which may be only nocturnal or activity related.[2] Provocative tests are helpful in identifying possible sites of compression.

A third cause of TOS is entrapment neuropathy. This is an impairment of the biomechanical aspects of the nerve's ability to glide through surrounding tissue and to tolerate tension.[2] It may occur secondary to intraneural or extraneural fibrosis associated with cervical or shoulder trauma or as a result of long-standing repetitive stress activities.[2]

The diagnosis of TOS is based not only on a thorough upper quarter evaluation but also on the exclusion of other pathologies (e.g., cervical disc disease, nerve root impingement, shoulder pathology, tendinitis). Patients with TOS (unless it is long-standing) rarely show objective test abnormalities, because their symptoms are often intermittent and provoked by arm elevation.[3] Also, it is not uncommon to find carpal and/or cubital tunnel syndromes associated with TOS because of double or multiple crush syndromes[4,5] (i.e., a proximal source of nerve compression renders the distal nerve segment more susceptible to additional sites of compression). The progression of TOS symptoms is the same as for any peripheral nerve compression problem and is dependent on the amount and duration of compression.

Initially, patients exhibit symptoms only with provocative or positional maneuvers (asymptomatic at rest). As progression increases, more severe stages of chronic nerve compression are evident (i.e., abnormal sensory changes and muscle atrophy). However, severe chronic stages of nerve compression in the brachial plexus are rare, because the patient learns to decrease discomfort and symptoms by modifying extremity position and posture.[6] These modifications in posture increase and exacerbate muscle imbalance in the upper back, neck, and shoulders. The following protocol offers guidelines for both evaluation and treatment of this complex and challenging syndrome.

DEFINITION

Thoracic outlet syndrome comprises symptoms of arterial insufficiency, venous engorgement, or nerve dysfunction that can be produced by compression or stretching of the subclavian artery, subclavian vein, or portions of the brachial plexus as they pass from the neck to the axilla.

I.   Types of compression[7]
  A. Arterial: 1% of all cases. Main symptom is unilateral vasospastic disease, with two distinct age groups
    1. Young adults, due to external compression of the subclavian artery, usually by a cervical rib
    2. Patients older than 40 years of age, in whom localized degenerative changes of the artery may result from turbulent flow caused by extrinsic pressure
  B. Venous: 2% of all cases
    1. Seen throughout adulthood.
    2. More prevalent in athletic men
  C. Neurological: 97% of all cases
    1. More prevalent in young or middle-aged adults
    2. Women outnumber men (2 or 3:1).
II. Cause of thoracic outlet syndrome
  A. Dynamic[1] (anatomic)
    1. Impingement at acromioclavicular joint or humeroscapular articulation
    2. Compression beneath the coracoid process and pectoralis minor during hyperabduction of the arm
  B. Static[1] (postural)
    1. Muscular hypertrophy or spasm (e.g., scalenus hypertrophy or spasm, omohyoid muscle hypertrophy) may reduce anatomic space for passage of neurovascular structures.
    2. Muscular atrophy: Reduction in muscle mass and tone may cause sagging of local structures. (Shoulder trauma or neurological disease could cause muscle weakness.)
    3. Postural abnormalities: Rounded shoulders and forward head are commonly seen and can contribute to neurovascular compression and possibly exacerbate any previously asymptomatic congenital factor. Also, guarded posturing of the upper extremity can decrease the size of the thoracic outlet.
  C. Congenital[8] (anatomic)
    1. Cervical ribs (most common factor) cause compression by narrowing the intrascalene triangle.

    2. Fascial bands behind anterior scalene or abnormal insertion of middle scalene on first rib

    3. Bifid clavicle

    4. Bony protuberance on first rib

    5. Enlargement of costal element of transverse process of seventh cervical vertebra

    6. Fibrous bands extending between cervical vertebra and first ribs

    7. Rudimentary first thoracic rib (rare condition)

    8. Scoliosis

D. Traumatic[9] (entrapment)

    1. Fibrous callus formation caused by fracture of clavicle or first rib

    2. Shoulder dislocation

    3. Crush injury or traction injury to upper thorax (may stretch brachial plexus and/or thrombose artery or vein)

    4. Whiplash

    5. Cumulative trauma through repetitive above-shoulder level movements

    6. Thoracoplasty surgery

E. Arteriosclerotic

F. Tumor in thoracic outlet: less common

TREATMENT PURPOSE

To increase the space in the thoracic outlet and relieve compression on neurovascular structures, through conservative therapy and/or surgical procedures.

TREATMENT GOALS

I. Modify postural habits and body mechanics that exacerbate the patient's symptoms.

II. Relieve muscle tension of shoulder girdle musculature.

III. Improve cervical and scapular alignment (restore muscle balance).

IV. Increase nerve gliding through surrounding tissue.

V. Return to optimal level of function.

VI. Prevent recurrence of symptoms.

NONOPERATIVE INDICATIONS/PRECAUTIONS FOR THERAPY

I. Indications

A. Symptoms of neurovascular compression are produced and are related to arm position and use.

B. The following is a list of other shoulder and neck conditions that may exhibit symptoms similar to those of TOS.[7,9,10]

    1. Cervical disc abnormality (i.e., nerve root impingement)

    2. Osteoarthritis

    3. Reflex sympathetic dystrophy

    4. Spinal cord tumors

    5. Arachnoiditis

    6. Multiple sclerosis

7. Visceral diseases (angina pectoris, esophageal diseases, gastric ulcer, pulmonary diseases)
8. Blockage of subclavian artery or vein
9. Bursitis, tendinitis, or capsulitis of the shoulder
10. Rotator cuff injuries
11. Acromioclavicular joint separation
12. Median nerve compression
13. Ulnar nerve entrapment
14. Radial nerve entrapment
15. Raynaud's syndrome
16. Pancoast's tumor of the lung
17. Metastasis of carcinoma to, or inflammation of, axillary lymph nodes

II. Precautions
   A. Infection
   B. Acute fracture
   C. Extreme discomfort
   D. Marked edema

NONOPERATIVE THERAPY

I. Pretreatment evaluation
   A. History
      1. Mechanism and site of injury (possible whiplash, traction injuries, clavicle fracture)
      2. Onset and duration of symptoms and other related injuries
      3. Detailed description of symptoms (e.g., pain versus paresthesias)
      4. Habits, work conditions, and stressful conditions
      5. Which positions aggravate the symptoms (e.g., overhead activities) and what relieves the symptoms
      6. Obtain results from referring physician's examination if possible.
         a. Radiographs of cervical spine and chest
         b. Pulse volume recordings (Doppler studies)
         c. Computed tomography (CT) scan
         d. Angiography
         e. Electrodiagnostic testing: nerve conduction studies (helpful if tested in both traditional resting position and position of provocation that would cause stress on lower trunk of brachial plexus).[5] Somatosensory evoked potentials (SSEP) may be tested, but their diagnostic value is still questionable.[11]
         f. Neurosensory testing (Pressure-Specified Sensory Device [PSSD]) and motor testing (digit–grip)[12]
         g. Magnetic resonance imaging (MRI)
         h. Social work evaluation: Minnesota Multiphasic Personality Inventory (MMPI) results and personality factors that may affect the patient's response to treatment
         i. Current medications
   B. Physical examination: upper quarter evaluation. Also, mobility and status of the lumbar spine and lower extremity need to be

evaluated to determine other coincidental postural problems that may contribute to the postural abnormalities in TOS.[13]

1. Visual inspection
   a. Postural assessment: rounded shoulders, uneven shoulders, forward head, head tilt, guarding posture of shoulder
   b. Atrophy: especially in hypothenar and intrinsic muscles, since C8 and T1 nerve roots are at greatest risk of compression
   c. Color, skin condition
   d. Edema
   e. Musculoskeletal deformity
   f. Breathing pattern (i.e., diaphragmatic versus accessory muscle respiration)
   g. Evaluation of cervical and thoracic spine[14-17]
2. Strength: grip and pinch measurements
3. Manual muscle testing
   a. Identify weak and overstretched muscles (frequently middle/lower trapezius and cervical extensors).
   b. Identify tight muscles and hypertrophy (frequently scalenes, sternocleidomastoid, upper trapezius, and pectoral muscles).
   c. Identify trigger points (palpate from origin to insertion for tenderness)
4. Range of motion (ROM) evaluation of glenohumeral, scapular, and cervical motion
5. Sensory evaluation[18]
   a. May need to perform sensory tests immediately after provocation of symptoms.
6. Pain: location, type, frequency, visual analog scale, McGill pain questionnaire, modified Hendler's pain evaluation, others
7. Skin temperature (for vascular component)
8. Supraclavicular Tinel's sign (positive when patient reports tingling sensation in the arm, and not only local tingling)[13]
9. Compression maneuvers used to attempt to localize vascular compression sites[1,7,8] (check bilaterally). *NOTE: These three tests should be used in conjunction with all other objective testing procedures; they are extremely technician sensitive and are frequently positive in normal, asymptomatic individuals.
   a. *Adson's maneuver:* Clinician holds arm in extension and external shoulder rotation as the patient holds a deep breath and rotates head toward the affected side. Repeat with head turned away from the affected side. Positive findings result in obliteration of the radial pulse and/or reproduction of symptoms, presumably because of subclavian artery compression by the scaleni (i.e., scalene triangle).
   b. *Costoclavicular maneuver:* Exaggerated military position with shoulders drawn downward and backward, used to check for compression occurring at costoclavicular region. Note obliteration of radial pulse and/or reproduction of symptoms.

      c. *Hyperabduction maneuver:* Arm held by clinician in fully abducted position to test for compression at pectoralis minor insertion (i.e., axillary region). Again note reproduction of symptoms and/or obliteration of radial pulse.

  10. Provocative maneuvers used to assess status of brachial plexus

      a. *Elevated arm stress test (EAST) or Roos test* (also indicative of vascular manifestation): Patient assumes the "stick-up" position (i.e., shoulders abducted and externally rotated to 90 degrees and forearms flexed to 90 degrees) and then opens and closes his hands for 3 minutes or until the symptoms are provoked.[7] A modification of the Roos test can also be used: Arms are elevated overhead with elbows extended (to avoid reproducing ulnar nerve symptoms) and wrists in neutral position (to avoid reproducing median nerve symptoms). This test position is maintained for 1 minute without opening and closing hands.[13]

         (1) *Arterial involvement:* demonstrates pallor with empty veins

         (2) *Venous involvement:* cyanosis and/or venous engorgement

         (3) *Neurologic involvement:* paresthesias and heaviness

      b. *Elvey's upper limb tension test (ULTT):* Tests mobility of brachial plexus and nerve roots. Clinician looks for provocation of symptoms by placing progressively increased tension in the nerve roots/peripheral nerve. Care must be taken to avoid placing excess traction on the plexus. Specific ULTT techniques have been described by Barbis and Wallace[9] and by Totten and Hunter.[19]

      c. *Hunter test—high:* Tests for ulnar nerve findings (involvement of C8-T1, lower trunk). For specific technique, see Totten and Hunter.[19]

      d. *Erb test:* Tests for radial nerve findings (involvement of posterior cord). Specific techniques can be found in MacKinnon and Dellon.[5]

      e. *Hunter test—low:* Tests for median nerve findings (involvement of C6-C7, upper trunk). Specific technique can be found in Totten and Hunter.[19]

      f. Provocative maneuvers to test for distal compression sites (i.e., cubital tunnel and carpal tunnel).

      g. *Medial clavicle compression:* Manual compression superior and posterior to the medial one third of the clavicle may also provoke symptoms.[20,21]

  11. *NOTE: Some of the provocative tests as well as some movements tested during ROM evaluation may not be tolerated by a patient with severe symptoms.

II. Treatment

  A. Progression[2]

    1. Stage I: Decrease and control patient's symptoms; increase comfort.

    2. Stage II: Treat tissues that are creating structural limitations of motion (e.g., soft tissue mobilization, nerve gliding, stretching exercises).

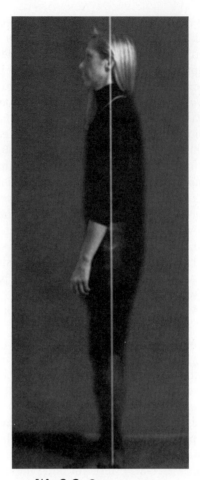

FIG. **9-2** Correct posture.

3. Stage III: Condition and strengthen muscles necessary to maintain postural correction; restore functional ROM of upper extremity for activities of daily living (ADL) and occupational activities.

B. Conservative management

1. Patient education to avoid symptom-producing postures and activities, which include occupational, recreational, and sleeping habits. Note irritability of symptoms and progress as tolerated toward proper posture. Orthotic devices have been advocated to support the upper body in an upright position. However, most of these devices are strapped anteriorly over the pectoral region and then cross over in a figure-of-eight pattern posteriorly, potentially increasing pressure on the brachial plexus and placing the patient in an extremely upright position to which he or she is unaccustomed.[13] Also, splinting may be needed to reduce tension or compression on more distal peripheral neuropathies. The following is a guideline for reducing the aggravation of symptoms (unpublished protocol).[20,21]

   a. Correct posture: The plumb line should fall anterior to the lateral malleolus and knee, through the femoral greater

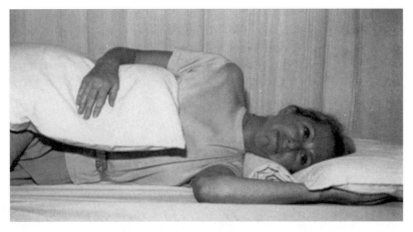

FIG. **9-3** Positioning for sidelying.

trochanter, and midway through the trunk, the shoulder
joint, the cervical vertebrae, and the earlobe. The patient
should look in mirror, front and side (Fig. 9-2).
  (1) Bring head and shoulder back to a relaxed position.
  (2) Small curve in low back
  (3) Weight distributed equally on both feet
  (4) Maintain correct posture when sitting, standing, or
      walking. (Note: ideal posture must be gradually
      approximated over time.)
b. Sleeping
  (1) Patient should avoid sleeping on affected side, in
      facelying position, or with arms overhead.
  (2) A position that decreases symptoms is sidelying on the
      unaffected side with one pillow or a cervical roll under
      the head and another pillow in the line of the trunk to
      support the upper arm (Fig. 9-3).[13]
  (3) Another position of comfort is lying on the back with
      one pillow under the head and shoulders and one
      pillow under each arm (Fig. 9-4).
c. Working (discomfort often associated with arm elevated
   positions or downward pull)
  (1) Patient should not lean over while standing or sitting.
      Be as erect as possible.

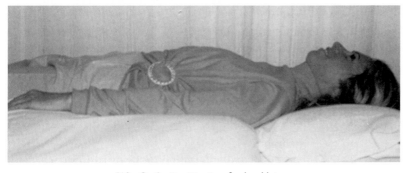

FIG. **9-4** Positioning for backlying.

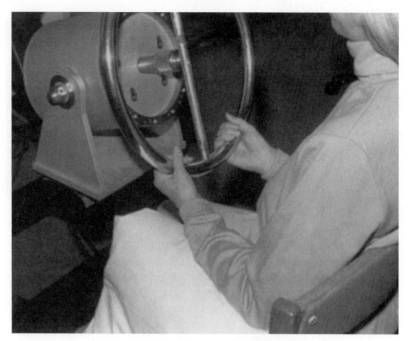

FIG. 9-5 Positioning for driving.

(2) When sitting at a desk or armchair, there should be
    a forearm-supporting surface that does not cause
    excessive elevation or depression of the shoulders and
    minimizes irritation of the cervicoscapular region.
(3) Patient should guard against working above shoulder
    level and should use a stepstool to reach high objects.
(4) Patient should avoid carrying heavy objects with affected
    arm. Heavy items (e.g., briefcases, purses, grocery bags)
    should be carried with unaffected arm or held close to
    body in both arms.
d. Driving (Fig. 9-5)
    (1) Hands should be kept low and relaxed on steering
        wheel.
    (2) A small pillow or arm rest should support the affected
        side.
    (3) If shoulder strap of seat belt crosses the clavicle on the
        affected side, the patient must not draw the strap too
        tightly.
e. General precautions
    (1) Stressful situations should be avoided. Stress leads to
        tension of the cervical musculature.
    (2) Affected arm should not hang at side while working or
        standing. The hand can rest in a pocket to avoid
        pulling down on the shoulder.
    (3) Obesity contributes to poor posture and continuation of
        symptoms.
    (4) For female patients with breast hypertrophy, brassieres
        with wider straps that cross at the back are suggested,

   to decrease stress on supraclavicular region and
   encourage upright posture.
   (5) Strenuous exercises that create labored breathing
       should be avoided, because this requires action of
       secondary respiratory muscles whose function is
       elevation of the ribs.
   (6) Patient should change activities or rest if symptoms
       arise.
   (7) Patient should have others remind him or her about
       correct posture.
   (8) Patients should wear several layers of light clothing
       during cold weather. (Heavy coats may weigh down
       the shoulders.) Cold weather creates shivering and
       hypertonicity of muscles, including the upper cervical
       musculature; hence, keeping warm is important.
2. Modalities to decrease pain (e.g., transcutaneous electrical
   nerve stimulation [TENS], moist heat): Begin with pain- and
   inflammation-reducing treatments (may need sling or
   postural support to help maintain rest position of brachial
   plexus—that is, abduction and elevation of scapula and
   internal rotation and adduction of shoulder).[9] Modalities
   should be used for temporary relief of pain or spasm to
   enhance the exercise program. As a primary treatment, they
   may reinforce patient dependency on therapy.
3. Management of muscle spasm and tension in shoulder girdle
   and cervical musculature
   a. Moist heat
   b. Ultrasound
   c. Cold packs (use cautiously on patients with trigger points)
   d. Massage (deep friction and relaxation)
   e. Spray and stretch technique to help inactivate tender
      trigger points[22]
   f. Occasionally analgesics and/or muscle relaxants are
      prescribed by physician
   g. *NOTE: Cervical traction, either static or intermittent,
      should be avoided, because it tends to increase rather than
      relieve patient's symptoms.
4. Manual therapy to restore or increase accessory joint movement
   a. Joint mobilizations of sternoclavicular, acromioclavicular,
      and scapulothoracic joints[20,23]
   b. Mobilization of the occiput on the atlas also facilitates axial
      extension movement.[21]
   c. Techniques of joint mobilization should be performed only
      by therapists with appropriate training in manual therapy.
5. Brachial plexus gliding exercises
   a. Use of the ULTT as an exercise for mobilizing the brachial
      plexus
   b. For specific exercise technique, see Barbis and Wallace[9]
      and Totten and Hunter.[19]
6. Postural exercises[2,8,9,21,24]
   a. Improve cervical and scapular alignment; include exercises
      to stretch pectoralis minor, scaleni, and cervical lateral flexors

and exercises to strengthen scapular adduction/depression and paracervical extension. Shoulder/glenohumeral joint exercises and thoracic flexion/extension exercises can be added as needed.

b. The following is a suggested exercise program. Exercises should be performed slowly, with 10 repetitions, two times a day to start. (If patient's tolerance is low or symptoms are aggravated, decrease number and frequency of exercises and/or change exercise position to minimize stress on injured tissues; for example, use gravity-assisted positions, supine with pillow support, or isometric exercises. Endurance, rather than power, is emphasized. Be aware of excess stretch on neural structures.)[3,13,25]

(1) *Shoulder girdle motion* (to emphasize shoulder retraction): Sit with shoulders relaxed; arms supported. Make small circles with shoulder joints, gradually increasing in size. Work in both directions.

(2) *Stretching of scalene muscles:* Stand erect; arms at sides, with shoulders internally rotated. (May also be done in supine position to maximize cervical relaxation.[2]) Bend the neck, trying to touch ear to shoulder, first to right then to left. Relax and repeat. (May add shoulder depression to increase stretch.) (See Fig. 9-6.)

(3) *Stretching of pectoral muscles* (begin pectoral stretches in a gravity-assisted position and progress to corner stretches as tissue irritability decreases if patient can tolerate): Corner stretches should be performed as follows: stand facing a corner of a room with one hand

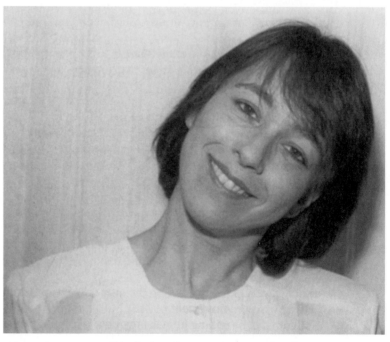

FIG. **9-6** Scalene stretch exercise.

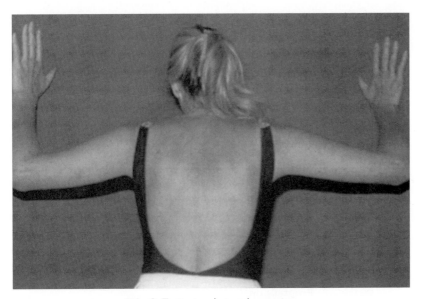

FIG. **9-7** Pectoral stretch exercise.

on each wall, hands at head level, palms forward, elbows bent. Do a standard push-up into corner and return to original position. Inhale as body leans forward, exhale on return. Repeat (Fig. 9-7).

(4) *Stretching of pectoralis minor:* Lie supine with knees bent. Keep arms level on bed surface. Slide affected arm up into abduction, attempting to reach ear.

(5) *Strengthening of scapular adductors:* Sit with shoulders relaxed; arms supported in lap. Gently squeeze shoulder blades together, hold for a count of 3, return to starting position and repeat (Fig. 9-8).

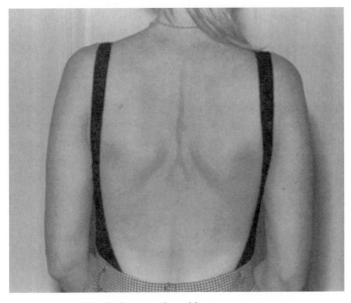

FIG. **9-8** Scapular adduction exercise.

(6) *Strengthening of cervical extensors:* Begin in supine position with a towel roll supporting the cervical spine in flexion. Perform gentle, repetitive cervical retraction exercises. Progress to gentle, gravity-resisted positions.

(7) *Diaphragmatic breathing* (to discourage overuse of accessory muscles for respiration, which elevates the rib cage, resulting in decreased thoracic outlet space): Assume backlying position with one hand on stomach and one hand on chest. Inhale—hand on stomach should rise; hand on chest should stay about same height. Exhale—hand on stomach should fall; hand on chest stays at same height. Perform for three inhalation/exhalation cycles. An aerobic, walking exercise program, which emphasizes proper breathing, is also suggested and helps improve the cardiovascular system.[13]

(8) Progression

(a) Increase frequency of home exercise program slowly to patient tolerance.

(b) Assess progress as often as needed (once or twice per week).

(c) Relief of symptoms should be achieved after at least 3 to 4 months of conservative management; otherwise an alternative method of treatment may be indicated (possibly surgery).

7. ROM exercises for cervical region and upper extremity

INDICATIONS/PRECAUTIONS FOR SURGERY

I.   Indications

A. Conservative treatment is not beneficial.

B. Patient requires narcotic medication and is unable to sleep or work.

C. Muscle atrophy

D. Marked edema

E. Arterial emboli or fingertip ulceration/gangrene

II. Precautions

A. Malignant conditions (especially with prior irradiation)

B. Alcohol abuse

C. Diabetes

D. Other neurological or vascular disease

OPERATIVE MANAGEMENT

I.   Surgical techniques

A. Cervical rib resection

B. Scalenectomy procedures

C. Transaxillary approaches for fascial band release

D. Arterial reconstructive procedures

E. Supraclavicular and infraclavicular approaches

POSTOPERATIVE THERAPY[7,9,26]

I. ROM exercises every 1 to 2 hours, as soon as possible after surgery, to maintain freedom of movement of the plexus
    A. Elvey's ULTT is helpful for nerve gliding, because the patient can perform forearm supination and wrist and finger extension without stressing the surgical wound.
    B. Cervical and shoulder ROM on first postoperative day
II. Continue gentle ROM exercises to shoulder and scapular area for 1 to 2 weeks postoperatively.
III. Mild use of shoulder 4 to 6 weeks postoperatively, with progressive strengthening exercises
IV. Full use of upper extremity 8 to 10 weeks postoperatively

POSTOPERATIVE COMPLICATIONS

I. Infection
II. Persistent painful paresthesias
III. Decreased muscle strength with atrophy
IV. Persistent numbness
V. Decreased circulation with possible ulceration of fingertips
VI. Nonunion of clavicle if clavicle is divided during surgery
VII. Lung collapse
VIII. Phrenic nerve injury

EVALUATION TIMELINE

I. Initial evaluation
    A. Postural assessment
    B. Edema
    C. Strength (grip and pinch measurement)
    D. Manual muscle test
    E. ROM evaluation
    F. Sensory evaluation
    G. Pain: location, type, frequency, and so on
II. Repeat evaluations every 4 weeks for progress assessment.

OUTCOMES

Very few outcome studies are available. Novak and colleagues[27] treated 42 patients with conservative management; at 1 year follow-up, 25 patients had 60% overall symptomatic relief. Lindgren[28] studied 119 patients managed conservatively with inpatient physical therapy for approximately 11 days, followed by a home exercise program; at 2 year follow-up, 88% were satisfied with their outcome and 73% had returned to work.

REFERENCES

1. Lord JW, Rosati LM: Clinical Symposia: Thoracic Outlet Syndromes. CIBA Pharmaceutical Co., Summit, NJ, 1971
2. Walsh MT: Therapist management of thoracic outlet syndrome. J Hand Ther 7: 131-144, 994

3. Novak CB, MacKinnon SE, Patterson GA: Evaluation of patients with thoracic outlet syndrome. J Hand Surg Am 18:292, 1993

4. Upton A, McComas AJ: The double crush in nerve-entrapment syndromes. Lancet 2:359, 1973

5. MacKinnon SE, Dellon AL: Surgery of the Peripheral Nerve. Thieme Medical Publications, New York, 1988

6. Mackinnon SE, Patterson GA, Novak CB: Thoracic outlet syndrome: a current review. Semin Thorac Cardiovasc Surg 8:176-182, 1996

7. Roos DB: Thoracic outlet syndrome. In Machleder HI (ed): Vascular Disorders of the Upper Extremity. Futura, Mount Kisco, 1983, p. 91

8. Wilgis EFS: Vascular Injuries and Diseases of the Upper Limb. Little, Brown, Boston, 1983

9. Barbis JM, Wallace KA: Therapists management of brachioplexopathy. In Hunter JM, Mackin EJ, Callahan AD (eds): Rehabilitation of the Hand: Surgery and Therapy. 4th Ed. Mosby, St. Louis, 1995, p. 923

10. Sheth RN, Belzberg AJ: Diagnosis and treatment of thoracic outlet syndrome. Neurol Clin North Am 12:295-309, 2001

11. Komanetsky RM, Novak CB, Mackinnon SE, et al.: Somatosensory evoked potentials fail to diagnose thoracic outlet syndrome. J Hand Surg Am 21:662-666, 1996

12. Howard M, Lee C, Dellon AL: Documentation of brachial plexus compression (in the thoracic inlet) utilizing provocative neurosensory and muscular testing. J Reconstr Surg 19:303-312, 2003

13. Novak CB, Mackinnon SE: Thoracic outlet syndrome. Orthop Clin North Am 27:747-762, 1996

14. Maitland G: Peripheral Mobilization. Butterworth, Boston, 1977

15. McKenzie RA: The Lumbar Spine: Mechanical Diagnoses and Therapy. Spinal Publications, Waikanae, New Zealand, 1981

16. McKenzie RA: Treat Your Own Neck. Spinal Publications, Waikanae, New Zealand, 1983

17. Cyriax J: Textbook of Orthopaedic Diagnosis of Soft Tissue Lesions: Vol. I. Balliere Tindall, London, 1980

18. Anthony MS: Sensory Evaluation. In Clark GL, Wilgis, EFS, Aiello B, et al. (eds): Hand Rehabilitation: A Practical Guide. 2nd Ed. Churchill Livingston, New York, 1997, p. 55

19. Totten PA, Hunter JM: Therapeutic techniques to enhance nerve gliding in thoracic outlet syndrome and carpal tunnel syndrome. Hand Clin 7:505, 1991

20. Smith KF: The thoracic outlet syndrome: a protocol of treatment. Am Phys Ther Assoc 1:89, 1979

21. Jaeger SH, Read R, Smullens SN, Breme P: Thoracic outlet syndrome: diagnosis and treatment. In Hunter JM (ed): Rehabilitation of the Hand: Surgery and Therapy. 2nd Ed. Mosby, St. Louis, 1984, p. 378

22. Travell JG, Simon DG: Myofascial Pain and Dysfunction: The Trigger Point Manual. Baltimore, Williams & Wilkins, 1983

23. Jackson P: Thoracic outlet syndrome: evaluation and treatment. Clin Manage Phys Ther 7:6, 1987

24. Klinefelter HF: Postural myoneuralgia. Int Angiol 3:191, 1984

25. Novak CB: Thoracic outlet syndrome. Clin Plastic Surg 30:175-188, 2003

26. Whitenack SH, Hunter JM, Jaeger SH, et al.: Thoracic outlet syndrome: a brachial plexopathy. In Hunter JM, Mackin EJ, Callahan AD (eds): Rehabilitation of the Hand: Surgery and Therapy. 4th Ed. Mosby, St. Louis, 1995, p. 857

27. Novak CB, Collins ED, Mackinnon SE: Outcome following conservative management of thoracic outlet syndrome. J Hand Surg Am 20:542-548, 1995

28. Lindgren KA: Conservative treatment of thoracic outlet syndrome: a 2-year follow-up. Arch Phys Med Rehabil 78:373-378, 1997

SUGGESTED READINGS

Adson AW: Surgical treatment for symptoms produced by cervical ribs and the scalenus anticus muscle. Surg Gynecol Obstet 85:687, 1947

Butler SD: Tension testing the upper limb. In Butler DS (ed): Mobilization of the Nervous System. Churchill Livingstone, New York, 1991, p. 141

Byron PM: Upper extremity nerve gliding: programs used at the Philadelphia hand center. In Hunter JM, Mackin EJ, Callahan AD (eds): Rehabilitation of the Hand: Surgery and Therapy. 4th Ed. Mosby, St. Louis, 1995, p. 951

Cailliet R: Neck and Arm Pain. FA Davis, Philadelphia, 1964

Cailliet R: Soft Tissue Pain and Disability. FA Davis, Philadelphia, 1977

Carroll RE, Hurst LC: The relationship of thoracic outlet syndrome and carpal tunnel syndrome. Clin Orthop 164:149, 1982

Edwards RH: Hypothesis of peripheral and central mechanisms underlying occupational muscle pain and injury. Eur J Appl Physiol 57:275, 1988

Elvey RL: Brachial plexus tension tests and the pathoanatomical origin of arm pain. In Glasgow EF, Twoney L (eds): Aspects of Manipulative Therapy. 2nd Ed. Churchill Livingstone, New York, 1985, p. 116

Hawkes CD: Neurosurgical considerations in thoracic outlet syndrome. Neurosurg Consid 207:24, 1986

Huffman JD: Electrodiagnostic techniques for and conservative treatment of thoracic outlet syndrome. Electrodiagn Tech 207:21, 1986

Kaltenborn FM: Manual Therapy for the Extremity Joints. Olaf Norlis Bokhandel, Oslo, 1976

Leffert RD: Thoracic outlet syndrome. J Am Acad Orthop Surg 2:317, 1994

Leffert RD, Graham G: The relationship between dead arm syndrome and thoracic outlet syndrome. Clin Orthop 223:20, 1987

Michlovitz SL: Thermal Agents in Rehabilitation. 2nd Ed. FA Davis, Philadelphia, 1990

Novak CB: Physical therapy management of thoracic outlet syndrome in the musician. J Hand Surg April-June:74-79, 1992

Novak CB, Collins D, MacKinnon SE: Outcome following conservative management of thoracic outlet syndrome. J Hand Surg Am 20:542, 1995

Novak CB, MacKinnon SE, Brownlee R, Kelly L: Provocative sensory testing in carpal tunnel syndrome. J Hand Surg Br 17:204, 1992

Osterman AL: Double crush and multiple compression neuropathy. In Gelberman R (ed): Operative Nerve Repair and Reconstructions. JB Lippincott, Philadelphia, 1991, p. 1919

Roos D: Thoracic outlet syndrome: update 1987. Am J Surg 15:568, 1987

Roos DB: Thoracic outlet syndromes in musicians. J Hand Surg April-June:65-72, 1992

Schwartzman RJ: Neurologist's approach to brachial plexopathy. In Hunter JM, Mackin EJ, Callahan AD (eds): Rehabilitation of the Hand: Surgery and Therapy. 4th Ed. Mosby, St. Louis, 1995, p. 837

Sessions RT: Recurrent thoracic outlet syndrome: causes and treatment. South Med J 75:1453, 1982

Silliman JF: Neurovascular injuries to the shoulder complex. J Orthop Sports Phys Ther 18:442, 1993

Sommerich CM: Occupational risk factors associated with soft tissue disorders of the shoulder: a review of recent investigations in the literature. Ergonomics 36:697, 1993

Sucher BM: Thoracic outlet syndrome—a myofascial variant: Part 1. Pathology and diagnosis. J Am Osteopath Assoc 90:686-696, 703-704, 1990

Travell JG, Simmons DG: Myofascial Pain and Dysfunction: The Trigger Point Manual. Williams & Wilkins, Baltimore, 1983

Tyson RR, Kaplan GF: Modern concepts of diagnosis and treatment of the thoracic outlet syndrome. Orthop Clin North Am 6:507, 1975

Urschel HC, Razzuk MA: The failed operation for thoracic outlet syndrome: the difficulty of diagnosis and management. Ann Thorac Surg 42:523, 1986

Whitenack SH, Hunter JM, Jaeger SH, Read RL: Thoracic outlet syndrome complex: diagnosis and treatment. In Hunter JM, Schneider LIH, Mackin EJ, Callahan AD (eds): Rehabilitation of the Hand: Surgery and Therapy. 3rd Ed. Mosby, St. Louis, 1990, p. 530

Wood VE, Frykman GK: Winging of the scapula as a complication of first rib resection: a report of six cases. Clin Orthop 149:160, 1980

Wright IS: The neurovascular syndrome produced by hyperabduction of the arms. Am Heart J 29:1, 1945

Nerve Repair 10

Linda Luca

Peripheral nerves activate the intricately balanced muscles and transmit sensory stimuli in the upper extremity that enable hand function. With nerve loss, this balance is lost and permanent hand deformities can occur. Understanding the anatomy of the peripheral nervous system, nerve regeneration, and surgical techniques to repair lacerated nerves is vital for rehabilitation after nerve repair.

Peripheral nerves are made up of groups of fascicles that contain numerous axons and an enveloping myelin sheath. Fascicles are surrounded with a dense outer coating called the **epineurium**. The epineurium is the site of suture placement in epineural repair, which is the most commonly used repair for nerve reconstruction. Group fascicular repair, the second most common technique, involves tedious coaptation of individual groups of fascicles.[1] Recovery after nerve repair is least successful when a nerve is repaired under tension. Therefore, if a gap is present after nerve injury, nerve grafting may be necessary.

Therapy after any type of nerve repair is critical for restoration of hand function. Care should be taken to avoid stretching of the repaired nerve ends, because tension leads to scarring and may prevent the regenerating axons from achieving functional reinnervation.[1] As the nerve is regenerating, the focus of therapy should be to maintain or promote full mobility of all joints and soft tissue, to continue patient education, and to prevent hand deformities from occurring. As sensory and muscle reinnervation becomes evident, a motor retraining, desensitization, and sensory reeducation program should be initiated.

The following protocol is a guideline for treating patients with peripheral nerve interruption. Appendix 10-1 describes the effects of nerve lesions on motor function.

DEFINITION

Nerve repair consists of approximation of the ends of an injured nerve via direct repair or nerve graft or tube (Fig. 10-1).

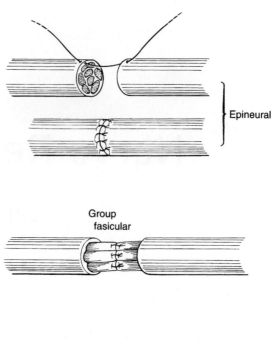

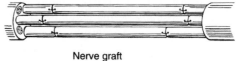

FIG. 10-1 Approximated ends of a lacerated nerve.

TREATMENT AND SURGICAL PURPOSE

To protect against damage and deformity within the defined territory of the injured nerve before its maximum recovery. The goal of surgery is to restore nerve continuity by direct repair or nerve grafting so that an optimum number of nerve fibers will reach their appropriate sensory and/or motor end organs. Modern nerve surgery includes use of nerve tubes to bridge nerve gaps. During the preoperative and postoperative periods, appropriate monitoring and therapy is required to optimize the final result. Patience on the part of both clinicians and patients is necessary because of the slow rate of nerve healing.

TREATMENT GOALS

   I. Maintain range of motion (ROM) of all upper extremity joints during nerve recovery period.
  II. Educate the patient.
III. Restore sensibility.
 IV. Minimize recovery time.
  V. Restore motor function.

VI. Maximize functional recovery. The expected rate of recovery for nerve repairs is 1 inch per month.[2]

VII. Provide appropriate preoperative care for delayed repairs or grafts. See later discussion for postoperative care with flexor tendon involvement.

OPERATIVE INDICATIONS AND PRECAUTIONS

I. Indications: severance of nerve

    A. Primary nerve repair: indicated for a clean, sharply cut nerve in which the damaged ends can be seen and approximated. This type of nerve repair is performed immediately after an injury or within 1 to 2 weeks.[3]

    B. Secondary nerve repair: usually indicated in the presence of a severely crushed or avulsed nerve. This surgery involves resection of the damaged segment of the nerve and removal of the neuroma at least 1 week after the injury.[3]

    C. Nerve grafts: usually performed when a direct repair cannot be done without tension or the nerve condition is poor. It is often done as a secondary procedure. Nerve tubes may also be used.

II. Precautions

    A. Fractures/dislocations

    B. Stretching of the nerve beyond its elastic limit

    C. Loss of sensation, which could cause secondary injury

POSTOPERATIVE THERAPY FOR PRIMARY OR SECONDARY REPAIR

Postoperative management of a nerve repair varies in the literature. "The exact tensile strength of nerve at various times during wound healing is not known."[4] According to Dagum,[4] axonal sprouts will have crossed the repair site at 3 weeks. In general, the time frame for immobilization after an isolated nerve repair varies in the literature from 2 to 4 weeks, followed by controlled ROM for 3 weeks. Millesi[5] says to begin "careful mobilization," following a nerve graft, after 8 days and gradually increase the motion over the following weeks, following the "rules that apply to any kind of nerve repair." Communication with the hand surgeon helps guide the postoperative care.

I. Ulnar and median nerve repairs at the wrist level

    A. 0 to 3 days: Rest hand in dressing with wrist flexed at 30 degrees. At postoperative day 3, remove dressings, examine wounds, and, after splint is made, educate patient on ROM of all uninvolved joints.[3]

    B. 3 to 7 days: Position hand in dorsal protection splint with wrist flexed at 30 degrees (Fig. 10-2). For lacerations within the proximal half of the forearm, the elbow is splinted in flexion also. Include a C-bar on the protection splint for median nerve injuries to prevent thumb adduction contracture and encourage active digital motion. Educate patient on insensate areas.

    C. 2 to 3 weeks: Remove sutures. Begin restricted ROM of involved joints. Begin friction massage on scar and encourage patient to perform this several times daily, gradually increasing intensity as tolerated. Apply a gel sheet or an elastomer mold to scar once wound is healed.

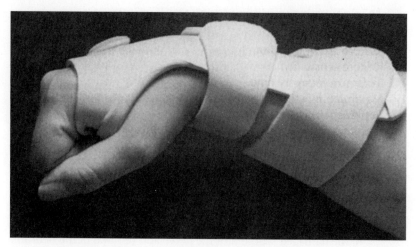

FIG. **10-2** Splinting for wrist-level lacerations of median or ulnar nerve.

D. 2 to 4 weeks: Progress ROM to active-assisted range of motion (AAROM) and then passive range of motion (PROM) if needed. This progression is dependent on the patient's progress. Some nerve repairs are protected for 4 weeks. If PROM is necessary, never perform aggressive stretching.[6] Also, adjust the splint weekly to increase extension of the wrist. The test to determine rate of extension splinting is to check for complaints of burning and tingling during gentle extension of the wrist. Once this has been determined, shape the splint before that point of extension. Continue to encourage patient protection of the insensate areas such as compensating visually when around heat or sharp objects and performing skin inspections for pressure areas. The hand should be kept warm in cold climates. When cooking, oven mitts and long-handled utensils should be used as well.

E. 4 weeks: Educate patient on the expected sensations that are associated with sensory return. They may be described as electrical, shocking, or moving sensations.[7] After the initial 3- to 4-week latency period, the nerve will begin to regenerate at approximately 1 to 3 mm/day.[6]

F. 5 weeks: Splint only at night and in crowds. Children need to be protected for about 1 week longer than adults. For ulnar nerve lesions, position the hand in a lumbrical block (antideformity) splint to wear during the day[8] (Fig. 10-3). For median nerve repair, if needed, the patient should wear a separate C-bar splint when not wearing a protective splint[7] (Fig. 10-4).

G. 6 weeks: Begin wrist extension with fingers extended. Evaluate sensibility. Begin sensory reeducation and desensitization program when appropriate (see Chapter 5).

H. 6 to 12 weeks: Motor retraining as appropriate. Once reinnervation is suspected, neuromuscular electrical stimulation (NMES) may be appropriate for proprioceptive feedback.[6] Functional activities and place-hold exercises are also very effective. Once muscle control has been gained, isotonic exercises are appropriate.

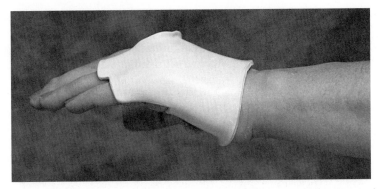

FIG. **10-3** An antideformity splint for an ulnar nerve injury. (From Coppard B, Lohman H: Introduction to Splinting. Mosby, St. Louis, 2001.)

  I. 7 to 8 weeks: Use dynamic splinting, if necessary, for joint tightness.
  J. 12 weeks to 1 year: Continue strengthening. A home exercise program should be well established and upgraded as appropriate. Continue sensory reeducation, progressing as appropriate. Reevaluate periodically.

II.   Radial nerve repair for forearm and above
  A. 0 to 3 days: Rest hand in dressing with wrist extended. At postoperative day 3, remove dressings, examine wound, and, after splint is in place, begin ROM on all uninvolved joints.
  B. 3 to 7 days: Position hand in forearm-based static wrist extension splint with dynamic extension outriggers for fingers and thumb.[8] If lesion is more proximal, the elbow should be immobilized. AROM of the digits in the splint is encouraged to prevent contractures. A prefabricated wrist cock-up splint may be adequate for nighttime wear, or a custom wrist cock-up splint with metacarpophalangeal (MCP) joint extension support may be more appropriate, leaving the dynamic splint for day wear.[6]
  C. 2 weeks: Remove sutures. Begin active and passive flexion and extension of interphalangeal (IP) joints, with MCP joints and

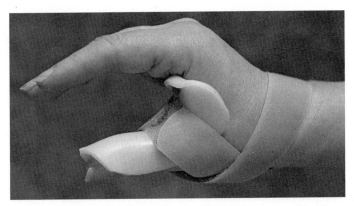

FIG. **10-4** A C-bar or web spacer splint for a median nerve injury. (From Coppard B, Lohman H: Introduction to Splinting. Mosby, St. Louis, 2001.)

wrist in extension. Begin restricted ROM of the wrist and elbow if applicable. Begin friction massage on scar, and encourage patient to perform this several times daily, gradually increasing intensity as tolerated. Apply a gel sheet or an elastomer mold to scar once wound is healed.

D. 2 to 5 weeks: Progress ROM of wrist and elbow to AAROM and then PROM, if needed, avoiding aggressive stretching. Educate patient on insensate areas, as noted earlier.

E. 6 to 12 weeks: Institute motor retraining as appropriate.

F. 7 weeks: Use dynamic splinting, if necessary, for tightness.

G. After 12 weeks: Depending on progress of the patient, begin advanced strengthening program and/or work rehabilitation.

PREOPERATIVE CARE FOR DELAYED PRIMARY REPAIR OR NERVE GRAFT

I.   Goals of therapy

A. Full PROM: Provide patient with home exercise program to be performed several times a day.

B. Minimal tendon adherence in the scar: Achieve through active movement and scar management techniques.

C. Promote good skin condition: Massage with cream several times a day.

D. Patient education to avoid injury from sharp objects, heat, pressure areas

1. Teach patient to compensate visually for loss of protective sensation.

2. Have patient wear warm gloves in winter.

3. Use long-handled cooking utensils.

POSTOPERATIVE THERAPY FOR NERVE GRAFTS

I.   Treatment

A. 0 to 9 days: Remove dressings, examine wound, and splint wrist in neutral position with elbow in slight flexion. Encourage ROM of all uninvolved joints. Begin patient education.

B. 10 to 14 days: Remove sutures, if needed. Begin restricted AROM of involved joints. Adjust splint weekly to accommodate for increased ROM. Begin scar management as tolerated.[8,9] Careful mobilization should increase over the following weeks, according to the usual rules of any nerve repair.[5]

C. 4 weeks: Expect an advancing Tinel's sign. Begin more progressive AROM and PROM.

D. 5 weeks: Treat as for a nerve repair (see earlier sections on nerve repair treatment).

POSTOPERATIVE CARE WITH FLEXOR TENDON INVOLVEMENT

Treatment recommendations in the literature are vague for combined tendon and nerve repairs. Chao and colleagues[10] found that some authors advise up to 3 weeks of immobilization. When treating a zone II combined tendon and nerve repair, Dagum[4] recommended following the same protocol as for an isolated zone II tendon laceration. As with a combined flexor tendon and median and ulnar nerve laceration, Dagum recommends following a protective passive mobilization protocol. The wrist is immobilized in 30 degrees flexion and the MCPs in 70 degrees flexion with PROM to the digits within the limits of the dorsal block splint.[4] Dagum's study with fresh cadavers supported use of the modified Duran mobilization protocol with combined digital nerve and tendon repairs. This study found that 100% of the 100 nerves repaired stayed intact with up to 5 mm of resection length. Early active motion of tendon repairs combined with digital nerve repairs should begin once the IP joints tolerate full extension with MCP joints at 60 degrees flexion.[11] The major postoperative complication in nerve repair with tendon involvement is flexor tightness of the wrist due to tendon adherence. To help overcome this complication, scar management techniques are emphasized. Also, finger flexion exercises should be stabilized and performed individually. If the nerve becomes adherent in scar, then the ability to extend the flexor tendons may be dependent on what the nerve can tolerate.[7]

POSTOPERATIVE COMPLICATIONS

    I. Severe edema
   II. Infection
  III. Neuromas
  IV. Secondary deformity
   V. Severe pain (if noted during ROM exercises, may indicate overstretching of the nerve)
  VI. Intraneural fibrosis
 VII. Hand burns or cuts due to loss of protective sensation

EVALUATION TIME LINE

    I. 0 to 3 days
       A. Wound condition
       B. ROM, uninvolved joints
   II. 5 to 7 days: Edema
  III. 2 to 4 weeks: ROM, involved joints
  IV. 6 to 8 weeks: Sensory
   V. 8 to 12 weeks: Manual muscle test
  VI. For sensory and manual muscle testing, reevaluate once every 6 to 8 weeks thereafter.

OUTCOMES

Establishment of anatomic motor and sensory reinnervation does not guarantee functional recovery.[4] Functional recovery can take up to 2 years, and improvement can occur from nerve injuries proximal to the wrist for up to 4 years. Table 10-1 shows that overall recovery of sensation varies but is likely to be excellent or good, although many of the studies had incomplete data.[12] Some generalities have been made: distal nerve injuries do better than proximal ones, younger patients do better than older patients, sensory or pure motor nerve repair does better than mixed nerve repair, and guillotine injury does better than a crush injury or an avulsion injury.[4]

TABLE **10-1** Compilation of Digital, Median, Ulnar, and Radial Nerve Repair Studies

Authors (ref. no.)	Year	n	Excellent S4 S2PD <6 mm	%	Good S3+/S3 S2PD 7-15 mm	%	Poor ≤S2 S2PD >15 mm	%
DIGITAL								
Sullivan (13)	1985	36	7	17	13	30	—	—
Goldie et al. (14)	1992	27	9	37	—	—	—	—
Efstathopoulos et al. (15)	1995	64	31	49	15	24	18	28
Wang et al. (16)	1996	74	36	49	—	—	—	—
MEDIAN AND ULNAR								
Mailander et al. (17)	1989	20	10	50	—	—	—	—
Hudson & deJager (18)	1993	15	2	13	2	13	9	60
Polatkan et al. (19)	1998	28	10	36	12	43	6	21
RADIAL								
Roganovic (20)	1996	100	—	85% were excellent or good	—	—	—	—

Data from Allan C: Hand Clin 16:67-72, 2000.

REFERENCES

1. Smith KL: Nerve response to injury and repair. In Hunter JM, Mackin EJ, Callahan AD (eds): Rehabilitation of the Hand: Surgery and Therapy. 4th Ed. Mosby, St. Louis, 1995, p. 609
2. Hopkins HL, Smith HD: Willard and Spackman's Occupational Therapy. 6th Ed. Lippincott-Raven, Philadelphia, 1983, p. 468
3. Dvali L, Mackinnon S: Nerve repair, grafting, and nerve transfers. Clin Plast Surg 30:203-221, 2003
4. Dagum AB: Peripheral nerve regeneration, repair, and grafting. J Hand Ther 11: 111-117, 1998
5. Millesi H: Techniques for nerve grafting. Hand Clin 16:73-91, 2000
6. Skirven T, Callahan A: Therapist's management of peripheral-nerve injuries. In Mackin EJ, Callahan AD, Skirven TM, et al. (eds): Hunter-Mackin-Callahan Rehabilitation of the Hand and Upper Extremity. 5th Ed. Mosby, St. Louis, 2002, p. 599
7. Bell Krotoski JA: Flexor tendon and peripheral nerve repair. Hand Surg 7:83-100, 2002
8. Wilgis EF: Nerve repair and grafting. In Green DP (ed): Operative Hand Surgery. 2nd Ed. Vol. 2. Churchill Livingstone, New York, 1988, p. 915
9. Omer GE, Spinner M: Management of Peripheral Nerve Problems. WB Saunders, Philadelphia, 1980
10. Chao RP, Braun SA, Ta KT, et al.: Early passive mobilization after digital nerve repair and grafting in a fresh cadaver. Plast Reconstr Surg 108:386-391, 2001
11. Brushart T: Nerve repair and grafting. In Green DP (ed): Operative Hand Surgery. 4th Ed. Vol. 2. Churchill Livingstone, New York, 1999, p. 1389
12. Allan C: Functional results of primary nerve repair. Hand Clin 16:67-72, 2000
13. Sullivan DJ: Results of digital neurorrhaphy in adults. J Hand Surg Br 10:41-44, 1985
14. Goldie BS, Coates CJ, Birch R: The long term result of digital nerve repair in no-man's land. J Hand Surg Br 17:75-77, 1992
15. Efstathopoulos D, Gerostathopoulos N, Misitzis D, et al.: Clinical assessment of primary digital nerve repair. Acta Orthop Scand Suppl 264:45-47, 1995
16. Wang WZ, Crain GM, Baylis W, et al.: Outcome of digital nerve injuries in adults. J Hand Surg Am 21:138-143, 1996
17. Mailander P, Berger A, Schaller E, et al.: Results of primary nerve repair in the upper extremity. Microsurgery 10:147-150, 1989

18. Hudson DA, de Jager LT: The spaghetti wrist: simultaneous laceration of the median and ulnar nerves with flexor tendons at the wrist. J Hand Surg Br 18:171-173, 1993
19. Polatkan S, Orhun E, Polatkan O, et al.: Evaluation of the improvement of sensibility after primary median nerve repair at the wrist. Microsurgery 18:192-196, 1998
20. Roganovic Z, Savic M, Petkovic S, et al.: Results of repair of severed nerves in war injuries [Serbian]. Vojnosanit Pregl 53:463-470, 1996

SUGGESTED READINGS

Arsham NZ: Nerve injury. In Ziegler EM (ed): Current Concepts in Orthotics: A Diagnosis-Related Approach to Splinting. Rolyan Medical Products, Chicago, 1984, p. iv

Boscheinen MJ, Davey V, Conolly WB: The Hand: Fundamentals of Therapy. Butterworth, Cambridge, 1985, p. 60

Lampe EW: Clinical Symposium: Surgical Anatomy of the Hand. New Jersey Pharmaceutical Division, CIBA-GEIGY Corporation, Summit, NJ, 1988, p. 10

MacKinnon SE, Dellon AL: Surgery of the Peripheral Nerve. Thieme Medical Publishers, New York, 1988

Sunderland S: Nerves and Nerve Injuries. 2nd Ed. Churchill Livingstone, New York, 1978

Tam AM: Nerves. In Kasch MC, Taylor-Mullins PA, Fullenwider L (eds): Hand Therapy Review Course Study Guide. Hand Therapy Certification Commission, Garner, NC, 1990, p. 12-1

Trombly CA: Occupational Therapy for Physical Dysfunction. 2nd Ed. Williams & Wilkins, Baltimore, 1983, p. 357

APPENDIX **10-1**

Effects of Nerve Lesion on Motor Function[6,7]

I.   High radial nerve lesion
  A. Wrist drop due to paralysis of wrist extensors
  B. Diminished abduction and extension of thumb due to paralysis of abductor pollicis longus (APL) and extensor pollicis brevis (EPB)
  C. Inability to extend metacarpophalangeal (MCP) joints due to paralysis of the long extensors
  D. Weak grasp and pinch due to inefficiency of the unopposed long flexors (shortened)
  E. Loss of sensation of the lateral two thirds of the dorsum of the hand and a portion of the thenar eminence area, as well as the dorsum of the proximal phalanges of the lateral three and one-half fingers
  F. Weakened supination due to paralysis of the supinator muscle
II. Posterior interosseus nerve: same effects as described earlier, except that sensation is not lost and wrist extension is present, although weakened
III. Ulnar nerve lesion at the wrist
  A. Loss of adduction and abduction of the fingers due to paralysis of interossei
  B. Hyperextension of fourth and fifth MCP joints with flexion of the interphalangeal (IP) joints due to unopposed action of the extensor digitorum communis (EDC)
  C. Weak thumb adduction due to paralysis of adductor pollicis (AdP)
  D. Loss of opposition of the fifth finger due to paralysis of the opponens digiti quinti
  E. Weak thumb opposition due to paralysis of the AdP
  F. Weak MCP flexion due to paralysis of the third and fourth lumbricals
  G. Weak pinch due to paralysis of the AdP, deep head of the flexor pollicis brevis (FPB), and the first dorsal interosseous
  H. Weak grasp due to paralysis of the interossei, the third and fourth lumbricals, and the flexor digitorum profundus (FDP) of the fourth and fifth fingers
  I. Sensory nerve loss of volar and dorsal aspects of the medial third of the hand, little finger, and ulnar half of the ring finger
IV. Ulnar nerve lesion in the proximal forearm involves these additional problems.
  A. Weak flexion of IP joints of fourth and fifth fingers due to paralysis of the ulnar half of the FDP
  B. Weak wrist flexion due to paralysis of the flexor carpi ulnaris (FCU)

 V. Median nerve (wrist level)
     A. Sensory loss of the central palm area and the palmar surfaces
        of the lateral three and one-half digits
     B. Weak MCP joint flexion of index and middle fingers due to
        paralysis of the first two lumbricals
     C. Weak pinch due to paralysis of opponens pollicis, abductor
        pollicis brevis (APB), and the superficial head of the FPB
     D. Loss of thumb palmar abduction due to paralysis of the APB
 VI. Anterior interosseous nerve (proximal one third of forearm)
     A. Loss of distal interphalangeal (DIP) joint flexion of the index and
        middle fingers due to paralysis of FDP to each of these digits
     B. Loss of thumb IP joint flexion due to paralysis of flexor pollicis
        longus (FPL)
     C. Weak forearm pronation due to paralysis of pronator quadratus
VII. Median nerve lesion in the proximal forearm
     A. Weak forearm pronation due to paralysis of pronator teres
     B. Weak wrist flexion due to paralysis of flexor carpi radialis (FCR)
     C. Weak finger flexion due to paralysis of flexor digitorum
        superficialis (FDS)

Desensitization and Reeducation

11

Rebecca N. Larson

The function of a healthy peripheral nerve is to provide sensory feedback through neural impulses to the peripheral nervous system. This sensory feedback is interpreted, and an appropriate motor response is generated. After a nerve lesion, the transmission of these impulses is disrupted. A nerve generates hundreds of feedback signals throughout the course of a single function. When the signal or impulse reaches the somatosensory cortex, it is matched with a memory profile stored in an "association" cortex. This profile is used to determine the characteristics of the stimulus and generate the appropriate response. If a profile cannot be identified, the altered profile may be ignored or misinterpreted and may illicit a painful or exaggerated response. Desensitization and reeducation can be initiated to reorganize residual sensory clues, helping the patient establish and respond to a new set of matching profiles.[1]

Desensitization and reeducation require a patient who is intelligent, motivated, and willing to participate in a daily home exercise program. The patient must also incorporate the hand into functional activities. In this way, through the use of higher cortical functions (attention, learning, and memory), a patient can learn to compensate for sensory deficits.[2]

The following treatment protocol is a guideline. There is no single technique that is documented to be superior. Although desensitization and reeducation cannot facilitate nerve regeneration, the ultimate goal is to allow the patient to reach his or her sensory potential and regain maximum function of the involved extremity.[3]

DEFINITION

I. **Desensitization:** the use of modalities and procedures to reduce the symptoms of hypersensitivity
II. **Dysesthesia:** a painful and persistent sensation induced by a gentle touch to the skin
III. **Allodynia:** Pain secondary to normally nonpainful stimuli

IV. **Hypersensitivity (hyperalgesia):** a condition of extreme discomfort or irritability in response to a normally non-noxious tactile stimulation.

V. **Sensory reeducation:** a method by which the patient learns to interpret the pattern of abnormal sensory impulses generated after an interruption in the peripheral nervous system

TREATMENT PURPOSE

After injury to peripheral nerves, the pattern of recovery is variable and seldom returns to normal. Only some sensory fibers reach their proper end organs. The territory of reinnervation therefore is incomplete. Feedback generated from this immature sensory area may be misleading or evoke a painful response. Sensory reeducation teaches the patient to recognize the altered sensory feedback to the brain and interpret the sensory stimulus.[3] Desensitization helps the patient build tolerance to and acceptance of stimulation to a hypersensitive area. This training may also prevent permanent pain pathways from forming within the central nervous system, thereby lessening the development of chronic pain disorders.[4,5]

TREATMENT GOALS

I. Desensitization
   A. Maximize patient's function by minimizing the painful response to touch in hypersensitive areas.
II. Sensory reeducation
   A. Achieve the highest sensory potential provided by nerve repair or other nerve recovery.
   B. Attain independence in activities of daily living (ADLs) and vocational pursuits through sensory and motor rehabilitation.

POSTINJURY INDICATIONS/PRECAUTIONS FOR THERAPY

I. Although surgical intervention is the most frequent antecedent to peripheral nerve disturbance, even minor injury can require desensitization and/or sensory reeducation (e.g., burn, frostbite, long-standing immobilization minimizing sensory input to the extremity). Although the mechanism of injury is often vastly different, the therapeutic intervention is similar.
II. Desensitization program: (Due to the variability of reactions to hypersensitivity, patients may need to undergo desensitization before the initiation of reeducation.)
   A. Indications
      1. Amputation
      2. Dysesthesia response to normally non-noxious stimuli
      3. Hypersensitive scar or surrounding area
      4. Neuroma (NOTE: Surgical excision is often required despite conservative treatment.)
   B. Precautions/Contraindications
      1. Active infection
      2. Diffuse/organic pain

   3. Open wounds
   4. Psychological aspect to pain
III.   Sensory reeducation program
   A. Indications
      1. Severely decreased sensibility as evidenced by inability to perceive potentially harmful stimuli (pinprick, deep pressure, hot/cold, repetitive low-grade friction).[2]
      2. Presence of protective sensibility with lack of discriminative sensation (i.e., localization, two-point discrimination, and tactile gnosis).[2]
   B. Precautions/Contraindications
      1. Hypersensitivity/hyperalgesia
      2. Joint stiffness
      3. Open wounds
      4. Severe edema

POSTOPERATIVE THERAPY (DESENSITIZATION)

   I.   Desensitization program development and implementation[6]: (Due to aversion response to stimulation, the hypersensitive area may require protection between desensitization treatments. Splinting, gel sheets, or scar molds may be indicated.)
   A. Complete a thorough evaluation, including sensibility, hypersensitivity, and pain, to establish a treatment baseline (see Chapter 5).
   B. Assess patient's tolerance to stimulation of hypersensitive area with texture, immersion particles and vibration (i.e., what is the most irritating stimulus the patient can tolerate?). The Three-Phase Hand Sensitivity Test is recommended[3] (Appendix 11-1).
   C. Instruct patient to organize stimuli in each category from least to most irritating.
   D. Begin desensitization of the hypersensitive area with a stimulus that is slightly irritating, but tolerable. Advance to the next stimulus when comfortable.
   E. End program when the most irritating stimulus is tolerated.
   F. Progress to sensory reeducation program (if not already implemented) and ADL simulation as appropriate.
   II.   Suggested techniques
   A. Texture (see Appendix 11-1)
      1. Use graded textures to stroke and tap the hypersensitive area.
      2. Suggested guideline for progression: cotton, lamb's wool, felt, orthopedic felt (1/8 inch), orthopedic felt (1/4 inch), terry cloth towel, Velcro loops, Velcro hooks or fine grades of sandpaper.
   B. Immersion particles (see Appendix 11-1)
      1. Immerse hand into particle media for bombardment of sensory input.
      2. Suggested particle media: cotton, Styrofoam pieces, sand, beans, popcorn, rice, and macaroni (Fig. 11-1).
   C. Vibration (see Appendix 11-1)
      1. Stimulate hypersensitive area with tuning fork and/or battery- or electric-powered vibrator. Vary attachment shape and speed of vibration as tolerated (Fig. 11-2).

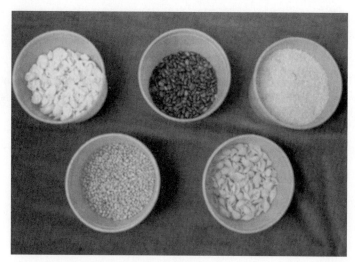

FIG. **11-1** Examples of particle media.

2. Progress from stimulation at periphery of hypersensitive area, to intermittent stimulation of actual area, to continuous contact with actual area.

D. Maintained pressure
   1. Apply continuous mild pressure with an Isotoner glove, gel sheet, or elastomer mold to increase comfort.
   2. Progress treatment using varying degrees of pressure over area, including weight-bearing pressure as patient tolerates.

E. Physical agent modalities[7]
   1. Transcutaneous electrical nerve stimulator (TENS): Frame point of hypersensitivity with electrodes to modulate pain

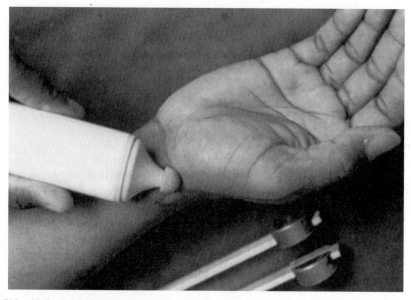

FIG. **11-2** Graded vibration can range from tuning fork to battery- or electric-powered vibrators.

at the spinal cord and endorphin-release level. Determine intensity of setting and frequency according to patient's report of pain response and desired outcome for treatment. Guidelines for application:

    a. Conventional/high rate (100 to 150 pulses per second [pps]): pain controlled only during application; safe for 24-hour use[7]

    b. Acupuncture/low rate (2 to 10 pps): pain controlled for 4 to 5 hours after application; used for a maximum of 30 minutes[7]

    c. Burst mode (10 pps): pain controlled for an unspecified time after application; often better tolerated than acupuncture/low rate[7]

2. Ultrasound: Apply directly over hypersensitive or surrounding area (as tolerated) to increase tissue extensibility, stimulate thermal receptors, change nerve conduction patterns, and alter transmission/perception of pain. Intensity and frequency depend on tissue depth.[7]

3. Fluidotherapy: Submerse extremity to "bombard" nerves with sensory stimulation and increase tissue extensibility.[4]

F. Therapeutic activities to regain confidence and restore function

    1. Initiate exercises for strengthening.

    2. Progress to ADLs and work simulation.

G. Additional modalities to decrease hypersensitivity: massage, paraffin and moist heat for relaxation.

H. Stimuli that may magnify pain symptoms and should be avoided in early desensitization include exposure to cold, emotional stress, and local irritants.[4]

III. Home program

A. Perform activity in 10- to 15-minute increments, four to five times daily in a quiet environment.[5]

B. Educate patient to discontinue activity if stimulation becomes too noxious or if fatigue is reached.[5]

C. Incorporate exercises into functional activity and use of the extremity as soon as it is safe and tolerable to do so.

POSTOPERATIVE THERAPY (SENSORY REEDUCATION)

I. Considerations in sensory reeducation program design

A. It is never too late to begin sensory reeducation. Early initiation of retraining exercises is recommended to lessen likelihood of development of hypersensitivity.

B. Educate patient on frequent inspection of skin in addition to protection of the insensate hand.[2]

C. Activities should be simple and able to be performed independently; they should accommodate limitations in manual dexterity or motion (e.g., seat objects in putty)[8] (Fig. 11-3).

D. The patient should not stimulate the involved hand directly with the uninvolved hand, because two sets of sensory information will be received.[1]

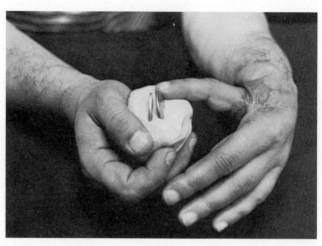

FIG. **11-3** Object seated in putty to accommodate decreased manipulation. (From Callahan AD: Methods of compensation and reeducation for sensory dysfunction. In Hunter JM, Mackin EJ, Callahan AD [eds]: Rehabilitation of the Hand: Surgery and Therapy. 4th Ed. St. Louis, Mosby, 1995.)

    E. Place emphasis on the fingertips, because they are most discriminative for ADL function.[2]

    F. Consider Dellon's recognized pattern of sensory return in program progression: pain, 30 cps vibration, moving touch, constant touch, and 256 cps vibration.[1] Use caution not to progress patient too quickly, to avoid feelings of frustration over failure.

    G. Be aware of progress plateau. When patient enters chronic phase of sensory loss, educate in strategies of compensation and adaptation.

  II.   Sensory reeducation program development and implementation

    A. Complete a thorough evaluation, including sensibility, hypersensitivity, and pain, to establish a treatment baseline (see Chapter 5).

    B. Begin reeducation within the appropriate phase to accommodate patient's sensory needs.

    C. Progress to complex tasks (combining sensory and motor components), ADL simulation, and vocational tasks as appropriate.

  III. Early-phase reeducation: Begin when 30 cps vibration and/or moving touch sensation has returned to an area, or when protective sensation is present and there is return of touch perception to the fingertips, within the range of 4.31 or lower as measured by the Semmes–Weinstein monofilaments.[2]

    A. Phase goal: Reeducate specific perceptions (e.g., movement versus constant touch) and correct inaccurate localization (in which the stimulus is perceived in reference to the site of stimulation).[2]

    B. Suggested techniques[2,3]

      1. With patient observing, perform initial stimulus (moving or constant touch) with eraser tip (Fig. 11-4).

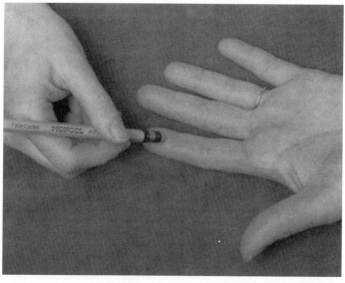

FIG. 11-4 Blunt surface used for early-phase sensory reeducation.

2. Repeat stimulus with patient's vision occluded; instruct patient to concentrate on what he or she is perceiving to match what was just observed.

3. Apply third stimulus with patient observing; advise patient to verbalize the perception (e.g., "I feel something moving up my index finger into my palm").[1]

4. If patient's response is incorrect, repeat process.

5. As perception improves, progress through each submodality (moving touch, constant touch, and 256 cps vibration) and include touch localization in poststimulus recognition ("Point to the area that was just touched").

C. Evaluate progress with accuracy of response, mapping of localization, Semmes–Weinstein monofilaments, static and two-point discrimination, and/or vibration testing (preferably vibrometer).

IV. Late-phase reeducation: Begin when moving and constant touch and/or 256 cps vibration is perceived at the fingertips with good localization (no later than when recovery reaches the proximal phalanx).[2,3]

A. Late-phase goal: Guide recovery of tactile gnosis or object recognition[2]

B. Suggested techniques

1. Sequence of stimuli/object introduction is similar to that in early-phase reeducation. The stimulus is manipulated by the patient, first with eyes open, then eyes shut with concentration of perception, and finally with eyes open (with verbalization of specific features detected) for reinforcement.

2. Grade exercises, beginning with the discrimination of larger objects, using objects with greater differences in size, shape, weight, temperature, and texture. Progress to more subtle differences (Fig. 11-5).

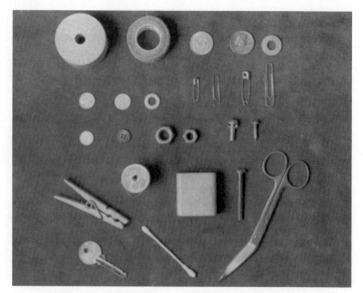

FIG. **11-5** Graded object discrimination to recover tactile gnosis.

3. Progress to function- and vocation-specific object recognition and manipulation.
C. Evaluate progress with accuracy and time of response and moving and/or static two-point discrimination.
V. Five-stage reeducation: Although the sensory reeducation strategies already described are more widely recognized, Nakada and Uchida[8] have developed a program specific to both sensory and motor function. The program uses residual proximal vibration and muscle tension senses to reeducate hands with sensory loss. Because no entry level criteria exist, five-stage reeducation can begin immediately.[8]
A. Suggested techniques
   1. Complete tasks with repetition.
   2. Correct failed responses with eyes open and closed.
   3. Progress as mastery is gained in each stage.
B. Stage 1: Feature detection and recognition of objects[8]
   1. Principle: Visual, tactile, and kinesthetic perception are used to scan an object during manipulation. When sensibility is impaired, a disruption occurs in the interaction between tactile and joint sensibility, making object recognition difficult. Proprioceptive input during joint movement can be used to establish certain characteristics of an object.
   2. Example task
      a. Cover tops of five Styrofoam cups with Coban, Dycem, theraband, moleskin, and hook Velcro. With vision occluded, ask the patient to identify characteristics of each cover (e.g., flexibility, rigidity, roughness).
      b. During exploration, encourage patient to use motor function (e.g., pressure, contour following) to combine joint and skin receptors for increased learning and recall.

(Moving touch recovers faster than constant touch; therefore, horizontal movement during object exploration is often preferred.)

c. As feature detection improves, progress to more subtle differences.

C. Stage 2: Correction of prehension patterns[8]

1. Principle: A pattern of prehension depends on the ability of the hand to detect the characteristics and contour of an object. This input is gathered by receptive fields of neurons along the hands and fingers. In normal function, the hand precisely fits an object. When sensibility is impaired, appropriate prehension is difficult to achieve due to poor input from the neuron fields.

2. Example task:

a. Cover ends of five clothespins with felt, hook/loop Velcro, sandpaper, and foam (texture will increase relevant receptors on sensory surfaces). Ask patient to open and close pins to practice prehension patterns.

b. As skill improves, progress to picking up objects with clothespins of varying size and weight (e.g., marbles, pegs, objects seated in putty).

D. Stage 3: Control of grasping force[8]

1. Principle: Control of grasp force is achieved through an intricate balance of motor control. This control is critical in ADL function to allow manipulation and dexterous handling of objects without dropping or crushing them.

2. Example task:

a. Cover a small cone with putty. Ask patient to grasp and release the cone and watch putty response to assess force of contact (with appropriate force, a minimal hand imprint should remain).

b. As skill improves in simple grasp and release, ask patient to progress to more skillful object handling (e.g., rotate cone in hand) with continued focus on material response.

E. Stage 4: Maintenance of grip force during proximal joint movement[8]

1. Principle: During functional activity, a patient must monitor and adapt grip force while executing movement at the proximal joints. When sensibility is impaired, this adaptation is altered, and objects are commonly dropped during multijoint motions.

2. Example task:

a. Using a Styrofoam cup, ask patient to maintain grasp and practice a single-joint movement (e.g., flex/extend wrist). Watch that cup is not dropped or showing signs of stress.

b. As skill improves, progress from single to multijoint movements (e.g., hold cup→flex/extend wrist while holding cup→without dropping cup, bring cup to mouth).

F. Stage 5: Manipulation of objects[8]

1. Principle: Skillful manipulation requires an equal balance of fine sensory and motor functions. Skills from each stage

are combined to achieve purposeful manipulation. With sensory loss, visual feedback is required to coordinate muscle contraction and maintain long sequences of motor actions to successfully manipulate objects.

   2. Example task:

     a. Combine all previous stages and activities in purposeful, work-specific tasks (Fig. 11-6).

VI. Additional techniques of reeducation

   A. Graphesthesia: Trace a number, letter, or geometric figure on involved area and ask patient to identify it.[2]

   B. Games: Ask patient to trace Velcro figures, string maze, or Braille letters with involved fingertip.

   C. Ask patient to pick out and identify an object in a bowl of sand, rice, or beans with vision occluded (Fig. 11-7).

   D. Include work-specific activities to practice sensory grips and prepare for return to work.

VII. Home program

   A. Program to be implemented with same frequency, duration, and protocol as for desensitization.

POSTOPERATIVE COMPLICATIONS

I. Complications that may require desensitization[2,3]

   A. Nerve regeneration without an intact endoneural tube.

   B. Scar formation of regenerating axons with or without constriction.

   C. Neuroma formation.

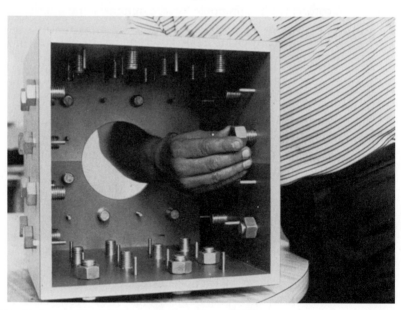

FIG. **11-6** Example of skillful manipulation in work-specific activity. (From Callahan AD: Methods of compensation and reeducation for sensory dysfunction. In Hunter JM, Mackin EJ, Callahan AD [eds]: Rehabilitation of the Hand: Surgery and Therapy. 4th Ed. St. Louis, Mosby, 1995.)

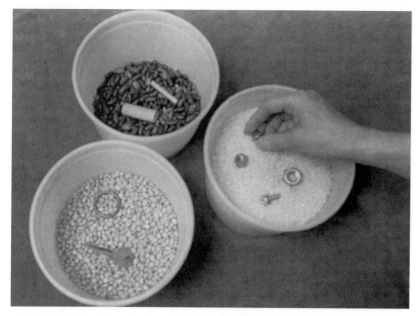

FIG. 11-7 Objects immersed in particle media for practice of prehension patterns.

   D. Adherence of nerve to its bed
   E. Constriction of blood flow causing ischemic pain
II. Complications that may require sensory reeducation
   A. Axons regenerate to an irreversibly degenerated end
      organ.
   B. Axon arrive at correct digital area but reinnervate the wrong
      end organ.
   C. Axons never reenter distal endoneurial sheath.
   D. Axons are misdirected to the wrong finger.

EVALUATION TIMELINE

Initially, the patient should be seen two to three times a week for treatment, assessment, and home program review. Gradually decrease the frequency of visits as the patient feels comfortable with the home program and shows improvement. If desensitization was required before sensory reeducation, progress the patient as tolerated into a program that combines both concepts. A thorough reevaluation should be completed once a month until discharge.

OUTCOMES

The concepts of desensitization and sensory reeducation after peripheral nerve injury are not new. As early as the 1600s, documentation exists of primitive forms of treatment for stump pain after amputation, including massage and percussion with various media.[4] Although no one technique is universally recognized to be superior, desensitization and sensory reeducation programs have become far more standardized since that time. Despite the long-standing existence of such programs, research continues to not only justify but also improve on current treatment strategies.

Imai and associates[9] conducted a controlled study of patients recovering from median nerve repair at the wrist. The reeducation group received sensory reeducation and was reevaluated between 1 and 2 years after repair. The repair group was retrospectively evaluated between 1 and 16 years after repair. Findings of statistical significance included decreased development of functionally limiting postoperative paresthesias ($P < 0.01$), improved two-point discrimination testing ($P < 0.0002$), and improved overall sensibility, as evidenced by increased object recognition ($P < 0.005$).[9,10]

Wei and Ma[11] evaluated the effect of delayed sensory reeducation on 13 patients with a total of 22 toe-to-hand transfers. Using Dellon's recommended protocol, reeducation was initiated at a mean of 38 months after transfer. Patients were monitored at monthly intervals for 3.3 months before the final sensibility measurement. Statistically significant findings included improvements in both static (7 mm average) and moving (6 mm average) two-point discrimination ($P < 0.0001$).[10,11]

Nakada and Uchida[8] developed a five-stage sensory reeducation program based on the neurophysiological findings of Iwamura and the work of Parry, Dellon, Callahan, Carter-Wilson, and Dannenbaum. The foundation of this program is based on restoration of hand function through sensory and motor reeducation. The effectiveness of this protocol was demonstrated in a case study of a 61-year-old woman with a long-standing history of leprosy. During an active phase of the disease process, she was diagnosed with neuritis in her left upper extremity which resulted in severe median, ulnar, and radial nerve loss. Despite routine rehabilitation for peripheral nerve damage, there were few functional gains. The five-stage sensory reeducation program was initiated 18 months after the diagnosis of neuritis was made. After 5 months of participation, the patient had improved in object recognition, body image, and functional use of the involved hand. No objective test results were provided.[8]

Moberg[5] stated, "Without sensation, the hand is blind." Poor sensibility is a severe functional hindrance; however, through the skillful development of desensitization and reeducation programs, patients recovering from peripheral nerve injuries can reach their full sensory potential and maximize their function.

REFERENCES

1. Dellon AL: Evaluation of Sensibility and Re-education of Sensation in the Hand. Williams & Wilkins, Baltimore, 1981
2. Callahan AD: Methods of compensation and reeducation for sensory dysfunction. In Hunter JM, Mackin EJ, Callahan AD (eds): Rehabilitation of the Hand: Surgery and Therapy. 4th Ed. Mosby, St. Louis, 1995
3. Dellon AL, Jabaley ME: Reeducation of sensation in the hand following nerve suture. Clin Orthop 163:75, 1982
4. Waylett-Rendall J: Desensitization of the traumatized hand. In Hunter JM, Mackin EJ, Callahan AD (eds): Rehabilitation of the Hand: Surgery and Therapy. 4th Ed. Mosby, St. Louis, 1995
5. Shieh SJ, Chiu HY, Lee JW, et al.: Evaluation of the effectiveness of sensory reeducation following digital replantation and revascularization. Microsurgery 16:578, 1995
6. Skirven TM, Callahan AD: Therapist's management of peripheral nerve injuries. In Mackin EJ, Callahan AD, Skirven TM, et al. (eds): Hunter-Mackin-Callahan Rehabilitation of the Hand and Upper Extremity. 5th Ed. Mosby, St. Louis, 2002
7. Cameron MH: Physical Agents in Rehabilitation from Research to Practice. WB Saunders, St. Louis, 2003
8. Nakada M, Uchida H: Case study of a five-stage sensory reeducation program. J Hand Ther 10:232, 1997

9. Imai H, Tajima T, Natsumi Y: Successful reeducation of functional sensibility after median nerve repair at the wrist. J Hand Surg Am 16:60, 1991

10. Fess EE: Sensory reeducation. In Mackin EJ, Callahan AD, Skirven TM, et al. (eds): Hunter-Mackin-Callahan Rehabilitation of the Hand and Upper Extremity. 5th Ed. Mosby, St. Louis, 2002

11. Wei FC, Ma HS: Delayed sensory reeducation after toe-to-hand transfer. Microsurgery 16:583, 1995

SUGGESTED READINGS

Anthony M: Sensory re-education. Adv Phys Ther 5:19, 1994

Brunelli G, Battiston B, Dellon AL: Gnostic rings: usefulness in sensibility evaluation and sensory reeducation. J Reconstr Microsurg 8:31, 1992

Callahan AD: Methods of compensation and reeducation for sensory dysfunction. In Hunter JM, Mackin EJ, Callahan AD (eds): Rehabilitation of the Hand: Surgery and Therapy. 3rd Ed. Mosby, St. Louis, 1990

Dannenbaum RM, Jones LA: The assessment and treatment of patients who have sensory loss following cortical lesions. J Hand Ther 6:130, 1993

Davis RW: Phantom sensation, phantom pain, and stump pain. Arch Phys Med Rehabil 74:79, 1993

Dellon AL: Techniques of sensory re-education. In Dellon AL: Somatosensory Testing and Rehabilitation. American Occupational Therapy Association, Silver Spring, MD, 1996

Hardy MA, Moran CA, Merritt WH: Desensitization of the traumatized hand. Va Med 109:134, 1982

Merzenich MM, Jenkins WM: Reorganization of cortical representations of the hand following alterations of skin inputs induced by nerve injury, skin island transfers and experience. J Hand Ther 6:89, 1993

Nakada M: Localization of a constant-touch and moving touch stimulus in the hand: a preliminary study. J Hand Ther 6:23, 1993

Shieh SJ, Chiu HY, Hsu HY: Long-term effects of sensory reeducation following digital replantation and revascularization. Microsurgery 18:334, 1998

Waylett-Rendall J: Sensibility evaluation and rehabilitation. Orthop Clin North Am 19:43, 1988

Waylett-Rendall J: Sequence of sensory recovery: a retrospective study. J Hand Ther 2:4, 1989

APPENDIX **11-1**

THREE-PHASE DESENSITIZATION RECORD FORM

1 NAME _John Doe_ _____ AGE _25_ SEX _M_ ___

2 DIAGNOSIS _Median Nerve Laceration (Partial)_ _____

3 SOURCE OF PAIN: AMPUTATION ____ SCAR ____ CRUSH ____ NEUROMA ____ BURN ____ OTHER _See above_ ___

4 DESCRIPTION OF PAINFUL AREA: INITIAL: _3/7/95_ _____

5   DISCHARGE: _____

6 DOMINANCE: RIGHT _X_ LEFT _____

7 HOW INJURY OCCURRED _____

8 DATE OF INJURY _12/5/94_ ____ DATE OF SURGERY _12/7/94_ ____ DATE OF 1ST RX: _12/30/94_

9 NO. OF WEEKS FROM D.O.I. OR SURGERY TO 1ST DESEN. RX: _3 weeks_ _____

10 NO. OF WEEKS BETWEEN 1ST AND LAST RX: _____ NO. OF TREATMENTS _____ REFERRING M.D. _____

11	DOWEL TEXTURES			CONTACT PARTICLES			VIBRATION	
12	LEVEL A	DATE BEGUN/COMMENTS		LEVEL B	DATE BEGUN/COMMENTS		LEVEL	DATE BEGUN/COMMENTS
13	1	1	12/30/94	1	3	12/30 tolerated	1	1/5/95
14	2	2	"	2	2	1/17/95 "	2	
15	3	3	"	3	1		3	
16	4	4	"	4	4		4	
17	5	5	"	5	5		5	
18	6			6	6		6	
19	7			7	8		7	
20	8			8	9		8	
21	9			9	7		9	
22	10			10	10		10	

(Form © LMB Hand Rehab Products, Inc.)

THREE-PHASE DESENSITIZATION TREATMENT PROTOCOL

Dowel Textures

1. Moleskin
2. Felt
3. Quickstick
4. Velvet
5. Semirough cloth
6. Velcro loops
7. Hard T-foam
8. Burlap
9. Rug back
10. Velcro hook

Contact Particles

1. Cotton
2. Terry cloth pieces
3. Dry rice
4. Unpopped popcorn
5. Pinto beans
6. Macaroni
7. Plastic wire insulation pieces
8. Small pebbles
9. Larger pebbles
10. Plastic squares

Vibration

1. Battery/no contact
2. Battery/near contact
3. Low cycle/near contact
4. Low cycle/intermittent contact
5. Low cycle contact
6. Low cycle continuous
7. High cycle/intermittent
8. High cycle/intermittent
9. High cycle/continuous
10. Vibration, not irritating

From Waylett-Rendall J: Desensitization of the traumatized hand. In Hunter JM, Mackin EJ, Callahan AD (eds): Rehabilitation of the Hand: Surgery and Therapy. 4th Ed. Mosby, St. Louis, 1995, with permission.

Tendon Transfers for Median Nerve Palsy 12

Michele A. Klein

Injury to the median nerve after trauma or long-standing carpal tunnel syndrome results in significant functional deficits for a patient. With low lesions, the major motor deficit is a loss of functional opposition, resulting in a loss of dexterity and difficulty with palmar grasp. With high median nerve injury, the most significant functional deficits are a result of denervation of the flexor pollicis longus (FPL) and of the flexor digitorum profundus (FDP) of the index finger (IF), and possibly of the middle finger. Patients also will have denervation of the radial two lumbricals and possibly of the flexor carpi radialis (FCR) and palmaris longus (PL); however, clinically and functionally these losses are not as significant.[1]

The functional deficits and severity of the loss of opposition are variable. However, with profound dysfunction and if it is evident that reinnervation is unlikely, patients may decide to undergo a tendon transfer to regain function.

Tendon transfers transmit the muscle power of one muscle to another by moving the tendon insertion from the original muscle to that of the denervated muscle. A wide range of transfers using different muscles for low- and high-level median nerve damage are used to restore functional opposition and pinch.

Success of tendon transfers requires a skilled and knowledgeable surgeon, a motivated and compliant patient, and a tenacious and dedicated therapist. Generally, the research indicates that success after tendon transfers is common; complications and failures are rare. Nevertheless, there are many things that can and should be done to enhance the outcome of the surgical procedure.

Careful planning and detailed preoperative evaluations must be completed. The patient should have a full understanding of what to expect in therapy and what is a realistic outcome. The therapist should be in close communication with the surgeon and may be helpful in deciding possible donor muscles and together determining the postoperative plan. For postoperative care, it is extremely helpful for the therapist to be present in the operating room.[2]

The results of tendon transfers can be enhanced in a number of ways. Arthrodesis or capsulodesis may be necessary if a transfer crosses several joints, if a joint is very unstable, or in combined nerve injuries. This allows the force to be transmitted across the newly stable joint to the joints at which the motion is desired. With a combined nerve injury, a tenodesis transfer may be necessary.[3]

DEFINITION

Tendon transfer is the transfer of an innervated muscle's power to a denervated or weaker muscle by way of transfer of its tendinous insertion.

SURGICAL PURPOSE

The goal of tendon transfer procedures is to restore balance and function to a hand that has been compromised through the loss of a muscle or group of muscles or irreplaceable loss of nerve innervation. This may occur through prolonged compression as in carpal tunnel syndrome, trauma, disease, infectious process, congenital anomalies, or spastic paralysis.[4-6]

This chapter addresses the most common transfer procedures indicated with an injury to the median nerve and the corresponding treatment techniques. The transfers that are covered in this chapter are for restoration of opposition/abduction (abductor pollicis brevis [APB]) and pinch (FPL). There are many exceptions to these guidelines, given the surgeon, therapist, patient, mechanism of injury, tissue integrity, comorbidities, and sociocultural and economic variables. Close communication with the surgeon is invaluable.

TREATMENT GOALS

I.   Preoperative goals
   A. Achieving and maintaining full passive range of motion (PROM) and active range of motion (AROM) if possible. It is not appropriate to address joint stiffness or contracture after the transfer procedure.[2,5]
   B. Achieving maximum strength of the donor muscle and antagonist muscles
   C. Maintaining supple, soft tissue by minimizing scar, edema, and adhesions and resolving intrinsic/extrinsic muscle tightness. Any scar tissue will increase drag on the transfer.[3-5] Use gel, elastomer molds, kinesiotape, and so on.
   D. Complete comprehensive evaluation, including sensory testing, functional assessments, ROM measurements, strength testing, and photographs for postoperative comparison
   E. Educate the patient about the therapy process, splinting demands, and realistic postoperative expectations.
   F. Establish good communication with the surgeon, schedule postoperative therapy, and arrange to observe the surgery, if possible. Review operative report when available.
II. Postoperative goals
   A. Protect transferred tendon.

B. Maintain ROM of uninvolved joints and involved joints as able.[1,3,4,7,8]

C. Control postoperative edema and pain.

D. Control scar tissue (skin and subcutaneous) and prevent adhesions to decrease drag on transfer.[3]

E. Progress patient to functional use of hand.

POSTOPERATIVE INDICATIONS/PRECAUTIONS FOR THERAPY

I. Indications

A. Surgical tendon transfers

II. Precautions

A. Acceptance of less than full PROM before transfer[6]

B. Overestimation of donor muscle strength[6]

C. "Drag" along transfer route secondary to scar[3]

D. Technical failures (e.g., rupture of juncture, too loose or too tight)

E. Be mindful of stretching out transfer. Wait until 6 weeks after surgery before addressing tightness of transfer. (Keep in mind the phases of wound healing.) (See Chapter 1.)

POSTOPERATIVE THERAPY: LOW MEDIAN NERVE INJURY

Opponensplasty

I. Postoperative day 10 to 14: Remove postoperative cast, have tension checked by surgeon, and immobilize patient in splint. Address wound care, edema reduction, and scar management if indicated.

A. FDS of ring finger (RF) or PL to APB (Camitz): long opponens splint (Figs. 12-1 and 12-2)

1. Wrist in 20 degrees flexion

2. Thumb in maximum palmar abduction under IF

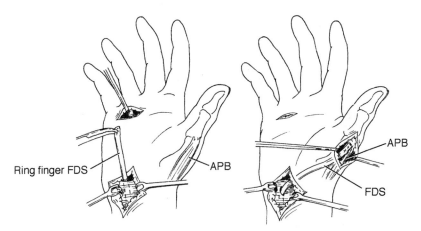

FIG. 12-1 Flexor digitorum superficialis *(FDS)* of ring finger to abductor pollicis brevis *(APB)*. The FDS of the ring finger is routed subcutaneously to the APB for opposition. (From Trumble T: Principles of Hand Surgery and Therapy. Saunders, St. Louis, 2001.)

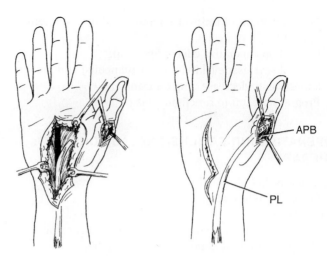

FIG. **12-2** Palmaris longus *(PL)* transfer to the abductor pollicis brevis *(APB)*—
Camitz transfer. The PL is routed subcutaneously to the tendon of the APB. (From
Trumble T: Principles of Hand Surgery and Therapy. Saunders, St. Louis, 2000.)

B. Extensor indicis proprius (EIP) to APB: long opponens splint
   (Fig. 12-3)
   1. Wrist in neutral to flexion/extension (depending on route
      of transfer)
   2. Thumb in maximum palmar abduction under IF
C. Abductor digiti minimi (ADM) to APB (Huber):
   hand-based or long opponens (Fig. 12-4)
   1. Wrist position insignificant
   2. Thumb in maximum palmar abduction under IF
II.   Week 3: Begin AROM of thumb in splint to activate transfer,
      six to eight times per day[9]

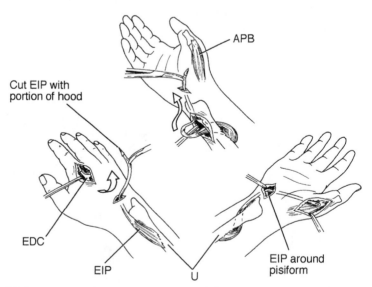

FIG. **12-3** Extensor indicis proprius *(EIP)* to abductor pollicis brevis *(APB)*. The EIP
is harvested and routed around the ulnar border of the forearm. Using the pisiform
as a pulley, the EIP tendon is then routed to the ABP insertion. (From Trumble T:
Principles of Hand Surgery and Therapy. Saunders, St. Louis, 2000.)

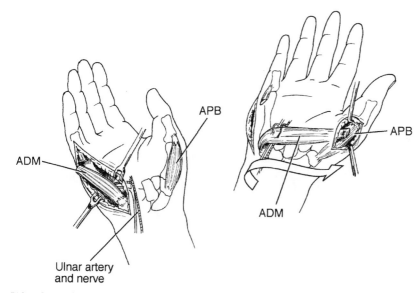

FIG. **12-4** Abductor digitorum minimus (ADM) to abductor pollicis brevis (APB)—Huber transfer. The ADM is rotated across the palm and inserted into the APB tendon. (From Trumble T: Principles of Hand Surgery and Therapy. Saunders, St. Louis, 2000.)

III. Week 4: Begin AROM of thumb and other joints out of splint. Focus on activation of transfer. May use light grasp and prehension tasks.

IV. Week 6: Discharge splint for protection and begin unrestricted A/PROM. May introduce light resistance.[7,10,11]

V. Week 8: Progressive resistive exercises. Preferably the patient should complete frequent low-resistance exercise sessions rather than occasional higher-resistive exercises. It is important not to fatigue the transfer.[11]

VI. Week 12: Resume unrestricted activities.

POSTOPERATIVE THERAPY: HIGH MEDIAN NERVE INJURY

Flexor Pollicis Longus

I. Postoperative day 10 to 14: Remove postoperative dressing; have surgeon check the tension of transfer. Splint for immobilization. Address wound care, edema reduction, and scar management if possible.

A. Brachioradialis/FDS to FPL: dorsal blocking splint (possibly long arm splint with elbow in 90 degrees flexion for brachioradialis) (Fig. 12-5)

1. Wrist in 20 degrees flexion
2. Thumb metacarpophalangeal (MCP) joint in 20 degrees flexion, interphalangeal (IP) joint in 20 degrees flexion, and carpometacarpal (CMC) joint in full palmar abduction

II. Week 3: AROM of MCP/IP within splint to activate transfer, six to eight times per day[9]

III. Week 4: AROM out of splint for transfer activation and light prehension

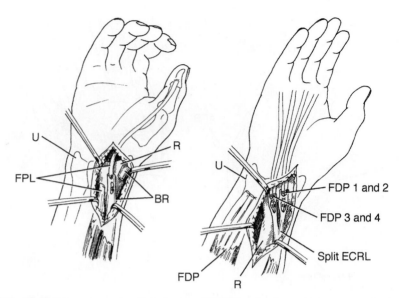

FIG. **12-5** Extensor carpi radialis longus (ECRL) to the flexor digitorum profundus (FDP). For high median nerve injury (or combined median/ulnar nerve injuries), the ECRL tendon is harvested, routed radially and volarly, and woven through the four FDP tendons. *BR,* Brachioradialis; *R,* radius; *U,* ulna. (From Trumble T: Principles of Hand Surgery and Therapy. Saunders, St. Louis, 2000.)

IV.   Week 6: Discharge splint; PROM and splinting to decrease tightness if present

V.   Weeks 7 to 8: Progressive resistive exercises

POSTOPERATIVE COMPLICATIONS

I.   Scarring of tendon to surrounding structures, particularly at sites of pulleys

II.   20% of patients will have an extension lag at IF with EIP-to-APB transfer[12]

III.   Palmar abduction is used to position thumb; true opposition/pronation is not always achieved[12,13]

IV.   Difficulty activating transfer. May need to use neuromuscular electrical stimulation (NMES) or biofeedback to assist patient in activation of transfer.

V.   Transfer too loose or too tight. Wait 6 weeks before doing any PROM or splinting against transfer.

VI.   Rupture

EVALUATION TIMELINE

I.   Postoperative day 10 to 14 (after tension has been checked by surgeon)
    A. Control of edema and pain, wound care
    B. ROM of uninvolved joints and protected ROM of involved joints as allowed
    C. Splint for protection and immobilization

II.   Week 3: AROM of joints and activation of tendon transfer in splint

III.   Week 4: AROM of all joints with splint removed; nonresistive activities in therapy, NMES for transfer activation
IV.   Weeks 6 to 8: Discharge protective splint. A/PROM and functional activities, splinting for tightness. Progressive resistive exercises at week 8.[2-5,7,12]

OUTCOMES

It has been written in the literature that subjective satisfaction is high after tendon transfer surgery.[1,3,4,11] However, "There is little available quantitative information on the relative merits of different types of transfers and of different methods of mobilizing stiff or adherent tendons."[4] New literature comparing rehabilitation after tendon transfers is sparse. "Despite the comparatively long history of tendon transfer surgery [1896] and a large volume of data on surgical procedures, little had been written specifically regarding rehabilitation after tendon transfer."[11]

A literature review found little research comparing rehabilitative techniques. In a 1995 article,[8] Silfverskiold and May expressed this same frustration. Despite the vast literature on early motion after primary tendon repair, other than early-restricted PROM, most authors indicate immobilization for 3 weeks to be the current standard of care.[8,11,14]

Two recent studies have compared early mobilization of tendon transfers versus immobilization. The first article was published by Silfverskiold and May in 1995 in the *Journal of Hand Surgery*. It was titled, "Early Active Mobilization After Tendon Transfers Using Mesh Reinforced Suture Technique."[8] Twenty patients underwent a total of 23 different tendon transfers using a mesh-reinforced suture technique and early mobilization within the first 3 postoperative days. Postoperative care included a resting splint/cast and intermittent controlled active flexion and extension within the splint. The patients were taught how to release the straps at home and complete the exercise program. Findings indicated that this suture technique was strong enough for early mobilization and that early AROM is a feasible and sound method with definite advantages. Few complications were seen, all but two patients were able to activate the transfer within 1 day after beginning exercises, adhesions were limited, and there was no atrophy of muscle. By 1 month after surgery, the patients had recovered 69% to 78% of final ROM measurements (Table 12-1).

TABLE 12-1   Mean of Final ROM Measurements at Discharge and Comparison of AROM of Tendon Transfer to ROM of the Unaffected Hand

	EPL		FPL			Wrist	
Reconstruction	At MCP	At IP	At MCP	At IP	**EDC**	Extension	Flexion
Mean AROM at discharge (degrees)	49	67	61	50	82 at MCP joints	50	24
AROM of unaffected hand (%)	95	95	100	75	92	78	34

From Silfverskiold KL, May EJ: J Hand Surg Br 20:291-300, 1995.

AROM, Active range of motion; *EDC,* extensor digitorum communis; *EPL,* extensor pollicis longus; *FPL,* flexor pollicis longus; *IP,* interphalangeal joint; *MCP,* metacarpophalangeal joint; *ROM,* range of motion.

TABLE **12-2** Active Range of Motion of Metacarpophalangeal (MCP) and Interphalangeal (IP) Joints during Treatment

Joint	Week 3	Week 4	Week 6	Week 8
MCP				
Immobilization	43	55	67	63
Dynamic	30	49	63	66
IP				
Immobilization	31	50	74	70
Dynamic	59	74	86	84

From Germann G, Wagner H, Blome-Eberwein S, et al: J Hand Surg Am 26:1111-1115, 2001.

The second article, by Germann and colleagues,[14] was titled, "Early Dynamic Motion Versus Postoperative Immobilization in Patients with Extensor Indicis Proprius Transfer to Restore Thumb Extension: A Prospective Randomized Study." It was published in *The Journal of Hand Surgery* in 2001. Twenty patients with EIP-to-extensor pollicis longus (EPL) transfers were selected; 10 were treated with immobilization and 10 with early dynamic motion. Both groups were immobilized in an extension thumb spica cast for 3 weeks. During that time, one group of 10 was allowed active flexion through dynamic extension of the IP joint with rubber band traction. At 3 weeks, both groups were allowed full function and began identical therapy programs with ROM and increasing resistance, stress loading, and PROM. At 3 weeks, the AROM of the metacarpophalangeal joint of the group with dynamic mobilization was better than that of the immobilized group; after 6 weeks, the groups were statistically identical. At 3 weeks, the IP AROM of the immobilized group was half that of the mobilized group, but at 6 to 8 weeks there was no statistically significant difference. Grip and pinch strength followed the same pattern. The most notable difference between the groups was duration of treatment and cost. The study demonstrated cost-effectiveness through use of fewer therapy appointments, less splinting materials, and less time off work (Tables 12-2 and 12-3).

TABLE **12-3** Cost-Effectiveness of Dynamic Motion and Immobilization with Respect to Physical Therapy (PT), Occupational Therapy (OT), and Splinting

Treatment	Number of Visits		Cost of Therapy ($)			Duration of Treatment Days Until Return to Work	Overall Cost ($)
	PT	OT	PT	OT	Splint		
Dynamic motion	10	7	200	140	100	55	440
Immobilization	13	11	260	220	40	65 = $500*	1020

From Germann G, Wagner H, Blome-Eberwein S, et al: J Hand Surg Am 26:1111-1115, 2001.

*Payment for health insurance, $20/session for PT and OT. Dynamic motion group saved $500/patient for the insurance companies, according to the German Social Security system (amount converted to dollars).

REFERENCES

1. Richards RR: Tendon transfers for failed nerve reconstruction. Clin Plastic Surg 30:223-245, 2003
2. Bell-Krotoski JA: Preoperative and postoperative management of tendon transfers after median and ulnar nerve injury. In Mackin EJ, Callahan AD, Skirven TM, et al. (eds): Hunter-Mackin-Callahan Rehabilitation of the Hand and Upper Extremity. 5th Ed. Mosby, St. Louis, 2002
3. Brand PW: Biomechanics of tendon transfers. In Hunter JM, Schneider LH, Mackin EJ (eds): Tendon Surgery in the Hand. Mosby, St. Louis, 1987
4. Brand PW: Mechanics of tendon transfers. In Mackin EJ, Callahan AD, Skirven TM, et al. (eds): Hunter-Mackin-Callahan Rehabilitation of the Hand and Upper Extremity. 5th Ed. Mosby, St. Louis, 2002
5. Riordian DC: Principles of tendon transfers. In Hunter JM, Schneider LH, Mackin EJ (eds): Tendon Surgery in the Hand. Mosby, St. Louis, 1987
6. Schneider LH: Tendon transfers: an overview. In Mackin EJ, Callahan AD, Skirven TM, et al. (eds): Hunter-Mackin-Callahan Rehabilitation of the Hand and Upper Extremity. 5th Ed. Mosby, St. Louis, 2002
7. Omer GE: Early tendon transfers as internal splints. In Hunter JM, Schneider LH, Mackin EJ (eds): Tendon Surgery in the Hand. Mosby, St. Louis, 1987
8. Silfverskiold KL, May EJ: Early active mobilization after tendon transfers using mesh reinforced suture techniques. J Hand Surg Br 20:291-300, 1995
9. Cannon N: Diagnosis and Treatment Manual for Physicians and Therapists: Upper Extremity Rehabilitation. 4th Ed. The Hand Rehabilitation Center of Indiana, Indianapolis, IN, 2001
10. Tubiana R: Tendon transfers for restoration of opposition. In Hunter JM, Schneider LH, Mackin EJ (eds): Tendon Surgery in the Hand. Mosby, St. Louis, 1987
11. Toth S: Therapist's management of tendon transfers. Hand Clin 2:239-246, 1986
12. Trumble T: Tendon transfers. In Trumble T: Principles of Hand Surgery and Therapy. Saunders, St. Louis, 2001
13. Kozin S: Peripheral nerve injuries of the upper quarter. In Kozin S: Tendon Transfers: Surgical Demonstration and Therapists Management (lecture). Drexel University, Philadelphia, March 2003
14. Germann G, Wagner H, Blome-Eberwein S, et al: Early dynamic motion versus postoperative immobilization in patients with extensor indicis proprius transfer to restore thumb extension: a prospective randomized study. J Hand Surg Am 26:1111-1115, 2001

Tendon Transfers for Ulnar Nerve Palsy

13

Michele A. Klein

Deficits resulting from trauma to the ulnar nerve are variable. With low lesions, the motor deficits are a result of the loss of intrinsic function; this causes a significant imbalance and deformity in the hand. Low lesions affect pinch and grip strength and manipulation and cause difficulty with the approach of objects due to a claw-hand deformity. With high ulnar nerve injury, denervation of the flexor digitorum profundus (FDP) to the ring finger (RF) and small finger (SF) complicates the deficits of intrinsic weakness by further weakening grasp.[1-6]

As with median nerve injury, if dysfunction is profound and it is evident that ulnar nerve reinnervation is unlikely, patients may decide to undergo a tendon transfer to regain function. Unfortunately, an isolated tendon transfer cannot restore all of the power requirements of an ulnar nerve palsy.[4] The signs indicative of ulnar nerve palsy are as follows:
- Froment's sign: hyperflexion of the thumb interphalangeal (IP) joint when loading the thumb for pinch due to loss of thenar musculature and first dorsal interossei (Fig. 13-1)
- Jeanne's sign: hyperextension of the thumb metacarpophalangeal (MCP) joint when attempting pinch (see Fig. 13-1)
- Duchenne's sign: clawing of the RF and SF due to the unopposed power of the flexor digitorum profundus (FDP)/flexor digitorum superficialis (FDS) and the extensor digitorum communis (EDC)/ extensor digiti quinti (EDQ) by the intrinsic muscles (Fig. 13-2)
- Wartenburg's sign: abduction of the SF due to the unopposed power of the extensor digiti quinti (EDQ) (Fig. 13-3).

In response to the loss of the intrinsic musculature with ulnar nerve palsy, tendon transfers are completed to rebalance the unopposed power of the extrinsic flexors and extensors. Various types of transfers are used for low- and high-level ulnar nerve damage to restore balance to the hand and give the patient functional pinch and grip.

As with all tendon transfer procedures, careful planning and detailed preoperative evaluations are necessary. The patient should have a full

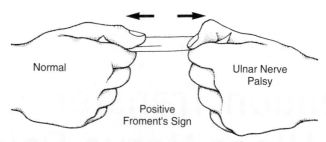

FIG. **13-1** Froment's sign: hyperflexion of the thumb interphalangeal (IP) joint due to an imbalance of the intrinsic and extrinsic muscles acting on the thumb. The pull of the flexor pollicis longus (FPL) overpowers the weak or atrophied intrinsics. Jeanne's sign: hyperextension of the thumb IP joint during pinch due to intrinsic weakness. (From Trumble T: Principles of Hand Surgery and Therapy. Saunders, St. Louis, 2000.)

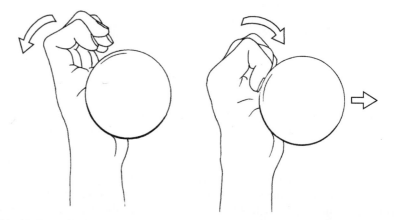

FIG. **13-2** Duchenne's sign: With the claw deformity of the hand, there is hyperextension of the metacarpophalangeal (MCP) joints and increased flexion of the distal interphalangeal (DIP) and proximal (PIP) joints to create a roll-up deformity due to the lack of flexion of the MCP joints that is provided by the lumbrical muscles. (From Trumble T: Principles of Hand Surgery and Therapy. Saunders, St. Louis, 2000.)

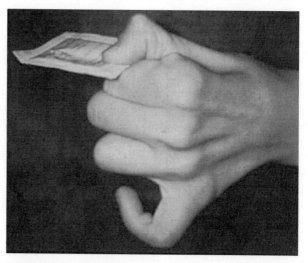

FIG. **13-3** Wartenburg's sign: Weakness or paralysis of the interosseous muscle causing an imbalanced pull of the extensor digiti quinti (EDQ). (From Trumble T: Principles of Hand Surgery and Therapy. Saunders, St. Louis, 2000.)

understanding of what to expect in therapy and what is a realistic outcome.[7] The therapist should be in close communication with the surgeon and may be helpful in deciding possible donor muscles and together determining the postoperative plan. For postoperative care, it is extremely helpful for the therapist to be present in the operating room if possible.[1]

DEFINITION

Tendon transfer is the transfer of the power of an innervated muscle to a denervated or weaker muscle or muscles by way of transfer of its tendinous insertion.

SURGICAL PURPOSE

The goal of tendon transfer procedures is to restore balance and function to a hand that has been compromised through the loss of a muscle or group of muscles, or through irreplaceable loss of nerve innervation. This may occur as a result of prolonged compression as in cubital tunnel syndrome, trauma, disease, infectious processes, congenital anomalies, or spastic paralysis.[7-9] Sometimes transfers are complemented by static procedures such as capsulodesis.

This chapter addresses the most common transfer procedures indicated with an injury to the ulnar nerve and the corresponding postoperative care. The transfers that are covered in this chapter restore grip (due to loss of MCP flexion and FDP of RF and SF) and restore pinch (due to loss of thumb flexion-adduction). There are various other techniques not mentioned here, and there are many exceptions to these guidelines. Differences among surgeons, therapists, patients, the mechanism of injury, tissue integrity, comorbidities, and sociocultural and economic status all may affect the outcome of surgery.

TREATMENT GOALS

I.   Preoperative goals
     A. Achieving and maintaining full passive range of motion (PROM) and active range of motion (AROM) if possible. It is not appropriate to address joint stiffness or contracture after the transfer procedure. Anti-claw splinting is usually helpful, and cylindrical casting for proximal interphalangeal (PIP) joint contractures may be indicated with long-standing claw-hand deformity.[1,6,9]
     B. Achieving maximum strength of the donor muscle and antagonist muscles[2]
     C. Maintaining supple, soft tissue by minimizing scar, edema, and adhesions and resolving intrinsic/extrinsic muscle tightness. Any scar tissue will increase drag on the transfer.[2] Use gel, elastomer molds, kinesiotape, and so on.
     D. Complete comprehensive evaluation, including sensory testing, functional assessments, ROM measurements, strength testing, and pictures for postoperative comparison
     E. Educate the patient about the therapy process, splinting demands, and realistic postoperative expectations. Patients with nerve

injuries may not be accustomed to using their hands functionally and are at risk for injury (e.g., burns).

F. Establish good communication with the surgeon, schedule postoperative therapy, and arrange to observe the surgery if possible.

II.   Postoperative goals

A. Protect transferred tendon or tendons.

B. Maintain ROM of uninvolved joints and involved joints as able.[2,4,5,8,10]

C. Control postoperative edema and pain.

D. Control scar tissue (skin and subcutaneous) and prevent adhesions to decrease drag on transfer.[2,10]

E. Progress patient to functional use of hand.

POSTOPERATIVE INDICATIONS/PRECAUTIONS FOR THERAPY

I.   Indications

A. Surgical tendon transfers

II.   Precautions

A. Acceptance of less than full PROM before transfer[7]

B. Overestimation of donor muscle strength[7]

C. "Drag" along transfer route secondary to scar[2]

D. Technical failures (e.g., rupture of juncture, too loose or too tight)

E. Be mindful of stretching out transfer. Wait until 6 weeks after surgery before addressing tightness of transfer. (Keep in mind phases of wound healing.) (See Chapter 1.)

F. Be careful of anesthetic skin in some of these patients.

POSTOPERATIVE THERAPY: LOW ULNAR NERVE INJURY

Intrinsic Rebalancing

FDS of middle finger (MF): The FDS is divided into two tails and routed between the neurovascular bundles and the intermetacarpal ligament, following the path of the lumbrical muscles. The tails are attached respectively to the RF/SF lateral bands or into the proximal phalanx (Fig. 13-4).

Zancolli lasso procedure: Similar to the FDS technique, but the slips of the FDS are passed through the interval between the A1 and A2 pulleys of the RF and SF. It is then folded over on itself, thus creating a "lasso" effect (Fig. 13-5).

I.   Postoperative day 10 to 14: Remove postoperative cast, have tension checked by surgeon, and immobilize patient in splint or recast. Immobilization in the cast for 3 to 4 weeks is common.[6,11] Apply wound care, edema reduction, and scar management measures if indicated.

A. Fit the patient with a dorsal blocking splint (DBS)[6,11,12]

1. Wrist is neutral or in 20 to 30 degrees flexion

2. MCP is in 60 to 70 degrees flexion

3. IP joints are in 0 degrees flexion

B. Gentle AROM and PROM within the restraints of the DBS

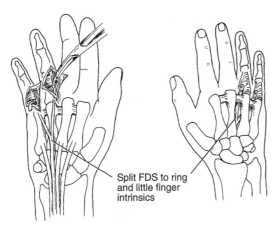

FIG. 13-4 The tendon of the flexor digitorum superficialis (FDS) is split and attached to the lateral bands or the proximal phalanx of the ring and small fingers. (From Trumble T: Principles of Hand Surgery and Therapy. Saunders, St. Louis, 2000.)

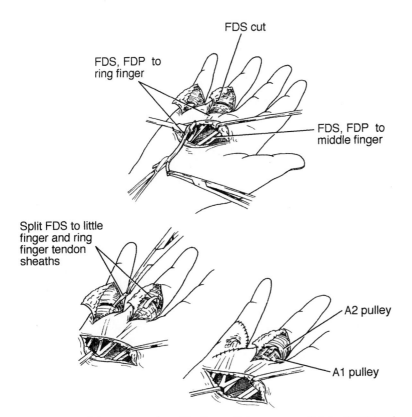

FIG. 13-5 Zancolli lasso procedure: The flexor digitorum superficialis (FDS) tendon is split and passed between the A1 and A2 pulleys of the ring and small fingers. It is then sewn back over on itself, creating a "lasso." (From Trumble T: Principles of Hand Surgery and Therapy. Saunders, St. Louis, 2000.)

II.   Week 4: Begin AROM out of splint, avoiding composite extension. Trumble[6] advocates at this time removing the DBS and fabricating a hand-based MCP block splint at 30 to 40 degrees flexion.

III.   Week 6: Discharge DBS splint and begin using hand-based MCP block splint. Complete unrestricted AROM/PROM, avoiding composite digital extension. May introduce light resistance.[11] Closely monitor MCP joint flexion; a slight flexion contracture is the goal of intrinsic rebalancing procedures, to provide an "internal splint."[4,6]

IV.   Week 8: Progressive resistive exercises. Preferably frequent low-resistance exercise sessions rather than occasional high-resistive exercises. It is important not to fatigue the transfer.[11]

V.   Week 12: The hand-based splint may be needed until this time. Resume unrestricted activities; continue to avoid composite digital extension with resistance.

Brand transfer of extensor carpi radialis longus (ECRL)/extensor carpi radialis brevis (ECRB) to intrinsics with tendon graft: If ECRL is used, the transfer is routed volarly through the carpal canal, then inserted into the radial, lateral bands of RF and SF or the proximal phalanx. If the ECRB is used, the transferred tendon is passed dorsally, passed through the intermetacarpal spaces, and inserted in the same fashion to provide MCP flexion[2,5,6,8,12] (Fig. 13-6).

Modified Stiles-Bunnel procedure: The distal end of the MF FDS is harvested, divided into two slips, and routed to the lateral bands of the RF and SF or into the proximal phalanx.[2,5,6,8,12]

I.   Weeks 3 to 4 (depending on insertion): Remove postoperative cast and fabricate dorsal block splint.
    A. ECRB: Wrist in 20 to 30 degrees flexion
       1. MCP in 60 to 70 degrees extension
       2. IP in 0 degrees extension
    B. ECRL/FDS: Wrist in 20 to 30 degrees flexion
       1. MCP in 60 to 70 degrees flexion
       2. IP in 0 degrees flexion
    C. Begin AROM to joints within the splint, with emphasis on long flexors. Passive IP joint extension with MCP joint flexion. Keep

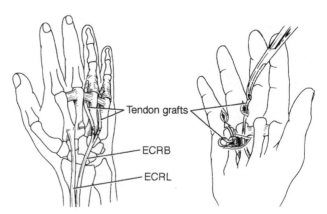

FIG. 13-6 Brand transfer of the extensor carpi radialis longus (ECRL)/extensor carpi radialis brevis (ECRB) routed to the lateral bands of the ring and small fingers or into the proximal phalanx using an interpositional tendon graft. (From Trumble T: Principles of Hand Surgery and Therapy. Saunders, St. Louis, 2000.)

the MCP joints in flexion with IP extension to avoid tension on the transfer with composite digital extension at this time.

D. Scar management

II.   Weeks 4 to 6: Some authors suggest discharge of the DBS[6] and fabrication of an MCP block splint in 30 to 40 degrees flexion with a palmar bar, given 0 PIPJ extension lag. Continue AROM, avoid full MCP extension, and work on functional use of the hand and activation of the transfer in splint.

III. Week 6: Discharge DBS and switch to hand-based MCP block splint at 30 to 40 degrees flexion. May begin PROM exercises in flexion and continue activities within the MCP block splint.

IV.   Weeks 8 to 12: May begin dynamic splinting as needed and gentle progressive resistive exercises. Monitor PIP extension lags closely. Slight MCP flexion contracture is a goal of this procedure. Continue MCP flexion splint to 12 weeks if warranted.

Restoration of Power Pinch

Smith-Hastings procedure: The ECRB is transferred to adductor pollicis (ADP) with graft. The ECRB is detached proximal to its insertion into the third metacarpal. Using an interpositional graft (the palmaris longus [PL]), the tendon is routed through the second and third metacarpals, and, using the third metacarpal as a pulley, it is then woven into the ADP[5,6] (Fig. 13-7).

FDS of RF to ADP: The FDS tendon is harvested distally, and at the level of the MCP crease it is passed subcutaneously and below the index finger (IF) and MF FDP. It is secured to the tendon of the ADP[6] or into the radial aspect of the proximal phalanx[3,5] (Fig. 13-8).

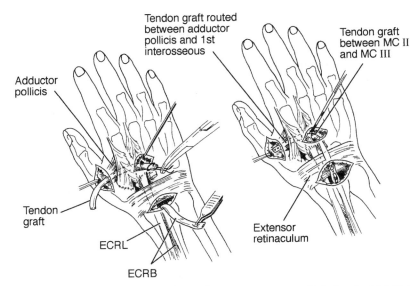

FIG. **13-7** Smith-Hastings procedure: The extensor carpi radialis brevis (ECRB) is transferred to the adductor pollicis (ADP) using a tendon graft. The ECRB is detached proximal to its insertion into the third metacarpal and then routed volarly, using the third metacarpal as a pulley, and woven into the adductor. (From Trumble T: Principles of Hand Surgery and Therapy. Saunders, St. Louis, 2000.)

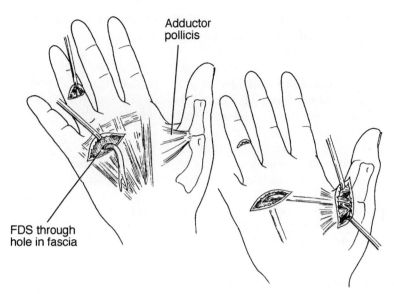

FIG. **13-8** Flexor digitorum superficialis (FDS) of ring finger to adductor pollicis (ADP): The FDS tendon is passed subcutaneously, at the level of the distal palmar crease, to the ADP tendon or into the radial aspect of the proximal phalanx. (From Trumble T: Principles of Hand Surgery and Therapy. Saunders, St. Louis, 2000.)

I.   Weeks 0 to 3: Keep the hand in the postoperative cast or, at 10 to 14 days, fabricate a protective splint and address wound, scar, and edema. No AROM until 3 weeks after surgery.

II. Week 3: Fabricate splint to allow for activation of transfer. Some authors suggest fabrication of the splint at 10 to 14 days postoperatively,[12] but even then AROM is not initiated until 3 weeks postoperatively. Fabrication of the splint early allows the therapist to address necessary scar and wound care.

   A. Smith-Hastings procedure: DBS
      1. Wrist in 20 to 30 degrees extension
      2. Thumb carpometacarpal (CMC) in 30 degrees palmar abduction

   B. FDS of RF: DBS
      1. Wrist in neutral position to slight flexion (15 to 20 degrees)
      2. Thumb CMC in 30 degrees palmar abduction

   C. AROM/PROM within the confines of the splint is initiated. Work on thumb adduction, abduction, and extension (to splint) and flexion.[3,4,6,12,13]

III. Week 4: Begin activation of transfer out of splint. For the ECRB transfer, emphasize adduction with simultaneous wrist extension. Splint is worn between exercise sessions and at night. At this time, Trumble[6] advocates a hand-based splint with the thumb in adduction

IV. Week 6: Discharge splint and address tightness of tissues. A web spacer or extension splint may be needed.[6,12] Emphasize use of the hand and transfer with activities for prehension and light pinch.

V.   Week 8: Progress resistance and wean from splints.

POSTOPERATIVE THERAPY: HIGH ULNAR NERVE INJURY

ECRL to FDP: Commonly used for combined median and ulnar nerve injuries. The tendon is mobilized and routed volarly, typically around the radial aspect of the forearm. After the FDP tendons are synchronized, the ECRL tendon is woven through the FDP tendons using a Pulvertaft weave (passing the tendon a minimum of three times). Tension is set with full digital flexion with the wrist at 30 to 45 degrees extension[5,6,14] (Fig. 13-9).

I. Postoperative day 10 to 14: Remove postoperative dressing; have surgeon check tension of transfer. Splint for immobilization. Address wound care, edema reduction, and scar management when able.
   A. DBS. Surgeon may request a long arm splint with elbow in 90 degrees flexion
      1. Wrist in neutral position to 20 degrees flexion
      2. MCP joints in 60 to 70 degrees flexion
      3. IP joints in 0 degrees flexion
   B. May begin PROM of the digits into flexion and extension within the confines of the DBS.
II. Week 3: AROM within splint to activate transfer, six to eight times per day
III. Week 4: AROM out of splint for transfer activation and light grasp. May need to use neuromuscular electrical stimulation (NMES) to activate transfer. Emphasize tenodesis activities. Consider sensory deficits for combined median and ulnar nerve injuries, and use a mirror or biofeedback during tasks.
IV. Week 6: Discharge splint and begin PROM. Splinting at end of active range in resting pan splint at night to decrease flexor tightness may be needed.

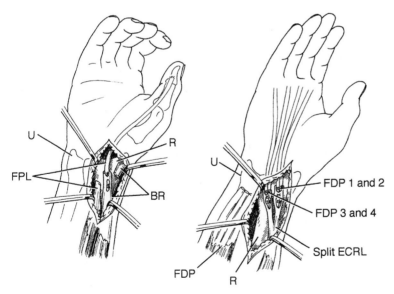

FIG. 13-9 Extensor carpi radialis longus (ECRL) to flexor digitorum profundus (FDP): For high ulnar nerve injuries (or combined median/ulnar nerve injuries), the ECRL tendon is harvested, routed radially and volarly, and woven through the four FDP tendons. *BR,* Brachioradialis; *R,* radius; *U,* ulna. (From Trumble T: Principles of Hand Surgery and Therapy. Saunders, St. Louis, 2000.)

V. Weeks 7 to 8: Progressive resistive exercises for hand and wrist; focus on tenodesis activities with resistance.

POSTOPERATIVE COMPLICATIONS

I. Scarring of tendon to surrounding structures, particularly at junction sites, causing "drag" on the transfer[2,8,9,10]
II. Difficulty activating transfer. May need to use NMES or biofeedback to assist patient in activation of transfer.
III. Transfer too loose or too tight. Wait 6 weeks before doing any splinting against transfer.
IV. Rupture of transfer repairs

EVALUATION TIMELINE

I. Postoperative day 10 to 14 (after tension has been checked by surgeon)
   A. Assess edema, pain, and incisional site
   B. ROM of uninvolved joints and protected ROM of involved joints as allowed
II. Week 3: AROM of joints involved in tendon transfer while in splint
III. Week 4: AROM of all joints with splint removed. Nonresistive activities in therapy, NMES for transfer activation.
IV. Weeks 6 to 8: Discharge protective splint. AROM/PROM and functional activities, splinting for tightness. Progressive resistive exercises at week 8.[1,2,5,6,9]

OUTCOMES

Please refer to Outcomes in Chapter 12.

REFERENCES

1. Bell-Krotoski JA: Preoperative and postoperative management of tendon transfers after median and ulnar nerve injury. In Mackin EJ, Callahan AD, Skirven TM, et al. (eds): Rehabilitation of the Hand and Upper Extremity. 5th Ed. Mosby, St. Louis, 2002
2. Brand PW: Biomechanics of tendon transfers. In Hunter JM, Schneider LH, Mackin EJ (eds): Tendon Surgery in the Hand. Mosby, St. Louis, 1987
3. Littler WJ: Restoration of thumb pinch strength with loss of flexion-adduction muscle function. In Hunter JM, Schneider LH, Mackin EJ (eds): Tendon Surgery in the Hand. Mosby, St. Louis, 1987
4. Omer GE: Early tendon transfers as internal splints. In Hunter JM, Schneider LH, Mackin EJ (eds): Tendon Surgery in the Hand. Mosby, St. Louis, 1987
5. Richards RR: Tendon transfers for failed nerve reconstruction. Clin Plastic Surg 30:223-245, 2003
6. Trumble T: Tendon transfers. In Trumble T: Principles of Hand Surgery and Therapy. Saunders, St. Louis, 2001
7. Schneider LH: Tendon transfers: an overview. In Mackin EJ, Callahan AD, Skirven TM, et al. (eds): Rehabilitation of the Hand and Upper Extremity. 5th Ed. Mosby, St. Louis, 2002
8. Brand PW: Mechanics of tendon transfers. In Mackin EJ, Callahan AD, Skirven TM, et al. (eds): Rehabilitation of the Hand and Upper Extremity. 5th Ed. Mosby, St. Louis, 2002
9. Riordian DC: Principles of tendon transfers. In Hunter JM, Schneider LH, Mackin EJ (eds): Tendon Surgery in the Hand. Mosby, St. Louis, 1987

10. Silfverskiold KL, May EJ: Early active mobilization after tendon transfers using mesh reinforced suture techniques. J Hand Surg Br 20:291-300, 1995

11. Schneider LH: Tendon transfers: an overview. In Mackin EJ, Callahan AD, Skirven TM, et al. (eds): Rehabilitation of the Hand and Upper Extremity. 5th Ed. Mosby, St. Louis, 2002

12. Toth S: Therapist's management of tendon transfers. Hand Clin 2:239-246, 1986

13. Cannon N: Diagnosis and treatment manual for physicians and therapists: upper extremity rehabilitation. 4th Ed. The Hand Rehabilitation Center of Indiana, Indianapolis, IN, 2001

14. Tubiana R: Tendon transfers for restoration of opposition. In Hunter JM, Schneider LH, Mackin EJ (eds): Tendon Surgery in the Hand. Mosby, St. Louis, 1987

Tendon Transfers for Radial Nerve Palsy

14

Arlynne Pack Brown

Injury to the radial nerve at the humerus results in limited forearm supination as well as absent wrist extension, metacarpophalangeal (MCP) joint extension, and thumb abduction and extension. These clinical limitations result in the functional limitation of decreased ability to open the hand to grasp.

If it is clear that the muscles are not likely to be reinnervated, tendon transfers are frequently performed. Tendon transfers transmit the muscle power of one muscle to another by moving the tendon insertion from the original muscle to that of the denervated muscle. There are multitudes of muscles available for transfer. The pronator teres muscle is usually the donor of choice to provide wrist extension. The flexor carpi ulnaris muscle is usually used for MCP joint extension. Raskin and Wilgis[1] substantiated that use of the flexor carpi ulnaris did not significantly impair wrist function. Thumb extension and abduction are commonly provided by the palmaris longus, one half of the flexor carpi radialis, and the ring finger sublimus muscles. The following rehabilitation guidelines are based on using these muscles as transfers.

The result of tendon transfers can be enhanced in a number of ways. If a transfer crosses several joints, one of which is unstable, the action of the tendon transfer can be improved with an arthrodesis of that joint. The arthrodesis allows the force to be transmitted across the newly stable joint to the joints at which the motion is desired. Another consideration is the phase of the original action of the donor muscle with the new desired action. It is typically easier to reeducate muscles transferred within phase. That is, a muscle that is originally a wrist flexor is best transferred to a digital extensor. Recall the tenodesis coordination between these motions during normal hand function: during wrist flexion, the extrinsic digital extensors, in phase with the wrist flexors, naturally cause digital extension.

DEFINITION

Schneider[2] defines **tendon transfers** as "the application of the motor power of one muscle to another weaker or paralyzed muscle by the transfer of its tendinous insertion."

SURGICAL PURPOSE

Loss of extensor muscle function is most commonly associated with radial nerve interruption. It is impossible for the patient with this condition to open the hand to grasp objects; therefore, the transfer of normally functioning muscle–tendon units is frequently used to overcome the deficit. The radial nerve supplies all of the wrist extensors and finger extensors, including the thumb. Depending on the level of nerve interruption, tendon transfer planning may or may not include wrist extension. Preoperative instruction and splinting may supplement postoperative rehabilitation if the patient is knowledgeable about the function of the transferred units.

Some surgeons perform tendon transfers (internal splints) during the nerve repair recovery phase (i.e., pronator teres to extensor carpi radialis brevis [ECRB]), so that patients do not have to wait for nerve recovery to have a functional hand.

Restoration of lost muscle action by the transfer of available and effective muscle units is the goal of this form of treatment.

TREATMENT GOALS

I. Preoperative goals
    A. Establish tissue equilibrium.[3,4]
    B. Educate patient about the new muscle–joint relationship.
    C. Maximize passive range of motion (PROM), particularly the thumb–index web space, and wrist extention.[3-5]
    D. Assess upper extremity muscle strength.
    E. Maximize strength and power of donor muscles.[2,3,5]
    F. Maintain strength of unaffected muscles.[3,5,6]
    G. Maintain function and discourage habit of using tenodesis between wrist and MCP joints for function.[4,6]
    H. Monitor sensation: If the median nerve distribution sensation is absent, the patient will be unlikely to use the transfer.[5,7]
II. Postoperative goals
    A. Protect transferred tendon.[3]
    B. Minimize edema.
    C. Maintain ROM of uninvolved joints.[3]
    D. Maximize functional ROM of involved joints (e.g., flex wrist to 20 degrees when digits are in composite flexion).
    E. Establish firm scar at juncture site that is able to glide through adjacent structures.[5]
    F. Return to functional use of hand.

PRECAUTIONS FOR THERAPY

Do not overstretch donor muscles.

PREOPERATIVE THERAPY

I. Minimize edema: elevation, active muscle pumping; intermittent compression via fluid flushing massage or Jobst compression; continuous compression via Coban wrapping, Ace wrapping, gloves, or air splints; and electrical stimulation.

II. Maximize active range of motion (AROM) and PROM[2-5]: individual joint AROM/PROM, intrinsic and extrinsic AROM/PROM, contract–relax, place-hold techniques; serial splinting, static progressive splinting,[7] and dynamic splinting techniques.

III. Assess strength and power of the uninvolved muscles of the upper extremity,[3,5] and strengthen as indicated through a progressive resistance exercise program.

IV. Assess strength and power of the possible donor muscles,[2,6] and strengthen as indicated through a progressive resistance exercise program.

V. Maximize scar mobility[3,5,6]: heat followed by friction massage, molds, gel sheets, and compression; low-load splinting; exercises promoting independent gliding between muscle/tendon tissue and surrounding tissue

VI. Provide splints: Use splints to promote normal function of the hand[6] (Figs. 14-1 and 14-2). Several types of splints are available to position the wrist and digits, preventing simultaneous composite wrist and digit flexion and promoting normal use of the hand.

VII. Monitor sensation.[7]

NONOPERATIVE COMPLICATIONS

Overstretched extensor tendons

POSTOPERATIVE INDICATIONS/PRECAUTIONS FOR THERAPY

I. Indications
   A. Surgical tendon transfers
II. Precautions
   A. Neuroma
   B. Overestimation of donor muscle strength
   C. Less than full ROM before surgical transfer[2]

POSTOPERATIVE THERAPY

I. Week 0 to week 3 or 4: Splint/cast. Immobilization of elbow at 90 degrees flexion (at option of surgeon), the forearm at 30 to 90 degrees pronation, wrist at 30 to 45 degrees dorsiflexion, MCP joints at 0 degrees flexion, proximal interphalangeal (PIP) joints free or at 20 to 45 degrees flexion, thumb at full abduction and extension or at slightly less than full abduction and extension (Fig. 14-3). Teach the patient exercises to be performed at home between therapy appointments.
   A. Maintain ROM of uninvolved joints: active range of motion of the neck, shoulder, and distal interphalangeal (DIP) joints.
   B. Protective ROM of individual joints: Extend all other joints while flexing one joint at a time. For example, be sure the wrist, PIP joints, and DIP joints are fully extended when flexing the MCP joints. The same full protective ROM to the elbow (maintaining full forearm pronation and digit extension) and

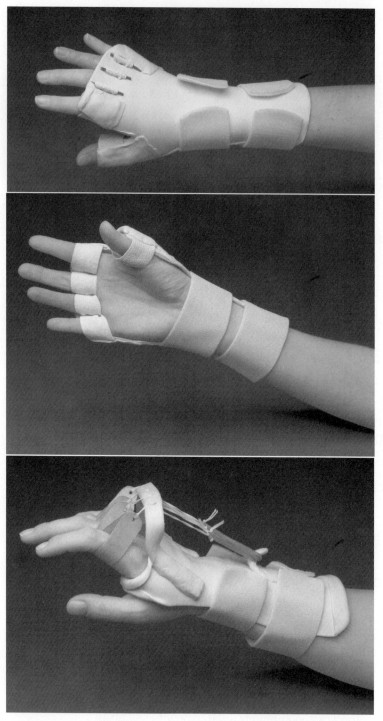

FIG. 14-1 Splints can promote normal use of hand by statically supporting the wrist in extension, dynamically supporting the metacarpophalangeal (MCP) joints in extension, and allowing active flexion of the digits.

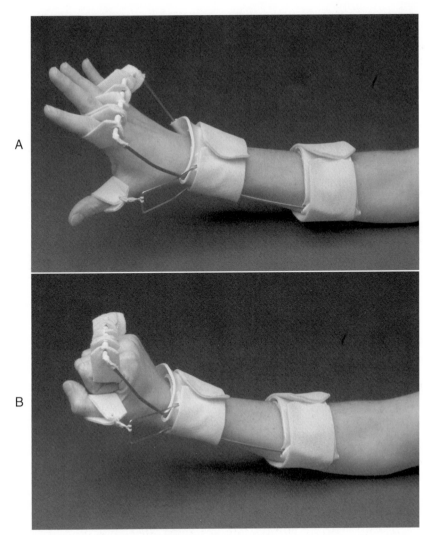

FIG. 14-2 This splint supports the proximal phalanges by a static loop. **A,** Wrist flexion results in digital extension. **B,** Digital flexion results in wrist extension.

protective ROM to the MCP and interphalangeal (IP) joints is permitted. Limit ROM to the wrist to within 10 to 30 degrees of dorsal flexion.[6]

C. Avoid composite wrist and digit flexion.

D. Edema management: While observing sterile technique, apply electrical stimulation, elevation, fluid flushing massage, and Coban and Ace wrapping.

E. Scar management: Use techniques to minimize edema, which will in turn minimize fibroblast infiltration and scar formation.

F. Desensitization techniques: gentle stroking, touching and tapping to tolerance and application of transcutaneous electrical nerve stimulation (TENS).

II. Week 3 or 4: Splint. Fabricate splint, according to surgeon's guidance, which may or may not include the elbow. Position the hand and wrist in same positions as in the original cast.

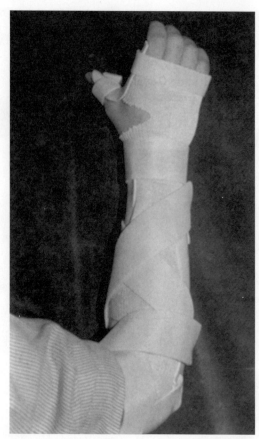

FIG. **14-3** Example of splint used for postoperative positioning.

    A. ROM: as above.

    B. Scar management: Use heat followed by friction massage, molds, gel sheets, and compression; low-load splinting; exercises promoting independent gliding between muscle/tendon tissue and surrounding tissue.

III.   Weeks 5 to 6: Muscle reeducation. Begin brief sessions of muscle contractions (place-hold techniques to gentle active contraction, palpation of tendon, biofeedback exercises) and education of transferred muscle. Progress to full ROM during light pick up–release activities for digits and twisting activities for thumb (e.g., nut and bolt assembly).[4] The physician should be contacted for approval to use functional electrical stimulation (FES) before using it to acquire gentle muscle stimulation. Timing of FES varies from surgeon to surgeon.

IV.   Week 7: Begin dynamic flexion splinting if extrinsic extensor tendon tightness is present.

V.   Week 8: Discontinue protective daytime splinting; introduce resistive exercises.[6] Begin passive wrist flexion to gain maximum pronator teres length.[8]

VI.   Week 12: Resume unrestricted activities.

POSTOPERATIVE COMPLICATIONS

I.   Scarring of tendon to surrounding structures, particularly at sites of pulleys
II. Bowstringing of transferred tendon
III. Rupture of tendon juncture[2,5]
IV. Overstretching of transferred tendon[2,3]
V.   Wrist postures in slight radial deviation when flexor carpi ulnaris is used as a donor muscle

EVALUATION TIMELINE

I.   Week 1
     A. ROM of uninvolved joints
     B. Evaluation of edema
     C. Protected ROM of individual involved joints
     D. Sensibility evaluation
II. Week 5: Composite AROM flexion and extension of joints involved in tendon transfer
III. Week 7: Composite PROM flexion and extension of joints involved in tendon transfer
IV. Week 10: Manual muscle testing and functional outcomes

OUTCOMES

The guidelines suggested here for therapeutic management of tendon transfers for radial nerve palsy are based on the science of soft tissue healing and years of clinical experience at The Curtis National Hand Center. There are no scientific outcome studies evaluating therapeutic intervention after radial nerve palsy tendon transfers. The only consistent details offered in therapeutic manuscripts are the types of splints used for full-time immobilization for the first 3 to 4 postoperative weeks, and for subsequent immobilization only at night for the fifth to sixth postoperative weeks, and some nondescript therapy.[9-12]

There are scant articles assessing patient satisfaction after surgical repair of radial nerve palsy using tendon transfer. Reliably, this surgery leaves patients with sufficient ROM to perform activities of daily living (ADLs).[1,8,11-13] However, Skoll and associates[12] cautioned that limited wrist ROM should not be accepted before sufficient time has passed and proper therapeutic techniques have been employed to maximize wrist ROM. Many patients can perform their original work with minimal complaints related to work simulation, power grip, and power of the wrist movement.[1,12] Reduction of power precludes the majority of heavy manual laborers from returning to their original employment.[11,12] In general, patients are satisfied with their function in terms of ADLs and non-heavy work employment after tendon transfers for treatment of radial nerve palsy.

REFERENCES

1. Raskin KB, Wilgis EFS: Flexor carpi ulnaris transfer for radial nerve palsy: functional testing of long-term results. J Hand Ther 20A:737, 1995
2. Schneider LH: Tendon transfers in the upper extremity. In Hunter JM, Schneider LH, Mackin EJ, et al. (eds): Rehabilitation of the Hand: Surgery and Therapy. 5th Ed. Mosby, St. Louis, 2002, pp. 792-798

3. Reid RF: Radial nerve palsy. Hand Clin 4:179, 1988

4. Omer GE: Tendon transfers in radial nerve paralysis. In Hunter JM, Schneider LH, Mackin EJ (eds): Tendon Surgery in the Hand. Mosby, St. Louis, 1987, p. 425

5. Riordan RC: Principles of tendon transfers. In Hunter JM, Schneider LH, Mackin EJ (eds): Tendon Surgery in the Hand. Mosby, St. Louis, 1987, p. 410

6. Reynolds CC: Preoperative and postoperative management of tendon transfers after radial nerve injury. In Hunter JM, Schneider LH, Mackin EJ, et al. (eds): Rehabilitation of the Hand: Surgery and Therapy. 5th Ed. Mosby, St. Louis, 2002, pp. 825-826

7. Bell-Krotoski J: Advances in sensibility evaluation. Hand Clin 7:527-546, 1991

8. Schreuders TA, Stam HJ, Hovius SE: Training of muscle excursion after tendon transfer. J Hand Ther 9:243, 1996

9. Tajima T: In Hunter JM, Schneider LA, Mackin EJ (eds): Tendon Surgery of the Hand. Mosby, St. Louis, 1987, pp. 432-438

10. Chotigavanich C: Tendon transfer for radial nerve palsy. Bull Hosp Jt Dis Orthop Inst 50:1-10, 1990

11. Kruft S, von Heimburg D, Reill P: Treatment of irreversible lesion of the radial nerve by tendon transfer: indication and long-term results of the Merle d'Aubigne procedure. Plast Reconstr Surg 100:610-616, 1997

12. Skoll PPJ, Hudson DA, de Jager W, et al.: Long-term results of tendon transfers for radial nerve palsy in patients with limited rehabilitation. Ann Plast Surg 45:122-126, 2000

13. Palmer AK, Werner FW, Murphy D, et al.: Functional wrist motion: a biomechanical study. J Hand Surg 10A:39-46, 1985

Brachial Plexus Injuries

15

Mark T. Walsh and Gregory K. Davis

Brachial plexus neuropathy (BPN) is a common upper extremity pain syndrome. Peripheral neuropathies of the involved upper extremity and cervical spine pathology complicate the diagnosis. As this pain syndrome becomes more ingrained within the central nervous system (CNS), accompanying alterations in the neural biomechanics of the brachial plexus and peripheral nerves occur, making the diagnosis and treatment more difficult. It is the intent of this chapter to communicate a clearer understanding of brachial plexopathy and its varied manifestations, allowing the clinician to develop a logical sequence of evaluation, assessment, and treatment.

There are three potential spaces for the development of BPN within the thoracic inlet. The first and most medial space is the interscalene triangle, which is located within the boundaries of the posterior cervical triangle. The presence of a prefixed (major contribution from C4) or postfixed (major contribution from T2) brachial plexus, along with other anatomic anomalies, may add to poor neurovascular mobility and tension attenuation. Injury to the shoulder girdle or repetitive trauma may lead to symptoms and pathology. The second potential space is the costoclavicular interval, located inferior to the clavicle and superior to the first rib. Moving laterally, the third potential space is the axillary interval. In this area the anterior structures—the deltopectoral fascia, the pectoralis minor, and the coracoid—have all been implicated as potential sources of compression of the neurovascular structures[1] (Fig. 15-1). Pathology at the scalene triangle may provoke neurological symptoms related to the brachial plexus trunks.

With upper trunk plexopathies (C5-C6 distribution), the pain may tend to be more proximal in nature, distributed over the anterior and lateral aspect of the cervical region, portions of the face, and the scapular and interscapular region. Distal paresthesia and pain may be distributed over what appears to be the median and/or ulnar nerve distribution or the C5-C6 dermatome. With lower trunk plexopathies (C8-T1 distribution), symptoms of pain and paresthesia are distributed mostly distally, over the medial aspect of the arm, forearm, and ulnar aspect of the hand, appearing to be related to the ulnar nerve. With middle trunk plexopathies

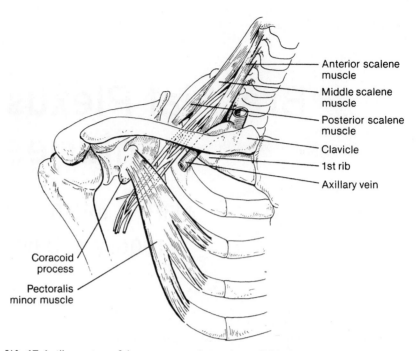

FIG. 15-1 Illustration of the anatomic relationships of the thoracic inlet. (From Pratt N: Clinical Musculoskeletal Anatomy. JB Lippincott, Philadelphia, 1991.)

(C7 distribution), symptoms may be distributed along the posterior/lateral arm and posterior forearm and distally into the middle finger.

At the costoclavicular interval, symptoms may be related to the anterior and posterior divisions of the brachial plexus. Generally, anterior division plexopathies tend to produce symptoms in the anterior compartments of the arm and forearm, along a median and ulnar nerve distribution. Posterior division plexopathies tend to produce symptoms in the posterior compartments of the arm and forearm, along a radial nerve distribution. At the axilla, the symptoms may follow a cord distribution. Medial cord plexopathies may produce symptoms along the medial arm and forearm and produce pain and paresthesia along a median and/or ulnar nerve distribution. Lateral cord plexopathies may produce symptoms distributed along the anterior arm and forearm. Distal pain and paresthesia may follow a median nerve distribution. Posterior cord plexopathies may produce symptoms along the posterior/lateral arm and posterior forearm. Distal pain and paresthesia may follow a radial nerve distribution. Based on these anatomic distributions of symptoms, it is easy to see how the patient's complaints may be distributed throughout the upper quarter.

It is also important to consider neural biomechanics. The ability of the nervous system to tolerate tension associated with movement results from an intraneural (within the nerve) and an extraneural (outside the nerve) anatomic design. Internally, the nerve has undulations of a tortuous nature[2] that allow the nerve to unfold as length increases. The nerve is also able to tolerate elongation through intraneural gliding[2-4]; the nerve's connective tissue allows for intraneural excursion interfascicularly and between individual nerve fibers. The intrafunicular plexus formation within the nerve also allows for internal elongation. Extraneural gliding provides for attenuation of tension via a gliding surface between the para-neurium and epineurium.[4] Another integral component to peripheral nerve gliding is the fact that the interfacing tissues surrounding the nerve along its entire course are required to have the ability to adapt in length in relation to joint motion.[4]

Finally, it is important to appreciate the principle of the peripheral nervous system (PNS), CNS, and autonomic nervous system (ANS) as a continuum.[5,6] This continuum is achieved electrically, chemically, and mechanically and is visually demonstrated in Fig. 15-2. This anatomic preparation, dissected by Rufus Weaver, MD, of Hahnemann Medical College in 1887, illustrates how placing tension on either the PNS or the CNS could have a potential effect on the nervous system at another location. If the nervous system is in a diseased and hyperirritable state, mechanical stresses such as compression or tension may provoke pain

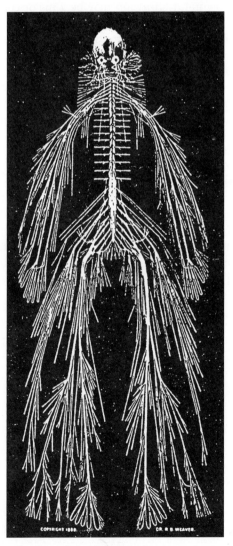

FIG. **15-2** Photograph of the dissected nervous system demonstrating the contin-uum. (Courtesy Drexel University, Philadelphia.)

syndromes and movement dysfunction within the nervous system and its interfacing tissues.

DEFINITION

There are two major types of brachial plexopathy to consider. The first, **compressive brachial plexus neuropathy (CBPN)** is the type classically described as thoracic outlet syndrome (TOS). It is considered a general term for compression neuropathies or vasculopathies of the brachial plexus and subclavian vessels.[7] A comprehensive discussion of TOS can be found in Chapter 9. The second type of brachial plexopathy, **brachial plexus traction injury (BPTI)**, is less understood. A result of a traction injury to the brachial plexus,[8,9] BPTI impairs neural tissue gliding and the ability to tolerate tension, possibly as a result of intraneural or extraneural fibrosis from direct trauma,[10] local pathology within the cervical or thoracic spine,[11] or long-standing compression or overuse.

Additionally, postural dysfunction may be a major component of both types of brachial plexopathies.[12,13] This limitation in the nerve's adaptability is called **adverse mechanical tension (AMT)**.[14,15] AMT occurs each time the individual uses the affected upper extremity and places traction on the involved nerve and its surrounding tissue bed. This can result in compromise of a nerve's vascularity, resulting in the release of chemical mediators such as histamine or bradykinins, potentially creating a state of inflammation in or around the connective tissues of the nerve and increasing its level of irritability.[16,17] Additionally, axoplasmic flow may be compromised, potentially altering the nerve's physiology and function. The contrasting features of TOS and BPTI are listed in Table 15-1.

I. The primary components identified in BPTI are the following
    A. Trauma associated with onset of symptoms,[8,9] involving either a traction injury directly to the brachial plexus or local soft tissue inflammation resulting in a compromise of adequate blood flow to the brachial plexus and the development of intraneural or extraneural fibrosis
    B. Delayed onset of intractable pain and/or paresthesia occurring several days, weeks, or months after injury

TABLE 15-1 Clinical Classification of Thoracic Outlet Syndrome (TOS) Versus Brachial Plexus Traction Injury (BPTI)

Thoracic Outlet Syndrome	Brachial Plexus Traction Injury
Postural relationship	Trauma related: shoulder, cervical spine
Insidious onset	Delayed onset
Transient symptoms: pain/paresthesia	Intractable pain/paresthesia
Provocation tests more reliable	Provocation tests not reliable
Adson's test: scalene triangle	Positive upper limb tension
Costoclavicular maneuver: retroclavicular space	Traction on plexus
Wright's test: axillary space	
Treatment: transient symptom provocation	Treatment: provokes symptoms, delayed response
Nonirritable	Irritable

From Mackin EJ, Callahan AD, Skirven TM, et al. (eds): Hunter-Mackin-Callahan Rehabilitation of the Hand and Upper Extremity. 5th Ed. Mosby, St. Louis, 2002.

TABLE **15-2** Common Myofascial Trigger Points That May Mimic Thoracic Outlet Syndrome or Brachial Plexus Traction Injury

Muscle	Area of Referral
Trapezius	Face and interscapular region
Scalene	Posterolateral arm/radial three digits
Supraspinatus	Lateral arm/forearm
Infraspinatus	Lateral arm/forearm and radial half of hand
Latissimus dorsi	Posteromedial arm, forearm, and ulnar half of hand
Pectoralis	Anterior shoulder, medial arm, and ulnar two digits
Subscapularis	Posteromedial arm and wrist
Serratus	Medial arm, forearm, and ulnar half of hand and digits

From Mackin EJ, Callahan AD, Skirven TM, et al. (eds): Hunter-Mackin-Callahan Rehabilitation of the Hand and Upper Extremity. 5th Ed. Mosby, St. Louis, 2002.

   C. Poor reliability of provocative tests for determining level or location of lesion

   D. Treatment may provoke symptoms, or the response may be delayed by several hours to 1 day.

   E. High level of irritability. Minimal upper quarter movement may provoke severe sustained response (hyperpathia).

   F. Pain is typically the primary complaint and can be categorized into two types
      1. Nerve trunk pain[18]: results from increased activity in nociceptive endings in nerve connective tissues. Described as deep, knifelike, or aching; overlies a specific nerve trunk or distribution.[19] Relieved with rest or reduced tension on involved nerve.
      2. Dysesthetic pain[18]: results from demyelinated, damaged, or regenerating afferent fibers. Described as burning or tingling; associated with sensory loss; poorly localized.[19]

II.   Differential diagnosis
   A. Classic TOS
   B. Myofascial trigger points[20] (Table 15-2)
   C. Cervical spine dysfunction or pathology
   D. Glenohumeral joint pathology ("dead arm syndrome")[21]
   E. Double or multiple crush syndromes[22,23]
   F. Carpal tunnel and/or ulnar nerve neuropathy[24,25]
   G. Visceral causes such as apical lung tumor, coronary artery pathology, or subclavian aneurysm
   H. Brachial neuritis: Parsonage-Turner syndrome

TREATMENT PURPOSE

Mitigate those factors responsible for producing adverse mechanical tension on the brachial plexus, using tools available to the therapist including patient education, manual techniques, nerve mobilization techniques, modalities, and exercise.

TREATMENT GOALS

    I. Attain symptom control and comfort.
    II. Demonstrate postural, positional, and behavioral awareness.
    III. Demonstrate proper diaphragmatic breathing pattern.
    IV. Minimize secondary system complaints in glenohumeral joint, cervical spine, and surrounding soft tissue structures.
    V. Restore proper upper quarter muscular balance and mobility.
    VI. Normalize neural mobility and tolerance of tensile loads.
    VII. Return to vocation or avocation with appropriate modifications as necessary.

NONOPERATIVE INDICATIONS/PRECAUTIONS FOR THERAPY

    I. Indications
        A. Patients whose upper quarter neurovascular symptoms appear to be provoked by adverse tensile loads to the neurovascular structures of the thoracic inlet
    II. Precautions
        A. Irritable conditions
        B. Spinal cord signs
        C. Nerve root signs
        D. Severe, unremitting night pain lacking a diagnosis
        E. Recent paresthesia, anesthesia, or complex regional pain syndrome type I or II
        F. Mechanical spine pain with paresthesia
    III. Contraindications
        A. Recently repaired peripheral nerve
        B. Malignancy
        C. Active inflammatory conditions
        D. Neurological: acute inflammatory/demyelinating disease

NONOPERATIVE THERAPY

    I. Evaluation
        A. History
            1. Determine mechanism of injury and/or date of onset of symptoms.
            2. Identify positions, postures, or activities that relieve, accentuate, or aggravate the symptoms.
            3. Determine prior upper quarter trauma such as motor vehicle accident with cervical spine injury or blunt trauma directly over the superior aspect of the shoulder and upper trapezius region.
            4. Determine concomitant medical conditions such as diabetes mellitus, hyperthyroidism or hypothyroidism, arthritis or other systemic neurological disease.
        B. Symptoms
            1. Upper trunk plexopathies (C5-C6) produce more proximal symptoms, including the face, scapular, and interscapular regions.[26] Distal paresthesia and pain in median or ulnar nerve distribution or C5-C6 dermatome.

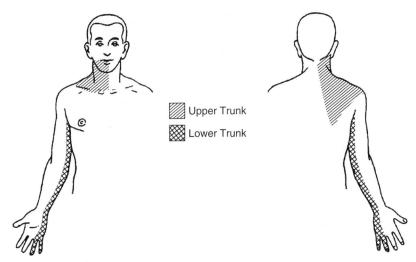

FIG. **15-3** Illustration of the distribution of symptoms that may involve the upper trunk or lower trunk of the brachial plexus. (From Mackin EJ, Callahan AD, Skirven TM, et al. [eds]: Hunter-Mackin-Callahan Rehabilitation of the Hand and Upper Extremity. 5th Ed. Mosby, St. Louis, 2002.)

    2. Lower trunk plexopathies (C8-T1) produce more distal symptoms over the medial aspect of the arm, forearm, and ulnar aspect of the hand (Fig. 15-3).

    3. Cord or division level plexopathies produce even greater variability of symptoms. The use of a body diagram may provide further insight.

    4. Early neurogenic symptoms: muscle performance deficits, altered sensibility, ANS changes (hyperhidrosis, vasomotor instability, burning pain),[27] headache.[28]

    5. Late neurogenic symptoms: pain, paresthesia, intrinsic muscle loss, sensory loss, and reflex changes.[13] Pencil pointing of digits of involved nerve.

C. Diagnostic tests

    1. Radiography: to detect presence of cervical rib or bony pathology

    2. Arteriography: to detect occlusion of subclavian or axillary artery

    3. Somatosensory evoked potentials[28,29]

    4. Electromyography (EMG)/nerve conduction velocity (NCV) studies of antebrachial cutaneous nerve to locate level of lesion[29-31]

D. Observation

    1. Postural examination in sitting and standing

       a. Fig. 15-4 demonstrates cervical asymmetry with rotation and lateral flexion to the involved side, accompanied by shoulder girdle elevation and increased upper trapezius muscle tone. This may suggest an attempt by the patient to alleviate tension on the brachial plexus.

    2. Edema in supraclavicular fossa or extremity, muscular atrophy, trophic changes, temperature or color changes

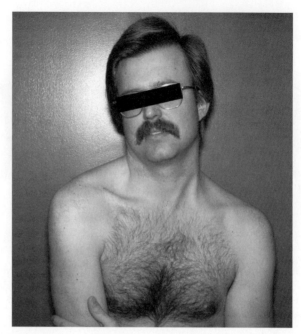

FIG. **15-4**   Patient attempting to reduce tension on the brachial plexus with ipsilateral cervical rotation and side bending and shoulder girdle elevation. (From Mackin EJ, Callahan AD, Skirven TM, et al. [eds]: Hunter-Mackin-Callahan Rehabilitation of the Hand and Upper Extremity. 5th Ed. Mosby, St. Louis, 2002.)

    3. Upper extremity positioning: shoulder adduction/internal rotation, elbow flexion, forearm neutral, and wrist and digital flexion may be used by patient to reduce neural tension via distal joints[32,33] (Fig. 15-5, *A*).

E. Upper quarter screening
    1. Cervical screen: include Spurling's test for foraminal encroachment[34] and vertebral artery test[35]
    2. Myotomal screen: reflex testing, grip and pinch strength
    3. Sensory evaluation using vibrometry and cutaneous pressure monofilaments. Look for dermatomal, brachial plexus, or peripheral nerve distributions.

F. Neural tissue examination
    1. Tinel's sign in supraclavicular fossa and peripheral nerve trunks to assess neural hyperalgesia or pathology
    2. Active motion dysfunction[36]: Determine whether imparting tension on the PNS in various locations alters active motion of the cervical spine or upper extremity.
       a. Observe resting posture for signs that the patient is attempting to reduce adverse neural tension (see Fig 15-5, *A*).
       b. Have patient move shoulder into comfortable coronal plane abduction and note range of motion (ROM) (see Fig. 15-5, *B*).
       c. Have patient move cervical spine into lateral flexion and rotation away from painful side and measure shoulder abduction or degree of elbow flexion. Repeat with the cervical

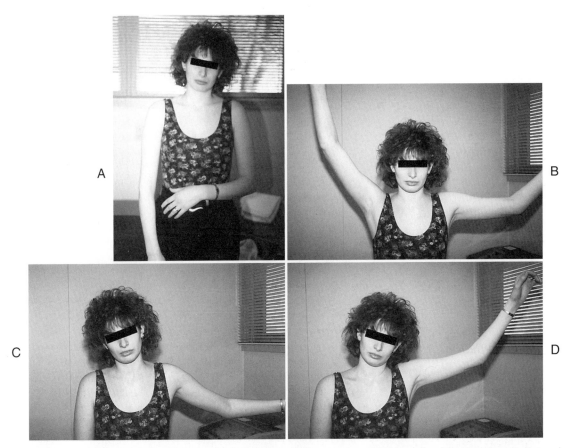

FIG. 15-5 Photographs of active motion dysfunction. **A,** Resting posture. **B,** Active shoulder elevation. **C,** Coronal plane abduction with contralateral cervical lateral flexion. **D,** Coronal plane shoulder abduction with ipsilateral cervical lateral flexion. Note the change in shoulder abduction with the change in cervical position. (From Mackin EJ, Callahan AD, Skirven TM, et al. [eds]: Hunter-Mackin-Callahan Rehabilitation of the Hand and Upper Extremity. 5th Ed. Mosby, St. Louis, 2002.)

   spine in flexion and rotation toward the painful side, and measure comfortable shoulder abduction or elbow flexion. A decrease in abduction or increase in elbow flexion with contralateral cervical motion and an increase in abduction or elbow extension with ipsilateral cervical motion may indicate a neurogenic component to the patient's pain complaint (see Fig. 15-5, *C* and *D*).

3. Passive motion dysfunction: Upper limb tension testing (ULTT) as first described by Elvey[9] and refined by Butler,[14,37] systematically places the neurovascular structures of the upper extremity into segmental tension.

   a. Do not move beyond encountered resistance (muscle guarding) or symptom provocation to avoid exacerbation. Perform on noninvolved side first to determine patient's normal response.

   b. For base maneuver with median nerve bias, patient is supine with therapist facing patient. Carefully bring shoulder into comfortable abduction, then external rotation, forearm supination, wrist/finger extension, and elbow extension in sequence. Measure final position of each joint when resistance or symptom provocation is encountered. If additional tension is required to provoke symptoms, shoulder girdle depression and/or contralateral cervical flexion may be added (Fig. 15-6). To bias the radial and ulnar nerves, see Table 15-3.

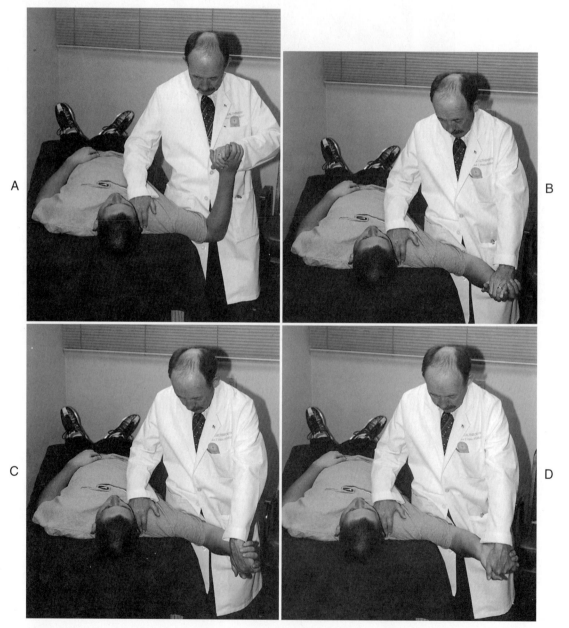

FIG. 15-6 Photographs of the successive application of the steps of the median nerve (base) upper limb tension test. **A,** Shoulder abduction. **B,** Shoulder external rotation. **C,** Forearm supination. **D,** Wrist/hand extension.

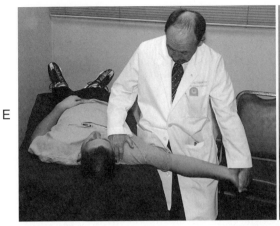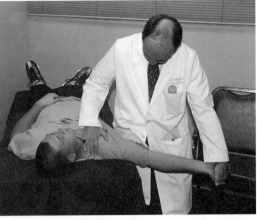

FIG. **15-6, cont'd E,** Elbow extension. **F,** Additional sensitizing motions of contralateral cervical flexion and scapular depression. (From Mackin EJ, Callahan AD, Skirven TM, et al. [eds]: Hunter-Mackin-Callahan Rehabilitation of the Hand and Upper Extremity. 5th Ed. Mosby, St. Louis, 2002.)

G. Provocative tests, including Adson's test[7], the stress hyperabduction test (Wright's test)[1], the costoclavicular maneuver,[38] and Roo's test,[39] may be performed. These provocative positions can potentially place adverse tension on the PNS or brachial plexus, exacerbating the patient's symptoms and creating false-positive findings.

H. Palpation: Pectoralis minor and deltopectoral fascia tightness, myofascial trigger points,[20] muscle spasm of cervical and shoulder girdle, sternoclavicular joint tenderness. Local tender points in tissues innervated by hypothesized involved nerve.[36]

II. Treatment

A. General considerations

1. Multisystem involvement (glenohumeral joint pathology, trigger points, double/multiple crush syndromes, and mechanical cervical or thoracic spine involvement) is often present and may necessitate longer-term conservative measures. These entities may need to be managed before the brachial plexus component of the patient's symptomatology is addressed.

TABLE **15-3** Upper Extremity Neural Tension Testing Components

Median Nerve	Ulnar Nerve	Radial Nerve
Shoulder abduction	Shoulder abduction	Shoulder abduction
Shoulder external rotation	Shoulder external rotation	Shoulder internal rotation
Forearm supination	Forearm supination or pronation	Forearm pronation
Wrist/finger extension	Wrist/finger extension	Wrist/index-thumb flexion
Elbow extension	Elbow flexion	Elbow extension
Shoulder depression	Shoulder depression	Shoulder depression
Cervical contralateral lateral flexion	Cervical contralateral lateral flexion	Cervical contralateral lateral flexion

From Mackin EJ, Callahan AD, Skirven TM, et al. (eds): Hunter-Mackin-Callahan Rehabilitation of the Hand and Upper Extremity. 5th Ed. Mosby, St. Louis, 2002.

2. The longer the duration of symptoms, the longer conservative care may be necessary.

3. BPTI patients who have more complex pain patterns involving the CNS and ANS along with affective and motivational issues may not attain complete symptom resolution. The goal for these patients may be an improved quality of life through symptom control and improved ROM allowing them to use their upper extremity in a more functional manner.

B. Stage I: Symptom Control Phase
   1. Primary goal is symptom control and relief.
   2. Behavior modification
      a. Proper extremity positioning to avoid tension across brachial plexus and vascular structures
         (1) Use opposite extremity to support involved extremity (Fig. 15-7).
         (2) Rest affected extremity on armrest of chair or pillow on lap.
         (3) Place hand in coat pocket or in belt loop while standing or walking.
      b. Avoid strenuous aerobic activity, which may create exertional breathing. This may increase accessory muscle activity, potentially compromising neurovascular structures in the thoracic inlet.

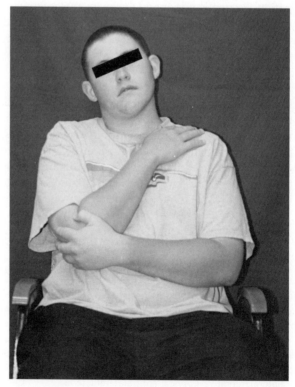

FIG. **15-7** Brachial plexus slack position, Note the posture of the head and cervical spine favoring the involved side. (From Mackin EJ, Callahan AD, Skirven TM, et al. [eds]: Hunter-Mackin-Callahan Rehabilitation of the Hand and Upper Extremity. 5th Ed. Mosby, St. Louis, 2002.)

    c. Implementation of a low-impact, tolerable aerobic exercise program

    d. Avoid all motions and activities that exacerbate symptoms.

    e. Avoid direct pressure over thoracic inlet, such as bra straps and automobile seat belts. Additional padding that increases the surface area of these items may help dissipate these forces.

    f. Avoid carrying heavy objects, including handbags, that increase shoulder depression and place tension across the neurovascular structures.

3. Postural and positional modifications

    a. Minimize postural faults, but avoid overcorrecting these postures, because this may exacerbate symptoms by placing additional adverse tension on the brachial plexus, peripheral nerves, or nerve roots. These postural changes may indicate long-standing tissue adaptations, and an attempt to correct them too quickly may adversely affect the patient's symptoms.

    b. Sleep with involved extremity supported to minimize tension on the brachial plexus. Support cervical spine in neutral position. May be beneficial to exchange sides of bed with significant other.

    c. Modification of workplace environment may be necessary. Avoid overhead activity as well as prolonged static positioning.

4. Diaphragmatic breathing allows for accessory muscle relaxation and improved circumferential excursion of the thoracic cavity.

5. Patient education must occur during each session to address and reinforce these concepts. Only if the therapist presents these concepts in a consistent and appropriate manner will the patient take them seriously. Involving family members in the educational process may also help increase patient awareness while at home.

6. Begin to address secondary problems such as trigger points and muscle spasm. Modulate pain through modalities and exercise, and address double or multiple crush problems.

7. Initiate general nerve mobilization techniques.

    a. Glide versus tension: Tension creates length changes within the nerve by simultaneously pulling on both ends of the nerve, causing it to unfold.[40,41] This has a profound effect on the nerves' neurophysiology because of alterations in vascular and axoplasmic flow. Glide refers to placing tension on a nerve at one point while releasing tension at another. In theory, the overall tension remains unchanged. In the irritable patient, glide may be the most appropriate approach. Box 15-1 summarizes the guidelines a clinician should consider when initiating a treatment strategy.

    b. Begin at a remote site away from the hypothesized location of injury, using the spine and lower extremities to glide the neural tissue in pain-free and tension-free range.

BOX **15-1** Treatment Guidelines

Working knowledge/understanding of the ULTT components
    Evaluation/reevaluation
        Response to treatment change
        Hypothesis of location and tissues at fault
    Tension versus glide (excursion)
        Tension: lengthens the nerve, stresses vascular supply
        Glide: tension in one location and release in another
    Irritable versus nonirritable
        Irritable: gliding (tissue barrier/muscle guarding), selected component
            distal to site (lower extremity or trunk), pain-free range, tension free
        Nonirritable: tension (+) symptoms (mild), rapid recovery, selected
            component/nerve directly involved
    Neural versus nonneural
        Treat nonneural tissues directly with neural tension eliminated (brachial
            plexus slack position)
        Treat nonneural tissues under neural tension (nonirritable)
    Intraneural versus extraneural fibrosis
        Intraneural: attempt to increase mobility away from the site
        Extraneural: treat interfacing tissue in conjunction with glide/tension

From Mackin EJ, Callahan AD, Skirven TM, et al. (eds): Hunter-Mackin-Callahan Rehabilitation of the Hand and Upper Extremity. 5th Ed. Mosby, St. Louis, 2002.

C. Stage II: Restoration Phase
1. Begin only after comfort and symptom control have been achieved.
2. Be mindful of any active motion dysfunction resulting from neurogenic involvement to avoid the end-ranges of motion, which may lead to adverse tension and exacerbation of pain.
3. Soft tissue mobilization, described by Smith,[42] may be instituted to restore normal tissue resting lengths and normal posture. Begin joint mobilization of the glenohumeral, scapulothoracic, acromioclavicular, and sternoclavicular joints and first rib. Begin to address cervical spine dysfunction. Avoid placing adverse tension on the brachial plexus during these techniques.
4. Progress nerve mobilization techniques as dictated by patient response and with continual clinical reasoning to avoid further exacerbation or injury. Any symptom provocation should be transient in nature.
    a. Nerve mobilization may be graded according to Maitland's gradation[43] for joint mobilization, using the first half (pain-free range) of the available ROM for symptom control and the last half (guarded or end-range) of the available ROM for restoration of mobility.
    b. Use components of the ULTT in the pain-free range. Begin at a remote site such as the wrist or forearm, and progress toward hypothesized involved site or nerve.

   c. There are no clear guidelines or research to support the most effective amplitude, dosage, or duration necessary to achieve the desired result. Elvey and colleagues[44] recommended that end-range grades not be used, and that the duration should be less than that for joint mobilization. Butler[37] recommended pain-free midrange and end-range mobilizations for an irritable disorder, lasting 20 to 30 seconds for an initial treatment.

  5. Home program

   a. Because of the long-standing nature of the problems faced by this patient population, a home program may be more important than specific hands-on techniques. It is only over an extended period that the adaptive tissue changes can be corrected and balances between the soft tissues and neurovascular structures restored.

   b. Many home exercises are designed to improve flexibility of the entire thoracic outlet. Examples of some common home exercises can be found in Chapter 9. These exercises may need to be modified to avoid placing tension on the brachial plexus, its vascular structures, and the peripheral nerves, by placing the distal limb segments in brachial plexus slack position while working proximal segments such as cervical spine or scapulothoracic articulation.

   c. Examples of home exercises for nerve gliding are pictured in Fig. 15-8, *A* and *B*.

  6. Scapulothoracic stabilization techniques in quadruped position or use of therapeutic ball may help optimize scapulothoracic motor control.

  7. Gradually advance a low-impact aerobic exercise program in the form of walking, stationary bicycling, or treadmill walking. Avoid activities that require excessive cervical or upper extremity motion, which may cause adverse tension on the brachial plexus.

  8. Handling these patients too aggressively with manual techniques or exercise may only result in restoring their initial level of tissue irritability.

 D. Stage III: Rehabilitative Phase

  1. Maximize aerobic capacity and fitness.

  2. Encourage proper nutritional habits, particularly for overweight patients, because obesity has been associated with TOS.[45]

  3. Strengthen postural muscles to restore proper muscle balance between weak, elongated posterior groups and tight anterior groups.

  4. Reversal of long-standing postural faults may not be a realistic expectation, but diligence in reversing the offending posture frequently throughout the day is.

  5. Perform work-conditioning exercises in the clinic that are task specific. Modify these tasks to avoid inappropriate stresses across the brachial plexus region. Continue to incorporate proper posture and breathing.

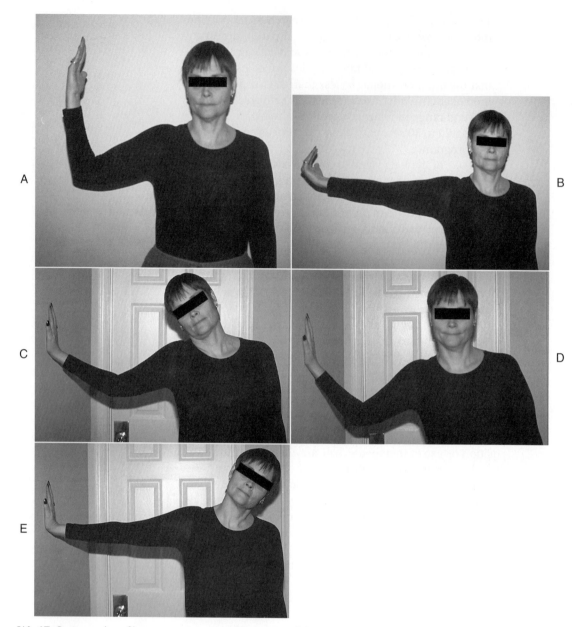

FIG. **15-8** Examples of home exercises used for nerve mobilization. **A** and **B,** Gliding: Note that as tension occurs in one location (elbow extension), it is released at another location (wrist flexion). **C** and **D,** Tension: Note that tension is added at one joint (cervical) while the positions of the other joints of the upper extremity are maintained. **E,** Progression of tension by adding cervical contralateral flexion and elbow extension. (From Mackin EJ, Callahan AD, Skirven TM, et al. [eds]: Hunter-Mackin-Callahan Rehabilitation of the Hand and Upper Extremity. 5th Ed. Mosby, St. Louis, 2002.)

6. Specific nerve gliding or "tensioning" maneuvers may be performed to address localized and secondary involvement of the PNS.
   a. Begin only after symptoms are mild and absent at rest and recovery from exacerbation is rapid.
   b. Institute end-range mobilizations where mild muscle guarding or symptom provocation is encountered.

Progress toward hypothesized location of involvement in an effort to recover mobility.
c. Examples of nerve-tensioning exercises used in a home program are pictured in Fig. 15-8, *C*, *D*, and *E*.
d. Periodic visits to the clinic may be needed to adjust the exercise prescription, to apply more specific exercise or nerve mobilization techniques.
e. Complete resolution of symptoms may not be seen.

NONOPERATIVE COMPLICATIONS

The predominant complication of conservative management of patients with BPN is exacerbation of their symptoms. If the manual intervention or exercise prescription is too aggressive, any progress made may necessitate a return to the stage I level of treatment to regain symptom control and comfort. It is also conceivable that aggravation of the patient's symptoms beyond the initial complaint may occur with treatment that is too aggressive.

SURGICAL INDICATIONS

I. First rib resection versus neurolysis of brachial plexus or cervical rib resection
II. Surgery after failure of conservative measures (3 months of therapy)

POSTOPERATIVE INDICATIONS/PRECAUTIONS FOR THERAPY

I. Indications
   A. Failure of conservative management
   B. Pain, edema, loss of motion, loss of function
II. Precautions
   A. Monitor wound for excessive drainage or infection.
   B. Protect extremity with an arm sling in crowded areas or while riding in a car.
   C. Avoid painful positions or activities.

POSTOPERATIVE THERAPY

There is a paucity of literature addressing postoperative care after thoracic outlet surgery. General postoperative guidelines have been suggested by some.[46,47]

I. Week 1: Pain-free active ROM (AROM) and active-assisted ROM exercises for shoulder, wound care, nerve mobilization of distal segments, and cervical AROM exercises
II. Weeks 2 to 3: Gentle, progressive AROM for shoulder complex; continue nerve gliding exercises for brachial plexus to minimize adhesion formation; begin scar mobilization and desensitization
III. Weeks 4 to 5: Progressive use of upper extremity for light activity; begin gentle strengthening exercise to cervical and shoulder girdle musculature

IV. Weeks 6 to 7: Ergonomic training, progression of strengthening program

V. Weeks 8 to 12: Progressive work-conditioning program and full use of involved extremity as tolerated

POSTOPERATIVE COMPLICATIONS[48]

I. Hematoma formation around the brachial plexus

II. Injury to the thoracic duct, which may leak proteinaceous fluid, resulting in dense scar formation around the plexus, if not repaired

III. Phrenic nerve injury

IV. Temporary motor dysfunction as a result of intraoperative traction during dissection of plexus from scar tissue

V. Injury to the long thoracic nerve

VI. Mild numbness and paresthesia, which may be accompanied by hypersensitivity along the peripheral nerve distribution due to manipulation of the plexus

VII. Horner's syndrome

VIII. Vascular injury

EVALUATION TIMELINE

The initial evaluation, as described earlier, is carried out on the patient's first visit to the clinic. Depending on the level of irritability, it may not be possible to collect all data due to symptom exacerbation. The remainder of the initial data collection can be carried out over the next several visits as symptoms allow.

Reevaluation is an ongoing process that occurs at each visit. Formal reports should be generated every 4 weeks and communicated to the referring physician. Minimal progress toward stated therapy goals or persistent exacerbation of symptoms requires a review of the appropriateness of goals, the interventions being used, and the likelihood of further clinical improvement.

OUTCOMES

There are numerous studies in the literature that support the use of conservative management of TOS and BPTI before surgical intervention is considered.[45,49-51] Therapeutic interventions in these studies included patient education, activity and postural modification, ergonomic intervention, diaphragmatic breathing, stretching of shortened muscles, strengthening of postural muscles, myofascial release, pain management, conditioning exercises, and a home exercise program. Outcomes reported have included subjective improvement ranging from 59% to 88.1%.

REFERENCES

1. Wright IS: The neurovascular syndrome produced by hyperabduction of the arm. Am Heart J 29:1, 1945

2. Sunderland S: The connective tissues of peripheral nerves. Brain 88:841, 1965

3. Lundborg G, et al.: Peripheral nerve: the physiology of injury and repair. In Woo S, Buckwalter J (eds): American Academy of Orthopedic Surgeons Symposium: Injury and Repair of the Musculoskeletal Soft Tissues. AAOS, Park Ridge, IL, 1998

4. Millesi H, Zoch T, Rath T: The gliding apparatus of peripheral nerve and its clinical significance. Ann Chir Main Memb Super 9:87, 1990

5. Lew PC, Morrow CJ, Lew AM: The effect of neck and leg flexion and their sequence on the lumbar spinal cord. Spine 19:2421, 1994

6. O'Connell JE: The clinical signs of meningeal irritation. Brain 69:9, 1946

7. Adson A, Coffey JR: Cervical rib: a method of anterior approach for relief of symptoms by division of the scalenus anticus. Ann Surg 85:839, 1927

8. Elvey R: Treatment of arm pain associated with abnormal brachial plexus tension. Aust J Physiother 32:225, 1986

9. Elvey R: Brachial plexus tension test and the pathoanatomical origin of arm pain. In Glasgow E, Tavomey L (eds): Aspects of Manipulative Therapy. Lincoln Institute of Health Sciences, Melbourne, Australia, 1979

10. Capistrant T: Thoracic outlet syndrome in whiplash injury. Ann Surg 185:175, 1977

11. Weinberg H, Nathan H, Magora F, et al.: Arthritis of the first costovertebral joint as a cause of thoracic outlet syndrome. Clin Orthop 86:159, 1972

12. Willshire WH: Supernumerary first rib clinical records. Lancet 2:633, 1860

13. Leffert R: Thoracic outlet syndrome. Hand Clin 8:285, 1992

14. Butler D, Gifford L: The concept of adverse mechanical tension in the nervous system: part 2. Examination and treatment. Physiotherapy 75:629, 1989

15. Shacklock M: Positive upper limb tension test in a case of surgically proven neuropathy: analysis and validity. Man Ther 1:154, 1996

16. Lundborg G: Intraneural microcirculation. Orthop Clin North Am 19:1, 1988

17. Mackinnon SE, Dellon AL: Experimental study of chronic nerve compression clinical implications. Hand Clin 2:639, 1986

18. Asbury A, Fields H: Pain due to peripheral nerve damage: an hypothesis. Neurology 34:1587, 1984

19. Bennett GJ: Neuropathic pain. In Wall PD, Melzack R (eds): Textbook of Pain. 3rd Ed. Churchill Livingstone, New York, 1994, p. 201

20. Travell J, Simmons D: Myofascial Pain and Dysfunction: The Triggerpoint Manual. Williams & Wilkins, Baltimore, 1983

21. Leffert R, Cumley G: The relationship between dead arm syndrome and thoracic outlet syndrome. Clin Orthop 223:20-31, 1987.

22. Upton A, McComas A: The double crush in nerve entrapment syndrome. Lancet 2:359-362, 1973

23. Urschel HC Jr, Razzuk MA, Wood RE, et al.: Objective diagnosis (ulnar nerve conduction velocity) and current therapy of the thoracic outlet syndrome. Ann Thorac Surg 12:608-620, 1979

24. Eurroll R, Hurst L: The relationship of thoracic outlet syndrome and carpal tunnel syndrome. Clin Orthop 164:149-153, 1982

25. MacKinnon S: Double and multiple "crush" syndromes: double and multiple entrapment neuropathies. Hand Clin 8:369-390, 1992

26. Jamieson WG, Chinnick B: Thoracic outlet syndrome: fact or fancy? A review of 409 consecutive patients who underwent operation. Can J Surg 39:321-326, 1996

27. Adson AW: Cervical ribs: symptoms, differential diagnosis, and indications for section of the insertion of the scalenus anticus muscle. J Int Coll Surg 14:546, 1951

28. Raskin NH, Howard MW, Ehrenfeld WK: Headache as the leading symptom of the thoracic outlet syndrome. Headache 25:208-210, 1985

29. Komanetsky RM, Novak CB, Mackinnon SE, et al.: Somatosensory evoked potentials fail to diagnosis thoracic outlet syndrome. J Hand Surg Am 21:662, 1996

30. LeForestier N, Moulonguet A, Maisonobe T, et al.: True neurogenic thoracic outlet syndrome: electrophysiological diagnosis in six cases. Muscle Nerve 21:1129, 1998

31. Yiannikas C, Walsh JC: Somatosensory evoked responses in the diagnosis of thoracic outlet syndrome. J Neurol Neurosurg Psychiatry 46:234, 1983

32. Quinter J: Stretch induced cervicobrachial pain syndrome. Aust J Physiother 36:99, 1990

33. Pollach W: Surgical anatomy of the thoracic outlet syndrome. Surg Gynecol Obstet 150:97, 1980

34. Spurling RG, Scoville WB: Lateral rupture of the cervical intervertebral discs: a common cause of shoulder and arm pain. Surg Gynecol Obstet 78:350, 1944

35. Hopenfield S (ed): Physical Examination of the Spine and Extremities. Appleton-Century-Crofts, New York, 1976.

36. Elvey R: Physical evaluation of the nervous system in disorders of pain and dysfunction. J Hand Ther 10:122, 1997

37. Butler D: Adverse mechanical tension in the nervous system: a model for assessment and treatment. Aust J Physiother 35:27, 1989
38. Falconer MA, Weddell G: Costoclavicular compression of the subclavian artery and vein: relation to the scalenus anticus syndrome. Lancet 2:539, 1943
39. Roos D, Owens C: Thoracic outlet syndrome. Arch Surg 93:71, 1966
40. Kleinrensink GJ, Stoeckart R, Mulder PG, et al.: Upper limb tension tests as tools in the diagnosis of nerve and plexus lesions: anatomical and biomechanical aspects. Clin Biomech 15:9, 2000
41. Wright T, Glowczewskie F, Wheeler D, et al: Excursion and strain of the median nerve. J Bone Joint Surg Am 78:1897, 1996
42. Smith K: The thoracic outlet syndrome: a protocol of treatment. J Orthop Sports Phys Ther 1:89-99, 1979
43. Maitland GD: Treatment of the glenohumeral joint by passive movement. Physiotherapy 60:3, 1983
44. Elvey R, Quinter J, Thomas A: A clinical study of RSI. Aust Fam Physician 15:1314, 1986
45. Novak C, Collins D, Mackinnon S: Outcome following conservative management of thoracic outlet syndrome. J Hand Surg Am 20:542, 1995
46. Anthony MS: Thoracic outlet syndrome. In Clark GL, Wilgis EFS, Aiello B, et al. (eds): Hand Rehabilitation: A Practical Guide. Churchill Livingstone, New York, 1993
47. Wishchuk JR, Dougherty CR: Therapy after thoracic outlet release. Hand Clin 20:87, 2004
48. Whitenack SH, Hunter JM, Read RL: Thoracic outlet syndrome: a brachial plexopathy. In Mackin EJ, et al. (eds): Rehabilitation of the Hand and Upper Extremity. 5th Ed. Mosby, St. Louis, 2002, p. 727
49. Ingesson E, Ribbe E, Norgren L: Thoracic outlet syndrome: evaluation of a physiotherapeutical method. Man Med 2:86, 1986
50. Sucher B: Thoracic outlet syndrome—a myofascial variant: part 2. Treatment Journal of the Osteopathic Association 90:810, 1990
51. Lindgren KA: Conservative treatment of thoracic outlet syndrome: a 2-year follow-up. Arch Phys Med Rehabil 78:373, 1997

Complex Regional Pain Syndrome

16

Romina P. Astifidis

DEFINITION

Complex regional pain syndrome (CRPS), formerly known as reflex sympathetic dystrophy (RSD), is generally a posttraumatic neuropathic syndrome, found in adults (rarely in children), that is characterized by pain and vasomotor/sudomotor changes in the involved limb or limbs. In 1993, during a conference of the International Association for the Study of Pain, terminology was established dividing CRPS into two types, type 1 and type 2, with the presence of a peripheral nerve insult distinguishing the two (Box 16-1).

The cause of CRPS has not been definitively established. Generally, theories involve some sort of neurogenic inflammation that perpetuates itself.

BOX 16-1 International Association for the Study of Pain (IASP) Criteria for Complex Regional Pain Syndrome (CRPS)

CRPS TYPE I (RSD)
Develops after an initiating noxious event
Spontaneous pain or allodynia/hyperalgesia occurs but is not limited to a single peripheral nerve
Pain is disproportionate to the inciting event
Evidence of edema, skin blood flow abnormality, or abnormal sudomotor activity in the region of the pain
Diagnosis is excluded by the existence of conditions that would otherwise account for the degree of pain and dysfunction

CRPS TYPE II (CAUSALGIA)
Develops after a nerve injury
Spontaneous pain or allodynia/hyperalgesia occurs and is not necessarily limited to the territory of the injured nerve
Evidence of edema, skin blood flow abnormality, or abnormal sudomotor activity in the region of the pain

---

From Stanton-Hicks M, Janig W, Hassenbusch S, et al.: Pain 63:127-133, 1995.

There may be no inciting event, or CRPS can occur after surgery, trauma, or local and systemic disease. Diagnosis of CRPS is primarily based on clinical findings that are listed in treatment indications.

Diagnostic testing, including vascular studies, electrodiagnostic studies, radiographic studies, and blood tests, should initially be geared toward ruling out other conditions. Other tests, including thermography, sweat testing, and sympathetic blocks, can be used to aid in the diagnosis of CRPS, although they are not always positive.

The key to successful treatment of CRPS, aside from prevention, is early diagnosis and intervention. Any symptoms that are recognized or suspected should be addressed immediately to ensure correction and restoration of maximum function.

TREATMENT PURPOSE

The various symptoms of CRPS can severely limit functional use of the extremity, altering the patient's ability to participate in activities of daily living (ADLs), leisure, or vocational activities. Treatment should include an aggressive multidisciplinary team approach that addresses not only the physical aspects of the disorder but also the emotional and psychosocial aspects. Treatment should also include extensive patient education, including information about the condition as well as activity modification and symptom management.

TREATMENT GOALS

    I.   To decrease or eliminate pain, edema and other symptoms
   II. To restore maximum mobility
  III. To restore maximum function
  IV. To restore patient confidence that he or she will get better

NONOPERATIVE INDICATIONS/PRECAUTIONS

Treatment is indicated after diagnosis of CRPS is made. Often, the therapist is the first clinician to observe symptoms indicative of CRPS. It is imperative to consult the physician immediately on suspicion of CRPS, because often both therapeutic and medical interventions are needed for appropriate management (Fig. 16-1).

    I.   Indications for immediate treatment include *abnormal* presentations of any of the following signs and symptoms.[1,2]
       A. Pain: often spreading beyond the area of original injury
          1. Described as burning, pressure, searing, stabbing
          2. Allodynia: pain from mechanical or thermal sources that usually do not cause pain
          3. Hyperalgesia: magnified response to a painful stimulus
          4. Hyperpathia: pain that persists after the removal of noxious stimulus; pain that is disproportionately increased by a stimulus, especially a repetitive stimulus
       B. Edema: initially soft, but can change to brawny and eventually to periarticular stiffness
       C. Stiffness, contracture, palmar fasciitis
       D. Discoloration: redness, mottling, cyanosis

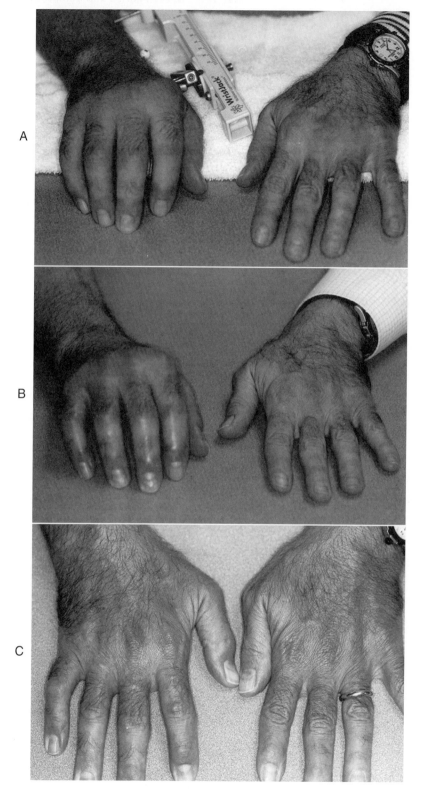

FIG. **16-1 A,** In this patient, symptoms of complex regional pain syndrome (CRPS) began 6 weeks after distal radius fracture treated with external fixation. **B,** Symptoms worsened after external fixation was removed. Discoloration, swelling, and stiffness were prominent features. **C,** Symptoms resolved after three stellate blocks and 5 months of therapy. Motion was restored except for recalcitrant proximal interphalangeal (PIP) joint contracture in small finger.

   E. Abnormal temperature
   F. Abnormal hair growth and texture
   G. Hyperhydrosis (early stage), anhydrosis (late stage)
   H. Hypertrophic or atrophic nails: usually in late stages
   I. Motor dysfunction, including tremor, dystonia, muscle spasms
      or weakness
   J. Osseous demineralization
   K. Palmar nodules (palmar fasciitis)
II.   Precautions
   A. Overly aggressive range of motion (ROM) by therapist and/or
      patient or modalities causing increased symptoms
   B. Overly aggressive manipulation or passive range of motion
      (PROM) on stiff joints under the influence of pain-altering
      treatments including medications and blocks

NONOPERATIVE TREATMENT (FIG. 16-2)

I.   Therapy: Treatment may include a combination of various
     techniques based on clinical reasoning, with modifications as
     needed if symptoms worsen.
   A. Pain management
      1. Transcutaneous electrical nerve stimulation (TENS)[3,4,6]
      2. Superficial heating modalities.[5,6] Cooling modalities can be
         considered if signs of vasodilation are noted and cold is well
         tolerated by the patient.[6]
      3. Contrast baths: use is controversial, because the bath may
         create (or worsen) an unstable vasomotor state.[5,6] Clinically,
         contrast baths are considered to promote desensitization and
         reduction of edema and to reset sensory thresholds, although
         there is no research to support these claims.[3,5,6]
   B. Edema management
      1. Elevation with and without gentle, pain-free active range of
         motion (AROM)[6]
      2. Sensory-level high-voltage pulsed current[7]
      3. Intermittent pneumatic compression[5]
      4. Compression gloves/stockings
      5. Massage: Avoid cyclic stimulation as provided in retrograde
         massage, because it may increase allodynia.[6]
   C. Sensory management: Protect sensitive areas between
      stimulation sessions.
      1. Vibration[3,6]
      2. Desensitization: including textures, immersion, pressure,
         fluidotherapy
      3. Sphygmomanometer cuff applied proximal to painful area to
         provide analgesia and allow desensitization[3]
   D. Vasomotor management
      1. Generalized aerobic exercise to increase circulation[4,6]
      2. Dietary changes to include avoidance of caffeine (causes
         vasoconstriction) and alcohol (causes vasodilation)
      3. Topical heat and ultrasound to increase blood flow[6]
      4. Stress-loading program with modifications, as needed, based
         on type of injury[8] (Fig. 16-3).
      5. Temperature biofeedback

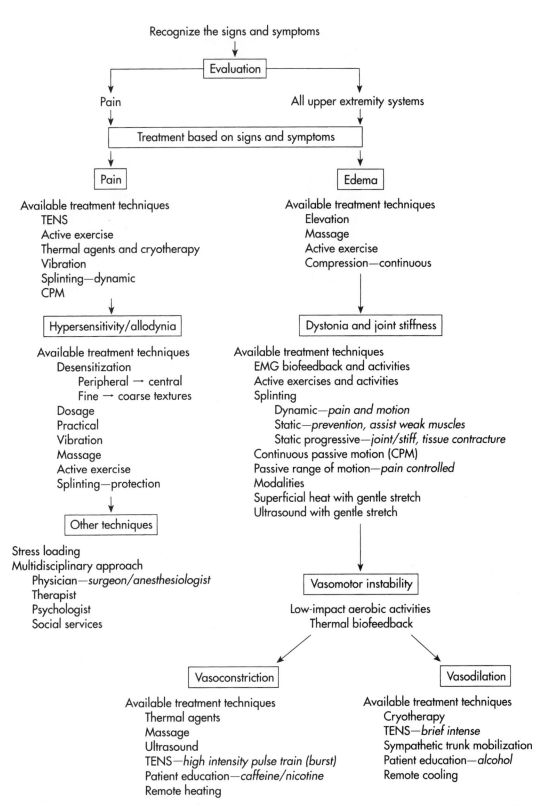

FIG. **16-2** Algorithm for evaluation and treatment. EMG, Electromyograph; TENS, transcutaneous electrical nerve stimulation. (From Walsh MT, Muntzer E: Therapist's management of complex regional pain syndrome [reflex sympathetic dystrophy]. In Mackin EJ, Callahan AD, Skirven TM, et al. [eds]: Hunter-Mackin-Callahan Rehabilitation of the Hand and Upper Extremity. 5th Ed. Mosby, St. Louis, 2002.)

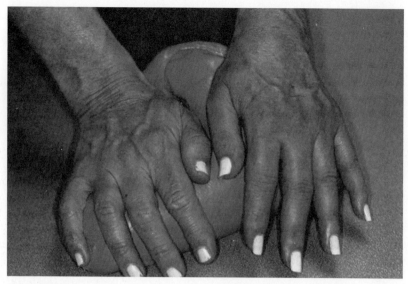

FIG. **16-3** Weight-bearing on putty with modified angle due to distal radius fracture that limits wrist extension.

E. Motion/strength
   1. Frequent gentle AROM of entire limb without increasing pain; PROM used with care if tolerated
   2. Blocked exercises and tendon gliding[1]
   3. Functional activities
   4. Continuous passive motion (CPM) machine[3-5]
   5. Splinting: Position in resting/safe position at night to limit nonfunctional contractures; use dynamic splint if tolerated to increase motion.[4,6]
   6. Strengthening: Begin with isometric and progress to isotonic as tolerated.
F. Patient education
   1. Symptom management
   2. Joint protection
   3. Work simplification/vocational rehabilitation
   4. Assistive devices to increase independence
   5. Support groups
   6. Psychological counseling, including relaxation techniques, imagery, hypnosis, and coping skills.[9]
G. Other clinical treatments
   1. Manual edema mobilization (MEM)[6]
   2. Kinesiotaping
   3. Neural mobilization[6]
H. Regional anesthesia
   1. Sympathetic block (Fig. 16-4)
      a. Stellate: blocks are often done in series, with longer-lasting medications in later blocks.[10] It is critical that a successful block be followed by therapy within 24 hours, to take advantage of pain reduction in order to increase motion.[3]
      b. Sympatholytic medication
      c. Sympathectomy[10,11]

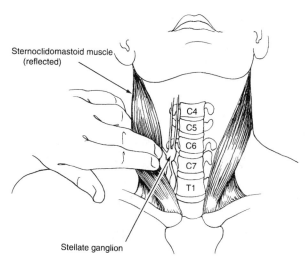

Sternoclidomastoid muscle
(reflected)

C4
C5
C6
C7
T1

Stellate ganglion

FIG. **16-4** Stellate ganglion block.

2. Somatic block (also blocks sympathetic nerves)
    a. Bier: intravenous regional block, often followed by therapy for motion exercises,[2] but may also receive manipulation while in operating room under anesthesia
    b. Intrathecal/epidural: indwelling or intermittent boluses of local anesthetic and opioid combinations[10]
    c. Local or regional somatic blocks
III. Pharmacological therapy[2,11]
    A. Oral steroids[1]: helpful early on to manage inflammation and stiffness
    B. Nonsteroidal antiinflammatory drugs[9,10]
    C. Antidepressant agents: to decrease pain, decrease depressive symptoms, and cause sedation to assist with sleeping patterns[9,11]
    D. Anticonvulsants[10]
    E. Topical analgesics: lidocaine transdermal patches
    F. Opiates[10]

NONOPERATIVE COMPLICATIONS

I.   Dystonia or contractions limiting function, even after CRPS is resolved
II. Persistent symptoms causing permanent impairment in function

POSTOPERATIVE THERAPY

Surgery is indicated if an inciting nerve lesion can be detected, such as a partial nerve injury or compressive disorder.

Surgical treatment (neuromodulation) is often beneficial if there is persistent pain, chronic in nature, not relieved by conservative measures. Therapy after surgical neuromodulation is similar to nonoperative therapy. The use of spinal cord stimulation,[2] peripheral nerve stimulation,[12] and intrathecal analgesia[2] decreases painful symptoms, allowing therapy to focus on improvement of motion and function.

POSTOPERATIVE COMPLICATIONS

I.   Persistent pain, dysfunction, and stiffness
II. Infection
III. Unsatisfactory positioning of stimulator[13]

EVALUATION TIMELINE[6]

I.   Initial evaluation: Some aspects may need to be adjusted or delayed based on patient tolerance.
   A. History, including mechanism of injury, previous treatment, and current symptoms
   B. Observation, including positioning, guarding of limb, and sudomotor, vasomotor, or trophic changes
   C. Initial AROM measurements in minimally symptomatic range
   D. Pain assessment, including standard quantitative measurements, body diagrams, McGill Pain Questionnaire, and pain patterns, including activities that improve or worsen pain
   E. Sensory screening, including monofilament discrimination and vibration testing. Delay if extreme hypersensitivity is present.
   F. Edema assessment, including volumetrics and circumferential testing
II. Additional evaluation as tolerated and if appropriate
   A. PROM, joint mobility, extrinsic/intrinsic tightness
   B. Strength measurements, including manual muscle testing, grip and pinch testing
   C. Pretreatment and posttreatment edema measurement
   D. Neural tension assessment
   E. Postural assessment
   F. Functional assessment, including ADLs, vocational and leisure activities.
III. Reevaluation with assessment of progress every 4 weeks

OUTCOMES

Outcome studies in the literature have been focused primarily on clinical features and epidemiology. The most important aspect found in outcome studies continues to be the importance of early intervention. Soucacos and colleagues, in a 1997 study,[14] demonstrated that with all types of RSD treatment is more effective if it is provided at an early stage, generally less than 4 months after the inciting event. Furthermore, Koman and co-workers[11] stated that 80% of patients treated within the first year after injury will show significant improvement, compared with only 50% of those treated after 1 year.

REFERENCES

1. Lankford LL: Reflex sympathetic dystrophy. In Hunter JM, Mackin EJ, Callahan AD (eds): Rehabilitation of the Hand: Surgery and Therapy. 4th Ed. Mosby, St. Louis, 1995
2. Rho RH, Brewer RP, Lamer TJ, et al.: Complex regional pain syndrome. Mayo Clin Proc 77:174-180, 2002
3. Hardy M, Hardy S: Reflex sympathetic dystrophy: the clinician's perspective. J Hand Ther 10:137-150, 1997

4. Hareau J: What makes treatment for reflex sympathetic dystrophy successful. J Hand Ther 9:367-370, 1996

5. Bengston K: Physical modalities for complex regional pain syndrome. Hand Clin 13:443-454, 1997

6. Walsh MT, Muntzer E: Therapist's management of complex regional pain syndrome (reflex sympathetic dystrophy). In Mackin EJ, Callahan AD, Skirven TM, et al. (eds): Hunter-Mackin-Callahan Rehabilitation of the Hand and Upper Extremity. 5th Ed. Mosby, St. Louis, 2002

7. Fedorczyk J: The role of physical agents in modulating pain. J Hand Ther 10:110-121, 1997

8. Watson HK, Carlson L: Treatment of reflex sympathetic dystrophy of the hand with an active "stress loading" program. J Hand Surg Am 12:779-785, 1987

9. Stanton-Hicks M, Janig W, Hassenbusch S, et al.: Consensus report. Complex regional pain syndromes: guidelines for therapy. Clin J Pain 14:155-166, 1998

10. Curran MJ, Astifidis R: Complex regional pain syndrome type 1 (formerly reflex sympathetic dystrophy). Orthop Phys Ther Clin North Am 10:649-665, 2001

11. Koman LA, et al.: Reflex sympathetic dystrophy (complex regional pain syndromes—types 1 and 2). In Mackin EJ, Callahan AD, Skirven TM, et al. (eds): Hunter-Mackin-Callahan Rehabilitation of the Hand and Upper Extremity. 5th Ed. Mosby, St. Louis, 2002

12. Cooney WP: Electrical stimulation and the treatment of complex regional pain syndromes of the upper extremity. Hand Clin 13:519-525, 1997

13. Kemler M, Barendse GA, van Kleef M, et al.: Spinal cord stimulation in patients with chronic reflex sympathetic dystrophy. N Engl J Med 343:618-624, 2000

14. Soucacos PN, Diznitsas LA, Beris AE, et al.: Reflex sympathetic dystrophy of the upper extremity. Hand Clin 13:339-354, 1997

SUGGESTED READINGS

Cooney WP, Schuind F (eds): Upper extremity pain dysfunction: somatic and sympathetic disorders. In: Hand Clinics. Vol. 13, No. 3. WB Saunders, Philadelphia, 1997

Stanton-Hicks M, Baron R, Boas R, et al.: Consensus report. Complex regional pain syndromes: guidelines for therapy. Clin J Pain 14:155-166, 1998

Walsh MT, Muntzer E: Therapist's management of complex regional pain syndrome (reflex sympathetic dystrophy). In Mackin EJ, Callahan AD, Skirven TM, et al. (eds): Hunter-Mackin-Callahan Rehabilitation of the Hand and Upper Extremity. 5th Ed. Mosby, St. Louis, 2002

PART **THREE**

Tendon Injuries

Flexor Tendon Repair

17

Mary Formby

The healing of the repaired flexor tendon is at least a 6-month process. The "best" way to manage the first 12-week period remains controversial despite significant research and clinical advances over the last 50 years. Effective communication among surgeon, therapist, and patient throughout the rehabilitation process is essential for achievement of a successful outcome.

DEFINITION

Tendon healing occurs by both intrinsic and extrinsic processes.[1] When **intrinsic healing** dominates, few adhesions form, and the result is more freely gliding tendons. Tendons with fewer adhesions must be carefully protected from resistive use, because they may be at greater risk for rupture. The rehabilitation timeline for such patients may need to be slowed. When **extrinsic healing** dominates, an increased inflammatory response occurs as the result of high-energy injury, postsurgical infection, or other factors. These patients have poorer tendon glide and may need their rehabilitation timeline advanced more quickly. Because each person's biological response to healing is different, a "pyramid-of-force" model[2] for flexor tendon rehabilitation was proposed by Groth in 2004. This model is based on a progression of force application that safely maximizes tendon excursion. Both time-based protocols and Groth's new rehabilitation model are presented in this chapter.

SURGICAL AND TREATMENT PURPOSE

The purpose of surgery and rehabilitation is to restore maximum active flexor tendon gliding, to ensure effective finger joint motion. The most common impediments to restoration of good tendon gliding are gap formation at the repair site, rupture of the tendon repair, and scarring with adhesions. The surgical technique requires gentle tendon handling; strong, effective suture material with grasping stitches; and meticulous

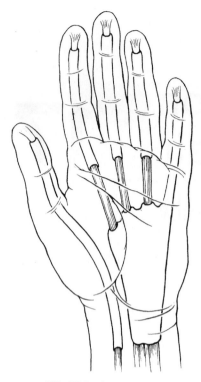

FIG. **17-1** Skin creases.

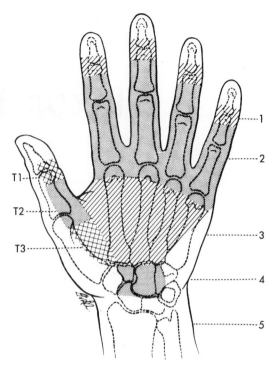

FIG. **17-2** Zones of injury. (From Kleinert HE, Schepel S, Gill T: Surg Clin North Am 61:267, 1981.)

postoperative management. The zone of tendon injury may not coincide with the level of skin laceration because of finger position when the cut occurs (Fig. 17-1). For surgeons, a critical distinction is whether the tendon is injured in zone II (Bunnell's "no-man's land") or another zone. The zone of injury dictates to some extent the therapeutic methods to be used (Fig. 17-2 and Table 17-1). The thumb flexor tendon lies alone in the digital sheath; in contrast, two intimately related tendons—profundus and superficialis—are in each digital sheath of the fingers. This fact alters some of the therapy requirements for the fingers compared with the thumb. The causes of flexor tendon injury are most commonly traumatic; however, rheumatoid arthritis may also bring it about.

TREATMENT GOALS

    I. Provide appropriate splint protection.
    II. Prevent development of excessive edema.
    III. Promote wound healing.
    IV. Maintain active range of motion (AROM) of all uninvolved joints—including neck, shoulder, elbow, and wrist.
    V. Maintain digital passive range of motion (PROM).
    VI. Prevent flexion contractures.
    VII. Restore digital tendon glide to achieve functional AROM.
    VIII. Provide guidance for functional use of hand at the appropriate time.

TABLE **17-1** Flexor Tendon Zones of the Hand

Zone Name	Zone Described	Therapy Concerns
Zone I	Distal to FDS insertion	40 degrees of DIP flexion is needed for satisfactory hand function. Evans' protocol[15] is specifically designed to preserve distal tendon glide.
Zone II	A1 pulley to FDS insertion	The FDS and FDP tend to develop adhesions, especially at the chiasma of Camper.[1] Hagberg and Selvik[23] showed active protocols to be more effective than passive protocols in achieving tendon excursion in zone II.
Zone III	Distal end of carpal tunnel to A1 pulley	Results of repair are better in this zone because of the absence of the retinacular sheath. Because scarring of the intrinsics may occur, attention must be paid to intrinsic stretching exercises.
Zone IV	Within carpal tunnel	The tight space of this zone can result in adhesions between tendons and median nerve compression. Tendon gliding and tenodesis exercises are important for differential glide of the tendons.
Zone V	Proximal to carpal tunnel	Tendon adhesions are less frequent here because the surrounding tissue is mobile.[1] Injuries here may be associated with median or ulnar nerve lacerations. Ring and little finger MCP joints should be splinted in 70 degrees of flexion if ulnar nerve is affected, because intrinsics will be unable to assist with PIP extension.[17] An injury in the muscle belly heals more quickly because of the good vascular supply.
Zone T-I	Distal to IP joint	Watch for compensatory MCP joint flexion instead of IP joint flexion—splint may need to limit MCP joint.
Zone T-II	A1 pulley to IP joint	Associated neurovascular injuries can affect the final outcome.[24]
Zone T-III	Thenar eminence	Better ROM may be expected.[24]

DIP, Distal interphalangeal joint; *FDP*, flexor digitorum profundus; *FDS*, flexor digitorum superficialis; *IP*, interphalangeal; *MCP*, metacarpophalangeal; *PIP*, proximal interphalangeal joint; *ROM*, range of motion.

    IX. Gradually strengthen the hand when appropriate.
    X. Return to previous level of function if possible. Guide patient toward vocational rehabilitation services if previous functional level cannot be achieved.

POSTOPERATIVE INDICATIONS/PRECAUTIONS FOR THERAPY

  I. Indications
    A. Surgical repair of flexor tendon laceration or rupture in fingers and/or thumb
  II. Precautions
    A. Infection: Notify surgeon if signs of infection appear.
    B. Concomitant injuries (e.g., extensor tendons, fractures, nerve or vessel repair): discuss with surgeon how these injuries will change the treatment approach.

C. Sympathetically mediated pain (more common with associated nerve injuries):
  1. Keep therapy gentle—use of transcutaneous electrical nerve stimulation (TENS) may help control pain.
  2. Surgeon may prescribe medications or nerve blocks.
D. Severe edema or joint stiffness—both conditions add to the "work of flexion"[4] and increase the force that is required to flex a digit through its range of motion. PROM should precede AROM to help decrease stiffness. AROM should be done only in the freely moving arc of motion, to avoid elongation at the repair site (gap formation). Gaps greater than 3 mm may be at increased risk for rupture throughout the rehabilitation process.[5]
E. Tendon rupture: If loss of normal postural "cascade" of digits and/or loss of AROM occurs, contact surgeon immediately.

BOX 17-1 Early Progressive Resistance Protocol*

WEEK 3

- DBS constructed with wrist neutral, MCP joints flexed to 50 degrees, IP joints neutral
- AROM and PROM measurements recorded
- Hourly PROM exercises inside splint per modified Duran protocol
- Hourly AROM tenodesis exercises out of splint
- Hourly AROM tendon gliding exercises out of splint

WEEK 4

- Remeasure AROM and PROM—if there is a 50-degree difference, initiate the early progressive resistance program—if not, continue week 3 exercises.
- Hourly manual blocking exercises to FDS and FDP
- Fabricate static volar night extension splint if needed to provide a prolonged stretch for flexion contractures and/or adherent tendons.

WEEK 5

- Remeasure AROM and PROM—if there is still a 50-degree difference, then continue to progress the program—if not, continue week 4 exercises. If there are signs of pain or inflammation due to the exercises, decrease the resistance or the repetitions.
- Begin therapy putty exercises for flexion and extension using light putty.
- Begin use of hand helper with one rubber band (full and hook fist gripping).
- Fabricate dynamic extension splint if needed for persistent joint contractures.
- Slowly increase functional use of hand out of splint as splint is weaned.
- Decrease frequency of home-exercise sessions to five to six times per day as functional use out of splint improves.

From Collins DC, Schwarze L: J Hand Ther 4:111-116, 1991.

AROM, Active range of motion; *DBS,* dorsal blocking splint; *FDP,* flexor digitorum profundus; *FDS,* flexor digitorum superficialis; *IP,* interphalangeal; *MCP,* metacarpophalangeal; *PROM,* passive range of motion.

*This protocol is used only for patients with substantial adhesion formation (defined as a 50-degree difference between total active and total passive digital flexion). It works well for patients who were treated with immobilization for the first 3 postoperative weeks.

POSTOPERATIVE THERAPY

In general, therapy protocols can be divided into three categories: immobilization, early passive mobilization, and early active mobilization. These protocols vary mainly in their management during the first 3 to 4 postoperative weeks. All protocols allow a gradual increase of active motion with splint protection from 3 to 6 weeks. A gradual increase of nonresistive functional use out of the splint is then allowed, with progression to resistance as needed for good tendon glide. Heavy resistive use is not recommended before 12 weeks postoperatively.

I. **Immobilization protocol**
    A. With this method there is no active or passive motion of the affected digits for at least 3 weeks.
    B. Immobilization is reserved for the following patients
        1. Those in whom the risk of noncompliance outweighs the benefits of early motion (e.g., young children, cognitively or behaviorly impaired adults)
        2. Those living under severely adverse environmental conditions
        3. Those with concomitant injuries that preclude motion (e.g., some bone and joint injuries, complex skin injuries, revascularizations, replantations)

Immobilization protocols have been shown in canine models to result in increased adhesion formation (extrinsic healing) and reduced ROM.[6] These patients will not be seen by the therapist until the surgeon removes the cast or immobilizing dressing. They will probably achieve better tendon glide if treated with a motion-driven progression of therapy after the first 3 weeks. They should be splinted in either a static or dynamic dorsal blocking splint when motion begins. Therapy management can proceed by either Collins' early progressive-resistance program[7] or Groth's pyramid-of-force application[2] (Boxes 17-1 and 17-2). Groth's exercise pyramid is shown in Fig. 17-3.

II. **Early passive mobilization protocols**
    A. This method uses passive flexion and passive/active extension of the affected digits. Motion is preferably initiated in the first few days postoperatively, but it can be started at any point during the first 3 weeks.
    B. Early passive mobilization is recommended for the following patients
        1. Those in whom surgical repair is inappropriate for AROM protocols—(e.g., less than four-strand core suture with epitendinous suture) or the type of surgical repair is unknown
        2. Those with significant postoperative edema
        3. Those who are unable to attend therapy sessions two to three times per week and are not capable of conducting an AROM protocol at home

Boyer and colleagues[8] and Strickland[9] have provided reviews of the science that has led to a better understanding of flexor tendon healing. This healing is facilitated by passive motion protocols that inhibit formation of intrasynovial adhesions and help restore tendon glide. These protocols can be grossly grouped as those that use.

BOX 17-2 Pyramid of Progressive Force Exercises*

Therapy consists of a series of exercise levels, demonstrated conceptually by a pyramid. The exercises at the bottom of the pyramid are used more frequently and with more repetitions than those at the top (see Fig. 17-3). Patients are seen in therapy one or two times per week. They are started on the lowest-level exercise on the first visit and on level 2 exercises when AROM is initiated. Further progression up the pyramid is determined by the response of tendon excursion to the force of exercise being used. On each visit, AROM is compared with PROM. The following criteria are used to determine whether the tendon is responsive or unresponsive to the force level being used:

  Absent (no adhesions): ≤5-degree difference between active and passive flexion

  Responsive: ≥10% resolution of active lag between therapy sessions
  Unresponsive: ≤10% resolution of active lag between therapy sessions

  If there is no significant discrepancy between AROM and PROM, then the patient remains at the same exercise level. If the tendon is unresponsive, then the patient is moved up one exercise level each therapy visit until the tendon is responsive. The patient remains at that level as long as the response continues to be favorable. The progression levels are as follows:

- Passive-protected digital extension—consists of passive flexion/extension of the PIP and DIP joints independently and in a composite fashion.[10] This level also includes passive-synergistic exercise using slight wrist extension. The frequency of first-level exercise is as often as feasible, but no less than four or five exercise sessions per day.
- Place-and-hold finger flexion—after a warm-up of slow passive flexion, the MCP, PIP, and DIP joints are held in a moderately flexed position.[27] This exercise is typically done in three to five sessions per day.
- Active composite fist—independent active digital flexion to the distal palmar crease with slight wrist extension. This exercise achieves maximum FDP glide and is the first level of exercise reserved for the unresponsive tendon. It may be prescribed as early as the third or fourth therapy session if needed to improve tendon glide.
- Hook and straight fist—hook fist achieves maximum differential glide; straight fist achieves maximum FDS glide.[28]
- Isolated joint motion—blocking exercises should be done carefully; the patient must not strain against the blocking mechanism.
- Discontinuation of protective splinting—considered to be a progression level because it results in increased functional use; wean from splint over 1 week's time.
- Resistive composite fist—begin with slow, minimally resistive exercises and grade up.
- Resistive hook and straight fist—vary the location of joint angles and wrist position.
- Resistive isolated joint motion—an external mode of resistance (dynamic splint) is applied to an adherent tendon. If the tendon remains unresponsive after 2 weeks, then surgical release may be needed.

From Groth GN: J Hand Ther 17:31-42, 2004.

AROM, Active range of motion; *DIP*, distal interphalangeal; *FDP*, flexor digitorum profundus; *FDS*, flexor digitorum superficialis; *MCP*, metacarpophalangeal; *PIP*, proximal interphalangeal; *PROM*, passive range of motion.

*This program can be used in conjunction with any of the protocols in this chapter. It is particularly helpful in treating patients with atypical tissue response patterns (tendon glide very poor or extremely good).

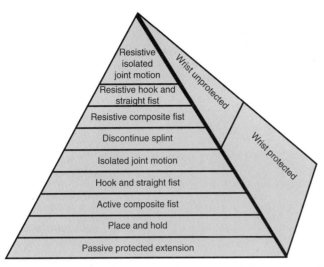

FIG. **17-3** Exercise pyramid. (From Groth GN: J Hand Ther 7:31-42, 2004.)

1. Manual passive flexion and passive/active extension in a dorsal blocking splint[10] (for splint positioning, see Figs. 17-4 through 17-7; for therapy protocols, see Boxes 17-3A, 17-3B, and 17-3C)
2. Dynamic flexion traction and active extension in a dorsal blocking splint[11] (for splint positioning, see Figs. 17-8 and 17-9; for therapy protocols, see Boxes 17-4A and 17-4B)

III. **Early active mobilization protocols**
   A. These protocols incorporate place-hold flexion and/or true active flexion of the affected digits. Motion must be initiated within the first 5 days postoperatively. Immediate mobilization (day 1 or 2) has been shown to be less effective than a delay of 3 to 5 days to allow inflammation to subside.[4] Adhesions inhibit tendon glide as early as 1 week postoperatively; therefore, the work of flexion

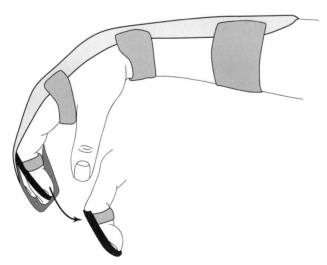

FIG. **17-4** Zone I static dorsal blocking splint.

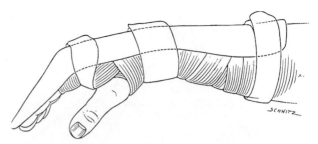

FIG. **17-5** Static dorsal blocking splint. (From Green DP [ed]: Green's Operative Hand Surgery. 4th Ed. Churchill Livingstone, New York, 1999.)

required to initiate active flexion after 7 days may be too great for the typical four-strand repair. Boyer and associates[12] showed that an eight-strand repair results in approximately 35% greater strength and rigidity than a four-strand repair. Such repairs may not need the same time restrictions for AROM initiation, but more research is needed to resolve this issue. Active protocols may offer the best opportunity to limit adhesion formation with increased tendon glide.

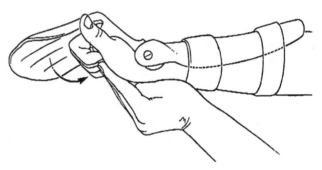

FIG. **17-6** Hinged splint. (From Cannon N: Post flexor tendon repair motion protocol. Indiana Hand Center Newsletter 1:13-18, 1993.)

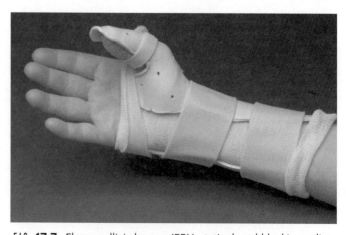

FIG. **17-7** Flexor pollicis longus (FPL) static dorsal blocking splint.

BOX **17-3A** Therapy Protocol for Zone I (Early PROM, Static Splint)*

ZONE I[15]
Week 1-3

Splint position: Wrist in 30 to 40 degrees flexion, MCP joint in 30 degrees flexion, DIP joint in 45 degrees flexion in separate splint taped over P2 (the middle phalanx of digit)
   At home (in splints)—perform 10 to 20 repetitions per waking hour
- Passive DIP joint flexion from 45 degrees to full flexion inside finger-based DBS
- Passive full fist
- Passive modified hook-fist
- Passive hyperflexion of MCP joint with full PIP extension to 0 degrees
- Gentle active place/hold of FDS tendon with other digits strapped in extension
   In therapy (in addition to above-mentioned exercises)—out of splint
- Passively flex digits into the palm while extending the wrist to 10 degrees.
- Passively hyperflex the wrist for passive hook-fist with MCP joint at 0 degrees.

Week 3
- Discontinue digital DBS.
- Continue forearm DBS and PROM exercises.
- Begin active place/hold exercises in DBS.
- Progress to active tenodesis wrist exercise, hook-fist, and gentle isolated FDP out of splint.

Week 4$\frac{1}{2}$
- Static digital extension is initiated to regain DIP joint extension.
- Continue progression as for zones II through V.

Modified from Duran RJ, Houser R: Controlled passive motion following flexor tendon repair in zones 2 and 3. In AAOS Symposium on Tendon Surgery in the Hand. Mosby, St. Louis, 1975.

DIP, Distal interphalangeal; *DBS,* dorsal blocking splint; *FDP,* flexor digitorum profundus; *FDS,* flexor digitorum superficialis; *MCP,* metacarpophalangeal; *PIP,* proximal interphalangeal; *PROM,* passive range of motion.

*A splint is pictured in Fig. 17-4 on p. 233.

BOX **17-3B** Therapy Protocol for Zones II through V (Early PROM, Static Splint)*

ZONES II THROUGH V[29]

Splint position: Wrist in 20 to 30 degrees flexion, MCP joints in 50 degrees flexion, IP joints fully extended

Week 1-3
At home (in splint)—perform 10 to 20 repetitions per waking hour
- Passive flexion/extension of DIP and PIP joints, and composite flexion
- Hyperflexion of MCP joint, with active/passive extension of PIP to 0 degrees
   In therapy (in addition to above-mentioned exercises)—out of splint
- Passively flex digits into the palm while extending the wrist to 20 degrees.
- Passively hyperflex the wrist for passive hook-fist with MCP joint at 0 degrees.
- Gentle active place/hold to FDS in digits with unrepaired FDS tendons.

Week 3
- Adjust DBS to bring wrist to neutral.
- Begin active place/hold flexion in splint.

Week 4
- Remove splint for AROM and tenodesis exercises at home.
- Evaluate tendon glide—if total passive motion (TPM) exceeds total active motion (TAM) by 50 degrees, begin active sustained flexion exercise (cones).

(Continued)

BOX 17-3B Therapy Protocol for Zones II through V (Early PROM, Static Splint)*—Cont'd

- **Week 6**
- Discontinue DBS.
- Begin active composite flexion and extension exercises.
- Begin gentle blocking exercises for PIP and DIP joints if needed for tendon glide.
- Begin stress progression (minimum needed for tendon glide progression): sustained flexion on cones; towel walking; light grasp and release; light putty).

Week 7
- Begin serial extension splinting as needed for flexion contractures.
- Continue stress progression as needed for improved tendon gliding.

Week 10-12
- Gradually progress to heavier gripping.
- Prepare for return to work.

Modified from Duran RJ, Houser R: Controlled passive motion following flexor tendon repair in zones 2 and 3. In AAOS Symposium on Tendon Surgery in the Hand. Mosby, St. Louis, 1975.

AROM, Active range of motion; *DBS,* dorsal blocking splint; *DIP,* distal interphalangeal; *FDS,* flexor digitorum superficialis; *IP,* interphalangeal; *MCP,* metacarpophalangeal joint; *PIP,* proximal interphalangeal; *PROM,* passive range of motion.

*A splint is pictured in Fig. 17-5 on p. 234.

BOX 17-3C Therapy Protocol for Flexor Pollicis Longus (Early PROM, Static Splint)*

FLEXOR POLLICIS LONGUS[29]

Splint position: Wrist in 30 degrees flexion, MCP joints in 15 degrees flexion, IP joints in 15 degrees flexion

Week 1-3
At home (in splint)—perform 10 to 20 repetitions per waking hour
- Passive flexion/extension of IP and MCP joints (separately)
- Composite passive flexion to the thumb joints
  In therapy (in addition to above-mentioned exercises)—out of splint
- Passively flex MCP and IP joints while extending the wrist to 20 degrees.
- Passively flex wrist while actively extending the thumb to neutral.

Week 3
Begin place/hold flexion in splint.

Week 4
Remove splint for AROM and tenodesis exercise.

Week 6
Discontinue DBS.

Week 8-12
Gradually progress strengthening.

Modified from Duran RJ, Houser R: Controlled passive motion following flexor tendon repair in zones 2 and 3. In AAOS Symposium on Tendon Surgery in the Hand. Mosby, St. Louis, 1975.

AROM, Active range of motion; *DBS,* dorsal blocking splint; *IP,* interphalangeal; *MCP,* metacarpophalangeal; *PROM,* passive range of motion.

*A splint is pictured in Fig. 17-7 on p. 234.

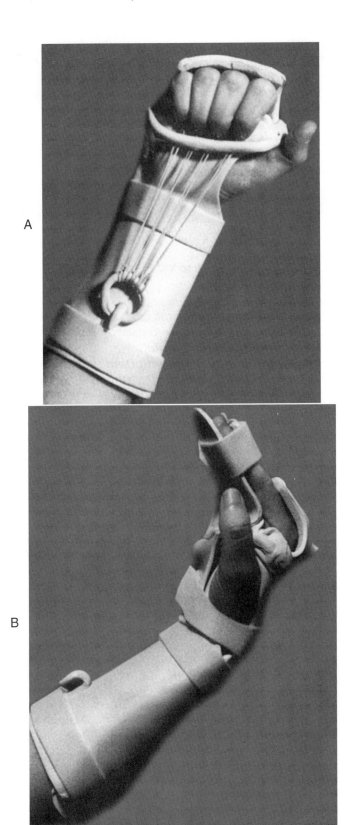

FIG. **17-8** **A,** Four-finger dynamic splint. **B,** Separate static night attachment.

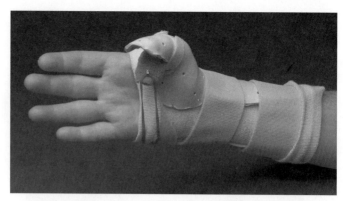

FIG. **17-9** Flexor pollicis longus (FPL) dynamic splint.

B. These protocols should be used exclusively for the following patients
   1. Those in whom a four-strand or greater core suture with epitendinous suture was performed by a surgeon who approves of an AROM protocol
   2. Those without significant postoperative edema
   3. Those who are compliant and able to attend therapy two to three times per week or able to conduct an AROM protocol safely with a home exercise program

---

BOX 17-4A Therapy Protocol for Zones I through V (Early PROM, Dynamic Splint)*

ZONES I THROUGH V[3,30-32]

Splint position:
    Day—Wrist in 30 to 45 degrees flexion, MCP joints in 50 to 70 degrees flexion, splint ends at PIP joints, dynamic pull from all four fingers through palmar pulley
    Night—Dynamic pull is disconnected, separate night attachment on palmar surface holds IP joints in full extension

Week 1-4 (in splint)
- Active extension with rubber bands unloaded (10 repetitions per waking hour)
- Passive flexion using unaffected hand after each extension repetition
- Rest IP joints in extension at night with supplemental splint

Week 4
Discontinue splint, begin AROM flexion/extension without resistance.

Week 6
Begin gentle resistive flexion exercises, splint for flexion contractures.

Week 8
Begin blocking and progressive resistance exercises.

Week 10-12
Return to unrestricted activity.

AROM, Active range of motion; *IP*, interphalangeal; *MCP*, metacarpophalangeal; *PIP*, proximal interphalangeal; *PROM*, passive range of motion.

*A splint is pictured in Fig. 17-8, *A* and *B* on p. 237.

BOX 17-4B Therapy Protocol for Flexor Pollicis Longus (Early PROM, Dynamic Splint)*

FLEXOR POLLICIS LONGUS[24,30,33]

Splint position: Wrist in 30 degrees flexion, MCP joint fixed so that tendon excursion will occur with IP joint motion, dynamic pull of IP joint across palm to ulnar side of splint.

Week 1-4 (in splint)
- Active extension of thumb with rubber band unloaded (10 repetitions per waking hour)
- Passive flexion using unaffected hand after each extension repetition
- Rest IP joint in slight flexion at night with supplemental splint.

Week 4
Begin AROM flexion/extension without resistance, continue splint wear.

Week 6
Discontinue splint

Week 8
Begin gentle resistive flexion exercises, splint for flexion contractures.

Week 10
Begin blocking and progressive resistance exercises.

Week 12
Return to unrestricted activity.

AROM, Active range of motion; *IP*, interphalangeal; *MCP*, metacarpophalangeal; *PROM*, passive range of motion.
*A splint is pictured in Fig. 17-9 on p. 238.

   C. For splint positioning see Figs. 17-5, 17-6, and 17-8. Early active
      therapy protocols can be found in Boxes 17-5A and 17-5B.

POSTOPERATIVE COMPLICATIONS

   I. Tendon rupture
   II. Minimal tendon gliding
   III. Flexion contractures
   IV. Excessive scar formation
   V. Extreme pain
   VI. Severe edema
   VII. Infection
   VIII. Triggering

EVALUATION TIMELINE

   I. First postoperative therapy session
      A. Wound—Determine appropriate dressing to be worn inside
         splint.
      B. Edema—Compare girth of affected digit to unaffected hand.
      C. Pain—scale from 0 to 10
      D. Sensibility—especially important with concomitant nerve
         injuries

BOX **17-5A** Therapy Protocol for Zones I through V (Early AROM, Static and/or Hinged Splint)*

ZONES I THROUGH V[34-36]

Splint position:
  Static splint—Wrist in 20 to 30 degrees flexion, MCP joints in 50 degrees flexion, IP joints fully extended
  Hinged splint—Wrist allowed to extend to 30 degrees and to fully flex, MCP joints in 60 degrees flexion,
    IP joints fully extended

Week 1-4

(In static splint)—perform 15 repetitions per waking hour—PROM flexion/extension of PIP and DIP joints, and composite flexion
  (In hinged splint)—perform 25 repetitions per waking hour—
  1. Passively flex digits and extend wrist to 30 degrees.
  2. Gently hold flexed position actively for 5 seconds.
  3. Allow wrist to drop back into flexion and extend digits to the limits of the splint.

Week 4

• Discontinue hinged splint.
• Continue use of DBS and PROM exercises.
• Remove splint hourly for AROM tenodesis exercises—no simultaneous wrist/finger extension.

Week 6

• Discontinue DBS.
• Begin blocking and passive-extension exercises.

Week 8

Gradual progressive strengthening is initiated.

This protocol has been modified at Curtis National Hand Center—only the static splint is used. The patient performs PROM, place/hold exercises, and gentle partial-range AROM exercises hourly (within the DBS). The therapist supervises passive tenodesis with active hold in the clinic until the patient seems able to perform the exercise safely at home out of the splint. The arc of AROM that the patient can perform gently should increase from about 50% range to almost full AROM within the first 3 weeks.

AROM, Active range of motion; *DBS*, dorsal blocking splint; *DIP*, distal interphalangeal; *IP*, interphalangeal; *MCP*, metacarpophalangeal; *PIP*, proximal interphalangeal; *PROM*, passive range of motion.

*Splints are pictured in Figs. 17-5 and 17-6 on p. 234. (No early AROM protocols are presented for the flexor pollicis longus due to increased risk of rupture.)

    E. Flexion PROM—assessed grossly (deficits in flexion to distal palmar crease)
    F. Extension deficit (inside dorsal blocking splint)
    G. Flexion AROM if early AROM protocol is being initiated
  II. 1 to 2 weeks postoperatively
    A. Reassess flexion AROM if using early active or place/hold protocol.
    B. Reassess pain, edema, and PROM.
  III. 3 weeks postoperatively
    A. Flexion AROM—Continue weekly reassessments to determine need for stress progression to facilitate tendon glide
    B. Scar—Assess need for elastomer mold and/or desensitization.
    C. Continue weekly reassessment of pain, edema, and PROM.
  IV. 10 weeks postoperatively—grip and pinch strength assessment
  V. 12 weeks postoperatively—provide data to surgeon for back-to-work assessment

---

BOX 17-5B Therapy Protocol for Zones I through V (Early AROM, Dynamic Splint)*

ZONES I THROUGH V[37]

Splint position:

    Day—Wrist in 30 to 45 degrees flexion, MCP joints in 50 to 70 degrees flexion, splint ends at PIP joints, dynamic pull from all four fingers through palmar pulley

    Night—Dynamic pull is disconnected, separate night attachment on palmar surface holds IP joints in full extension

Week 1-4

- Perform 10 repetitions per waking hour
  1. Actively extend the digits while manually unloading the tension of the rubber band with the other hand.
  2. Allow passive flexion of the digits by the rubber band.
  3. Provide manual assistance with the other hand to bring into full flexion.
  4. Gently contract the flexor muscles to hold the flexed position for 2 to 3 seconds.
- Instruct patient to sleep without dynamic traction—the separate night attachment splint holds the IP joints in extension.

Week 4

Patient removes splint for unassisted active flexion/extension exercises.

Week 6

Discontinue DBS—splint as needed to correct extension deficits.

Week 8

Initiate progressive resistance exercises.

Week 10-12

Return to work.

AROM, Active range of motion; *DBS*, dorsal blocking splint; *IP*, interphalangeal; *MCP*, metacarpophalangeal; *PIP*, proximal interphalangeal.

*Splints are pictured in Figs. 17-8, *A* and *B* on p. 237. (No early AROM protocols are presented for flexor pollicis longus due to increased risk of rupture.)

OUTCOMES

ROM is the criterion set to determine successful outcomes after flexor tendon repair. Several methods of evaluating ROM results have been developed. Two of these methods are presented in Tables 17-2 and 17-3. Strickland's method includes only proximal interphalangeal (PIP) and distal interphalangeal (DIP) joint motion (although the measurements are made while the patient attempts to make a full fist). Kleinert's method includes all three joints of the digit. Outcome information specific to the zone of injury follows.

Zone I: Guinard and colleagues[13] reported that patients' subjective assessments of functional outcome after zone I repairs were less favorable than would be indicated by Strickland's method of outcome assessment. Moiemen[14] reported the results of 102 zone I injuries treated with an early active therapy protocol. The results were compared with earlier zone I reports by Evans[15] and by Gerbino and associates.[16] They suggested that

TABLE **17-2** Outcomes of Flexor Tendon Repair: Strickland Method

Group	PIP + DIP Return (%)	PIP + DIP Minus Extension Loss (Degrees)
Excellent	85-100	150+
Good	70-84	125-149
Fair	50-69	90-124
Poor	<50	<90

$$\frac{\text{Active PIP} + \text{DIP flexon} - \text{extension lag}}{175} \times 100 = \text{percent of normal active PIP and DIP motion}$$

From Strickland JW, Glogovac SV: J Hand Surg Am 5:537-543, 1980.
DIP, distal interphalangeal joint; *PIP*, proximal interphalangeal joint.

a revision of Strickland's method would be more appropriate for zone I outcomes. The revised method would include only DIP joint motion (measured while attempting to make a full fist). Evans[15] suggested that a minimum of 40 degrees of DIP joint flexion is needed for good patient satisfaction.

Zone II: Elliot[17] surveyed the literature and found a 5% rate of both rupture and tenolysis after zone II repairs, regardless of suture technique used. Strickland[9] stated that good or excellent function may be expected more than 80% of the time if a strong repair is followed by an early postrepair motion protocol. Riaz and coworkers[18] performed a 10-year review of patients who had been treated with an early active-motion protocol. The original results had been published by Small and associates.[19] Riaz reported that 77% of the patients treated with early AROM continued to have good or excellent outcomes by Strickland's criteria, and 75% by Kleinert's criteria. Grip strength was 95.5% of that of the uninjured hand. Cold intolerance was a problem for 47% of these patients, although only 20% had associated nerve injuries.

Flexor pollicis longus (FPL): Elliot and associates[20] reported higher rupture rates for FPL repairs than for flexor digitorum superficialis (FDS) or flexor digitorum profundus (FDP) repairs among 233 patients treated with an early AROM protocol. More recently, Elliot and colleagues[17] explained why the FPL rupture rate may be higher. Because the FPL glides alone within its sheath, fewer adhesions form during healing. The FPL also retracts proximally after laceration, making delayed repairs more difficult.

TABLE **17-3** Outcomes of Flexor Tendon Repair: Kleinert Method

Group	Pulp to Distal Palmar Crease (cm)	Extension Deficit (Degrees)
Excellent	<1	1-15
Good	1-1.5	16-30
Fair	1.6-3	31-50
Poor	>3	>50

From Lister GD, Kleinert HE, Kutz JE: J Hand Surg Am 2:441-451, 1977.

Noonan and Blair[21] did a long-term (mean 6.8 years) follow-up of FPL repairs. The conclusion was that the method used to rehabilitate FPL repairs (static splint, dynamic splint, or immobilization) did not statistically affect the outcome.

Children: Outcomes in children seem to be better than in adults, possibly because of a better blood supply to the flexor tendons and a greater capacity for remodeling.[22]

REFERENCES

1. Wang ED: Tendon repair. J Hand Ther 11:105-110, 1998
2. Groth GN: Pyramid of progressive force exercises to the injured flexor tendon. J Hand Ther 7:31-42, 2004
3. Kleinert HE, Schepel S, Gill T: Flexor tendon injuries. Surg Clin North Am 61:267-286, 1981
4. Halikis MN, Manske PR, Kubota H, et al.: Effect of immobilization, immediate mobilization, and delayed mobilization on the resistance to digital flexion using a tendon injury model. J Hand Surg Am 22:464-472, 1997
5. Gelberman RH, Boyer MI, Brodt MD, et al.: The effect of gap formation at the repair site on the strength and excursion of intrasynovial flexor tendons. J Bone Joint Surg Am 81:975-982, 1999
6. Gelberman RH, Vande Berg JS, Lundborg GN, et al.: Flexor tendon healing and restoration of the gliding surface. J Bone Joint Surg Am 65:70-80, 1993
7. Collins DC, Schwarze L: Early progressive resistance following immobilization of flexor tendon repairs. J Hand Ther 4:111-116, 1991
8. Boyer MI, Strickland JW, Engles DR, et al.: Flexor tendon repair and rehabilitation. J Bone Joint Surg Am 84:1684-1706, 2002
9. Strickland JW: Development of flexor tendon surgery: twenty five years of progress. J Hand Surg Am 25:214-235, 2000
10. Duran RJ, Houser R: Controlled passive motion following flexor tendon repair in zones 2 and 3. In AAOS Symposium on Tendon Surgery in the Hand. Mosby, St. Louis, 1975
11. Kleinert HE, Kutz JE, Ashbell TS, et al.: Primary repair of lacerated flexor tendons in "no man's land." Proceedings of the American Society for Surgery of the Hand. J Bone Joint Surg Am 49:577, 1967
12. Boyer MI, Gelberman RH, Burns ME, et al.: Intrasynovial flexor tendon repair. J Bone Joint Surg Am 83:891-899, 2001
13. Guinard D, Montanier D, Thomas D, et al.: The Mantero flexor tendon repair in zone I. J Hand Surg Br 24:148-151, 1999
14. Moiemen NS, Elliot D: Primary flexor tendon repair in zone I. J Hand Surg Br 25: 78-84, 2000
15. Evans R: A study of the zone 1 flexor tendon injury and the implications for treatment. J Hand Ther 3:133-146, 1990
16. Gerbino PG, Saldana MJ, Westerbeck P, et al.: Complications experienced in the rehabilitation of zone I flexor tendon injuries with dynamic traction splinting. J Hand Surg Am 16:680-686, 1991
17. Elliot D: Primary flexor tendon repair: operative repair, pulley management, and rehabilitation. J Hand Surg Br 7:507-513, 2002
18. Riaz M, Hill C, Khan K, et al.: Long term outcome of early active mobilization following flexor tendon repair in zone 2. J Hand Surg Br 24:157-160, 1999
19. Small JO, Brennen MD, Colville J: Early active mobilization following flexor tendon repair in zone 2. J Hand Surg Br 14:383-391, 1989
20. Elliot D, Moimen N, Fleming A, et al.: The rupture rate of acute flexor tendon repairs mobilized by controlled active mobilization. J Hand Surg Br 19:607-612, 1994
21. Noonan KJ, Blair WF: Long-term follow up of primary flexor pollicis longus tenorrhaphies. J Hand Surg Am 16:653-662, 1991
22. Grobbelaar AO, Hudson DA: Flexor tendon injuries in children. J Hand Surg Br 19: 696-698, 1994
23. Hagberg L, Selvik G: Tendon excursions and dehiscence during early controlled mobilization after flexor tendon repair in zone II: an x-ray stereophotogrammetric analysis. J Hand Surg Am 16:669-680, 1991

24. Nunley JA, Levin LS, Devito D, et al.: Direct end-to-end repair of flexor pollicis longus tendon lacerations. J Hand Surg Am 17:118-121, 1992

25. Strickland JW, Glogovac SV: Digital function following flexor tendon repair in zone II: a comparison of immobilization and controlled passive motion techniques. J Hand Surg Am 5:537-543, 1980

26. Lister GD, Kleinert HE, Kutz JE: Primary flexor tendon repair followed by immediate controlled mobilization. J Hand Surg Am 2:441-451, Nov. 1977

27. Evans RB, Thompson DE: The application of force to the healing tendon. J Hand Ther 6:266-284, 1993

28. Wehbe MA, Hunter JM: Flexor tendon gliding in the hand: II. Differential gliding. J Hand Surg Am 10:575-579, 1986

29. Cannon N: Post flexor tendon repair protocol. Indiana Hand Center Newsletter 1:13, 1993

30. Silfverskiold KL, May EJ, Tornvall AH: Flexor digitorum profundus tendon excursions during controlled motion after flexor tendon repair in zone II: a prospective clinical study. J Hand Surg Am 17:122-131, 1992

31. May EJ, Silfverskiold KL, Sollerman CJ: Controlled mobilization after flexor tendon repair in zone II: a prospective comparison of three methods. J Hand Surg Am 17:942-952, 1992

32. Chow JA, Thomes LJ, Dovelle S, et al.: A combined regimen of controlled motion following flexor tendon repair in "no man's land." Plast Reconstr Surg 79:447, 1987

33. Percival NJ, Sykes PJ: Flexor pollicis longus tendon repair: a comparison between dynamic and static splintage. J Hand Surg Br 14:412-415, 1989

34. Evans RB, Thompson DE: Immediate active short arc motion following tendon repair. In Hunter JM, Schneider LH, Mackin EJ (eds). Tendon and Nerve Surgery in the Hand: A Third Decade. Mosby, St. Louis, Mosby, 1997, pp. 363-393

35. Klein L: Early active motion flexor tendon protocol using one splint. J Hand Ther 16:199-206, 2003

36. Strickland JW: The Indiana method of flexor tendon repair. In Taras JS, Schneider LH. Atlas of the Hand Clinics. WB Saunders, Philadelphia, 1996, pp. 77-103

37. Silfverskiold KL, May EJ: Flexor tendon repair in zone II with a new suture technique and an early mobilization program combining passive and active flexion. J Hand Surg Am 19:53-60, 1994

Flexor Tendon Reconstruction

18

Barbara Wilson

Although primary flexor tendon repair is usually the best postinjury treatment for flexor tendon lacerations, there are times when this is neither possible nor indicated. For example, the wound or the patient's general condition may disallow direct repair[1]; a flexor tendon injury may be missed at the time of injury[1]; or there may be a late referral for definitive care that makes it impossible for the surgeon to perform an end-to-end repair.[1]

Flexor tendon reconstruction can be accomplished with the use of single-stage procedures (primary tendon grafting) or two-stage procedures. Therapy for two-stage flexor tendon reconstruction consists of three parts: preoperative, postoperative stage I, and postoperative stage II. Therapy for single-stage tendon grafting is essentially the same as that for postoperative stage II of two-stage tendon reconstruction.

In cases of severe trauma, Frakking and colleagues[2] believed that easier solutions, such as arthrodesis or even amputation, should be considered as alternatives. They further stated that patients should be fully informed about the complexity of the problem, their chances for a good final result, and the possibilities of additional procedures after two-stage tendon reconstruction.

At the preoperative phase of two-stage tendon grafting, patient education is a major component. The purpose of patient education is twofold. The first purpose is to educate the patient regarding the surgical and rehabilitative requirements of these procedures. The second purpose is to monitor the patient's compliance with preoperative therapy, to help assess the patient's willingness and ability to follow through with postoperative therapy.

Therapist-surgeon communication regarding surgical details is indicated after stage I and stage II procedures. After stage I, the therapist should be made aware of any other procedures performed, such as pulley reconstruction or joint releases. After stage II, the therapist should be made aware of the amount of tension on the graft, the type of suture used (Pulvertaft weave versus stronger attachments such as the mesh-reinforced suture used by Silfverskiold and May[3]) and the potential active motion of the digit.

Three basic postsurgical treatment approaches are possible for stage II flexor tendon reconstruction and single-stage flexor tendon grafting: immobilization, early controlled passive mobilization, and early active motion. Early immobilization is rarely used today. However, if the surgeon chooses this approach secondary to potential patient noncompliance or if the patient is lost to follow-up for the first 3 or 4 weeks, this protocol may be used.

Early passive mobilization may be accomplished with[4] or without rubber band or elastic traction. If dynamic traction into flexion is used, it is important to monitor and carefully treat to prevent flexion contractures.

Early active mobilization after flexor tendon grafting is done in some centers. The protocol used needs to reflect the strength of the tendon graft. Khan and associates[5] presented the least aggressive early active motion protocol. This protocol may be used with the standard Pulvertaft weave, which has been used since 1956. Hunter and Mackin[4] presented an early active motion protocol that requires strong graft junctures during surgery, with the tendon bed being in excellent condition. Silfverskiold and May[3] used a more aggressive postoperative protocol after a mesh-reinforced tendon graft. It is crucial to consult with the surgeon to be sure that tendon graft strength is sufficient for the specific early active motion protocol to be used.

With both stage I and stage II of two-stage tendon reconstructions, it is necessary to adjust the progression of treatment according to the "feel" of the tendon graft as it is healing. If early recovery of active range of motion (AROM) is seen and the tendon is gliding well, protective splinting is continued longer and treatment progresses more slowly, because the risk of tendon rupture is greater in these patients. Conversely, if little active tendon glide is noted when AROM is initiated, progression may need to be faster (in consultation with the surgeon), to decrease the effect of tendon adhesions while preventing tendon rupture. Groth[7] published an article that helps the therapist better quantify when and how to progress more quickly or more slowly (see Box 17-2 in Chapter 17). Judgment must also be used, in educating the more active or impulsive patient as well as the more reluctant, to facilitate patient compliance in achieving the best result with the fewest complications.

DEFINITION

I.   **Primary tendon grafting:** removal of injured tendon and replacement with palm-to-fingertip tendon graft (Fig. 18-1)
II. Staged tendon reconstruction
     A. Two-stage tendon graft procedure
        1. Stage I: implantation of Silastic rod to establish a smooth-walled channel[8,9]
        2. Stage II: removal of the implant and placement of a free tendon graft within the neosheath (Figs. 18-2 and 18-3).

SURGICAL PURPOSE

I.   Primary tendon grafts: After flexor or extensor tendon injuries or conditions that cause scarring that prevents tendon gliding, primary tendon grafting may be indicated. The tendon graft is used to bridge a gap between the muscle unit and the insertion of the tendon into bone. It is most commonly used for flexor tendons that

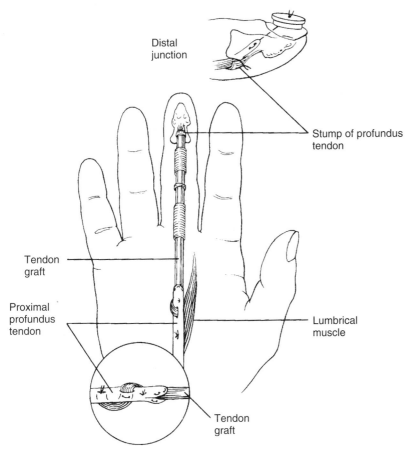

Distal
junction

Stump of profundus
tendon

Tendon
graft

Proximal
profundus
tendon

Lumbrical
muscle

Tendon
graft

FIG. **18-1** Primary tendon grafting. The injured tendon is removed and replaced with
a tendon graft.

have been interrupted between the origin of the lumbrical muscles
and their distal insertion.

II.   Staged tendon reconstruction: Staged tendon reconstruction is used
most often for the flexor units, although the technique also may be
used for the extensors. It is used when there is a scarred bed through
which the tendons are required to glide. Pulley reconstruction
may also be necessary. A passive tendon prosthesis is placed in
the finger to the palm or the wrist, to create a new tendon sheath
through which an autologous tendon is later passed. The method
is used primarily for salvage operations if other alternatives are not
available.

PREOPERATIVE TREATMENT GOALS

I.   Primary tendon grafts
A. Loss of both flexor digitorum superficialis (FDS) and flexor
digitorum profundus (FDP) function
1. Full passive range of motion (PROM) of the proximal
interphalangeal (PIP) and distal interphalangeal (DIP) joints

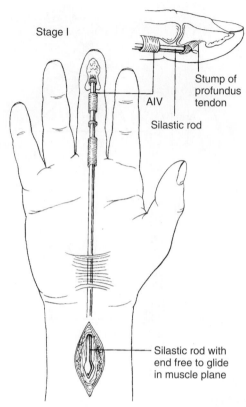

FIG. **18-2** Digit with Silastic rod embedded during stage I of a two-stage graft procedure.

       2. Soft, pliable tissues
       3. Patient education regarding preoperative and postoperative therapy
     B. FDS intact/FDP absent
       1. Same as for loss of both FDS and FDP function
       2. Normal FDS AROM and PROM
 II.   Staged tendon reconstruction
     A. Restore PROM with fingertip passively touching distal palmar crease
     B. Maintain or reestablish supple, soft tissues
     C. Maintain or reestablish strength of proximal muscles
     D. Promote balanced flexion-extension system

INDICATIONS FOR PREOPERATIVE THERAPY

  I.   Decreased range of motion (ROM)
 II. Adherent scar
III. Weak proximal muscle units

PREOPERATIVE THERAPY

  I.   Patient education regarding complexity of rehabilitation and necessary patient compliance

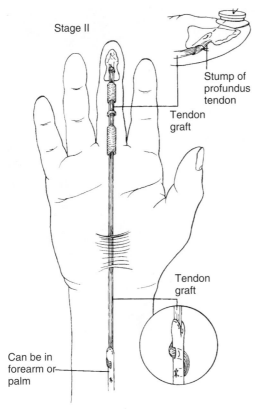

FIG. **18-3** Digit with graft placed within neosheath at stage II of a two-stage graft procedure.

II. Scar management
III. Exercise
　　A. PROM
　　B. "Finger trapping"
　　C. Active flexion of PIP joint if FDS is uninvolved
IV. Splinting
　　A. Flexion limited
　　　　1. Buddy-taping (Fig. 18-4)
　　　　2. Intrinsic stretch splinting (Fig. 18-5)
　　　　3. PIP/distal phalangeal (DIP) joint flexion straps (Fig. 18-6)
　　B. Extension limited
　　　　1. Three-point extension splint (Fig. 18-7)
　　　　2. Serial casting (Fig. 18-8)
　　　　3. Serially applied thermoplastic splints (Fig. 18-9)
V. Strengthening
　　A. Proximal flexor tendon units
　　B. Extrinsic/intrinsic extensors

POSTOPERATIVE TREATMENT GOALS

I.　Postoperative stage I of two-stage tendon reconstruction
　　A. Continue with staged tendon reconstruction goals previously
　　　　listed.

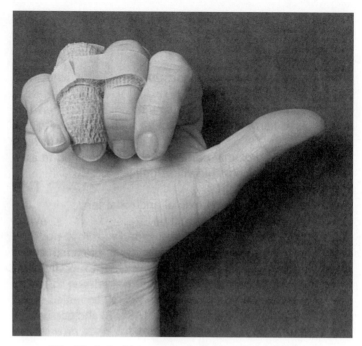

FIG. **18-4** Buddy-taping to facilitate increased flexion.

        B. Facilitate proximal portion of sheath formation in as
           lengthened a position as possible via splinting.[10]
  II.   Postoperative primary tendon grafts and stage II tendon
      reconstruction
      A. FDS and FDP absent
        1. Prevent rupture at proximal and distal tendon
           junctures.

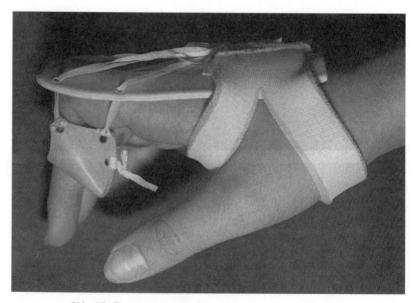

FIG. **18-5** Intrinsic stretch splinting to increase flexion.

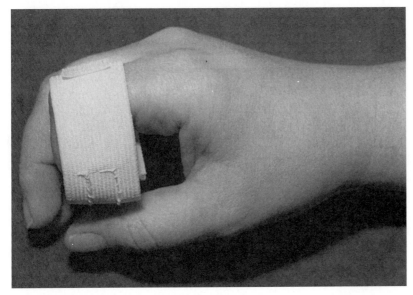

FIG. **18-6** Proximal interphalangeal (PIP)/digital interphalangeal (DIP) flexion strap for improving flexion.

   2. Minimize adhesion formation.
   3. Prevent flexion contractures.
   4. Prevent hyperextension deformity at PIP joint, which can occur with absent FDS.
   5. Promote tendon healing.
   6. Encourage tendon gliding.
   7. Restore AROM and PROM.
   8. Maintain full AROM of all uninvolved joints of affected upper extremity.
   9. Return to previous level of function.

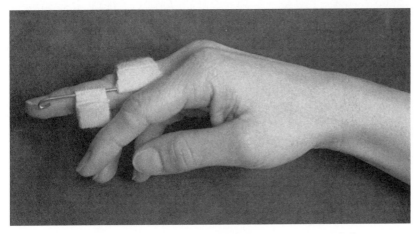

FIG. **18-7** Three-point extension splint to increase extension.

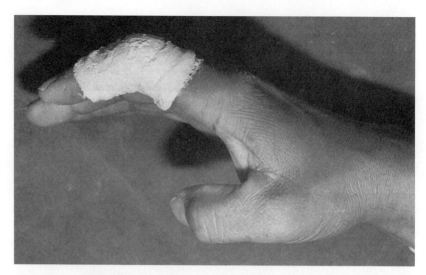

FIG. **18-8** Serial casts can help increase extension.

    B. FDS intact/FDP absent
       1. Same as for loss of both FDS and FDP function
       2. Regain active FDS function while protecting
          FDP graft.

INDICATIONS/PRECAUTIONS FOR POSTOPERATIVE THERAPY

I.   Stage I of two-stage tendon reconstruction[4]
    A. Avoid overexercising, which can lead to synovitis.
    B. Avoid attenuation of extensor tendon at DIP joint, by stressing
       active DIP extension and gentle passive DIP flexion.
    C. Protect reconstructed pulleys (if present).

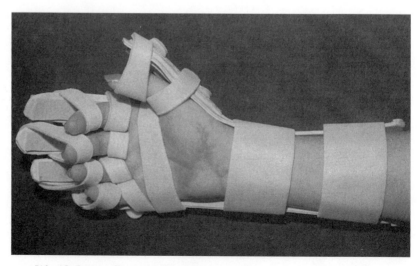

FIG. **18-9** Serially applied thermoplastic splints can increase extension.

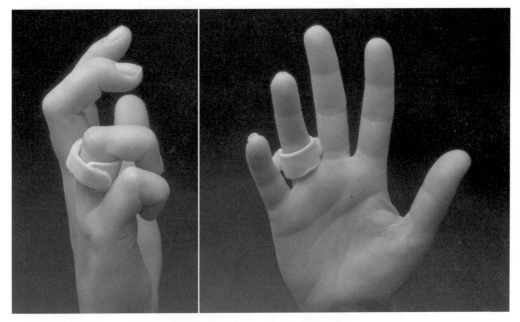

FIG. **18-10** Thermoplastic pulley ring.

II. Primary tendon grafts and stage II of two-stage tendon
    reconstruction
    A. Protect reconstructed pulleys, if indicated, via pulley ring for
       10 to 12 weeks[8] (Fig. 18-10).
    B. Avoid strengthening until 9 to 10 weeks after surgery due to the
       avascular nature of the free tendon graft.[11]

POSTOPERATIVE THERAPY

I. Primary tendon grafts
    A. Same as for stage II of two-stage tendon reconstruction; see
       appropriate guidelines
II. Staged tendon reconstruction
    A. Stage I
       1. Immediately after surgery
          a. Splint: dorsal protective splint with wrist in 30 degrees
             flexion, metacarpophalangeal (MCP) joints in 60 to
             70 degrees flexion, and interphalangeal (IP) joints in
             full extension (Fig. 18-11)
       2. Day 1 to 3 weeks after surgery
          a. PROM
          b. Wound care
          c. Edema control
          d. Scar management
       3. 3 to 6 weeks after surgery
          a. Splint
             (1) Protective splint is discontinued unless signs of
                 synovitis are present
             (2) Initiate splint or splints to facilitate full PROM

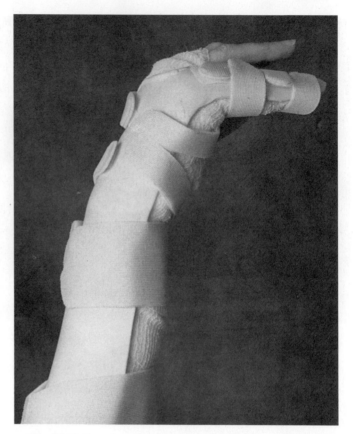

FIG. **18-11** Dorsal protective splint used after stage I surgery.

(3) Figure of 8 splint for PIP joint if "swan-neck" deformity
is present or developing (Fig. 18-12). Continue until
volar plate is strong enough to support PIP joint or
until stage II surgery is performed.
b. Exercise, wound care, edema control, and scar management continue.
4. 6 weeks after surgery
a. Return to normal activities
b. Treatment is continued until stage I goals are met.
B. Stage II
1. If both FDS/FDP are absent preoperatively, there are three
approaches. In all approaches, progression can be fine-tuned
with the use of Groth's "Pyramid of Progressive Force
Exercises to the Injured Flexor Tendon"[7] (see Box 17-2 in
Chapter 17).
a. Early immobilization
(1) Week 0 to week 3 or 4
(a) Splint: posterior plaster or thermoplastic splint with
wrist in 20 to 30 degrees flexion, MCP joints in
60 to 70 degrees flexion, and IP joints in extension.
(2) Weeks 3 to 4
(a) Splint: Worn between exercise programs for
1 to 2 additional weeks

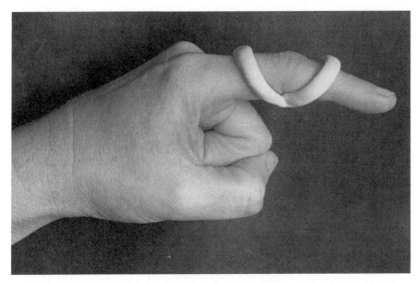

FIG. **18-12** Figure of 8 splint is used if "swan-neck" deformity is present or develops.

          (b) Exercise: See Boxes 17-1, 17-2, and 17-3B in
             Chapter 17.
    (3) Weeks 4 to 14: same as for early passive mobilization
  b. Early passive mobilization
    (1) Weeks 0 to 8: same as for primary flexor tendon
       grafting, except delay strengthening (see Box 17-3B in
       Chapter 17)
    (2) Weeks 9 to 10: Initiate graded strengthening.
    (3) Weeks 12 to 14: normal unrestricted use of hands
  c. Early active mobilization (three options given according to
    strength of graft junctures)
    (1) Standard surgical technique (Pulvertaft wave) used
       intraoperatively[5,6]
       (a) Postoperative splint position: wrist in midflexion,
          MCP joints at or slightly less than 90 degrees flexion,
          IP joints straight
       (b) 48 hours after surgery
          [1] Exercise is done at intervals of 2 hours throughout
            the day.
          [2] Two PROM into flexion exercises, followed by two
            AROM exercises
          [3] Gentle protected IP extension to help prevent
            flexion contractures
       (c) End of first week
          [1] Goal of PROM: full flexion and extension of IP
            joints
          [2] Goal of AROM: PIP actively flexed to about
            30 degrees, DIP actively flexed to 5 to 10 degrees
       (d) Weeks 2 through 5
          [1] Gradually increase flexion AROM of each joint.
          [2] PIP: 80 to 90 degrees flexion
          [3] DIP: 50 to 60 degrees flexion

(e) 4 weeks: If active flexion less than satisfactory, remove splint and begin more vigorous exercises. Progression can be fine tuned using Groth's Pyramid of Progressive Force Exercises to the Injured Flexor Tendon (see Box 17-2 in Chapter 17).

(f) 6 weeks: Discontinue protective splint

   [1] To prevent extension lag, use gentle passive stretching of IPs

   [2] If extension deficit is greater than 20 degrees beyond the 7th week, a dynamic three-point extension splint may be used

(g) Weeks 6 to 12: same as for early passive mobilization

(2) Strong graft junctures with tendon bed in excellent condition[4]

(a) Splinting: Protective dorsal splint with wrist at 30 degrees flexion, MCPs at 70 degrees flexion, and IPs at full extension

(b) First postoperative week: Active flexion protocol may be initiated without the use of elastic band; "passive hold" exercises in dorsal splint

   [1] Passive hold defined

      [a] Patient relaxes forearm muscles of involved extremity.

      [b] Patient gently presses fingers into flexion with the uninvolved hand and then tries to actively, lightly hold the fingers in flexion.

   [2] Rationale for passive hold: It takes less force to maintain an already flexed finger in flexion than to actively pull the finger into flexion from an extended position. The benefits of tendon excursion are the same as those derived from active flexion.

      [a] Patient is asked to perform this exercise in full flexion and at two ranges of partial flexion (e.g., slight flexion, midflexion, full flexion).

      [b] Three repetitions are performed at each range, three to four times per day.

      [c] Gentle passive flexion of IP joints is performed several times per day within the dorsal splint.

(c) 2 weeks: If the patient begins to glide the tendon very early and excellent tendon pull-through is demonstrated, therapy is slowed down at 2 weeks by applying elastic band traction. The patient can still perform the passive hold exercise, but the elastic band traction program adds protection.

(d) 6 to 12 weeks: Essentially the same as that described for early passive mobilization, including wristlet and graded strengthening.

(e) The therapist continues to devote attention to the prevention of flexion contractures.

(3) Mesh-reinforced graft[3] allows more aggressive postoperative treatment (see Box 17-5B in Chapter 17).

2. FDS intact with FDP absent preoperatively[12]: same as any of the above protocols, except that active isolated FDS flexion begun during the first postoperative week with wrist and MCPs flexed while holding unaffected digits (PIPs/DIPs) in passive extension.

POSTOPERATIVE COMPLICATIONS

I. Stage I of two-stage tendon reconstruction
   A. Hematoma
   B. Infection
   C. Extreme pain
   D. Severe edema
   E. Synovitis
   F. Swan-neck deformity
   G. Limited ROM
   H. Skin breakdown at distal insertion of implant
   I. Implant "kinking" or disruption
II. Primary tendon grafts and stage II of two-stage tendon reconstruction
   A. Infection
   B. Extreme pain
   C. Severe edema
   D. Adhesions limiting tendon gliding
   E. Tendon rupture
   F. Flexion contracture
   G. Pulley ruptured or attenuated
   H. Suboptimal graft length

EVALUATION TIMELINE

I. Preoperative
   A. Primary tendon grafts and staged tendon reconstruction
      1. Wound and skin condition
      2. Edema
      3. Pain
      4. Sensibility
      5. AROM/PROM
      6. Strength
II. Postoperative
   A. Stage I of two-stage tendon reconstruction
      1. Wound
      2. Edema
      3. Pain
      4. Sensibility
      5. Passive flexion
      6. Active PIP/DIP extension with wrist and MCP flexed
   B. Primary tendon grafts and stage II of two-stage tendon reconstruction
      1. First postoperative visit general assessment
         a. Wound and skin condition
         b. Edema
         c. Pain
         d. Passive flexion/protected active/passive extension

2. Week 6
   a. Active flexion and passive extension
   b. Sensibility
3. Week 12: strength

OUTCOMES

Tonkin and co-workers[13] found postgrafting total active motion (TAM) to be 76% of pregrafting total passive motion (TPM). This included both one-stage and two-stage flexor tendon reconstructions. All original injuries were in zone II. Final motion was independent of postoperative immobilization compared with gentle immediate controlled motion (Kleinert technique). Complications were higher in the group with immobilization compared with the immediate controlled motion group. One hundred forty five tendon grafts were performed in 127 patients, with 49 being one-stage and 83 two-stage reconstructions. Graft rupture was noted in 9 of the immobilized tendons versus 4 in the early controlled motion group. Tenolysis was done for 16 tendons in the immobilized group versus 8 in the early controlled motion group.

Amadio and colleagues[14] presented a study using 117 fingers in 89 patients including zones I through V. Postoperative treatment included both early immobilization and early passive motion. Fifty-five percent of the subjects had good to excellent results by the TAM/TPM method.[14] Only 19% had final TAM greater than 180 degrees. Poor results were associated with zone I or II injury and with patients younger than 10 years of age. Better results were associated with zone IV or V injury. Postoperative flexion contractures greater than 30 degrees were associated with patient dissatisfaction, despite significant increase in TAM.

Frakking and associates[2] presented a study of two-stage tendon grafting. The sample included 30 fingers and 10 thumbs in 38 patients. Based on the Buck-Gramcko score,[2] 70% of fingers had excellent or good results. None of the thumbs had excellent results, but 40% of thumbs had good results. Complications included infection in one patient. Additional procedures included tenolysis in 12 patients, repeat two-stage reconstruction in one patient, arthrodesis in one patient, and graft revisions in five patients secondary to graft rupture, bowstringing, and incorrect length of graft.

Khan and assocaites[5] presented a study of 9 two-stage tendon grafts in 9 patients. The standard Pulvertaft weave was used. The early active motion protocol was that described by Small and colleagues.[15] Results using Buck-Gramcko scoring were 3 excellent, 2 good, 2 satisfactory, and 2 poor. Using the criteria of Kleinert,[16] there was 1 excellent, 2 good, 5 fair, and 1 poor result. Regarding complications, there were no cases of tendon graft rupture or dehiscence at the junction between tendon and graft.

Silfverskiold and May[3] presented a study of 10 two-stage tendon grafts performed in 9 patients. A mesh-reinforced weave was used rather than the standard Pulvertaft weave, and this was followed by a more aggressive early active motion protocol. Using Strickland's[17] formula of composite IP TAM/175 (see Table 17-2 in Chapter 17), 50% had excellent results, 0% had good results, 30% had fair results, and 30% had poor results secondary to rupture. Regarding complications, 3 of 10 (30%) ruptured. One rupture occurred early in the series, before the importance of scraping the palmaris tendon clean of paratenon in the area where the mesh was to be applied was understood. It was later determined that when scraping was not done, the mesh attached to the paratenon rather than the tendon proper and could easily be pulled off the paratenon when tension was applied. The other two ruptures were secondary to falls on outstretched hands, one at 3 weeks and one at 3 months after surgery. Excluding the ruptured digits, active composite IP motion levels at 6 weeks and 6 months were, respectively, 79% and 76% of the AROM of the corresponding digit in the opposite hand.

REFERENCES

1. Schneider LH, Hunter JM: Flexor tendons: late reconstruction. In Green DP (ed): Operative Hand Surgery. Vol. 3. Churchill Livingstone, New York, 1988, p. 1969
2. Frakking TG, Depuydt KP, Kon M, et al.: Retrospective outcome analysis of staged flexor tendon reconstruction. J Hand Surg Br 25:168-174, 2000
3. Silfverskiold KL, May EJ: Early active mobilization of tendon grafts using mesh reinforced suture techniques. J Hand Surg Br 20:301-307, 1995
4. Hunter JM, Mackin EJ: Staged flexor tendon reconstruction. In Mackin EJ, Callahan AD, Skirven TM, Schneider LH, Osterman AL (eds): Rehabilitation of the Hand and Upper Extremity. 5th Ed. Mosby, St. Louis, 2002, pp. 469-497
5. Khan K, Riaz M, Murison MSC, et al.: Early active mobilization after second stage flexor tendon grafts. J Hand Surg Br 22:372-374, 1997
6. Pulvertaft RG: Tendon grafts for flexor tendon injuries in the fingers and thumb: a study of technique and results. J Bone Joint Surg Br 38:175-194, 1956
7. Groth GN: Pyramid of progressive force exercises to injured flexor tendon. J Hand Ther 17:31-42, 2004
8. Cannon NM, Strickland JW: Therapy following flexor tendon surgery. Hand Clin 1:156, 1985
9. Mackin EJ, Hunter JM: Pre- and Post-Operative Hand Therapy Program for Patients with Staged Tendon Implants (Hunter Design). Hand Rehabilitation Foundation, Philadelphia, 1986
10. Stanley BG: Flexor tendon injuries: late solution therapist's management. Hand Clin 12:140, 1986
11. Cannon NM: Therapy following flexor tendon surgery. Hand Clin 1:156, 1985, p. 147
12. McClinton MA, Curtis RM, Wilgis EFS: One hundred tendon grafts for isolated flexor digitorum injuries. J Hand Surg 7:224, 1982
13. Tonkin M, Hagberg L, Lister G, et al.: Post-operative management of flexor tendon grafting. J Hand Surg Br 13:277-281, 1988
14. Amadio PC, Wood MB, Cooney III WP, et al.: Staged flexor tendon reconstruction in the fingers and hand. J Hand Surg Am 13:559-562, 1988
15. Small JO, Brennen MD, Colville J: Early active mobilization following flexor tendon repair in zone 2. J Hand Surg Br 14:383-391, 1989
16. Kleinert HE, Vedon C: Report of the Committee on Tendon Injuries (International Federation of Societies for Surgery of the Hand). J Hand Surg Am 8:794-798, 1983
17. Strickland JW, Glogovac SV: Digital function following flexor tendon repair in zone II: a comparison of immobilization and controlled passive motion techniques. J Hand Surg Am 5:537-543, 1980

Flexor Tenolysis 19

Barbara Wilson

Flexor tenolysis is an elective surgical procedure that may be performed after primary tendon repair, grafting, or staged tendon reconstruction. It may be indicated if active range of motion (AROM) is significantly less than passive range of motion (PROM) secondary to scar adhesions.[1] This situation may arise despite optimal surgery and postsurgical therapy.

Close surgeon-therapist communication is helpful in optimizing postoperative therapy. The therapist needs to be aware of the quality of the tendon lysed and the need for any ancillary procedures. If the therapist is able to observe the surgery, this communication is greatly facilitated.

After surgery, two different treatment approaches may be used during the first 4 to 6 weeks. Both approaches involve early mobilization. With a good-quality tendon and good-quality pulleys (as noted by the surgeon intraoperatively), the more progressive approach may be used.[1,2] The "frayed tendon" protocol[1] is used with a poor quality tendon and/or pulley reconstruction. The frayed tendon guideline is used to decrease demands on the involved tendon or pulley while maintaining the tendon excursion achieved during surgery. If crepitus is noted during use of the more progressive approach, it is important to use the frayed tendon guideline, because this may be a sign of impending rupture.[1]

Initial AROM is ideally begun in the operating room or in the recovery room on the day of surgery, followed by daily formal hand therapy during the first postoperative week.

DEFINITION

Flexor tenolysis is a secondary surgical procedure in which adhesions or other obstacles that impede normal flexor tendon gliding are released (Fig. 19-1).

SURGICAL AND TREATMENT PURPOSE

To restore flexor tendon function if tendon gliding has been compromised or lost because of scar adhesions. The surgical approach may be very localized

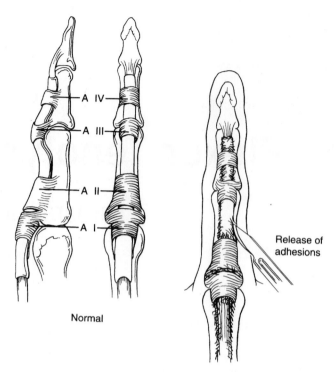

FIG. **19-1** Adhesions are released in tenolysis surgery.

or very extensive, depending on the preoperative and intraoperative assessments. Sharp dissection is used to minimize tissue trauma. Care is taken to preserve the critical portions of the digital pulley systems. Adequacy of the tendon release may be assessed by two intraoperative methods. In an awake patient and with the use of local anesthesia, active excursion may be demonstrated by the patient. If general anesthesia is used, the surgeon may test excursion by retracting the tendons proximal to the zone of scarring addressed. Early therapy is used to minimize subsequent development of tendon adhesions. Extensive surgical release may weaken the tendon or compromise blood supply to the newly freed tendon. These conditions create a risk of postoperative tendon rupture. Careful and attentive postoperative care is required to achieve an optimal goal while avoiding complications.

I. Week 1
   A. Achieve intraoperative AROM/PROM before binding adhesions can form.
   B. Prevent flexion contracture via splinting.[3]
   C. Minimize pain. An intraoperative catheter allows the patient to self-administer pain medication or transcutaneous electrical nerve stimulation (TENS).
   D. Minimize edema.
   E. Protect poor-quality or reconstructed pulleys.
II. Weeks 2 to 3
   A. Initiate functional use of involved hand.
   B. Initiate scar management.
III. Weeks 4 to 6
   A. Increase grip and pinch strength as tendon integrity allows.[3]

IV. Weeks 7 to 8
   A. Initiate job simulation in preparation for return to work at 8 to 12 weeks, depending on job demands.
   B. Initiate heavy resistance at week 8 if tendon quality permits.[3]

POSTOPERATIVE INDICATIONS/PRECAUTIONS FOR THERAPY

I. Indications
   A. Digits that have undergone flexor tenolysis surgery
II. Precautions
   A. Pulley reconstruction
   B. Capsulectomy
   C. Poor-quality or badly scarred tendon as reported by the surgeon after the procedure

POSTOPERATIVE THERAPY

I. Consult with surgeon regarding intraoperative AROM/PROM, condition of the tendon, status of the pulley system, as well as any additional procedure performed (e.g., pulley reconstruction, capsulectomy).
II. Pulley reconstruction protection[4]
   A. Identify areas of pulley reconstruction.
   B. Protect by circumferential Velcro/thermoplastic ring until edema is under control, and then with a thermoplastic ring (Fig. 19-2).
III. Program for good-quality tendons
   A. Hours 12 to 24 through first postoperative week (inflammation phase of wound healing)
      1. Splint
         a. Forearm-based progressive extension or static extension (Fig. 19-3) is worn day and night for 2 weeks, removed for exercise and wound care.
         b. Indications[3]
            (1) To prevent flexion contractures
            (2) To protect weakened tendons
            (3) To rest tissues between exercise sessions.
         c. Precautions[3]
            (1) Caution patient to avoid pulling or flexion against splint, to avoid early resistance and possible tendon rupture.
      2. Exercise
         a. Passive
            (1) Perform 10 repetitions per hour to loosen joints before active motion.[1]
            (2) Gentle, protected PROM of all joints
            (3) Technique
               (a) With wrist in passive extension, passively manipulate the digit into the fully flexed position with the uninvolved hand.
               (b) Patient actively maintains the digit in this position.

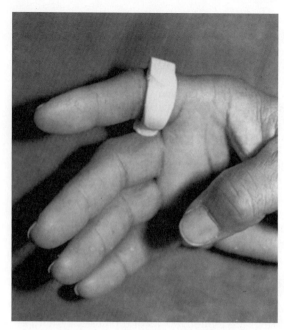

FIG. **19-2** Pulley reconstruction is protected by circumferential thermoplastic ring.

(c) Manipulation hand is released and lysed tendons are maintained in flexion with their own muscle power, confirming active muscle contraction. This is followed by active extension of the digit or digits.

(d) Additional protection can be achieved by maintaining some element of wrist flexion, although full excursion of the tendon is not achieved in this position.

(e) The patient's discomfort level determines the beginning number of repetitions; frequency is maintained every waking hour, working up to 10 repetitions per hour.

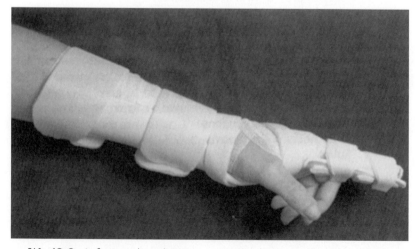

FIG. **19-3** A forearm-based static extension splint is used postoperatively.

b. Active
    (1) Perform 5 to 10 repetitions of each exercise hourly.
    (2) Place and hold.
        (a) Passively flex other digits and wrist while passively extending in turn the metacarpophalangeal (MCP), proximal interphalangeal (PIP), and distal interphalangeal (DIP) joints.
    (3) Finger blocking
        (b) Block MCP and PIP joints into extension, allowing isolated active DIP flexion.
        (c) Block MCP into extension, allowing isolated PIP flexion.
    (4) Finger extension
3. Edema control
4. Pain management
B. 2 to 3 weeks postoperative (initiation of proliferative phase of wound healing)
1. Splint
    a. Static or progressive extension
        (1) Decrease use in day as AROM achieved intraoperatively is maintained pain free.
        (2) Continue use at night to prevent/decrease flexion contracture and/or extrinsic flexor tendon tightness.
    b. Dynamic extension for flexion contractures may be used with surgeon's approval, for short periods during the day (Fig. 19-4).
2. Exercise
    a. Continue exercises as above.
        (1) PROM
        (2) Place and hold

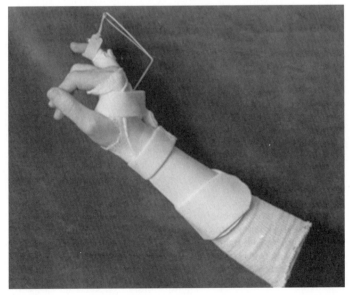

FIG. 19-4 Dynamic extension for contractures may be used with doctor's approval.

        (3) Finger blocking
        (4) Finger extension
     b. Add active tendon gliding (3 to 10 repetitions per hour)
  3. Activities of daily living (ADLs)
     a. Light ADLs
     b. Nonresistive grasp and release.
C. 4 to 6 weeks postoperative (proliferative phase of wound healing ending as scar remodeling phase begins)
  1. Splint
     a. Static or progressive extension. Wear in daytime only if needed.
     b. Dynamic extension to assist with extension as needed. May leave on for most of the day. Patient may exercise into flexion against resistance of splint.
  2. Exercise
     a. Continue exercises as above as needed
        (1) PROM
        (2) Place and hold
        (3) Finger blocking
        (4) Finger extension
        (5) Tendon gliding
           (a) Hook-fist: Begin with the fingers in full extension. With MCP joints in extension, actively flex PIP and DIP joints. Flexor digitorum superficialis (FDS) and flexor digitorum profundus (FDP) independently glide over each other most in this position[5] (Fig. 19-5).
           (b) Full fist: Beginning in hook-fist position, flex MCP, PIP, and DIP joints fully, touching distal palmar crease. (FDP reaches its maximum excursion with respect to bone in this position.) End with fingers in full extension[5] (see Fig. 19-5).
           (c) Straight fist: Begin with fingers in full extension. Actively flex MCP and PIP joints while maintaining DIP joints in extension. (FDS reaches its maximum excursion in respect to bone in this position)[5] (see Fig. 19-5).

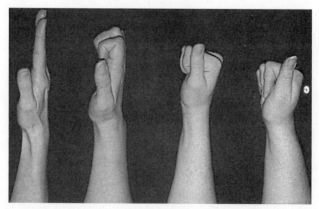

FIG. **19-5** Tendon gliding exercises. (From Mackin EJ, Callahan AD, Skirven TM, et al.: Hunter-Mackin-Callahan Rehabilitation of the Hand and Upper Extremity. 5th Ed. Mosby, St. Louis, 2002.)

        (d) Wrist flexion with finger flexion[6] (Fig. 19-6)

        (e) Wrist extension with finger extension[6] (see Fig. 19-6)

    b. Graded isometric grip strengthening with physician approval. Monitor closely.

  3. ADLs

    a. ADLs

    b. Graded ADLs

D. 8 to 12 weeks postoperative (scar remodeling continues)

  1. Gradually increase resistive exercises and activities to no restriction at 12 weeks.

IV. "Frayed tendon" program[1,2,7]

  A. Indications

    1. Surgical finding of poor-quality tendon

    2. Pulleys reconstructed

    3. Tendons with auditory or palpable crepitation during uncomplicated early mobilization program

  B. First 4 to 6 weeks postoperative

    1. Splint: same as for uncomplicated, good-quality tendons

    2. Exercise

      a. Protected PROM: Perform 10 repetitions every hour before place and hold.

      b. Place and hold: Perform 5 to 10 repetitions per hour.

  C. 7 to 12 weeks postoperative: same as for good-quality tendon program.

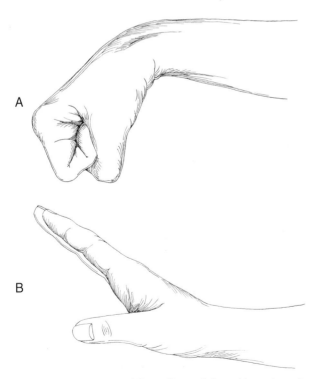

FIG. **19-6** **A** and **B,** Active wrist and finger flexion followed by active wrist and finger extension maximizes the potential excursion of the flexor digitorum superficialis (FDS) and flexor digitorum profundus (FDP), with 49 mm to the FDS and 50 mm with FDP. (Modified from Cannon NW: J Hand Ther 2:122, 1989, p. 126.)

POSTOPERATIVE COMPLICATIONS

    I. Pain
   II. Edema
  III. Bleeding
  IV. Infection
   V. Patient's inability to tolerate postoperative therapy
  VI. Excessive scar formation
 VII. Auditory or palpable crepitation
VIII. Tendon rupture
  IX. Flexion contractures
   X. Reconstructed pulley rupture

EVALUATION TIMELINE

   I. Preoperative
     A. AROM and PROM (blocked and full excursion)
     B. Fingertip to distal palmar crease (active and passive)
     C. Strength
     D. Circumferential measurements
     E. Sensibility
  II. First postoperative therapy session (12 to 24 hours postoperative)
     A. Assessment
       1. Wound
       2. Edema
       3. Pain
     B. Measurement
       1. AROM and PROM
       2. Fingertip to distal palmar crease (active and passive)
 III. Reevaluate AROM/PROM and scar weekly for first 8 weeks and then every 4 weeks.
  IV. Take strength measurements at 4 to 6 weeks with good-quality tendons and surgeon's approval,[3] at 8 weeks for both good-quality and "frayed" tendons, then at 4-week intervals.[3]
   V. Reevaluate sensibility at 4 weeks, and then at 4-week intervals.

OUTCOMES

Tenolysis outcome studies have demonstrated a wide range of results, although the general conclusions are similar. Digits that are most damaged before tenolysis perform the most poorly, whereas digits with the least damage due to injury and previous surgeries demonstrate the best outcome.[8,9]

REFERENCES

1. Cannon NW, Strickland JW: Therapy following flexor tendon surgery. Hand Clin 1:147, 1985
2. Strickland JW: Flexor tenolysis: a personal experience. In Hunter JM, Schneider LH, Mackin EJ (eds): Tendon Surgery in the Hand. Mosby, St. Louis, 1987
3. Schneider LH, Feldscher SB: Tenolysis: dynamic approach to surgery and therapy. In Mackin EJ, Callahan AD, Skirven TM, et al. (eds): Hunter-Mackin-Callahan Rehabilitation of the Hand and Upper Extremity. 5th Ed. Mosby, St. Louis, 2002

4. Sotereanos DG, Goitz RJ, Mitsionis GJ: Flexor tenolysis. In Taras JS, Schneider LH: Atlas of the Hand Clinics. WB Saunders, Philadelphia, 1996, pp. 105-120
5. Wehbe MS: Tendon gliding exercises. Am J Occup Ther 41:164, 1987
6. Cannon NW: Enhancing flexor tendon glide through tenolysis and hand therapy. J Hand Ther 2:122, 1989
7. Strickland JW: Flexor tenolysis. Hand Clin 1:121, 1985
8. Jupiter JB, Pess GM, Bour CJ: Results of flexor tendon tenolysis after replantation in the hand. J Hand Surg Am 14:1, 1989
9. Birnie RH, Idler RS: Flexor tenolysis in children. J Hand Surg Am 20:2, 1995

Management of Extensor Tendon Repairs

20

Rebecca J. Saunders

The anatomy and physiology of the extensor apparatus is complex and has been well described in the literature.[1-3] A thorough knowledge of the anatomy and the complex interplay between the extrinsic and intrinsic extensors is necessary for effective management of injuries to the extensor system (Figs. 20-1 and 20-2). Because of the dynamic interplay of the extrinsic and intrinsic systems and the intertendinous connections (of the extensor digitorum communis [EDC] via the juncturae tendinum), partial tendon injuries may not be apparent initially. Imbalance in the extensor system, if left untreated, can lead to the development of later-stage deformities (i.e., boutonniere or swan-neck deformities). Please refer to Chapter 21 for management of these deformities.

The superficial locations of the extensor tendons and minimal subcutaneous tissue on the dorsum of the hand predispose the extensor tendons to injury. Extensor tendon injuries frequently are associated with concurrent injuries to skin, bone, and joints. The reported incidence of such complex injuries varies from 66% to 80%.[4,5] The extent of the injury, the timing, and the type of repair influence selection of the rehabilitation technique for each patient. The patient's level of understanding of his or her injury and ability to comply with the selected technique are also factors to consider. Recent studies using static splinting have demonstrated results comparable to those obtained with early motion protocols,[6-8] and static management can be more cost-effective in some cases. Static management is recommended for children and for uncooperative patients.

Extensor tendon trauma is classified according to anatomical zones of injury; there are varying characteristics in different areas of the hand (Fig. 20-3). These zones will be referred to in the discussion of the rehabilitation techniques. In general, tendon injuries occurring between the joints (e.g., zone II) are managed similar to the next most distal level (e.g., zone I).[9]

Many of the advances in rehabilitation of extensor tendon injuries have been based on basic science and clinical research involving the synovial

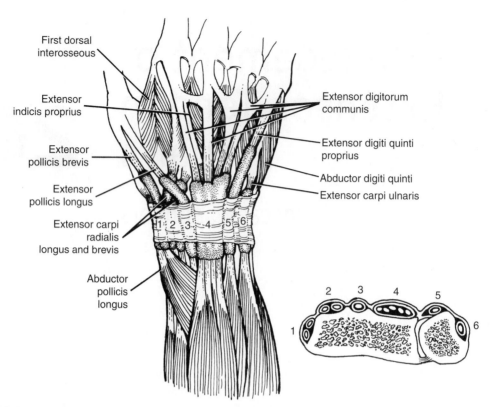

First dorsal
interosseous

Extensor
indicis proprius

Extensor
pollicis brevis

Extensor
pollicis longus

Extensor carpi
radialis
longus and brevis

Abductor
pollicis
longus

Extensor digitorum
communis

Extensor digiti quinti
proprius

Abductor digiti quinti

Extensor carpi ulnaris

FIG. 20-1 Extensor anatomy of the dorsum of the hand and wrist. 1 through 6, dorsal compartments through which extensors travel. (From Fess EE, Gettle K, Philips C, Janson JR: Hand and Upper Extremity Splinting: Principles and Methods. 3rd Ed. Mosby, St. Louis, 2005.)

flexor tendon system.[10,11-22] The benefits of early controlled motion, including decreased adhesion formation, improved tensile strength, and improved synovial diffusion, have been demonstrated by many studies.[11,14-16,21,23]

Although there are histological and nutritional differences between the flexor and extensor tendon systems, the basic work requirement of the tendon is the same. The tendon must glide relative to the surrounding tissues in order to transmit the force of muscle contraction.

Early passive range of motion (PROM) and active range of motion (AROM) protocols have been designed to reduce the complications associated with immobilization, including tendon adherence, extension lag, joint stiffness or contracture, and prolonged duration of treatment. Evans and Burkhalter[24] were among the early researchers of controlled PROM protocols for extensor tendon management. Using a review of literature along with biomechanical and intraoperative studies, they established the amount of metacarpophalangeal (MCP) joint flexion needed to create 5 mm of EDC glide in zones V through VII (28.3 degrees for the index finger, 27.5 for the middle finger, 40.9 for the ring finger, and 38.33 for the small finger).[24] This amount of tendon glide was beneficial and effective in restoring functional motion in simple and complex tendon injuries.[24,25]

Minamikawa and colleagues[26] studied the effect of wrist position on extensor tendon excursion after repair. In a cadaveric study, they measured the amount of glide that occurred in zones III to VIII with simulated active

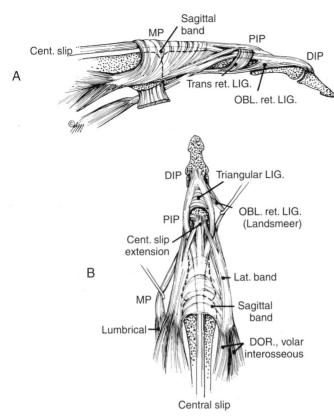

FIG. 20-2 **A,** The extensor tendon at the metacarpophalangeal (MP) joint level is held in place by the transverse lamina or sagittal band, which tethers and centers the extensor tendons over the joint. This sagittal band arises from the volar plate and the intermetacarpal ligaments at the neck of the metacarpals. Any injury to this extensor hood or expansion may result in subluxation or dislocation of the extensor tendon. **B,** The intrinsic tendons from the lumbrical and interosseous muscles join the extensor mechanism at about the level of the proximal and midportion of the proximal phalanx and continue distally to the distal interphalangeal (DIP) joint of the finger. The extensor mechanism at the proximal interphalangeal (PIP) joint is best described as a trifurcation of the extensor tendon into the central slip, which attaches to the dorsal base of the middle phalanx, and two lateral bands. The lateral bands continue distally to insert at the dorsal base of the distal phalanx. The extensor mechanism is maintained in place over the PIP joint by the transverse retinacular ligaments. (From Doyle JR: Extensor tendons: acute injuries. In Green DP, Hotchkiss RN, Pederson WC: Green's Operative Hand Surgery. 4th Ed. Churchill Livingstone, New York, 1999, p. 1953.)

grip and passive extension of the digits with the wrist in various degrees of extension. They found that gliding occurred with little or no tension in zones V and VI, through full simulated grip to full extension, if the wrist was positioned at 30 degrees or more extension. They believed that the digital flexion blocks limiting MCP excursion are not necessary if the wrist is extended 30 degrees and there is no debridement or shortening of the tendon. Browne and Ribik[27] reported excellent results using a dynamic extension splinting protocol allowing full flexion, but the patients in this group were carefully selected. Crosby and Wehbe[28,29] also used a dynamic

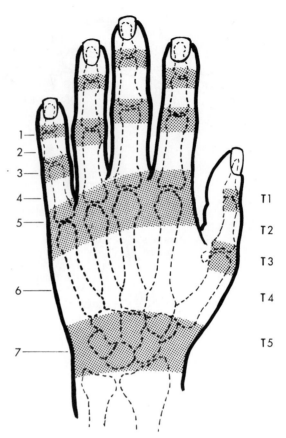

1
2
3
4
5
6
7

T1
T2
T3
T4
T5

FIG. 20-3 Extensor tendon zones as defined by the Committee on Tendon Injuries for the International Federation of the Society for Surgery of the Hand. (From Kleinert HE, Verdan C: J Hand Surg Am 8:794-798, 1983.)

extension splinting protocol that allowed active fisting. They advocated determining the need for a flexion block intraoperatively for postoperative management in any zone of injury.

Researchers have questioned the actual tendon excursion created with PROM protocols.[22,26] The belief that some degree of AROM may be necessary to create proximal migration of the repair site has led to the development of early AROM protocols in extensor tendon management.[4,30-34] Tendon excursion in the early phase of healing must be great enough to stimulate biochemical and mechanical changes but not so great as to create tendon gapping or rupture at the repair site. To apply controlled stress safely to the repair site, hand therapists need to understand tendon excursions as related to motion at each joint, as well as tensile strength as related to various suture techniques and the healing sequence.[4,35] Early controlled ROM, whether by passive or active means, can improve clinical and functional results. When selecting a method of rehabilitation for a patient, the hand therapist must communicate with the physician about the type of repair performed, associated injuries, and the appropriate rehabilitation technique. It is recommended that therapists read the original references before attempting early AROM techniques.

Timing is a crucial component in the early AROM protocols. Ideally, AROM protocols are initiated within 24 to 48 hours after surgery.

Immobilized tendon has been shown to lose tensile strength during the first 2 weeks after repair and to have decreased gliding function by 10 days postoperatively.[4,13,14] A late referral for early AROM protocols should be discussed with the referring physician before proceeding.

DEFINITION

Extensor tendon repair is primary repair of complete rupture or laceration of any digital extensor tendon in zones III through IX or of thumb extensors in zones TI through TV.

SURGICAL PURPOSE

To restore continuity and maintain gliding of the extensor mechanism from the PIP joints proximally toward the wrist level. Tendon gliding is critical beneath the retinacular ligaments covering the fibroosseous compartments at the wrist. Scarring over the dorsal surface of the hand is a problem because of scant soft tissue protection between the skin's surface and the underlying skeletal structures. Tendon suturing techniques vary depending on the zone in which the actual juncture is placed. The zone of tendon division may not coincide with that of the actual skin laceration. Other than lacerations, extensor tendon continuity may be lost secondary to attrition from sharp bone fragments after fracture, rheumatoid arthritis, tendinitis, or developmental absence.

TREATMENT GOALS

    I. Prevent tendon rupture.
    II. Promote tendon healing.
    III. Encourage tendon gliding while minimizing tendon gapping and extensor lag.
    IV. Restore AROM and PROM.
    V. Edema control
    VI. Pain control
    VII. Scar management
    VIII. Maintain full range of motion (ROM) of all uninvolved joints of the affected upper extremity.
    IX. Return to previous level of function.

POSTOPERATIVE INDICATIONS/PRECAUTIONS FOR THERAPY

    I.   Indications: surgical repair of extensor zones III through IX and thumb zones TI through TV
    II. Precautions
        A. Infection
        B. Combined flexor tendon repair
        C. Associated injures: fractures, nerve repairs, vessel repairs
        D. Type and strength of repair; degree of tendon shortening
        E. Extreme pain
        F. Severe edema
        G. Patient's level of understanding of his or her injury and ability to comply with protocol.

H. Extensor lag: The patient's ability to extend needs to be monitored closely as activities into flexion progress; the flexors are three to four times as strong as the extensors,[36] and an increase in extensor lag may require reinstitution of splinting and/or a decrease in flexion excursion. The goal is to maintain or improve extension as flexion progresses. It is much easier to prevent an extension lag than to fix one.

POSTOPERATIVE THERAPY

I.   Zones I and II: Formal repair at this level is difficult because of the size and nature of the terminal tendon in the digits. Newport[37] advocated tenodermodesis as the most reliable method of repair. In this technique, the skin and tendon are sutured as a single layer. A transarticular Kirschner wire is frequently used to supplement the repair and is left in place for 6 weeks. The repair is also protected via splinting. For therapy after K-wire removal, refer to management of mallet finger injury in Chapter 21.

II. Zones III and IV: Extensor tendon injuries in this area are challenging to treat because of the broad tendon-bone interface over the proximal phalanx and the complex interplay between the intrinsic and extrinsic tendon systems at this level. Injuries in this area are frequently complex. Numerous authors have reported this area to have the highest percentage of poor results.[38,39] Early PROM and AROM protocols were developed to help limit the problems associated with prolonged immobilization of the PIP joint. As with all protocols, it is recommended that the reader review in depth the theory and clinical application of the technique to ensure correct and safe use.

A. Early Active Short Arc Motion (SAM) protocol, as developed by Evans and Thompson[4,30-32]: Therapy begins as early as 24 hours after surgery.

1. The involved digit is splinted with the PIP and DIP at 0 degrees in a volar thermoplastic splint at all times excluding exercise.

2. Two template splints are used during active exercises to control the excursion of the repaired tendon and the application of stress.

a. Template splint no. 1 (Fig. 20-4, A and B) allows 30 degrees of PIP flexion and 20 to 25 degrees of DIP flexion

b. Template splint no. 2 (Fig. 20-5, A to C) supports the PIP at neutral and allows DIP flexion.

(1) Full DIP flexion is allowed in template splint no. 2 if the lateral bands were not repaired.

(2) DIP flexion is limited to 30 to 35 degrees if the lateral bands were repaired; active DIP extension is emphasized.

3. Exercises are performed every waking hour for 20 repetitions each session. The patient should be instructed to perform each exercise slowly and to hold the digit briefly in the extended position. Emphasis should be placed on supporting the PIP at neutral in splint no. 2 during DIP flexion.

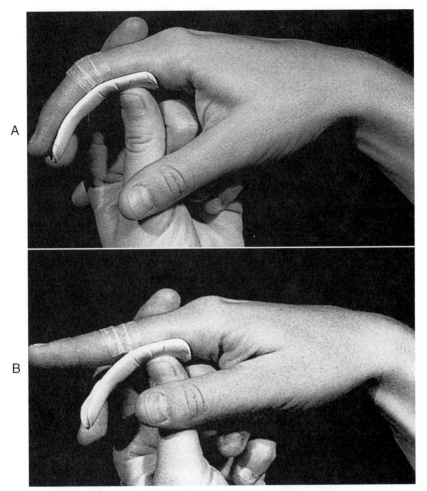

FIG. 20-4 **A,** Template splint 1 allows 30 degrees flexion at the proximal interphalangeal (PIP) joint and 20 to 25 degrees flexion at the distal interphalangeal (DIP) joint, preventing the patient from stretching the repair site by allowing only precalculated excursion of the central slip. The wrist is positioned in 30 degrees flexion, and the metacarpophalangeal joint at 0 degrees; the digit is supported at the proximal phalanx by the contralateral hand. **B,** The PIP joint is actively flexed and extended in a controlled range. (From Evans RB: J Hand Surg Am 19:992, 1994.)

       a. The wrist is positioned at 30 degrees flexion, and the MCP joint is at neutral or slight flexion during the performance of exercises. This position reduces the resistance of the flexors and facilitates assistance of the interossei in PIP extension.

4. Progression of PIP excursion
    a. If no PIP extension lag develops after 2 weeks of controlled motion at 30 degrees of flexion, template splint no. 1 is adjusted to allow 40 degrees flexion; 50 degrees flexion is allowed at 4 weeks postoperatively.
    b. If a PIP extension lag develops, continue limiting excursion at 30 degrees flexion and contact the referring physician to discuss further progression.

5. Splinting usually is discontinued at 6 weeks, and full AROM is begun.

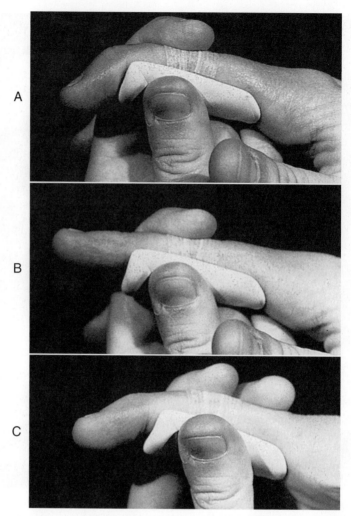

FIG. **20-5** **A** through **C,** Template splint 2 immobilizes only the proximal interphalangeal joint, allowing isolated distal joint motion to create gliding of the lateral
bands. If the lateral bands are not repaired, the distal joint is fully flexed and
extended **(A, B)**. If the lateral bands are repaired, the distal interphalangeal joint is
flexed only to 30 to 35 degrees **(C)**. (From Evans RB: J Hand Surg 19A:993, 1994.)

6. Begin light use of the hand and progress to strengthening at
   8 weeks. The degree of extension lag needs to be monitored
   closely as activities and use of the hand are progressed.

B. Early mobilization for repaired zone III and IV tendons, as
   described by Thomes and Thomes[40]: This protocol uses a hand-
   based dynamic splint to provide PIP extension and promote
   tendon gliding passively. It can be initiated as early as the same
   day of surgery. Some patients may require initial immobilization
   with the PIP at neutral during the early inflammatory phase.
   Thomes and Thomes recommended initiation of the dynamic
   splint no later than 2 to 4 days after surgery.

   1. A static hand-based splint with the PIP at neutral is
      recommended for night use. Patients in the study wore
      the dynamic splint at all times.

   2. A hand-based dynamic PIP extension splint is fabricated with
      the MCP at 20 degrees flexion (Fig. 20-6). Traction is adjusted

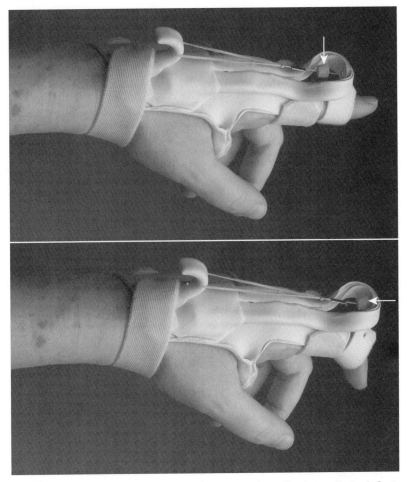

FIG. 20-6 The hand-based dynamic extension splint allowing a limited flexion excursion.

   to allow PIP extension to neutral or slight hyperextension
   (compared with the patient's normal PIP extension). The
   DIP is left free.
3. A stop bead limits PIP excursion
   a. PIP excursion is limited to 30 degrees during the first
      week, 40 degrees during the second week, and 50 degrees
      during the third week. The stop bead is removed at 4 weeks.
   b. Patients are instructed to perform flexion within a
      pain-free range 10 to 20 times hourly within the limits
      of the splint.
4. After completion of 4 weeks of dynamic splinting, the traction
   line is removed and the splint is worn as a protective bumper
   and to remind the patient not to overuse the hand.
5. Begin AROM without resistance (gentle blocking exercises)
6. Patients are instructed to perform reverse blocking exercises
   hourly to ensure full PIP extension (Fig. 20-7).
7. Protective splinting is discontinued at 6 weeks.
8. Gentle flexion strapping can be initiated at 6 weeks. The
   patient's ability to maintain PIP extension needs to be
   monitored closely.

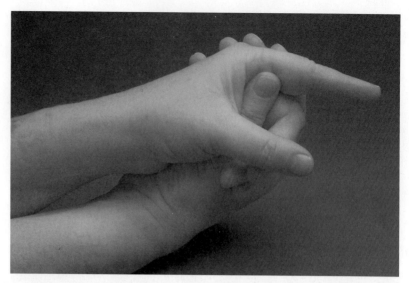

FIG. **20-7** Reverse blocking exercise. PIP extension is performed with the MP manually supported in flexion.

     9. Little detail is given regarding progression of resistive exercises. There were no reported ruptures or secondary surgeries.

III. Finger and wrist extensors, zones V, VI, and VII: With all methods of management, splints need to be monitored during the treatment phase to ensure proper fit as the edema subsides.

   A. Immobilization method: Management by immobilization may be indicated for simple injuries and in children and noncompliant patients.

     1. 0 to 21 days postoperatively

       a. Splinting: volar with wrist in 30 degrees extension, MCP in 0 degrees extension; interphalangeal (IP) joints may be left free for ROM in a blocking splint (Fig. 20-8). A removable pan to support IPs in extension may be used intermittently during the day and at night to prevent PIP flexion contractures.

         (1) Variation for simple injury of extensor indicis proprius (EIP) or extensor digiti minimi (EDM): Only the repaired tendon or digit needs to be immobilized.

         (2) Variation for simple injury of single extensor digitorum communis (EDC)

            (a) If repair site is *proximal* to interconnecting juncturae tendinum, all fingers need to be splinted in extension.

            (b) If repair site is *distal* to interconnecting juncturae tendinum, the affected digit is splinted in full MCP extension and the adjacent digits in 30 degrees MCP flexion with IPs free (Fig. 20-9).

       b. Therapy

         (1) Wound care

         (2) Edema control

         (3) MCP joint protective ROM: Therapist supports wrist and IPs in full extension while gently moving the *index* and *middle* finger MCPs from slight hyperextension to 30 degrees flexion and the *ring* and *small* finger MCPs from slight hyperextension to 40 degrees flexion.

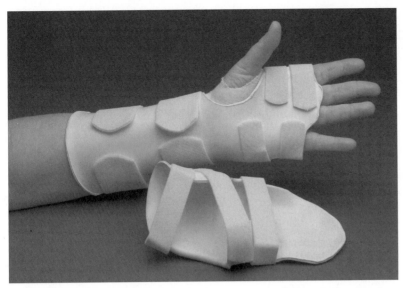

FIG. **20-8** Volar protective splint with the MPs in full extension allowing IP PROM. Removable pan component is used at night and intermittently during the day to rest IPs at neutral.

       (4) PIP/DIP joint protective ROM: Therapist supports wrist and MCPs in full extension while passively moving each individual PIP and DIP joint through complete ROM.

       (5) If patients demonstrate excessive stiffness with PROM, discuss switching to a dynamic passive mobilization protocol with the referring physician.

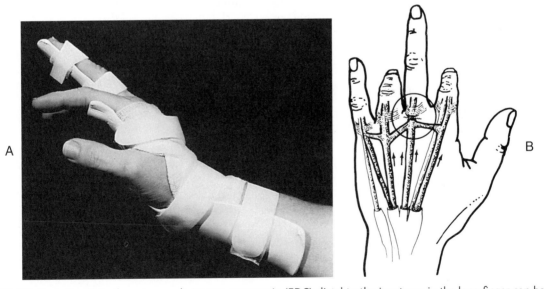

FIG. **20-9** **A,** Repair to the extensor digitorum communis (EDC) distal to the juncturae in the long finger can be adequately protected with splinting that rests the long finger metacarpophalangeal (MCP) joint at 0 degrees and adjacent MCP joints at 30 degrees flexion. This position relieves tension at the repair site while maintaining some extensibility of the collateral ligaments of the uninvolved fingers. **B,** Tension can be reduced on the anastomosis of the EDC when the repair site is distal to the juncturae tendinum if the adjacent fingers are held in mild flexion. This position advances the proximal end of the severed tendon by a force of the intertendinous connection. (From Beasley RW: Hand Injuries. WB Saunders, Philadelphia, 1981.)

2. 3 weeks postoperatively
   a. Splinting: volar, with wrist in 20 degrees extension, MCPs
      in 0 degrees extension; protective splinting is continued at
      all times excluding exercise periods.
   b. Therapy: begin protected AROM.
      (1) MCP AROM and active-assisted range of motion
          (AAROM) with tenodesis: MCP extension with wrist in
          neutral to slight flexion, MCP flexion (40 to 60 degrees)
          with wrist in full extension
      (2) IP AROM, AAROM, and PROM through complete
          range, while wrist and MCPs are supported in full
          extension
3. 4 weeks postoperatively
   a. Splinting: Dynamic MCP flexion may be needed if motion
      is limited in the range of 50 to 60 degrees.[4] Extension
      needs to be monitored closely; if an extension lag develops,
      stop MCP flexion splinting.
   b. Therapy
      (1) Composite MCP/IP flexion with wrist extension
      (2) Individual finger extension
      (3) Isolated EDC extension
4. Between 4 and 5 weeks postoperatively
   a. Splinting: A combination of MCP and IP flexion
      splinting may be initiated to decrease extrinsic
      extensor tightness.
   b. Therapy: same as for 3 and 4 weeks postoperatively
5. 6 to 10 weeks postoperatively
   a. Splinting: only as needed. The patient's ability to extend
      needs to be monitored closely as activities are progressed.
   b. Therapy
      (1) Composite finger and wrist flexion, initiated when no
          extension lag is present
      (2) Mild progressive strengthening including wrist
          flexion/extension and forearm pronation/supination
6. 10 to 12 weeks postoperatively: strong resistive exercise
B. Early passive motion method[4]
   1. 24 hours to 3 days postoperatively
      a. Splinting (Fig. 20-10): two-part dynamic splint
         (1) *Dorsal component*: dynamic MCP extension splint with
             MCPs supported at neutral; wrist is positioned at
             30 degrees extension.
         (2) *Interlocking volar component*: Wrist in 30 degrees
             extension; MCPs permitting active flexion of 30 degrees
             for index and middle fingers and 40 degrees for ring
             and small fingers
      b. Therapy
         (1) Wound care
         (2) Edema control
         (3) Splint adjustments
         (4) Controlled IP PROM: see immobilization method,
             PIP/DIP joint protective ROM—0 to 21 days
             postoperatively

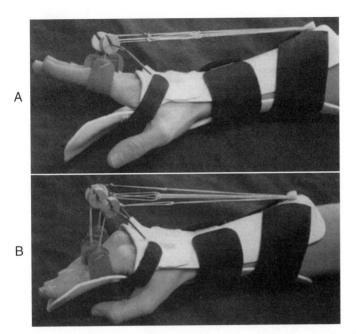

FIG. **20-10** **A,** Dynamic extension splint using an outrigger with rubber band traction to allow active flexion of the digits with passive extension to neutral. **B,** Dynamic extension splint with full flexion of the digits blocked by both a thermoplastic volar block and bead blocks on the outrigger lines (only one type of flexion block per splint is necessary in practice. (From Carney KL, Griffin-Reed N: Rehabilitation after extensor tendon injury and repair. In Berger RA, Weiss AC [eds]. Hand Surgery. Vol. 1. Lippincott Williams & Wilkins, Philadelphia, 2004, p. 774.)

(5) Patient performs exercise each waking hour
   (a) While maintaining IP extension, patient actively flexes digits at MCP joints until fingers touch volar splint. Patient releases digits, allowing extension loops to passively extend MCPs to 0 degrees.
   (b) For zone VII, while loops support other digits in extension, the patient individually flexes each digit to the limit of the splint, after which traction passively extends the digit; this is done to promote gliding under the retinaculum.
(6) Wrist tenodesis
   (a) Zones V and VI: simultaneous wrist extension with 30 degrees flexion of index and middle finger MCPs and 40 degrees flexion of ring and small finger MCPs, followed by simultaneous wrist flexion to 20 degrees with all digital joints held at 0 degrees
   (b) Zone VII *without* wrist tendon involvement: as above, except that when digits are placed in 0 degrees, wrist is in no less than 10 degrees extension
   (c) Zone VII *with* wrist tendon involvement: as above, except that when digits are placed in 0 degrees, wrist is in no less than 20 degrees extension

2. 3 weeks postoperatively
   a. Splinting
      (1) Day: Volar block splint is removed; continue with dorsal dynamic splint.
      (2) Night: Wear volar static splint (adjusted to 30 degrees wrist extension and 0 degrees MCP/IP extension).
   b. Therapy
      (1) Begin protected gradual active motion of MCP and IP joints within dynamic extension splint.
      (2) Dynamic splinting and exercise are the same as for management by immobilization from the 3 week period onward.
3. 4 to 5 weeks postoperatively: Initiate composite finger flexion with wrist in extension. Splinting continues between exercise sessions and at night until 6 to 8 weeks postoperatively, depending on the tendons involved and the patient's ability to maintain extension.
4. 6 to 12 weeks postoperatively: same as for immobilization method.
   a. Wrist extensors *without* finger extensor involvement (zone VII)
      (1) Splinting: wrist in 30 degrees extension, with MCPs and IPs free; continue protective splinting up to 8 weeks due to the loading requirements of these tendons.
      (2) Therapy
         (a) 3 weeks postoperatively: Gravity-eliminated active motion from 0 degrees to full wrist extension
         (b) 4 to 8 weeks postoperatively: Slowly add increments of wrist flexion, radial and ulnar deviation.
         (c) 8 to 12 weeks postoperatively: progressive strengthening

IV. Zones VIII and IX. Repairs in these zones involve more muscle than tendon.[37] These injuries may be managed with the dynamic extension splinting protocol, as outlined for zones V through VII, if a strong tendinous repair was possible. Consult with the attending surgeon. More proximal repairs in zone IX may require temporary splinting of the elbow at 90 degrees of flexion.

V. Thumb zones TI and TII: The extensor pollicis longus (EPL) in zone TI is more substantial than the terminal tendon in the digit and may tolerate a formal repair.
   A. Static splinting, zone TI: The IP is splinted in neutral or slight hyperextension for 5 to 6 weeks. Compare to patient's uninjured thumb for optimum positioning.
      1. At 3 weeks postoperatively, protected active IP extension is initiated, and flexion should gradually increase no more than 20 degrees per week.
      2. Protective splinting is continued at all times, excluding exercise periods, for an additional 2 to 3 weeks
      3. Light resistive pinch and grip exercises can begin at 6 to 8 weeks.
   B. Static splinting, zone TII: Injuries at this level are immobilized in a hand-based splint with the MCP and IP at neutral and the thumb radially extended; the IP may be in slight hyperextension.

1. Protective active motion can be initiated at 3 weeks: 25 to 30 degrees of flexion is recommended initially, with motion progressing slowly over the next 3 weeks. Splint protection continues between exercises and at night for a total of 6 weeks.

VI. Thumb zones TIII through TV

A. Immobilization method[4]

1. 0 to 21 days postoperatively
   a. Splinting: volar protective splint with wrist in 30 degrees extension, carpometacarpal (CMC) joint in slight abduction, and MCP and IP joints at 0 degrees.
   b. Therapy
      (1) Wound care
      (2) Edema control
      (3) MCP joint protective ROM: Therapist supports wrist and IP in full extension, while gently moving MCP from full extension to 30 degrees flexion. Check splint to be sure thumb MCP is not hyperextended.
      (4) IP joint protective ROM: Therapist supports wrist and MCP in full extension, while gently moving thumb IP from full extension to 60 degrees flexion.

2. 3 to 4 weeks postoperatively
   a. Splinting: all of the time except for exercise and showering. Shorten splint to allow active flexion and extension of IP joint
      (1) Variation for IP extensor lag: Add removable volar component.
      (2) Variation for MCP extension contracture: intermittent gentle dynamic MP flexion splinting while supporting wrist and first metacarpal in extension
   b. Therapy
      (1) Initiate supervised thumb abduction and MCP/IP flexion.
      (2) Home program:
         (a) MCP mobility: While supporting wrist and IP in full extension, gently move MCP from full extension to 30 degrees flexion.
         (b) IP mobility: While supporting wrist and MCP in full extension, gently move thumb IP from full extension to 60 degrees flexion.

3. 5 weeks postoperatively
   a. Splinting: A combination of thumb abduction and MCP and IP flexion may be initiated if needed.
   b. Therapy: Add a combination of thumb abduction and MCP and IP flexion to the home program.

4. 6 to 10 weeks postoperatively
   a. Splinting: as needed
   b. Therapy
      (1) Composite thumb and wrist flexion
      (2) Mild progressive strengthening including wrist flexion/extension and forearm supination/ pronation

5. 10 to 12 weeks postoperatively
   a. Therapy: strong resistive exercise

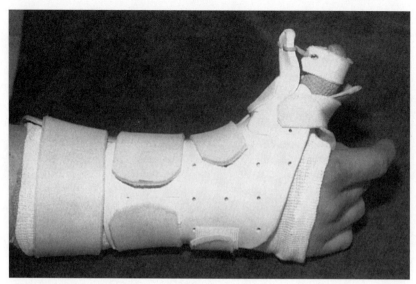

FIG. **20-11** Splint for dynamic treatment of thumb extensor repair in zones TIV and TV.

   B. Early passive motion method[4]
      1. 0 to 21 days postoperatively
         a. Splinting (Fig. 20-11)
            (1) Dorsal: wrist in 30 degrees static extension; MCP/IP in
                0 degrees dynamic extension
            (2) Volar: static splint allowing 60 degrees of IP motion
         b. Therapy
            (1) By patient: active flexion to volar splint with passive
                extension via dynamic traction
            (2) By therapist: maximal wrist extension with simultaneous
                MCP joint flexion to 30 degrees
            (3) Wrist tenodesis: wrist to 0 degrees extension with
                simultaneous thumb CMC, MCP, and IP extension,
                alternating with full wrist extension with thumb CMC,
                MCP, and IP relaxed.
      2. 3 to 4 weeks postoperatively
         a. Splinting: all of the time except during exercise and
            showering
         b. Therapy: Add the therapist-performed exercises of the first
            3 weeks to the home program.
      3. 5 to 12 weeks postoperatively: splinting and exercise
         essentially the same as in the early immobilization method
         from 5 to 12 weeks

POSTOPERATIVE COMPLICATIONS

   I.   Infection
   II. Tendon rupture
   III. Excessive scar formation
   IV. Active extensor tendon lag and tendon adherence
   V.   Extrinsic extensor tendon tightness limiting composite
        flexion

EVALUATION TIMELINE

I.   ROM: reevaluate weekly
A. At 3 to 4 weeks: AROM of MCP and IP joints
B. At 5 weeks: AROM of wrist
C. At 7 weeks: PROM and AROM of wrist, MCP, and IP joints

II. Strength: at 10 weeks; reevaluate strength measurements every 4 weeks.

OUTCOMES

Comparison of reported results is difficult because of variations in the degree of immobilization provided by the splint and variations in the timing and rate of application of the controlled stress applied to the tendons. Newport and colleagues[39] advocated the use of Miller's classification as being more discriminative and accurate (Table 20-1). TAM, as calculated by Strickland and Glogovac,[41] and Dargan's criteria[42] (Table 20-2) are also frequently used as assessment tools. Grip and pinch strength are frequently reported and are accepted measures of hand function, but they do not assess extensor function. Newport and colleagues[39] found that most patients achieve 85% to 100% of normalized strength.

Newport's group[39] performed a retrospective analysis of the long-term results of extensor tendon repairs treated with static splinting. They found that the percentage of digits losing flexion was greater than the percentage of digits losing extension. The average degree loss of flexion also was greater than the average degree loss of extension. The rate of rupture has been reported from zero to 2%.[24,27,39,43] Early removal of a splint and noncompliance are factors frequently cited.

Newport and colleagues[39] found that the more distal zones (I through IV) had a significantly higher number of poor results than did the more proximal zones (V through VIII). In zones III and IV, the results from static splinting were only 33% good to excellent . Thomes and Thomes[40] reported 86% excellent and 14% good results with their protocol using a dynamic PIP extension splint. Evans and Thompson's[30-32] results with the SAM protocol are summarized in Table 20-3.

In zone V injuries without associated fractures, Newport and colleagues[39] found 83% good to excellent results. If tendon injury was associated with fracture the rate of good to excellent results dropped to 50%.

Numerous outcome studies have been reported for zones V through VII treated with a passive mobilization program using dynamic splinting.[25,27-29,43-48] Overall, there has been a high rate of good to excellent results, a low incidence of extensor tendon lag, and a low rate of rupture.

TABLE 20-1 Miller's Classification of Results

Results	Total Extensor Lag (Degrees)	Total Flexion Loss (Degrees)
Excellent	0	0
Good	≤10	≤20
Fair	11-45	21-45
Poor	≥45	≥45

From Miller H: Surg Gynecol Obstet 75:693-698, 1942.

TABLE **20-2** Dargan's Classification of Results

Excellent	No extensor lag and with flexion of pulps to midpalm
Good	Extensor lag ≤15 with flexion of pulps to midpalm
Fair	Extensor lag 16 to 45 degrees or pulp-to-palm distance ≤2 cm
Poor	Extensor lag ≥45 degrees or pulp-to-palm distance ≥2 cm

From Dargan EL: Surg Gynecol Obstet 128:1269-1273, 1969.

There are not as many outcome studies that evaluate results of thumb repairs. Newport and colleagues[39] found that 60% of patients achieved good to excellent results with static splinting. Crosby and Wehbe[29] reported good to excellent results for all zones of the thumb using a dynamic extension splint and early passive mobilization. They found no difference in outcome in regard to extension lag, grip strength, or time to full recovery when comparing results by zone.

Recently, the results of early active mobilization programs have been reported. Sylaidis and associates[34] described a method of controlled active mobilization of extensor tendon repairs without dynamic splinting referred to as the Norwich regimen. Their prospective study of primary tendon repair in zones IV to VII included simple and complex tendon injuries. After surgery, the repairs were protected with a palmar splint that positioned the wrist in 45 degrees extension with the MCP joints flexed to 50 degrees and the IP joints extended. Controlled active mobilization exercises were begun on the first postoperative day. The patients performed two exercises actively: combined active MCP joint and IP joint extension and MCP joint extension with IP joint flexion (hook-fist). These exercises were performed for the first 4 weeks postoperatively at a rate of four repetitions of each exercise, four times daily. Daytime splinting was discontinued at 5 weeks but was continued at night for an additional 2 weeks. After the fifth postoperative week, exercises were upgraded to gentle composite flexion,

TABLE **20-3** Final Results and Analysis Comparing Group I and Group II

Results	Group I (Immobilization)	Group II (SAM)	Statistical Significance (*t* Test)	Statistical Significance (Chi Square Test)
No. digits	38	26		
Mean age (yr)	39.9	42.2	>.5 NS	
% Male gender	86.8	80.8		>.5 NS
% Complex injury	76.3	76.9		>.5 NS
Day motion initiated (mean)	32.9	4.59	<.001 S	
Days from injury to D/C (mean)	76.07	51.38	<.001 S	
PIP extension lag on first motion day (degrees)	13	3	<.01 S	
PIP extension lag at D/C (degrees)	8.13	2.96	<.01 S	
PIP motion at 6 wk (degrees)	44	88	<.001 S	
PIP motion at D/C (degrees)	72	88	<.01 S	
TAM (PIP and DIP) at D/C (degrees)	110.7	131.5	<.01 S	
DIP motion at D/C (degrees)	37.63	45	<.01 S	

From Evans RB: J Hand Surg Am 19:994, 1994.
D/C, Discharge; *DIP*, distal interphalangeal joint; *NS*, not statistically significant; *PIP*, proximal interphalangeal joint; *S*, statistically significant; *TAM*, total active motion.

increasing to full flexion and power grip. Patients with an extension lag of greater than 30 degrees at 4 weeks were progressed more slowly and continued splint use during the day until 6 weeks after surgery. These patients performed the original exercises, but fisting was delayed until the end of the seventh week. Results were assessed at 4 and 6 weeks using the Dargan criteria[42] (see Table 20-2). At 6 weeks postoperatively, 92% of patients in the simple injury group had excellent or good function, and 85% of patients in the complex injury group achieved excellent or good function. The average time for return to work was 6.5 weeks for the simple injury group and 8.5 weeks for the complex injury group. There were no reported ruptures. The authors believed their results were consistent with studies of dynamic splinting for simple tendon injuries and preferred to use the Norwich regimen for early active mobilization of simple and complex tendon injuries.

Khandwala and co-workers[33] performed a prospective, randomized study comparing dynamic extension splinting and controlled active mobilization of complete simple extensor tendon injuries in zones V and VI. Their study included 100 patients randomly assigned to rehabilitation in either a dynamic extension splint or a static palmar blocking splint. After surgery, patients were immobilized in a palmar plaster splint with the wrist in 45 degrees extension, MCP joints at 30 degrees flexion, and IP joints at neutral until their appointment with a hand therapist 3 to 4 days later. The patients were monitored weekly unless problems with their splint or hand were encountered. Splints were to be worn continuously for 4 weeks, then only at night or in crowds for an additional 2 weeks. Patients judged to be at risk for rupture continued splint use for another 2 weeks. The dynamic extension splint group followed a regimen similar to the one originally described by Chow and colleagues,[49] with the exception that motion was delayed for 3 to 4 days. The dynamic extension splint limited MCP joint flexion but allowed free movement of the IP joints at all times. During the first 2 weeks, patients performed active flexion and extension of the IP joints, then active flexion and passive extension of the MCP joints via the dynamic splint 10 times every hour. Composite flexion of all three joints was initiated within the limits of the splint at weeks 3 and 4. At the end of 4 weeks, the splint was removed for active composite flexion and extension exercises.

The regimen for the active mobilization group differed from that in previous active mobilization studies[4,31,34] in that it allowed composite flexion of all three joints from the onset of rehabilitation. The palmar blocking splint for this group positioned the wrist at 30 degrees extension and the MCP joints at 45 degrees flexion. Splint support ended proximal to the PIP joint, allowing free movement of the IP joints. During the first 2 weeks, patients performed composite flexion and extension of the MCP and IP joints within the limits of the splint. Active extension was limited to neutral; exercises were performed 10 times hourly. At 3 weeks, the palmar blocking splint was modified to allow 70 degrees of MCP flexion. At weeks 3 and 4, composite flexion within the splint and hook-fist exercise with MCP joints fully extended were added. At the end of 4 weeks, the splint was removed for composite flexion and extension exercises. For both groups, patients returned to light work at 4 weeks, driving at 8 weeks, and heavy manual work at 12 weeks postoperatively. ROM was assessed at 4 and 8 weeks postoperatively. If ROM was not equal to the contralateral joint at either time, the frequency of therapy was increased.

The results of treatment were assessed using the Miller[50] classification (see Table 20-1) and TAM.[41] By both types of assessment, there was no statistically significant difference in outcome for either group. Dynamic splinting yielded 95% excellent or good results, and palmar blocking (early active mobilization) yielded 93% excellent or good results. The authors[33] reported three ruptures in their study, which occurred in both groups. All three patients underwent immediate re-repair and later achieved two good and one fair result based on TAM.

The magnitude of the soft tissue trauma and skeletal injury must be taken into account when selecting the technique used in tendon rehabilitation. Before the initiation of therapy, the hand therapist should communicate with the physician about the extent of injury, the type of repair performed, and the appropriate rehabilitation technique for each patient.

REFERENCES

1. Agee J, Guidera M: The functional significance of the juncturae tendineae in dynamic stabilization of the metacarpophalangeal joints of the fingers. ASSH Proceedings. J Hand Surg 5:288, 1980
2. Rosenthal EA: The extensor tendons. In Hunter JM: Rehabilitation of the Hand. 2nd Ed. Mosby, St. Louis, 1984, pp. 324-352
3. Tubiana R: Extensor apparatus of the fingers. In Hunter JM, Schneider LH, Mackin EJ (eds): Tendon Surgery in the Hand. Mosby, St. Louis, 1987, pp. 319-324
4. Evans RB: An update on extensor tendon management. In Hunter JM, Mackin EJ, Callahan AD (eds): Rehabilitation of the Hand: Surgery and Therapy. 4th Ed. Mosby, St. Louis, 1995, pp. 565-603
5. Newport ML, Williams D: Biomechanical characteristics of extensor tendon suture techniques. J Hand Surg Am 17:1117-1123, 1992
6. Purcell T, Eadie S, Murugan M, et al.: Static splinting of extensor tendon repairs. J Hand Surg Br 25:180-182, 2000
7. Slater RR, Bynum DK: Simplified functional splinting after extensor tenorrhaphy. J Hand Surg Am 22:445-451, 1997
8. Walsh MT, Muntzer E, Patel J, et al.: Early controlled motion with dynamic splinting versus static splinting for zones III and IV extensor tendon lacerations. J Hand Ther 7:223-236, 1994
9. Wilson RL: Management of acute extensor tendon injuries. In Hunter JM, Schneider LH, Mackin EJ (eds): Tendon Surgery in the Hand. Mosby, St. Louis, 1987, pp. 336-343
10. Amiel D, Gelberman R, Harwood F, et al.: Fibronectin in healing flexor tendons subjected to immobilization or early controlled passive motion. Matrix 11(3):184-189, 1991
11. Freehan LM, Beauchene JG: Early tensile properties of healing chicken flexor tendons: early controlled passive motion versus post-operative immobilization. J Hand Surg Am 15:63-68, 1990
12. Gelberman RH, Khabie V, Cahill CJ: The revascularization of healing flexor tendons in digital sheath: vascular injection study in dogs. J Bone Joint Surg Am 73:868-881, 1991
13. Gelberman RH, VandeBerg JS, Manske PR, et al.: The early stages of flexor tendon healing: a morphologic study of the first 14 days. J Hand Surg Am 10:776-784, 1985
14. Gelberman RA, Botte RH, Spiegelman JJ: The excursion and deformation of repaired flexor tendons treated with protected early motion. J Hand Surg Am 11:106-110, 1986
15. Gelberman RH, Manske PR: Effects of early motion on the tendon healing process: experimental studies. In Hunter JM, Schneider LH, Mackin EJ (eds): Tendon Surgery in the Hand. Mosby, St. Louis, 1987, pp. 170-177
16. Gelberman RH, Nunley JA, Osterman AL: Influences of the protected passive mobilization interval on flexor tendon healing: a prospective randomized clinical study. Clin Orthop 264:189-196, 1991
17. Gelberman RH, Siegel DB, Woo SL: Healing of digital flexor tendons: importance of time between injury and operative repair. A biomechanical, biochemical, and morphological study in dogs. J Bone Joint Surg Am 73:66-75, 1991

18. Gelberman RH, Steinberg D, Amiel D: Fibroblast chemotaxis after repair. J Hand Surg Am 16:686-693, 1991
19. Gelberman RH, Vande Berg JS, Lundborg GN: Flexor tendon healing and restoration of the gliding surface: an ultrastructural study in dogs. J Bone Joint Surg Am 65:70-80, 1993
20. Gelberman RH, Woo SL, Lothringer K: Effects of intermittent passive mobilization on healing canine flexor tendons. J Hand Surg Am 7:170-175, 1982
21. Hitchcock TF, Light TR, Bunch WH: The effect of immediate constrained digital motion on the strength of flexor tendon repairs in chickens. J Hand Surg Am 12:590-595, 1987
22. Horii E, Lin GT, Cooney WP: Comparative flexor tendon excursions after passive mobilization: an in vitro study. J Hand Surg Am 17:559-566, 1992
23. Woo SL, Gomez MA, Amiel D: The effects of exercise on the biomechanical and biochemical properties of swine digital flexor tendons. J Biomech Eng 103:51-56, 1981
24. Evans RB, Burkhalter WE: A study of the dynamic anatomy of extensor tendons and implications for treatment. J Hand Surg Am 11:774, 1986
25. Evans RB: Clinical application of controlled stress to the healing extensor tendon: a review of 112 cases. Phys Ther 68:1041-1049, 1989
26. Minamikawa Y, Peimer CA, Yamaguchi T: Wrist position and extensor tendon amplitude following repair. J Hand Surg Am 17:268-271, 1992
27. Browne EZ, Ribik CA: Early dynamic splinting for extensor tendon injuries. J Hand Surg Am 14:72-76, 1989
28. Crosby CA, Wehbe MA: Early motion after extensor tendon surgery. Hand Clin 12: 57-64, 1996
29. Crosby CA, Wehbe MA: Early protected motion after extensor tendon repair. J Hand Surg Am 24:1061-1070, 1999
30. Evans RB: Early active short arc motion for the repaired central slip. J Hand Surg Am 19:991-997, 1994
31. Evans RB, Thompson DE: An analysis of factors that support early active short arc motion of the repaired central slip. J Hand Ther 5:187-201, 1992
32. Evans RB: Immediate active short arc motion following extensor tendon repair. Hand Clin 11:483-512, 1995
33. Khandwala AR, Webb J, Harris SB, et al.: A comparison of dynamic extension splinting and controlled active mobilization of complete divisions of extensor tendons in zones 5 and 6. J Hand Surg Br 25:140-146, 2000
34. Sylaidis P, Youatt M, Logan A: Early active mobilization for extensor tendon injuries. J Hand Surg Br 22:594-596, 1997
35. Evans RBI, Thompson D: The application of force to the healing tendon. J Hand Ther 6:266-284, 1993
36. Brand PW, Hollister A: Clinical Mechanics of the Hand. 2nd Ed. Mosby–Year Book, St. Louis, 1993
37. Newport MA: Early repair of extensor tendon injuries. In Berger RA, Weiss AC: Hand Surgery. Vol. 1. Lippincott Williams & Wilkins, Philadelphia, 2003, pp. 737-752
38. Lovett WL, McCalla MA: Management and rehabilitation of extensor tendon injuries. Orthop Clin North Am 44:811-826, 1983
39. Newport ML, Blair WF, Steyers CM: Long-term results of extensor tendon repair. J Hand Surg Am 15:961-966, 1990
40. Thomes L, Thomes B: Early mobilization method for surgically repaired zone III extensor tendons. J Hand Ther 8:195-198, 1995
41. Strickland J, Glogovac S: Digital function following flexor tendon repair in zone II: a comparison of immobilization and controlled passive motion techniques. J Hand Surg Am 5:537-543, 1980
42. Dargan EL: Management of extensor tendon injuries of the hand. Surg Gynecol Obstet 128:1269-1273, 1969
43. Chow JA, Dovelle S, Thomes LJ, et al.: A comparison of results of extensor tendon repair followed by early controlled mobilization versus static immobilization. J Hand Surg Br 14:18-20, 1989
44. Chester DL, Beale L, Beveridge J: A prospective, controlled randomized trial comparing early active extension with passive extension using a dynamic splint in the rehabilitation of repaired extensor tendons. J Hand Surg Br 27:283-288, 2000
45. Hung LK, Chan A, Chang J, et al.: Early controlled active mobilization with dynamic splintage for treatment of extensor tendon injuries. J Hand Surg Am 15:251-257, 1990

46. Ip WY, Chow SP: Results of dynamic splintage following extensor tendon repair. J Hand
    Surg Br 22:283-287, 1997
47. Kerr CD, Burczak JR: Dynamic traction after extensor repair in zones 6,7,8: a retrospective
    study. J Hand Surg Br 14:21-22, 1989
48. Thomas D, Moutet F, Guinard D: Postoperative management of extensor tendon repairs
    in zones V, VI, and VII. J Hand Ther 9:309-314, 1996
49. Chow JA, Dovelle S, Thomas L: Postoperative management of repair of extensor
    tendons of the hand: dynamic splinting versus static splinting. Orthop Trans 11:
    258-259, 1987
50. Miller H: Repair of severed tendons of the hand and wrist: statistical analysis of 300
    cases. Surg Gynecol Obstet 75:693-698, 1942

SUGGESTED READINGS

Allieu Y, Ascenio G, Rouzaud JC: Protected passive mobilization after suturing the extensor
    tendons of the hand: a survey of 120 cases. In Hunter JM, Schneider LH, Mackin EJ
    (eds): Tendon Surgery in the Hand. Mosby, St. Louis, 1987, pp. 344-348
Murphy MS, Astifidis R, Saunders R: Current management of tendon injuries in the hand.
    Orthop Phys Ther Clin North Am. 10:567, 2001
Savage R: The influence of wrist position on the minimum force required for active
    movement of the interphalangeal joints. J Hand Surg Br 13:262-268, 1998
Von Schroeder HP, Botte MI: Anatomy and functional significance of the long extensors to
    the fingers and thumb. Clin Orthop 29:74-83, 2001

Extensor Tendon Imbalance: Mallet Finger, Swan-Neck Deformity, Boutonniere Deformity

21

Jason A. Willoughby,
Juan Martin Favetto, and
William L. O'Neill, Jr

MALLET FINGER

Mallet finger injury is a traumatic disruption of the terminal tendon that results in a loss of active extension of the distal interphalangeal (DIP) joint. This may or may not be associated with a fracture of the articular surface. Names synonymous with mallet finger injury are "baseball finger" and "drop finger."[1] The primary goal of rehabilitation is to promote healing of the tendon so as to maximize function and range of motion (ROM) of the injured DIP joint with no loss of flexion of the proximal interphalangeal (PIP) joint.

Conservative treatment of the mallet finger consists of continuous immobilization of the involved joint, with regular exercises being performed to maintain the ROM of the uninvolved joints. At the conclusion of the initial immobilization period, the splint is removed and the integrity of the terminal tendon is evaluated. If the tendon is unable to maintain extension and the joint droops into flexion, a splint is reapplied and the tendon is tested periodically thereafter for healing and strength. After the tendon is "healed" enough, active flexion and extension are begun, with close monitoring for extension lag. ROM and strengthening exercises are initiated as indicated.

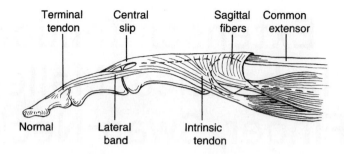

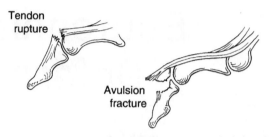

Potential for swan-neck deformity

FIG. 21-1 Normal anatomy and two variations of mallet finger injury.

Definition

Mallet finger injury is a traumatically induced loss of active extension of the DIP joint caused by avulsion, rupture, or laceration of the terminal tendon[2] or by a fracture of the base of the distal phalanx with tendon insertion attached (Fig. 21-1).

Treatment and Surgical Purpose

To restore extension to the DIP joint where there has been disruption of the terminal portion of the extensor tendon. If the injury is closed and tendon continuity is lost, splinting of the DIP joint is preferred. If there has been a laceration of the tendon, a surgical repair by suture may be indicated. An avulsion fracture of the distal phalanx without DIP dislocation may be treated by splinting with the joint in extension. If there is an avulsion fracture with volar subluxation of the distal phalanx, reduction (closed or open) and internal fixation is considered. These treatment regimens frequently provide a good result; however, a permanent extension lag at the DIP joint may be anticipated. In some patients, a concurrent hyperextension posture of the PIP joint (swan-neck deformity) is observed.

Treatment Goals

  I. Promote healing of terminal tendon.
 II. Maintain full ROM of all uninvolved joints of the upper extremity.
III. Prevent or correct swan-neck deformity and DIP joint flexion contracture.

IV. Maximize ROM of DIP joint and PIP joint; in particular, maximize active DIP joint extension.
V. Return to previous level of function.
VI. Prevent reinjury.

Nonoperative Indications/Precautions for Therapy

I. Indications
   A. Mallet finger deformity (loss of active DIP extension)
II. Precautions
   A. Extreme pain
   B. Extreme edema
   C. Tape allergy[3]
   D. Wound or skin breakdown

Nonoperative Therapy

I. Management of closed treatment with full passive DIP extension available. (If full passive DIP extension is not available, static progressive splinting will be necessary before initiating this timeline.)
   A. Weeks 0 to 8: Continuous splinting in 0 degrees or slight hyperextension[4] (see Splints). Change adhesive tape and check skin regularly.
   B. Weeks 8 to 10: Continue day and night splinting. Begin active flexion up to 25 to 30 degrees. May use a volar template to limit flexion during exercise.
   C. Weeks 10 to 12: If there is no extension lag, discontinue day splint but continue night splint. If extension lag persists, balance splinting and exercise to minimize lag.
   D. Week 12: Begin unrestricted use. Continue to monitor for extension lag; if lag returns, reinstitute appropriate level of splinting (night only versus day and night) for additional 2 weeks (return to step C).
II. Splints[4-6]
   A. Position DIP joint at 0 degrees or slight hyperextension. Hyperextend DIP joint without blanching dorsal skin.[5]
   B. Splints may be on dorsal surface, on volar surface, or circumferential. A gutter splint for the PIP joint may also be indicated if significant swan-neck deformity coexists (Fig. 21-2).
   C. Splint types (Fig. 21-3)
      1. Custom thermoplastic
      2. Alumafoam
      3. Stack
   D. Splint fasteners
      1. Adhesive tape
      2. Velcro: May not provide enough security against axial rotation and distal slippage of splint
      3. Coban

Nonoperative Complications

    I.   Maceration or necrosis of skin[3]
   II.   Maceration or necrosis of nailbed[5]
 III.   Swan-neck deformity[4]
 IV.   Tape allergy[3]
  V.   Extension lag at DIP joint[1]
 VI.   Loss of motion at PIP joints

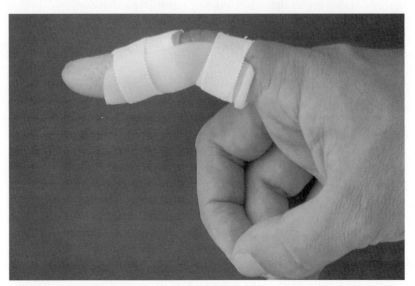

FIG. 21-2   Mallet finger with proximal interphalangeal (PIP) hyperextension; custom stack with PIP flexion splint.

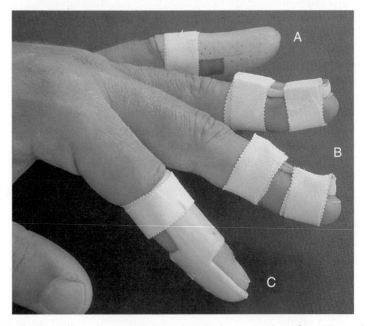

FIG. 21-3   Mallet splints. **A,** Custom thermoplastic. **B,** Alumafoam. **C,** Stack.

Postoperative Indications/Precautions for Therapy

I.   Indications: mallet finger deformity that fails to respond
     to conservative treatment
II. Precautions
     A. Infection
     B. Extreme pain
     C. Extreme edema

Postoperative Therapy

I.   General care
      A. Edema control
      B. Wound care
      C. Scar management
      D. Pain management
      E. Maintain ROM of uninvolved digits.
      F. Protect surgical repair.
II.   Weeks 0 to 6
      A. K-wire or button intact
      B. ROM of uninvolved joints
      C. Pin site care
III. Weeks 6 to 8
      A. K-wire removed
      B. Begin active range of motion (AROM) and follow closed
         treatment as described earlier (see Nonoperative Therapy).
      C. Extension splinting for 2 weeks

Postoperative Complications

I.   Infection
II.   Necrosis of nailbed[4]
III. DIP joint extension lag
IV.   Swan-neck deformity
V.   Osteomyelitis

Evaluation Timeline

I.   Week 1
      A. AROM and passive ROM (PROM) of all upper extremity
         joints except involved DIP joint
      B. Sensibility
II.   Week 8: Active extension of DIP joint
III. Week 10: Active flexion of DIP joint
IV.   Week 12
      A. Grip and pinch strength
      B. Passive flexion of DIP joint

SWAN-NECK DEFORMITY

Swan-neck deformities occur through extrinsic, intrinsic, or abnormal articular anatomic factors.[7] The causes of these factors include rheumatologic disease, extensor terminal tendon injuries (mallet finger), spastic

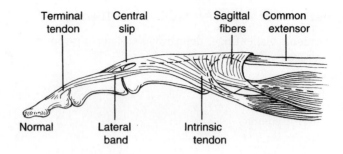

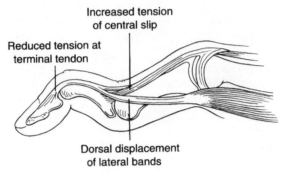

FIG. 21-4 Normal finger anatomy and dorsal subluxation of the lateral bands.

conditions, severe intrinsic tightness, injuries that cause volar plate laxity, fractures to the middle phalanx that heal in hyperextension, and generalized ligamentous laxity.[7] The deformity may also occur secondary to surgical procedures such as a flexor digitorum profundus (FDP) graft in which the flexor digitorum superficialis (FDS) is absent. The deformity is one in which function decreases as the proximal interphalangeal (PIP) joint loses its flexibility. The lateral bands become dorsally displaced, and tension to extend the distal interphalangeal (DIP) joint is reduced (Fig. 21-4). Treatment of the condition depends on the etiologic status of the PIP joint and its related anatomic structures. Successful treatment of swan-neck deformity depends on careful examination and determination of contributing factors.

Classification of the deformity may help determine the treatment method. Four classifications have been described: (1) PIP flexion remains supple in all positions; (2) PIP flexion is limited by intrinsic tightness; (3) PIP flexion is limited in all positions by articular factors and the joint remains good radiographically; (4) PIP flexion is limited in all positions by intraarticular factors as noted radiographically.[8]

Definition

Swan-neck deformity is a deformity in which the PIP joint is hyperextended and the DIP joint is flexed (Fig. 21-5).

Treatment and Surgical Purpose

Splinting of the PIP joint in a flexed posture may be used temporarily to prevent fixed contractures and restore extensor tendon and joint capsule balance by promoting volar plate tightening. Active therapy may be beneficial in

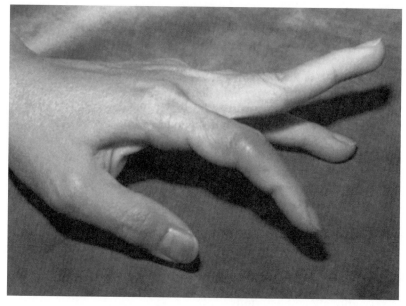

FIG. **21-5** Swan-neck deformity.

regaining balance in soft tissue structures that may be contributing to the condition. Surgical correction may be necessary for restoration of the extensor balance, including central slip tenotomy, PIP joint arthroplasty, and PIP joint arthrodesis.

Treatment Goals

I.   Nonoperative
    A. Promote balance of the extensor mechanism.
    B. Reduce intrinsic tightness.
    C. Maximize joint ROM.
    D. Maintain ROM of wrist and uninvolved digits.
II. Postoperative
    A. Promote wound healing.
    B. Control edema.
    C. Promote adhesion-free tendon gliding.
    D. Prevent attenuation or rupture of surgical procedure.
    E. Limit PIP extension and encourage full DIP extension.
    F. Promote full active flexion.
    G. Maintain ROM of uninvolved digits.

Nonoperative Indications/Precautions for Therapy

I.   Indications
    A. Digital posture of PIP hyperextension with DIP flexion
    B. Supple deformities in which prevention of PIP hyperextension restores DIP extension
II. Precautions
    A. Volar plate laxity
    B. Intrinsic tightness

C. Dynamic imbalance originating at other joints or caused by systemic or neurological conditions

Nonoperative Therapy

I.   AROM/PROM
II. Intrinsic stretching exercises
III. Splint to balance finger extension. A tripoint splint prevents PIP joint hyperextension and restores DIP joint extension. This type of splint places dorsal pressure proximal and distal to the PIP joint and volar pressure at the PIP joint. It allows full active flexion (Fig. 21-6).
     A. Custom figure 8 splint
     B. Silver ring splint
     C. Oval 8 splint

Nonoperative Complications

I.   Continuation of deformity
II. Reducible deformity becomes fixed
III. Reduction of hand function

Postoperative Indications/Precautions for Therapy

I.   Indications
     A. After surgical procedures designed to relieve the deformity. Review operative note or communicate with surgeon before treatment. Therapy varies depending on the extent of operative treatment.

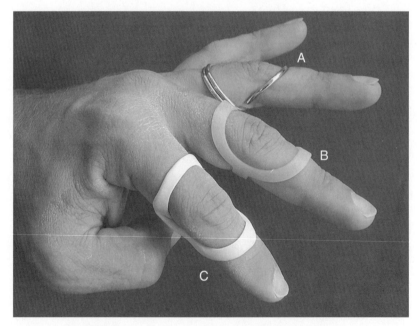

FIG. 21-6 Tripoint splints. A, Silver ring. B, Oval 8. C, Custom.

II. Precautions
A. Excessive exercise that could cause attenuation or rupture of tenodesis procedures
B. Procedures that involve joint fusions
C. Procedures that involve joint arthroplasty
D. Surgical treatment that requires capsulectomy
E. Surgical treatment that requires tenolysis
F. Procedure that requires intrinsic release or metacarpophalangeal (MCP) joint surgical treatment

Postoperative Therapy

I. General care
A. Edema control
B. Wound care
C. Scar management
D. Pain management
E. Maintain ROM of uninvolved digits.
F. Protect surgical repair.
II. Treatment after passive procedures for PIP joint flexion
A. Weeks 0 to 6 postoperatively
1. The PIP joint is splinted at 30 degrees flexion with the DIP joint at 0 degrees.
2. Active motion that allows full flexion and limits extension of the PIP joint to 30 degrees begins 3 to 14 days postoperatively.[7-9] A Kirschner wire (K-wire) or splint may be used to hold the DIP joint in extension to facilitate maximal PIP joint flexion.[7]
3. Splinting to improve PIP joint flexion may be initiated, if necessary, at 3 weeks postoperatively.
B. Weeks 6 to 10 postoperatively
1. The splint is gradually adjusted to allow increased active extension, or the patient is permitted to decrease use of the splint.
2. Passive extension exercises for the PIP joint are rarely necessary, because PIP joint extension typically increases gradually over several months. (A slight limitation in PIP joint extension is acceptable and expected.)
3. Dynamic extension splinting may be initiated at 8 weeks for PIP extension limitation greater than 30 degrees.
4. Strengthening for flexion may begin at 6 to 8 weeks.
III. Other procedures: Swan-neck deformity in rheumatoid arthritis commonly requires treatment by PIP joint arthroplasty. Details concerning rehabilitation after this procedure are presented in Chapter 50.

Operative Complications

I. Infection
II. Excessive edema
III. Pain
IV. Rupture of tenodesis

V.   Attenuation of tenodesis
VI.   Excessive scarring
VII.   Limited ROM

Evaluation Timeline

I.   Nonoperative
   A. Initial evaluation
     1. AROM/PROM: Determine limiting factors if present.
     2. Strength
   B. Reevaluate in 4 weeks.
II.   Operative: review operative note
   A. Initial postoperative visit
     1. Condition of surgical sites
     2. Edema
     3. Sensation
     4. Pain
     5. Management of activities of daily living (ADL)
   B. Weeks 1 to 4
     1. Active flexion and extension to limit of splint
     2. Passive flexion of PIP joint and MCP joint
   C. Week 6: passive flexion and extension of all joints
   D. Week 8: grip strength/pinch strength

BOUTONNIERE DEFORMITY

The boutonniere or "buttonhole" deformity occurs when the central slip of the common extensor tendon is damaged at its insertion onto the base of the middle phalanx. Volar subluxation of the lateral extensor bands palmar to the axis of motion of the PIP joint occurs secondary to the force imbalance. The PIP joint eventually herniates through the extensor mechanism, with resultant stretching of the spiral fibers and transverse fibers. Progression of the deformity may lead to compensatory MCP joint hyperextension. The distal phalanx also becomes involved as the oblique retinacular ligament undergoes adaptive shortening and the DIP joint is held in hyperextension[10-12] (Fig. 21-7).

The boutonniere deformity can result from injuries caused by division, rupture, avulsion, laceration, or closed trauma to the central extensor tendon inserting onto the middle phalanx. Dorsal burns, rheumatoid arthritis, Dupuytren's contracture, and congenital disease are other causes.[10,11,13,14]

Despite different classifications and numerous surgical techniques for correction of the boutonniere deformity, it appears that most authors' treatment of choice is conservative long-term hand therapy to increase PIP joint extension and DIP joint active full flexion through the use of splinting. Only if an acute, open injury occurs should immediate surgery be performed.

Definition

A **boutonniere deformity** is a deformity in which a digit assumes a posture of conjoint PIP joint flexion and DIP joint hyperextension (Fig. 21-8).

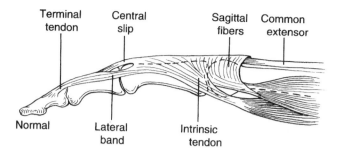

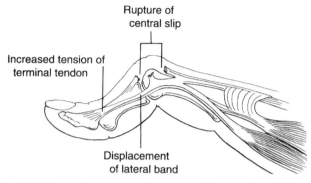

FIG. 21-7 Normal anatomy and anatomy of boutonniere deformity.

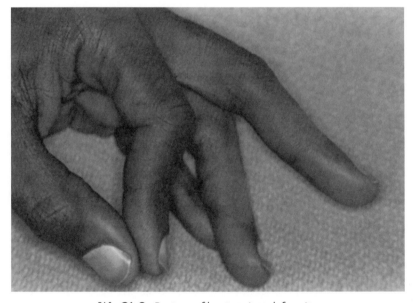

FIG. 21-8 Posture of boutonniere deformity.

Treatment and Surgical Purpose

To restore extensor tendon balance when there has been a laceration or tear of the central slip near its insertion into the middle phalanx at the PIP level. Nonsurgical treatment is directed toward splinting, either dynamic or static, that allows the central slip to heal while permitting DIP joint motion.

Active DIP joint flexion during the splinting process facilitates lengthening of the oblique retinacular ligaments and promotes adhesion-free gliding of the lateral bands while placing slack in the central slip. Various surgical repair and reconstructive methods have been described, all of which seek to restore the extensor mechanism function at the PIP joint. Full passive mobility of the PIP and DIP joints is paramount to ensure a surgical success.

Treatment Goals

    I. Prevent extensor tendon complete rupture.
    II. Reduce swelling and pain.
    III. Prevent PIP joint flexion contracture.
    IV. Prevent lateral band subluxation.
    V. Prevent oblique retinacular ligament contracture.
    VI. Restore AROM/PROM of MCP, PIP, and DIP joints.
    VII. Maintain ROM of uninvolved joints of the upper extremity.
    VIII. Return to previous level of function.

Nonoperative Indications/Precautions for Therapy

    I. Indications
        A. Limitation in PIP joint extension (may be active and passive)
        B. Secondary limitation in DIP joint flexion
    II. Precautions
        A. Rheumatoid arthritis
        B. Burns
        C. Diabetes
        D. Steroid use

Nonoperative Therapy

    I. Management of deformity with full passive PIP joint extension available (If not available dynamically, static progressive splinting or serial casting is required to regain full PIP joint extension before initiating this timeline.)
        A. Weeks 0 to 8: continuous splinting with PIP joint at 0 degrees and DIP joint free (see Splints)
            1. Regular performance of DIP joint flexion exercises within splint
            2. Monitor skin integrity regularly
            3. Joint mobilization may be necessary to maintain capsular mobility without allowing flexion of the PIP joint.
        B. Weeks 8 to 10: Continue day and night splinting.
            1. Begin active flexion of 30 to 40 degrees, with 10- to 20-degree increase weekly as tolerated. May use a volar template to limit flexion during exercise (Fig. 21-9).
            2. Continue with DIP joint flexion exercises in splint.
            3. Continue to monitor skin integrity.

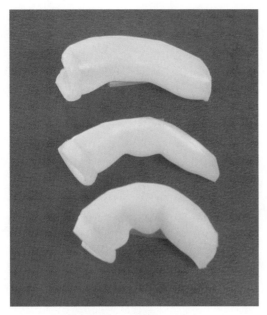

FIG. **21-9** Template splints.

C. Weeks 10 to 12: If no PIP joint extension lag exists, discontinue splinting; if extension lag persists, balance splinting and exercise to minimize lag.
D. Week 12: Begin unrestricted use. Continue to monitor for extension lag; if lag returns, reinstitute appropriate level of splinting (night only versus day and night) for additional 2 weeks (return to step C).
E. Incorporate strengthening and dynamic flexion splinting only as necessary.
II. Splints
A. Corrective splints to regain full passive extension
1. Dynamic (Fig. 21-10, *A, B*; Fig. 21-11)
2. Static progressive or serial casting (Fig. 21-12)
B. Static splints: Position PIP joint at 0 degrees and allow full motion at the MCP and DIP joints (see Fig. 21-10, *C*).
C. Splint fasteners
1. Adhesive tape
2. Velcro (limited control against rotation and distal slippage)
3. Coban

Nonoperative Complications

I. Oblique retinacular ligament tightness
II. Inability to achieve full active extension
III. Capsular stiffness secondary to immobilization
IV. Problems with skin integrity secondary to splinting

Operative Indications/Precautions

I. Indications
A. Failure of conservative treatment for longer than 6 months

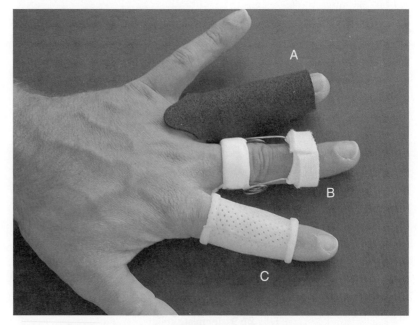

FIG. **21-10**   Extension splints. **A,** Tube. **B,** Capener. **C,** Custom.

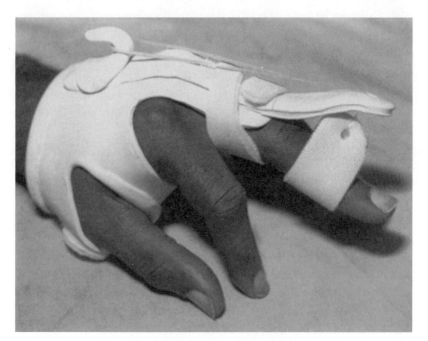

FIG. **21-11**   Short dorsal outrigger.

II.   Precautions
    A. Complicated wounds
    B. Infection
    C. Fractures
    D. Maximal pain
    E. Severe edema

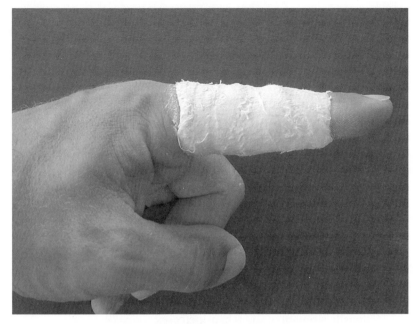

FIG. **21-12** Serial cast.

F. Previous failed surgical attempt
G. PIP joint contracture greater than 40 degrees

Postoperative Indications/Precautions

I. Indications
A. If K-wire is used, protect with splint
B. Wound care
C. Edema reduction
D. Restore DIP joint flexion

Postoperative Therapy

Depending on the stage of deformity and the surgical procedure, as described by Curtis and colleagues[15] and by Burton,[16] postoperative treatment may vary significantly. It is important to discuss the operation performed as well as specific restrictions with the physician before initiation of a therapy program.

I. Weeks 0 to 4
A. Splint or K-wire is used to maintain full PIP joint extension.
B. Active DIP joint flexion is encouraged to promote adhesion-free gliding of the lateral bands through the postsurgical scar.
C. Scar management
II. Weeks 4 to 6
A. PIP joint extension splinting continues at all times (except during exercise).
1. Dynamic extension splinting during the daytime (may use check-rein to control flexion limit)
2. Static extension splinting at night

B. Gentle AROM of the PIP joint into flexion is initiated along with active-assisted or passive extension (depending on surgical procedure).

C. Scar management

III. Weeks 6 to 8

A. Gradually wean from the splint during the day, with continued nighttime use as needed to control extension lag.

B. Closely observe for PIP joint lag. If lag resumes, splinting is continued during the day as well as at night for an additional 2 weeks.

C. Continue to advance AROM through activity and exercise.

IV. Weeks 8 to 12

A. Splinting at night if lag persists. Dynamic or static PIP flexion assistance may be initiated as needed (must be monitored closely as not to increase PIP joint extension lag).

B. AROM continues; may initiate gentle strengthening exercises to facilitate PIP joint flexion.

V. Weeks 12+

A. Night splinting may be necessary for several months as the tensile strength of the repair increases.

B. Initiate progressive strengthening activities as needed.

Postoperative Complications

I. Infection

II. Severe edema

III. Maximal pain

IV. Rupture of the repair

Evaluation Timeline

I. Nonoperative

A. AROM/PROM and strength measurements are performed at initial evaluation. Swelling and pain should also be noted.

B. Reevaluation should continue every 4 weeks.

II. Postoperative

A. Depending on the surgery performed, measurements can be performed beginning at 3 to 4 weeks for extensor tendon release from the dorsal capsule.

B. For other surgeries performed, AROM/PROM measurements are performed 8 weeks after surgery.

C. At 10 to 12 weeks, AROM/PROM and strength measurements can be performed.

D. Every 4 weeks until discharge, AROM/PROM and strength measurements should be performed.

REFERENCES

1. Clement RC, Wray RC Jr: Operative and nonoperative treatment of mallet finger. Ann Plast Surg 16:136, 1986

2. Elliott RA: Splints for mallet and boutonniere deformities. Plast Reconstr Surg 52:282, 1973

3. Stern PJ: Complications and prognosis of treatment of mallet finger. J Hand Surg Am 13:329, 1988

4. Evans RE: Clinical management of extensor tendon injuries. In Mackin EJ, Callahan AD, Skirven TM, et al. (eds): Rehabilitation of the Hand and Upper Extremity. 5th Ed. Mosby, St. Louis, 2002

5. Rosenthal EA: The extensor tendons: anatomy and management. In Mackin EJ, Callahan AD, Skirven TM, et al. (eds): Rehabilitation of the Hand and Upper Extremity. 5th Ed. Mosby, St. Louis, 2002

6. Patel MR, DeSai SS, Bassini-Lipson L: Conservative management of chronic mallet finger. J Hand Surg Am 11:570, 1986

7. Tubiana R: The swan neck deformity. In Tubiana R (ed): The Hand. Vol. III. WB Saunders, Philadelphia, 1988, p. 125

8. Nalebuff EA: The rheumatoid swan neck deformity. In Feldon P: Rheumatoid Arthritis. Hand Clin 5:203, 1989

9. Burton RI: Extensor tendons: late reconstruction. In Green DP (ed): Operative Hand Surgery. 2nd Ed. Vol. 3. Churchill Livingstone, New York, 1988, p. 2073

10. Tubiana R: The boutonniere deformity. In Tubiana R (ed): The Hand. Vol. III. WB Saunders, Philadelphia, 1988, p. 106

11. Schneider LH, Hunter JM: Swan-neck deformity and boutonniere deformity. In Green DP (ed): Operative Hand Surgery. 2nd Ed. Churchill Livingstone, New York, 1988, p. 2041

12. Froehlich JA, Akelmand E, Hendon JH: Extensor tendon injuries at the proximal interphalangeal joint. Hand Clin 4:25, 1988

13. Wynn Parry CB, Salter M, Millar D, et al.: Rehabilitation of the Hand. Butterworth, London, 1981

14. Ferlic D: Boutonniere deformities in rheumatoid arthritis. Hand Clin 5:215, 1989

15. Curtis RM, Reid RL, Provost JM: A staged technique for the repair of the traumatic boutonniere deformity. J Hand Surg 8:167, 1983

16. Burton RI: Extensor tendons: late reconstruction. In Green DP (ed): Operative Hand Surgery. 2nd Ed. Churchill Livingstone, New York, 1988, p. 2100

SUGGESTED READINGS

Caroli A, Zanasi S, Squarzina PB, et al.: Operative treatment of the post-traumatic boutonniere deformity. J Hand Surg Br 15:410, 1990

Semple JC: The Boutonniere injury [editorial]. J Hand Surg Br 15:393, 1990

Extensor Tendon Tenolysis 22

Rebecca J. Saunders

Extensor tenolysis may become necessary if tendon adhesions and joint stiffness occur as a result of trauma, infection, or inflammatory reactions.[1] The frequency of tenolysis following tenorrhaphy has decreased as the use of early mobilization protocols after acute injury has evolved. Metacarpal and phalangeal fractures often damage the extensor mechanism, resulting in adhesion formation during fracture healing.[1-4] The flexor tendons may develop adherence as well. If adherence is suspected in both the flexor and extensor systems, the dorsal adherence is usually addressed first (Fig. 22-1).[1]

Extensor tenolysis is indicated if tendon adhesions limit active and passive range of motion (AROM and PROM, respectively). Joint contractures frequently occur and require surgical remediation if the tenolysis alone does not restore full PROM (Fig. 22-2).

Before surgery, patients should have had at least a 3-month trial period of therapy including AROM/PROM, splinting, and resistive exercise. After 3 months, if progress in ROM has reached a plateau or if the range obtained is inadequate, the patient should be evaluated as a candidate for surgery.

Many authors advocate the use of local anesthesia with intravenous sedation during the procedure.[1,2,4-6] This allows the patient to participate and visualize the gains in ROM made, and to demonstrate whether the tenolysis alone was effective in restoring ROM (Fig. 22-3).

DEFINITION

Extensor tenolysis is surgical excision of scar tissue binding the tendon to surrounding tissues.

TREATMENT GOALS

I. Restore AROM to PROM available after the surgical release.
II. Improve hand function and return patient to prior level of function

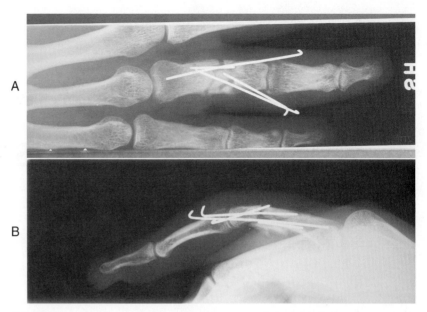

FIG. **22-1 A,** Anterior/posterior view of comminuted proximal phalanx fracture post K-wire fixation. **B,** Lateral view.

OPERATIVE INDICATION/PRECAUTIONS FOR THERAPY

I.   Extensor tenolysis is frequently performed in combination with other procedures such as capsulectomy. It is always advisable to speak to the referring physician before the first postoperative visit to obtain information on the quality of tendons lysed, other anatomic structures involved, the available ROM after release, and ROM goals.

II. The healing extensor tendons need to be protected from over-stretching during active motion for the first few weeks for two

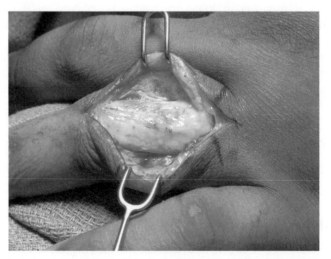

FIG. **22-2** Extensive scarring over the proximal phalanx secondary to a comminuted fracture.

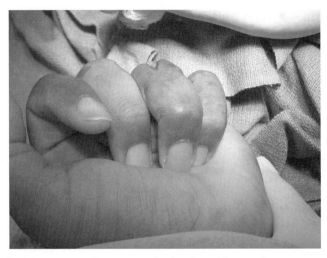

FIG. **22-3** Active range of motion under local anesthesia after extensor tenolysis and dorsal capsulotomy of the ring finger.

reasons. (1) The tendon may have been weakened from being stretched before surgery (i.e., extension lag at the metacarpophalangeal [MCP] or interphalangeal [IP] level) or from the procedure itself, and (2) the extensor tendons are significantly weaker than the opposing flexors.

III.   Active extension needs to be monitored closely throughout all phases of therapy. If patients are gaining flexion but losing extension, the splints supporting extension may need to be used more frequently and the AROM into flexion may need to be temporarily limited.

POSTOPERATIVE THERAPY

I.   General treatment principles for extensor tenolysis and/or capsulectomies

A. Edema control: as with acute hand injuries, effective management of edema is critical to a successful outcome. Postoperative edema needs to be monitored closely. Edema control includes elevation of the hand above the level of the heart to reduce limb dependency, use of light compressive dressings, and exercise. Cold packs applied with the extremity in elevation for 15- to 20-minute periods may be used as long as the dressing is kept dry and sterile and there is no vascular compromise. Postoperative edema should gradually subside over 2 to 3 weeks.

B. Pain management: Patients' experience of pain postoperatively varies widely. Some patients require narcotic analgesia for a short time. Pain, if present, needs to be managed effectively so that patients can participate in therapy and in their home exercise programs. Transcutaneous electrical nerve stimulation (TENS), high-voltage galvanic stimulation (HVG), and other types of electrical stimulation can be helpful in reducing postoperative discomfort.

C. Wound care: universal precautions should be used when performing dressing changes and exercises.

D. Initiation of AROM according to the orders of the physician (usually within 24 to 48 hours after surgery). If possible, speak to the surgeon directly before the first visit, to provide adequate protection and treatment of the involved structures. Active exercise should emphasize full excursion of the lysed tendons (Fig. 22-4). Extrinsic extensor tightness is frequently associated with MCP joint stiffness and intrinsic tightness, and these conditions need to be addressed through active exercise and splinting. Patients should be instructed to perform 10 repetitions of each exercise, holding the stretch at end range for 5 to 10 seconds. Exercise sessions should be performed every $1^1/_2$ to 2 hours during the day.

E. PROM, instruction in gentle passive stretching.

F. Scar management

G. Splinting

1. An appointment for postoperative therapy should be made when the surgery is scheduled.

2. Dynamic splints are used during the day as an adjunct to the patient's active exercise program and to protect weakened structures. Patients undergoing tenolysis in zone V and proximal may benefit from a dynamic MCP extension splint during the day to allow full excursion flexion while supporting the extensors. The splint should be removed periodically during the day for wrist ROM. After tenolysis of zones III and IV, a dynamic hand-based proximal interphalangeal (PIP) joint extension splint may be useful if the skin condition allows it. If a dynamic splint is not tolerated, the PIP joint should be supported at neutral between exercise sessions.

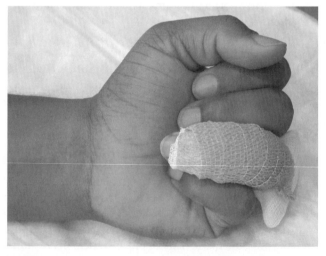

FIG. 22-4 Active range of motion available at 24 hours after surgery.

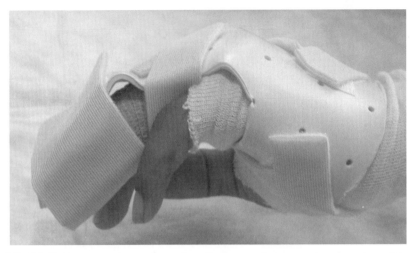

FIG. **22-5**   Postoperative resting splint allowing static progressive extension of the interphalangeal joints.

3. Static progressive splints or resting splints are used at night to maintain gains in ROM and provide a prolonged gentle stretch to the involved tissues (Fig. 22-5).
4. All splints need to be monitored and adjusted frequently, as the soft tissues respond to the stresses applied through active and passive exercise. The patient should be provided with detailed wearing instructions and precautions.
5. Splinting is continued until the patient is able to maintain the ROM present postoperatively with AROM and PROM (approximately 3 to 5 months) (Fig. 22-6).
6. If passive motion exceeds active motion, the emphasis on active exercise should be increased to overcome tendon weakness or adherence.

H. Functional activities and light use of the hand should be incorporated early to promote use of available ROM and to increase strength. Pain and edema need to be monitored closely as activities are incorporated.

I. Grip strengthening can be initiated 6 weeks postoperatively[3] if the tendon is of "good quality." If an extension lag is present, it may be advisable to start with extensor strengthening first and gradually proceed with resistive activities in flexion.

J. Most patients are able to return to work on average at 3 to 4 months postoperatively.[1]

POSTOPERATIVE COMPLICATIONS

 I.   Hematoma: Notify physician immediately if present; this condition may require physician treatment
 II. Infection: Notify physician immediately.
 III. Limited ROM secondary to edema and pain
 IV. Weakness of previously adherent tendons

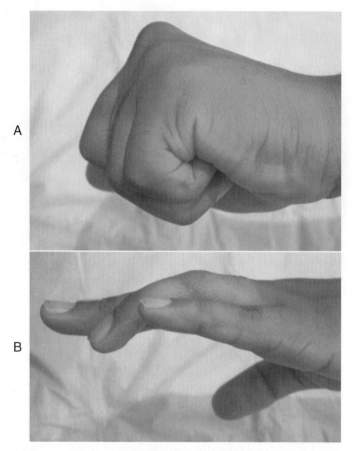

FIG. **22-6** **A,** Active flexion at 8 weeks after surgery. **B,** Active extension at 8 weeks after surgery.

V.   Tendon rupture
VI.   Complex regional pain syndrome

EVALUATION TIMELINE

I.   Preoperative evaluation at 1 to 2 weeks before surgery
      A. AROM/PROM
      B. Grip and pinch strength
      C. Sensation
      D. Functional assessment of activities of daily living (ADL), vocational and avocational activities

II.   Postoperative evaluation
      A. Initial AROM postoperatively: Available AROM should be monitored closely at each treatment session; splinting and exercise programs require frequent adjustment as ROM progresses.
      B. Weekly reevaluation of AROM/PROM
      C. Strength may be assessed at 8 weeks if the tendon was of "good quality" postoperatively; testing is delayed until 10 to 12 weeks if the tendons were "frayed."

OUTCOMES

Creighten and Steichen[3] reported on their series of extensor tenolysis procedures performed after phalangeal fractures. Patients were evaluated at an average of 6 months postoperatively. These authors found that total active motion (TAM) improved an average of 54 degrees (31%) from the preoperative TAM level, and active extension lag improved by 50% in patients requiring tenolysis alone. No improvement in active extension was noted in patients requiring tenolysis and dorsal capsulotomies, although TAM improved 34 degrees (21%).

Landi and colleagues[1] reported on their series of tenolysis procedures performed after tenorrhaphy, grafting, and closed trauma. Patients were evaluated at an average of 2.8 years postoperatively. To evaluate the results, these authors considered AROM and the patient's subjective judgment of improvement. Excellent results were achieved in 19.35% of the cases, defined as MCP active flexion greater than 80 degrees, PIP flexion greater than 90 degrees, and no extension deficit. Good results (MCP greater than 70 degrees, PIP greater than 90 degrees, extension deficit less than 30 degrees) were achieved by 32.25%; satisfactory results (MCP greater than 50 degrees, PIP greater than 60 degrees, extension deficit less than 30 degrees) by 22.5%; and poor results (MCP greater than 50 degrees, PIP less than 60 degrees, and extension deficit greater than 30 degrees) by 6.5%.

Patients undergoing extensor tenolysis need to be cautioned that some loss of extension with the recovery of flexion is not uncommon.[6] This is not necessarily negative if the arc of motion is more functional. All authors agree that a cooperative, compliant patient is necessary to achieve optimal results.

REFERENCES

1. Landi A, Saracino A, Giuseppe C, et al.: Complex tenolysis of the hand. In Hunter J, Schneider L, Mackin E (eds): Tendon and Nerve Surgery in the Hand: A Third Decade. Mosby, St. Louis, 1997
2. Uhl RL: Salvage of extensor tendon function with tenolysis and joint release. Hand Clin 11:461-470, 1995
3. Creighton JJ, Steichen JB: Complications in phalangeal and metacarpal fracture management: results of extensor tenolysis. Hand Clin 10:111-116, 1994
4. Creighton JJ, Steichen JB: Extensor tenolysis. In Strickland JB (ed): Master Techniques in Orthopaedic Surgery: The Hand. Lippincott-Raven, Philadelphia, 1998
5. Schneider LH, Feldscher SB: Tenolysis: dynamic approach to surgery and therapy. In Mackin EJ, Callahan AD, Skirven TM, et al. (eds): Hunter-Mackin-Callahan Rehabilitation of the Hand and Upper Extremity. 5th Ed. Vol. 1. Mosby, St. Louis 2002
6. Schneider LH: Tenolysis and capsulectomy after hand fractures. Clin Orthop 327: 72-78, 1996

SUGGESTED READINGS

Fess EE, McCollum M: The influence of splinting on healing tissues. J Hand Ther 11: 157-161, 1998
Hume MC, Gellman H, MCKellop H, et al.: Functional range of motion of the joints of the hand. J Hand Surg Am 15:240-243, 1990
Merritt WH: Written on behalf of the stiff finger. J Hand Ther 11:74-79, 1998
Skoff HD: Extensor tenolysis: a modern version of an old approach. Plast Reconstr Surg 93:1056-1060, 1994

Complex Extensor Reconstruction 23

Rebecca J. Saunders

Dorsal hand injuries with extensor tendon and soft tissue loss are a reconstructive challenge (Fig. 23-1). These injuries occur as a result of industrial or motor vehicle accidents, burns, crush injuries, severe infections, or subcutaneous extravasation of caustic intravenous solutions.[1,2] Patients require wound coverage with a flap and/or graft and extensor tendon reconstruction with tendon grafts. Donor graft sources include the palmaris longus, plantaris, and extensor digitorum longus of the second through fifth toes.[2] Tendon transfers are frequently necessary if the reconstruction has been performed in stages and there has been muscle contracture.[2-5] The flexor carpi radialis and flexor carpi ulnaris are frequently used for tendon transfer. Wrist flexion is synergistic with digital extension, and the use of these motors facilitates the patient's ability to activate the transfer.

These reconstructive procedures present the surgeon and therapist with a dilemma: how can digital extension be regained without losing flexion? Most authors recommend that tendon transfers and grafts be immobilized in a protected position for 3 to 5 weeks after surgery.[3,4,6-9] This lengthy

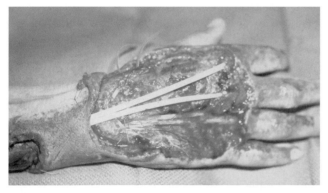

FIG. **23-1** Dorsal hand trauma with extensive soft tissue loss requiring flap coverage and staged extensor tendon reconstruction with Hunter rods.

period of immobilization can lead to tendon adherence, secondary joint stiffness, and the need for additional surgical procedures to regain digital joint motion. Pulvertaft cited graft adherence as the most common cause of failure after tendon grafting.[6]

Most of the research on tendon repairs and tendon grafting has been performed on a flexor tendon model.[10-14] The application of early controlled motion to the extensor tendon system has been based on flexor tendon studies and was proved clinically effective by Evans and Burkhalter,[15,16] Browne and Ribik,[17] and Chow and colleagues.[18] The following protocol for management of extensor tendon reconstruction in zones V through VII via tendon transfer with multiple intercalated grafts was developed based on these applications of applying controlled stress to healing tendons.[15-19]

DEFINITION

Complex extensor reconstruction is required for extensor tendon injuries with skin loss. Often these patients have fractures and segmental tendon loss.

SURGICAL PURPOSE

Complex extensor tendon injuries are seen in an upper extremity trauma practice. Multiple tissues need repair, including extensor tendons, metacarpals or phalanges, and overlying soft tissue. Traditionally, the skin and bone injuries are repaired first, leaving the extensor tendons for a second stage. Increasingly, use of free tissue transfer for wound coverage and stable fixation techniques for bone repair allows the surgeon to repair the extensor tendons at the time of wound closure, eliminating secondary operations.

TREATMENT GOALS

To restore active extension of the metacarpophalangeal (MCP) joints and to improve hand function and strength.

POSTOPERATIVE INDICATIONS/PRECAUTIONS FOR THERAPY

I. The initial splint is constructed without direct pressure over the tendon grafts (Fig. 23-2).
II. A separate resting splint is recommended for night use to maintain the wrist in 30 to 35 degrees extension and the MCP joints and interphalangeal (IP) joints at neutral.
III. The volar component of the daytime dynamic splint allows 30 degrees of MCP flexion. If the patient is overpowering the volar splint during the performance of exercises, an additional flexion stop can be added to the outrigger line.

POSTOPERATIVE THERAPY

I. Therapy is initiated at 2 to 3 days postoperatively.
II. Splinting: A dynamic MCP extension splint is fabricated with an interlocking volar component that limits MCP flexion to 30 degrees.

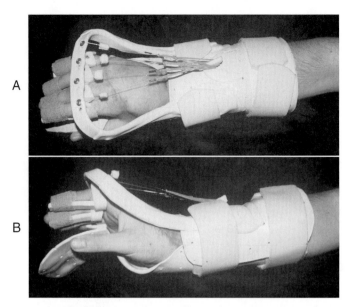

FIG. **23-2** **A** and **B,** Dynamic metacarpophalangeal (MCP) extension splint with interlocking volar component and limited MCP flexion excursion.

The wrist is positioned in 30 to 35 degrees of extension.[19] The splint is worn continuously during the day and is used for 6 to 8 weeks. A resting splint with the wrist at 30 to 35 degrees and the MCP and IP joints at neutral is used at night for a total of 10 to 12 weeks. Patients with an extension lag may require longer periods of splinting with both the dynamic and static components.

III.   Exercises

   A. 1 to 3 weeks: Active range of motion (AROM). The patient performs 10 repetitions of blocked MCP flexion within the limits of the splint every 1.5 to 2 hours during the day. The IP joints are allowed flexion within a pain-free range with the MCP joints supported at neutral in the dynamic splint, unless the surgeon believes that the distal suture site needs to be protected. If the distal repair needs to be protected, the IP joints are splinted in extension for 3 weeks.

   B. 4 weeks: Active, protected MCP extension is inititated. Initial attempts at extension should be gentle and include performance of wrist tenodesis exercise allowing up to 20 to 30 degrees of flexion. The dynamic MCP extension splint continues to be used at all times during the day, excluding the active exercise sessions.

   C. 5 weeks: The MCP excursion in the splint may be increased to 50 degrees, and the patient may perform gentle composite flexion when out of the dynamic splint, with the wrist well supported manually in extension.

   D. 6 weeks: The limitations in excursion of the dynamic splint are removed, and the emphasis on wrist ROM is increased.

   E. 8 weeks: Light resistive exercise is initiated if there is no significant extension lag (greater than 20 to 25 degrees). Strengthening of the digital extensors is initiated first (Fig. 23-3).

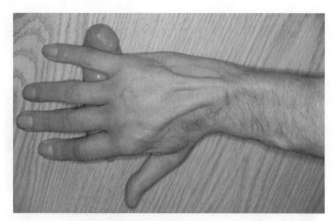

FIG. **23-3** Strengthening extensors.

POSTOPERATIVE COMPLICATIONS

I.   Hematoma: notify physician immediately; this condition may require treatment by the physician and modification of the planned postoperative therapy regimen.
II. Infection: notify physician immediately.
III. Limitations in ROM secondary to edema and/or pain
IV. Tendon adherence
V.   Tendon rupture
VI. Limitations in extension due to excessive length in the transfers and/or grafts

EVALUATION TIMELINE

I.   Preoperative evaluation 1 to 2 weeks before surgery
     A. AROM and passive range of motion (PROM)
     B. Grip and pinch strength
     C. Sensation
     D. Functional assessment of activities of daily living, vocational, and avocational activities.
II. Postoperative evaluation
     A. Initial blocked MCP ROM in splint within the limited excursion allowed
     B. AROM of IP joints with the wrist and MCP joints supported in extension, measured after this motion is approved by the physician and reassessed weekly
     C. Active MCP extension at 4 weeks, AROM of affected hand. As with all extensor tendon injury rehabilitation, active MCP extension needs to be monitored closely as exercise and activities progress.
     D. Active wrist ROM; AROM/PROM of affected hand
     E. Grip strength can be assessed at 10 to 12 weeks postoperatively.

OUTCOMES

Saldana[1] reported on the use of postoperative dynamic extension splinting for both primary and staged extensor tendon reconstruction. Tendon grafting resulted in an extension lag when the dynamic splint was removed, but with time, usually over the course of 6 months, the residual extensor lag was reduced to zero.

Cautilli and Schneider[20] reported on their series of seven patients in whom a total of 23 tendons were reconstructed. Four of the patients underwent staged reconstruction with silicone tendon implants. The other patients underwent grafting in a single stage after the flap coverage had healed and they recovered sufficient PROM. After grafting, the wrist and hand were immobilized in extension for 3 to 4 weeks. IP joint ROM was allowed at 10 days postoperatively. Little detail was given on postoperative management after the 4 weeks of immobilization. The reported restoration of extension was successful, and more difficulty was noted in the recovery of flexion. Two patients required tenolysis to improve flexion. At an average of 2 years of follow-up, most of the patients had achieved good to excellent ROM. One case was reported as a failure because of severely limited MCP flexion (less than 30 degrees).

Scheker and co-workers[21] reported on primary extensor reconstruction of dorsal hand defects requiring free flaps. Their postoperative protocol included use of a dynamic extension outrigger at 48 hours after surgery. The outrigger allowed active flexion and protected extension. The patients used the splint for 6 weeks and then began therapy to improve ROM and strength. Maximum improvement took approximately 3 months. Nine patients were treated with this method. Subsequent procedures included tenolysis, flap defatting, a Swanson arthroplasty, plate removal, and regrafting of a donor graft site. The authors reported results based on MCP ROM. Four patients were reported as having good results (73 degrees), four fair (42 degrees), and one poor (25 degrees).

The results of the six patients in our own series are summarized in Tables 23-1 and 23-2. Six patients (total of 23 digits) underwent late extensor tendon reconstruction for zones V through VII via multiple intercalated grafts. Five of the patients required tendon transfer. The flexor carpi ulnaris was transferred in three cases, and the flexor carpi radialis in two cases. Donor grafts included the palmaris and the extensor digitorum longus. The average age was 43 years. Patients were initially seen two times per week for the first 8 to 10 weeks, and then with variable frequency until discharge. Only one patient required dynamic flexion splinting to regain

TABLE 23-1 Characteristics of Patients Undergoing Complex Extensor Reconstruction with Early Controlled Motion

Patient	Age (yr)	Mechanism of Injury	Digits Involved	Associated Injuries	Flap Coverage	Hunter Rods
Case 1	43	Crush	IF, MF, RF	Capitate and fourth metacarpal fractures; second-degree burns	Yes	Yes
Case 2	28	MVA	IF, MF, RF, LF	—	Yes	No
Case 3	32	MVA	IF, MF, RF, LF	Intraarticular fracture IP thumb	Yes	Yes
Case 4	60	Infection	IF, MF, RF, LF	—	Yes	No
Case 5	47	Infection	IF, MF, RF, LF	—	Yes	No
Case 6	48	Saw injury	IF, MF, RF, LF	Metacarpal fractures of fingers 2-5 requiring ORIF/bone grafting	No	No

IF, Index finger; *IP*, interphalangeal; *LF*, little finger; *MF*, middle finger; *MVA*, motor vehicle accident; *ORIF*, open reduction with internal fixation; *RF*, ring finger.

TABLE **23-2** Results–Metacarpophalangeal Joint Extension after Complex Extensor Reconstruction with Early Controlled Motion

	Preoperative MP Extension				12-14 wk Postoperative MP Extension				26-28 wk Postoperative MP Extension			
	IF	MF	RF	LF	IF	MF	RF	LF	IF	MF	RF	LF
Case 1	−40	−40	−35	N/A	0	0	0	N/A	0	0	0	N/A
Case 2	−70	−75	−75	−75	−5	−5	0	0	0	0	+5	+10
Case 3	Unk.	Unk.	Unk.	Unk.	−3	−7	−5	+5	0	−10	0	0
Case 4	−65	−75	−75	−80	−20	−25	−10	−15	−10	−20	0	−5
Case 5	Unk.	Unk.	Unk.	Unk.	−5	0	0	+10	−5	0	0	+10
Case 6	−55	−50	−55	−50	−55	−50	−50	−55	−35	−30	−30	−25

IF, Index finger; *LF,* little finger; *MF,* middle finger; *N/A,* not applicable; *RF,* ring finger; *Unk.,* unknown.

digital flexion postoperatively. The average length of follow-up was 27 weeks (range, 2 to 9 months). Patients who had greater limitations in digital flexion preoperatively required more postoperative care. Five of the six patients achieved good to excellent MCP extension while using little or no wrist flexion (Fig. 23-4) Digital flexion was normal or restored to their preoperative ROM by 8 weeks postoperatively. All of the patients in this series

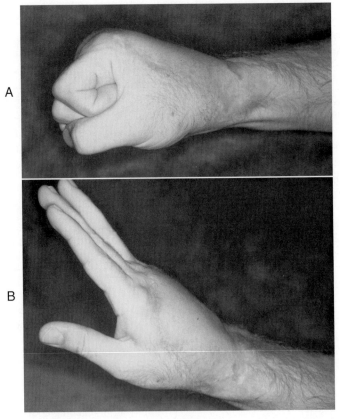

FIG. **23-4** **A,** Active flexion after staged extensor reconstruction of digits 2 through 5 with a flexor carpi ulnaris (FCU) transfer. **B,** Active extension of metacarpophalangeal joints performed in wrist extension.

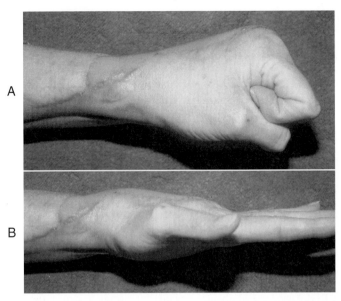

FIG. **23-5 A,** Active flexion after staged reconstruction of digits 2 through 5 with tendon transfer. **B,** Active metacarpophalangeal extension.

continued to gain active MCP extension for 7 to 9 months postoperatively. The patient with a "poor" result at 8 weeks improved to a "fair" result at 9 months postoperatively. This patient elected to have a tenolysis to improve extension. There were no tendon ruptures. All six patients recovered functional wrist ROM and strength. Three patients were able to return to work at 12 to 16 weeks from the date of surgery. Early controlled motion of complex extensor reconstruction proved to be a safe and effective method of postoperative management for the patients in this series (Fig. 23-5).

The mechanism of healing in tendon grafts remains controversial.[14] Further research is needed to elucidate the differences in healing between primary repairs and tendon grafts. We believe that the application of controlled stress to the healing grafts in our series improved excursion, decreased adhesions, and decreased the magnitude of secondary joint stiffness.

REFERENCES

1. Saldana MJ: Primary extensor grafts in zones 5 to 7. In Blair WF: Techniques in Hand Surgery. Williams & Wilkins, Baltimore, MD, 1996
2. Newport ML: Staged extensor grafts in zones 5 to 8. In Blair WF: Techniques in Hand Surgery. Williams & Wilkins, Baltimore, MD, 1996
3. Burton RI, Melchior JA: Extensor tendons: late reconstruction. In Green DP: Operative Hand Surgery. 2nd Ed. Vol. 2. Churchill Livingstone, New York, 1988, p. 2021
4. Smith RJ: Tendon transfers: postoperative care. In Smith RJ: Tendon Transfers of the Hand and Forearm. Little, Brown and Company, Boston, 1987, pp. 313-316
5. Lubahn JD, Cermak MB: Extensor mechanism reconstruction. In Peimer C: Surgery of the Hand and Upper Extremity. Vol. 1. McGraw-Hill, New York, 1996
6. Pulvertaft RG: Indications for tendon grafting. In Hunter JM, Schneider LH, Mackin EJ, et al. (eds): Rehabilitation of the Hand: Surgery and Therapy. 3rd Ed. Mosby, St. Louis, 1990
7. Reynolds C: Preoperative and postoperative management of tendon transfers after radial nerve injury. In Hunter JM, Schneider LH, Mackin EJ, et al. (eds): Rehabilitation of the Hand: Surgery and Therapy. 3rd Ed. Mosby, St. Louis, 1990

8. Karev A: Principles of tendon transfers. In Peimer C: Surgery of the Hand and Upper Extremity. Vol 1. McGraw-Hill, New York, 1996

9. Davis TC: Extensor tendon reconstruction after chronic injuries. In Berger RA, Weiss AP: Hand Surgery. Vol. 1. Lippincott Williams & Wilkins, Philadelphia, 2004

10. Gelberman RH, Menon J, Gonsalves M, et al.: The effects of mobilization on the vascularization of healing flexor tendons in dogs. Clin Orthop 153:283-289, 1980

11. Gelberman RH, Woo S, Lothringer K, et al.: Effects of early intermittent passive mobilization of healing canine flexor tendons. J Hand Surg Am 7:170-175, 1982

12. Gelberman RH, Botte MJ, Spiegelman JJ, et al.: The excursion and deformation of repaired flexor tendons treated with protected early motion. J Hand Surg Am 11: 106-110, 1986

13. Gelberman RH, Nunly JA, Osterman AL, et al.: Influences of the protected passive mobilization interval on flexor tendon healing: a prospective randomized clinical study. Clin Orthop 264:189-196, 1991

14. Flynn JE, Graham JUH: The role of tendon in healing with primary repair of tendon and tendon transplants. In Jupiter J (ed): Flynn's Hand Surgery. 4th Ed. Williams & Wilkins, Baltimore, 1991

15. Evans RB, Burkhalter WE: A study of the dynamic anatomy of extensor tendons and implications for treatment. J Hand Surg Am 11:774-779, 1986

16. Evans RB: Clinical application of controlled stress to the healing extensor tendon: a review of 112 cases. Phys Ther 69:1041-1049, 1989

17. Browne EZ, Ribik CA: Early dynamic splinting for extensor tendon injuries. J Hand Surg Am 14:72-76, 1989

18. Chow JA, Dovell S, Thomas LJ, et al.: A comparison of results of extensor tendon repair followed by early controlled mobilization vs static immobilization. J Hand Surg Br 89: 14B:18-20

19. Minamikawa Y, Peimer C, Yamaguchi T, et al.: Wrist position and extensor tendon amplitude following repair. J Hand Surg Am 17:268-271, 1992

20. Cautilli D, Schneider LH: Extensor tendon grafting on the dorsum of the hand in massive tendon loss. Hand Clin 11:423-429, 1995

21. Scheker LR, Langley SJ, Martin D, et al.: Primary extensor tendon reconstruction in dorsal hand defects requiring free flaps. J Hand Surg Br 18:568-575, 1993

SUGGESTED READINGS

Adams BD: Staged extensor tendon reconstruction in the finger. J Hand Surg Am 22: 833-837, 1997

Cyr LM, Ross RG: How controlled stress affects healing tissues. J Hand Ther 11:125-130, 1998

Desai SS, Chwei-Chin D, Levin LS: Microsurgical reconstruction of the extensor system. Hand Clin 11:471-482, 1995

Hung LK, Chan A, Chang J, et al.: Early controlled active mobilization with dynamic splintage for treatment of extensor tendon injuries. Hand Surg 15:251-257, 1990

Newport ML, Blair WF, Steyers CM Jr: Long-term results of extensor tendon repair. J Hand Surg Am 15:961-966, 1990

Quaba AA, Elliot D, Sommerlad BC: Long term hand function without long finger extensors: a clinical study. J Hand Surg Br 13:66-71, 1988

Quaba AA, Elliot D, Sommerlad BC: Functional deficit following loss of continuity of the long extensors of the fingers: a method of assessment. J Hand Surg Br 13:282-283, 1988

Walsh MT, Rinehimer W, Muntzer E, et al.: Early controlled motion with dynamic splinting vs. static splinting for zones III and IV extensor tendon lacerations: a preliminary report. J Hand Ther 7:232-236, 1994

PART **FOUR**

Shoulder

Shoulder Tendonitis   24

Mary Schuler Murphy

Understanding shoulder anatomy is of paramount importance in the rehabilitation of the shoulder. Tytherleigh-Strong and colleagues[1] stressed that shoulder stability is dependent on the soft tissues that surround the shoulder. The glenoid labrum and the capsular ligament provide static stability while the rotator cuff, biceps, deltoid, and scapulothoracic musculature provide dynamic stability. The importance of the balance among the rotator cuff, biceps, deltoid, and scapulothoracic muscles for normal shoulder movement is cited frequently in the literature.[1-19]

Shoulder impingement is thought to be caused by multiple factors. Posture requires assessment and remediation if it is found to be a possible contributor to shoulder impingement. Krabak and associates[11] emphasized the importance of stabilization of the trunk and hip in rehabilitation, reporting that 54% of the force and 51% of the kinetic energy transmitted through the shoulder are generated through the lower extremity and trunk. Tempelheh and co-workers[20] studied 411 volunteers without shoulder symptoms and reported that 23.4% of the participants had a full-thickness rotator cuff tear. Perhaps these patients remained asymptomatic because of good anatomic biomechanics.

Posterior capsular tightness is also thought to contribute to dysfunction of normal scapulothoracic and glenohumeral rhythm. Conroy and Hayes[8] suggested that abnormal scapular and clavicular elevation may indicate a problem with posterior capsular tightness and glenohumeral weakness leading to scapulothoracic compensation. Matsen and Arntz[21] also reported the effect of tight posterior joint capsule on decreased shoulder mobility and its role in shoulder impingement.

Primary subacromial impingement, popularized by Neer[22] in 1972, was defined as a mechanical encroachment of the rotator cuff beneath the coracoacromial arch against the anterior and undersurface of the anterior third of the acromion, the coracoacromial ligament, and perhaps the acromioclavicular joint, in the subacromial space. Bigliani and colleagues[23] found a hooked acromion in 70% of cadavers with a full-thickness rotator cuff tear. Other encroachment causes might include, but are not limited to, osteophytes, thickening of the coracoacromial ligament, or an enlarged humeral head secondary to fracture.

Secondary impingement syndrome is associated with overuse of the rotator cuff muscles secondary to possible problems with glenohumeral instability or with scapulothoracic muscle weakness. Warner and associates[24] reported that 68% of patients with anterior shoulder instability in their study showed signs of impingement. Kamkar and co-workers[10] hypothesized that proper sequencing of scapulothoracic joint motion with glenohumeral joint motion decreases the risk of impingement. They advocated strengthening of the scapulothoracic muscles for any therapy treatment protocol for secondary shoulder impingement syndrome.

Bang and Deyle[2] proposed that glenohumeral instability and weakness of either glenohumeral or scapulothoracic stabilizers can cause excessive humeral head migration into the subacromial space. Their study provided evidence that supervised therapeutic exercises, especially combined with manual therapy, decreased pain, increased strength, and improved function in patients with shoulder impingement syndrome.

Brox and colleagues[5] reported that supervised therapy exercises in their clinical trial were as effective as surgical subacromial decompression combined with postoperative therapy in the treatment of patients diagnosed with stage 2 primary shoulder impingement. Furthermore, in the 30-month follow-up of these subjects, the difference between those patients with arthroscopic surgery and supervised therapeutic exercises was not significant.

The therapist must address any problems with pain and inflammation, decreased ROM, instabilities, poor posture, and muscle weakness in the rotator cuff, biceps, deltoids, and scapulothoracic musculature through careful and ongoing evaluation and remediation based on findings. Patient participation and education is paramount to successful rehabilitation. Patients must not only participate in their individualized home exercise program but also avoid or modify offending activities. Failure to resolve the patient's pain and dysfunction may be a reflection of the inability to conservatively overcome either the primary or the secondary causes of the impingement process, necessitating the need for further physician intervention.

DEFINITION

Primary subacromial impingement is compression of the rotator cuff muscles, the long head of the biceps, and/or the subacromial bursa against the acromion and coracoacromial ligament. This is usually secondary to some form of anatomic encroachment on the undersurface of the coracoacromial arch resulting in ischemia, inflammation, and pain. Over time, this compression can lead to degradation of the tendon, predisposing it to calcification and rupture (Figs. 24-1 and 24-2). Secondary impingement is thought to be caused by an imbalance of the static and/or dynamic mobilizers of the shoulder (e.g., subtle glenohumeral instability, ligamentous laxity). Internal impingement involves contact of the undersurface of the rotator cuff with the superior glenoid and labrum; it frequently is seen in athletes who participate in overhead sports.

TREATMENT PURPOSE

The purpose of therapy is to reduce soft tissue inflammation and pain and to promote healing of the involved soft tissues while regaining the normal glenohumeral and scapulothoracic rhythm needed for normal shoulder function.

TREATMENT GOALS

I. Restore normal, pain-free use of the involved extremity.
II. Resolve the chronic inflammatory process.

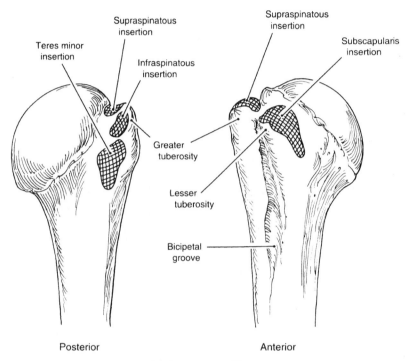

FIG. **24-1** Rotator cuff insertion.

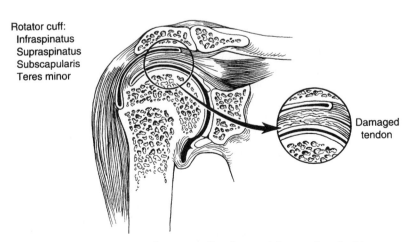

FIG. **24-2** Anatomy of rotator cuff and potential area of tendonitis.

III. Restore normal musculotendinous flexibility and strength.
IV. Correct postural imbalance and restore normal scapulothoracic/ glenohumeral rhythm.
V. Prevent recurrences through patient education. (Patient education and active participation in the therapy program is essential to successful rehabilitation.)

NONOPERATIVE INDICATIONS/PRECAUTIONS FOR THERAPY

I. Indications
   A. Pain on palpation of specific tendons (e.g., rotator cuff, biceps tendons)
   B. Pain on resisted motions for specific muscle actions (e.g., resisted external rotation testing for infraspinatus involvement)
II. Precautions
   A. Allergy to nonsteroidal antiinflammatory drugs (NSAIDs)

NONOPERATIVE THERAPY

I. Acute
   A. Transcutaneous electrical nerve stimulation (TENS), high-voltage galvanic stimulation (HVG), or an interferential electrical stimulation combined with cold application for control of pain and swelling can be used in therapy and at home if cold application alone is not sufficient in controlling pain.
   B. Positioning of the painful shoulder for circulation and healing
      1. Sitting: Rest the affected shoulder in approximately 30 to 45 degrees scaption.
      2. Standing or walking: Support affected shoulder by placing the hand in a pocket.
      3. Sleeping: Do not sleep on the affected side or with the shoulder positioned above 90 degrees; the arm should be positioned at approximately 30 to 45 degrees of scaption on a pillow.
   C. Activity modification (i.e., restrict offending activities)
      1. The patient may be instructed in the modification of particular tasks to be performed by reduction of repetitions and/or changing how the task is performed (e.g., reducing the amount of time allowed in the performance of an activity and keeping shoulder elevation below the impingement range). The patient may need to stop or restrict activities known to contribute to shoulder impingement during the early rehabilitation period.
      2. Active use of the affected upper extremity should be restricted to below the ROM level of impingement. (This may be at 70 degrees of shoulder elevation and not the frequently reported 90 degrees.)
   D. Iontophoresis
   E. Ultrasound/phonophoresis: There are limited studies as to effectiveness of these treatments for shoulder tendonitis, except for some studies reporting positive results for calcification tendonitis with the use of ultrasound.[2,6,25]
   F. NSAIDs

G. Exercise
1. Address and remediate any posterior capsule tightness, as well as ROM deficits. The use of manual therapy (passive accessory or passive physiological joint mobilization Maitland grades I through V) combined with a shoulder exercise program has been found to be more effective than a supervised exercise therapy program alone.[2]
2. Initiate postural exercises to open the glenohumeral space (Fig. 24-3, *A*).
3. Initiate program of AROM, active assisted range of motion (AAROM), and PROM with respect to pain to maintain ROM.
4. May use manual isometric scapular strengthening and/or closed kinetic chain exercises for scapular stabilization strengthening. Once pain is resolved and ROM and strength are restored, closed- and open-chain exercise may be incorporated into the therapy program for more specific return to the patient's normal activities. See Fig. 24-3, *A* through *H* for examples of scapular stabilization exercises.
5. Initiate submaximal isometric rotator cuff strengthening as tolerated (initially in approximately 20 degrees abduction and with progressive elevation in the plane of the scapula).
6. Initiate submaximal isometric deltoid strengthening as tolerated (initially performed at side and progressed to positions away from body).
7. Progress strengthening throughout functional ROM as pain diminishes, using isotonic, isokinetic, concentric, and eccentric exercises. Proprioceptive neuromuscular facilitation (PNF) patterns of strengthening are useful in the reestablishment of functional AROM. See Fig. 24-4, *A* through *H* for an example progression of rotator cuff strengthening.
II. Chronic
A. Heat modalities are typically used before ROM, joint mobilizations, and stretching. Cold modalities can be helpful after exercises to alleviate postexercise inflammation or pain.
B. Steroid injections
C. Ultrasound/phonophoresis
D. Iontophoresis
E. Deep transverse friction massage
F. Stretching
G. Education for prevention of recurrence, including possible modification in the affected upper extremity use in ADLs (including self-care, work, and vocational interests).
H. Exercise
1. Depending on evaluation findings, any of the exercises described from the acute phase may be used. Remediate any capsular tightness or ROM deficits.
2. Progressive program of rotator cuff, biceps, scapulothoracic, and deltoid strengthening, moving from nonprovocative to provocative positions (See Figs. 24-3, *A* to *H* and 24-4, *A* to *H*)
3. Postural exercises to increase the glenohumeral space
4. Include isolated exercises for specific muscle weaknesses; can also use patterned exercises for combination movement (e.g., proprioceptive neuromuscular facilitation, closed-chain exercises).

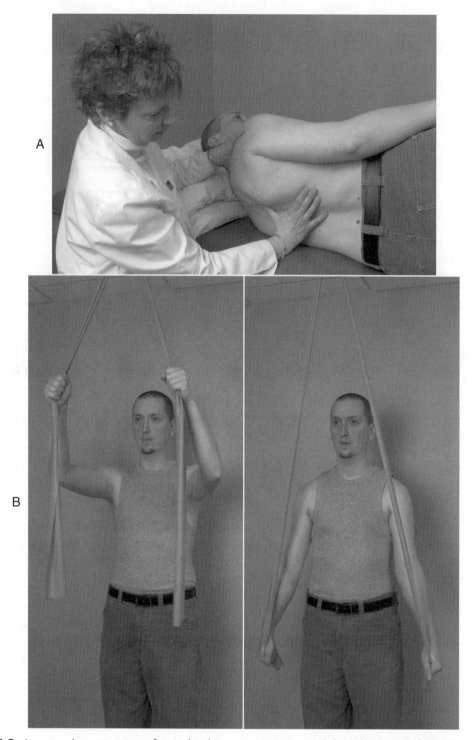

FIG. **24-3** An example progression of scapular depression exercises with lateral rotation of the inferior angle (**A** through **D**) and scapular protraction exercises (**E** through **H**). **A,** Active lower trapezius action performed with or without therapist's manual guidance. Manual resistance may also be applied by the therapist. **B,** Standing downward punch using Theraband.

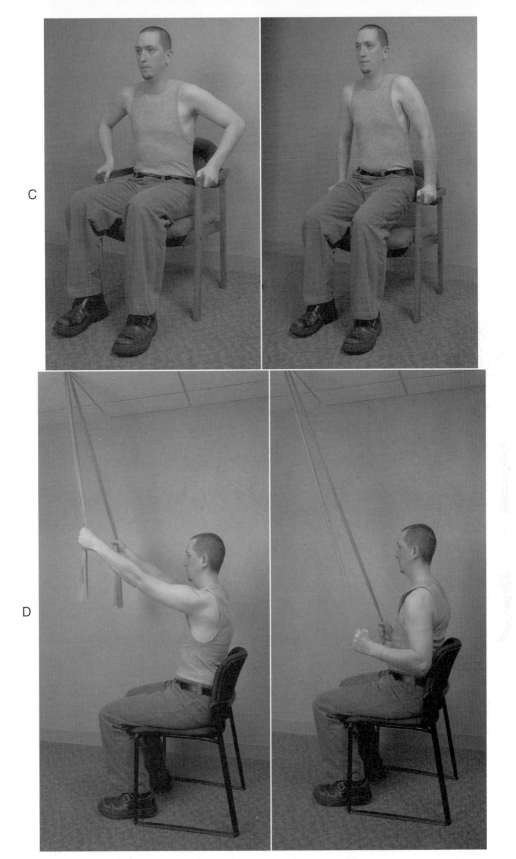

FIG. **24-3 Cont'd C,** Partial chair push-ups with lower extremity assistance. **D,** Seated downward row may also be performed standing, using Theraband.

(Continued)

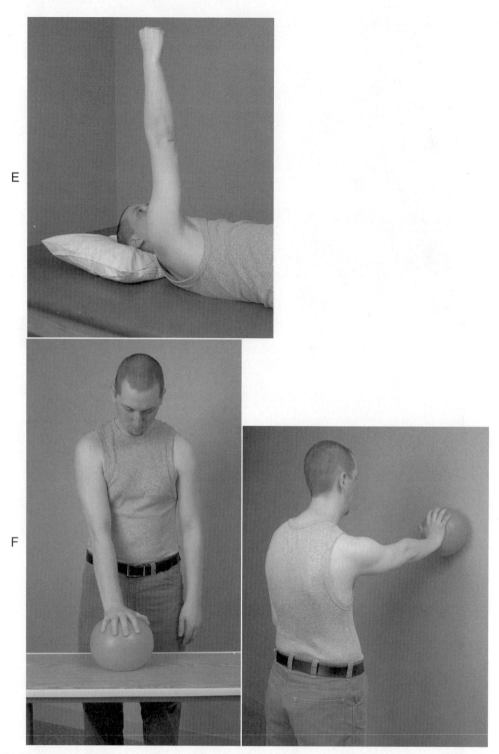

FIG. 24-3 Cont'd E, Supine serratus anterior punch without resistance. F, Shoulder protraction with a ball on a table; progress providing some resistance to wall.

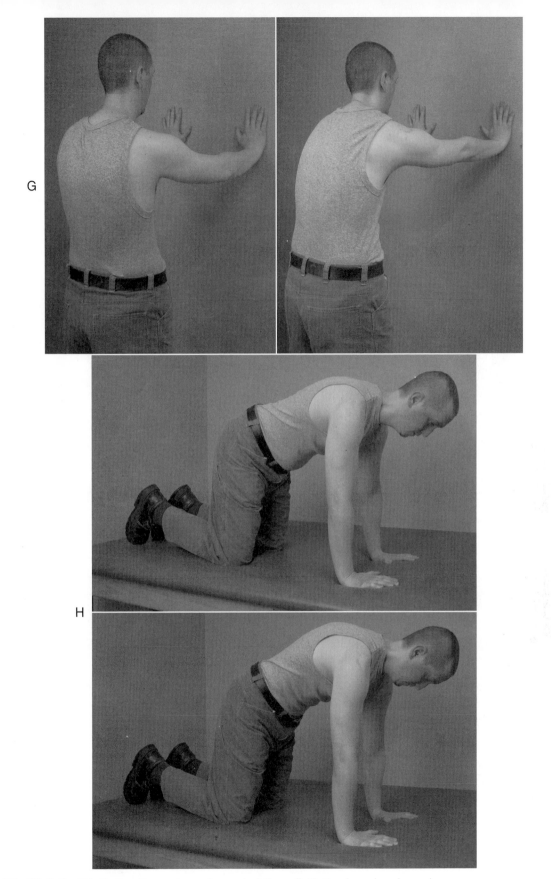

FIG. **24-3 Cont'd G,** Standing push-up plus against the wall. **H,** Quadruped push-up plus.

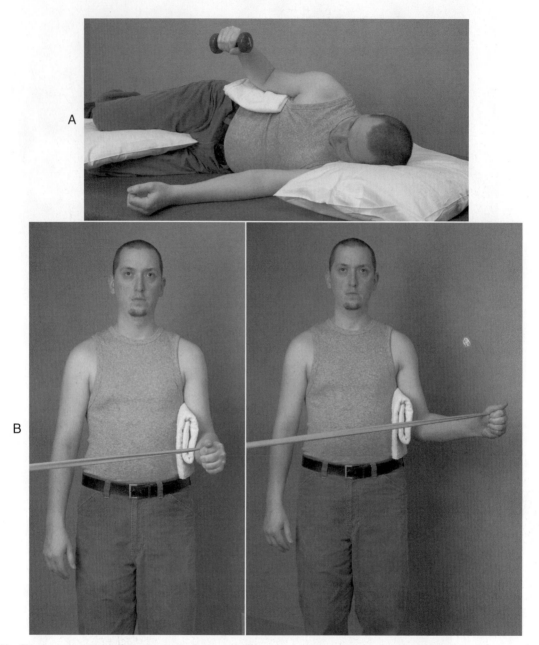

FIG. 24-4 An example of progression of rotator cuff exercises. **A,** Sidelying external rotation strengthening with a light weight. **B,** Standing external rotation strengthening exercises performed at the side with Theraband.

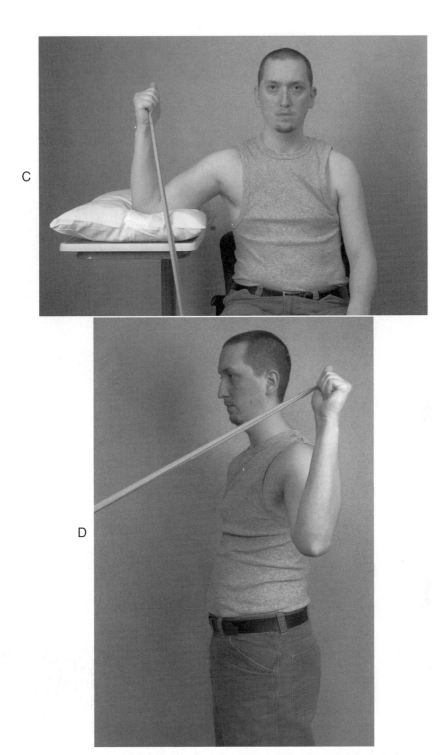

FIG. **24-4 Cont'd C,** Sitting external rotation with shoulder supported in abduction below 90 degrees using Theraband. **D,** Standing external rotation below 90 degrees abduction with Theraband.

(Continued)

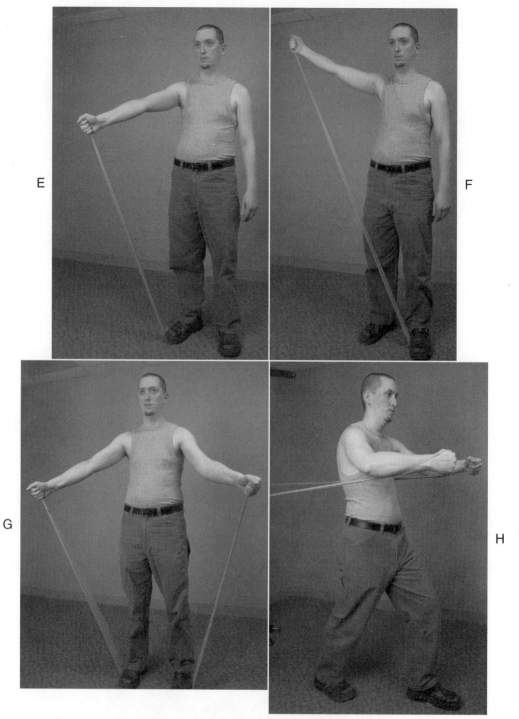

FIG. 24-4 Cont'd **E,** Standing scaption with external rotation using Theraband below 90 degrees. **F,** Standing horizontal abduction with external rotation above 90 degrees using Theraband. **G,** Standing bilateral scaption with external rotation using Theraband. **H,** Forward flexion with internal rotation followed by a step forward.

NONOPERATIVE COMPLICATIONS

I.   Continued pain
II. Calcification of tendons
III. Tendon rupture
IV. Development of adhesive capsulitis

POSTOPERATIVE INDICATIONS/PRECAUTIONS FOR THERAPY

I.   Indications
     A. Failure to respond to conservative treatment. The literature supports a trial of conservative treatment for approximately 6 to 12 months.
     B. Unresolved pain with decreased function
     C. Tendon calcification
II. Precautions
     A. Tendon rupture
     B. Repeat ossification
     C. Development of adhesive capsulitis

POSTOPERATIVE THERAPY (DECOMPRESSION)

I.   Day 1: Initiate cold application and high-voltage electrical stimulation for pain and edema management. The use of TENS, HVG, or interferential stimulation with cold is recommended in the patient's home program for control of postsurgical pain and inflammation.
II. Days 2 to 3: Add scapular and postural exercises, pendulum exercises (see Fig. 25-1 in Chapter 25), maintenance of PROM within pain tolerance.
III. Days 5 to 7: Progress to AAROM/AROM in gravity-eliminated planes. Follow nonsurgical progression of exercise sequencing.
IV. Days 7 to 14: Progress AAROM as tolerated to full pain-free ROM. Initiate submaximal isometric rotator cuff, scapulothoracic, and deltoid strengthening. Follow nonsurgical progression of exercise sequencing.
V.   Days 14 to 21: Progress strengthening according to conservative care, with emphasis on return to normal functioning.

POSTOPERATIVE COMPLICATIONS

I.   Infection
II. Potential rotator cuff tear
III. Unresolved pain
IV. Failure to regain adequate muscle functioning
V.   Adhesive capsulitis

EVALUATION TIMELINE

I.   Nonoperative
     A. Day 1
        1. Pain (e.g., pain questionnaire, palpation)

2. AROM and PROM (to pain tolerance), joint mobility
3. Posture
4. Special test (e.g., empty can test, Speed test, instability testing) only if the patient can be positioned for testing without pain
5. Upper quadrant screen as tolerated by the patient (e.g., cervical spine ROM, neurovascular status)
6. Strength testing as tolerated (e.g., isometrics at side)
7. ADLs (e.g., questionnaire)

II. Operative (consult physician as to surgery performed)
   A. Week 1: PROM within the precautions of surgical procedure and pain tolerance
   B. Week 2: AAROM, AROM
   C. Week 3: Isometric strength testing

OUTCOMES

Rahme and colleagues[26] studied pain in 42 patients who underwent either open anterior acromioplasty with postoperative physiotherapy or physiotherapy alone. The criterion for a successful outcome was a 50% reduction of the initial pain score using the visual analog scale. Comparisons of the two groups at 1 year indicated a significantly higher success rate in the combined surgery and therapy group (76%) compared with the physiotherapy group alone (19%).

In a study by Winters and associates,[27] 172 patients were placed into two diagnostic groups: a shoulder girdle group and a synovial group. In the shoulder girdle group, the duration of pain complaints was significantly shorter after manipulation compared with "classic physiotherapy." In the synovial group, three different interventions were compared: "classic physiotherapy," manipulation, and corticosteroid injections. All interventions resulted in significantly less pain, but pain duration was significantly shorter among those patients treated with corticosteroid injections.

Anderson and co-workers[28] reported no significant difference after arthroscopic subacromial decompression in their patients who underwent supervised physiotherapy compared with self-training exercises.

Bang and Deyle[2] compared supervised physical therapy exercises with manual therapy (i.e., passive accessory or passive physiological joint mobilization Maitland grades I through V) with supervised physical therapy alone. Both groups significantly improved their visual analog pain scale scores. However, the manual therapy group demonstrated a 70% decrease in pain, compared with 35% for the exercise group.

Brox and associates[4,5] reported that supervised therapy was as effective as surgical subacromial decompression combined with physiotherapy in the treatment of patients diagnosed with stage 2 primary shoulder impingement. They also reported that the difference between the two groups was not significant after 30 months of follow-up.

Conroy and Hayes[8] studied the impact of "comprehensive" therapy with or without joint mobilizations on function, pain, and ROM. The only significant difference found between the two treatment groups was in the area of pain, with the joint mobilization group doing significantly better. Both groups improved in ROM and function without significant differences.

REFERENCES

1. Tytherleigh-Strong G, Hrahara A, Miniaci A: Rotator cuff disease. Curr Opin Rheumatol 13:135, 2001
2. Bang MD, Deyle GD: Comparison of supervised exercise with and without manual physical therapy for patients with shoulder impingement syndrome. J Orthop Sports Phys Ther 30:126, 2000
3. Brewster C, Moynes Schwab DR: Rehabilitation of the shoulder following rotator cuff injury. J Orthop Sports Phys Ther 18:422, 1993
4. Brox JI, Gjengedal E, Uppheim G, et al.: Arthroscopic surgery versus supervised exercises in patients with rotator cuff disease (stage II impingement syndrome): a prospective, randomized, controlled study in 125 patients with a $2^1/_2$ year follow up. J Shoulder Elbow Surg 8:102, 1999
5. Brox JI, Staff PH, Ljunggren AE, et al.: Arthroscopic surgery compared with supervised exercises in patients with rotator cuff disease (stage II impingement syndrome). BMJ 307:899, 1993
6. Burke WS, Vangsness CT, Powers CM: Strengthening the supraspinatus. Clin Orthop 402:292, 2002
7. Cohen RB, Williams GR: Impingement syndrome and rotator cuff disease as repetitive motion disorders. Clin Orthop 351:95, 1998
8. Conroy DE, Hayes KW: The effect of joint mobilization as a component of comprehensive treatment for primary shoulder impingement. J Orthop Sports Phys Ther 28:3, 1998
9. Jobe CM: Superior glenoid impingement. Orthop Clin North Am 28:137, 1997
10. Kamkar A, Irrgang JJ, Whitney SL: Nonoperative management of secondary shoulder impingement syndrome. J Orthop Sports Phys Ther 17:212, 1993
11. Krabak BJ, Sugar R, McFarland EG: Practical nonoperative management of rotator cuff injuries. Clin J Sport Med 13:102, 2003
12. Readdy AS, Mohr KJ, Pink MM, et al.: Electromyographic analysis of the deltoid and rotator cuff muscles in persons with subacromial impingement. J Shoulder Elbow Surg 9:519, 2000
13. Roe C, et al.: Muscle activation after supervised exercises in patients with rotator tendinosis. Arch Phys Med Rehab 81:67, 2000
14. Rubin BD, Kibler WB: Fundamental principles of shoulder rehabilitation: conservative to post operative management. Arthroscopy 18:29, 2002
15. Ruotolo C, Nottage WM: Surgical and nonsurgical management of rotator cuff tears. Arthroscopy 18:527, 2002
16. Schmitt L, Synder-Mackler L: Role of scapular stabilizers in etiology and treatment of impingement syndrome. J Orthop Sports Phys Ther 29:31, 1999
17. Struhl S: Anterior internal impingement and arthroscopic observation. Arthroscopy, January 2002
18. Wilk KE, Arrigo C: Current concepts in the rehabilitation of the athletic shoulder. J Orthop Sports Phys Ther 18:365, 1993
19. Uhl TL, Carver TJ, Mattacola CG, et al.: Shoulder musculature activation during upper extremity weight-bearing exercise. J Orthop Sports Phys Ther 33:109, 2003
20. Tempelheh S, Rupp S, Seil R: Age-related prevalence of rotator cuff tears in asymptomatic shoulders. J Shoulder Elbow Surg 8:296, 1999
21. Matsen FA, Arntz CT: Subacromial impingements. In Rockwood CD, Matsen FA (eds): The Shoulder. WB Saunders, Philadelphia, 1990
22. Neer CS: Impingement lesions. Clin Orthop 173:17, 1983
23. Bigliani LU, Morrison DS, April EW: The morphology of the acromion and its relationship to the rotator cuff tears. Orthop Trans 10:228, 1986
24. Warner JJ, Micheli LJ, Arslanian LE, et al.: Patterns of flexibility, laxity and strength in normal shoulders and shoulders with instability and impingement. Am J Sports Med 18:366, 1990
25. van der Heijden GJ, van der Windt DA, de Winter AF: Physiotherapy for patients with soft tissue disorder: a systematic review of randomized clinical trials. BMJ 315:25-30, 1997
26. Rahme H, Solem-Bertoft E, Westerberg CE, et al.: The subacromial impingement syndrome: a study of results of treatment with special emphasis on predictive factors and pain-generating mechanisms. Scand J Rehabil Med 30:253-262, 1998
27. Winters JC, Sobel JS, Groenier KH, et al.: Comparison of physiotherapy, manipulation, and corticosteroid injection for treating shoulder complaints in general practice: randomized, single blind study. BMJ 314:1320, 1997

28. Anderson NH, Sojbjerg JO, Johannsen HV, et al.: Self training versus physiotherapist-supervised rehabilitation of the shoulder in patients treated with arthroscopic subacromial decompression: a clinical randomized study. J Shoulder Elbow Surg 8:99, 1999

SUGGESTED READINGS

Brotzman SB, Wilk KE: Clinical Orthopaedic Rehabilitation. 2nd Ed. Mosby, St. Louis, 2003

Calis M, Akgun K, Birtane M, et al.: Diagnostic values of clinical diagnostic tests in subacromial impingement syndrome. Ann Rheum Dis 59:L44, 2000

Decker MJ, Tokish JM, Ellis HB, et al.: Subscapularis muscle activity during selected rehabilitation exercise. Am J Sports Med 31:126, 2003

Desmeules F, Cote C, Fremont P: Therapeutic exercise and orthopedic manual therapy for impingement syndrome: a systematic review. Clin J Sport Med 13:176, 2003

Donatelli R, et al.: Physical Therapy of the Shoulder. 4th Ed. Churchill Livingstone, St. Louis, 2004

Ebenbichler GR, Erdogmus CB, Resch KL, et al.: Ultrasound therapy for calcific tendonitis of the shoulder. N Engl J Med 340:1533, 1999

Hatakeyama Y, Itoi E, Pradhan RL, et al.: Effect of arm elevation and rotation on the strain in the repaired rotator cuff tendon: a cadaveric study. Am J Sports Med 29:788, 2001

Moncrief SA, Lau JD, Gale JR, et al.: Effect of rotator cuff exercise on humeral rotation torque in healthy individuals. J Strength Cond Res 16:262, 2002

Near CS: Anterior acromioplasty for the chronic impingement syndrome of the shoulder. J Bone Joint Surg Am 54:41, 1972

Philadelphia Panel: Philadelphia Panel evidence-based clinical practice guidelines on selected rehabilitation interventions for shoulder pain. Phys Ther 81:1719-1730, 2001

Rockwood CA, Matsen III FA: The Shoulder. 2nd Ed. Saunders, Philadelphia, 1998

Ryu RK, Dunbar WH 5th, Kuhn JE, et al.: Comprehensive evaluation and treatment of the shoulder in the throwing athlete. Arthroscopy 18:70-89, 2002

Takeda Y, Kashiwaguchi S, Endo K, et al.: The most effective exercise for strengthening the supraspinatus muscle. Am J Sports Med 30:374, 2002

Wilk KE, Arrigo CA, Andrews JR: Closed and open kinetic chain exercise for the upper extremity. J Sport Rehabil 5:88-102, 1996

Zimmerman JM, et al.: Rehabilitation and nonoperative treatment. In Warren RF, Craig EV, Altchek DW (eds): The Unstable Shoulder. Lippincott-Raven, Philadelphia, 1999

Rotator Cuff Repairs 25

Mary Schuler Murphy

The rotator cuff is important for both mobility and stability of the gleno-humeral joint, as well as nourishment of the articular surface of the gleno-humeral joint. Studies have suggested that the rotator cuff provides 45% of the power in shoulder abduction and at least 90% of the power in external rotation.[1] The rotator cuff acts as a dynamic stabilizer, allowing the powerful deltoid to perform as the primary mover of the glenohumeral joint. In addition to the rotator cuff, scapulothoracic stability and mobility are essential for normal shoulder movement. A major goal of shoulder reconstruction is to preserve or restore the balance between the rotator cuff and the deltoid and scapulothoracic musculature. According to Neer,[2] the most common etiological cause of rotator cuff tears is impingement (approximately 95%, primarily in those older than 40 years of age). Normal aging of rotator cuff tendons, with decreased cellularity and vascularity, combined with repetitive microtrauma, predisposes the tendons to progressive deterioration and possible acute rupture.[3] According to Neer,[2] the most common cause of impingement is decreased space beneath the anterior acromion and acromioclavicular joint. An anterior acromioplasty is frequently performed in conjunction with the rotator cuff repair to alleviate this problem. In the presence of a massive rotator cuff tear, the coracoacromial arch acts as a passive stabilizer against humeral head anterior and superior subluxation. Gartsman and Burkhart[4,5] advocated that acromioplasty not be performed with rotator cuff tears that are not fully repairable.

The most common cause of rotator cuff injury in the active young adult is instability with excessive humeral head migration into the subacromial space.[6] Strengthening of the muscle forces acts to offset this excessive humeral head elevation.[7] The role of subtle anterior shoulder instability in internal impingement is caused by problems with the balance of the dynamic and static stabilizers and mobilizers of the shoulder.[3] Not all rotator cuff tears are symptomatic. Tempelheh and colleagues[8] studied 411 asymptomatic shoulders using magnetic resonance imaging; 23.4% of the participants were found to have a full-thickness rotator cuff tear. As indicated earlier, the causes of shoulder impingement vary, necessitating different approaches to the medical management. Not all rotator cuff tears require surgery. Ruotolo and Nottage[9] reported that approximately 50% of patients with rotator cuff tears improve with nonoperative treatment. Although pain is the primary reason for surgery, incapacitating weakness in large cuff deficits may also be an indication. Faryniarz and Craig[10] warned that some tears, in active patients, may progress to larger tears. Furthermore, those patients who choose nonoperative management should be monitored for decreasing strength. Conservative management of rotator cuff tears may follow the same type of program as described in Chapter 24 for rotator cuff tendonitis.

To understand the advancements made in the treatment of rotator cuff repairs, the therapist must appreciate the significant advances made in the recognition of the various causes of impingement, the recognition of different tear patterns with improved surgical repair techniques, and the use of arthroscopic evaluation and repair of the rotator cuff. Arthroscopic evaluation has provided the surgeon with the ability to explore and find lesions sometimes not identified with an open approach, with minimal disruption to the deltoid. According to Lo and Burkhart,[11] and others, arthroscopic rotator cuff repairs appear to be as good if not better than open repairs. The advantages of arthroscopic surgery include relative deltoid preservation, the identification and repair of intraarticular lesions, release of rotator cuff adhesions, and mobilization of the retracted rotator cuff tendons. According to Yamaguchi and colleagues,[12] as arthroscopic techniques have progressed to include large tear repairs, results are equal to or better than with open repair techniques. They also reported on the ability to repair massive rotator cuff tears arthroscopically using side-to-side repairs, margin convergence, and partial repairs. Burkhart[5] reported the importance of tear pattern type recognition. He maintained that most rotator cuff tears can be classified into crescent-shaped tears and U-shaped tears. Crescent-shaped tears do not retract far and may be directly repaired to bone. U-shaped tears usually extend much further medially, and side-to-side sutures of the tear are placed before attachment of tendon to bone.

Rehabilitation of the rotator cuff requires a basic understanding of the surgical procedure and the physician's expectation of outcome. The progression of the rehabilitation program depends on the patient's age, compliance, tissue quality, and type of tear, as well as the type of surgery performed. Regardless of the type of repair performed, tendon healing requires time, during which protection of the repair must be carefully monitored to prevent damage to the repaired tendon or other structures. Only the surgeon knows the integrity of the repair, so close communication with the surgeon is imperative to successful rehabilitation.

DEFINITION

Rotator cuff repair is the surgical repair of a partial or complete rupture of one or several of the tendons that comprise the rotator cuff (supraspinatus, infraspinatus, teres minor, and subscapularis).

Anterior acromioplasty is the surgical decompression of the rotator cuff through enlargement of the supraspinatus outlet by beveling of the anterior edge and the undersurface of the anterior third of the acromion and acromioclavicular joint.

I.   Neer's cuff tear terminology[2]
      A. Partial tear: incomplete tear that does not extend through
         the complete tendon thickness
      B. Complete tear: extends through the complete thickness of
         the tendon
      C. Massive tear: tear of more than one rotator cuff tendon
      D. Degenerative tear: nutritional or metabolic factors could be
         indicated as well as wear or injury
      E. Traumatic tear: implies an injury tearing a healthy tendon
      F. Acute extension: implies an injury suddenly enlarging an
         impingement tear
II.   Esch's categories of rotator cuff tears (according to size)[13]
      A. Small: less than 1 cm
      B. Moderate: 1 to 3 cm
      C. Large: 3 to 5 cm
      D. Massive: greater than 5 cm

Mini-open repair or **arthroscopic-assisted open rotator cuff repair** is
an arthroscopic subacromial decompression followed by an open repair
through a deltoid splitting procedure, or the arthroscope may also be used
to release adhesions and place tagging sutures with a mini-open approach
to obtain tendon-to-bone fixation. A **complete arthroscopic repair** is all of
the above-described procedures performed through the arthroscope.

Cuff tear arthropathy is a degeneration of the glenohumeral joint secondary to the effect of massive rotator cuff tears over time.

Margin convergence is the mechanical advantage that occurs with side-
to-side closure of large cuff tears, reducing strain on the repair to bone.

Crescent-shaped tears typically pull away from bone but do not retract
and are therefore repaired directly to bone with minimal tension.

U-shaped tears require side-to-side sutures that converge the free
margin of the cuff toward the bone, followed by repair to the bone with
suture anchors.

SURGICAL PURPOSE

Surgery is performed for rotator cuff tears to restore the continuity of the
tendon and relieve the subacromial impingement. This is often difficult to
achieve, and predictability of success depends on the quality of the tendon
substance, the length of time since the injury occurred, and the underlying
pathology that brought on the disruption. Successful rehabilitation of these
injuries requires full knowledge of these factors.

TREATMENT GOALS

I.   Repair of incomplete or small tears (less than 1 cm) and open and
      major tear repairs (1 to 5 cm)
      A. Short-term goals
         1. Prevent the formation of adhesions while protecting the
            repair.
         2. Maintain passive range of motion (PROM) within limits set
            by the physician.
         3. Patient education (i.e., precautions to allow for healing)

    4. Maintain full active range of motion (AROM) and strength in elbow, forearm, wrist, and hand of involved extremity.
  B. Long-term goals
    1. Restore full PROM.
    2. Restore pain-free AROM and return to functional active abduction and external rotation.
    3. Return to preinjury activity status.
II.   Massive repairs (repairs greater than 5 cm) with significant loss of deltoid function, rotator cuff function, or bone
  A. Long-term goals
    1. Restore pain-free limited but functional AROM, with emphasis on use of the extremity at the side.
    2. Return to as near previous levels of functioning as possible.
    3. Independent home exercise program stressing stability and the avoidance of excessive mobility.

POSTOPERATIVE INDICATIONS/PRECAUTIONS FOR THERAPY

I.   Indications
  A. A rehabilitation program is indicated for all types of repairs if the surgeon indicates that rotator cuff quality and glenohumeral joint stability are adequate.
II. Precautions
  A. Communication with the surgeon is of paramount importance. The therapist must know the type and quality of the repair. Severe loss of deltoid muscle function, rotator cuff, or bone requires a limited goal program with lesser ROM and increased stability.

POSTOPERATIVE THERAPY

I.   Incomplete or small tear repairs (less than 1 cm)
  A. Days 1 to 3
    1. Pain management including high-voltage galvanic stimulation (HVG) for pain and edema control. May use a sling for comfort for approximately 1 week. When sleeping, protect with sling, rest shoulder in approximately 45 degrees scaption on a pillow. Either transcutaneous electrical nerve stimulation (TENS), HVG, or an interferential unit combined with cold application for control of pain and swelling is recommended as part of the patient's home program.
    2. Initiate pendulum exercises (Fig. 25-1), to be performed four to six times a day for approximately 5 minutes each session.
    3. Initiate active scapulothoracic stabilization exercises, to be performed four to six times a day for 5 minutes each session (see Fig. 24-3, A in Chapter 24).
    4. Gentle AROM and PROM at the elbow and wrist
  B. Day 3 to 3 weeks
    1. Pain-free PROM of shoulder, including forward elevation in the plane of the scapula and internal and external rotation in the scapular plane. At the end of the third week, PROM should be within functional limits (approximately 150 degrees flexion/scaption, 60 degrees external rotation).

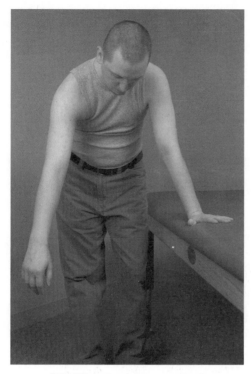

FIG. **25-1** Pendulum exercises.

    2. Progress to AAROM of the shoulder in supine in
       gravity-eliminated planes (e.g., place-hold in 90 degrees
       flexion with assistance) (Fig. 25-2). Initiate external AAROM
       rotation at the side and progress in the plane of the scapula.
    3. Progress to pain-free isometric scapulothoracic stabilization
       strengthening exercise (e.g., resist patient's protracted shoulder
       positioned in 90 degrees flexion in supine) (Fig. 25-3), and
       pain-free submaximal rotator cuff and deltoid isometric
       strengthening. Distal strengthening.

C. Weeks 3 to 6
    1. Supported AROM on tabletop, progressing to unsupported
       AROM (Fig. 25-4, *A* and *B*). Continue with AROM in supine,
       increasing the movement out of the gravity-eliminated plane
       into gravity-challenged planes. For example, the patient starts
       moving out of the place-hold position of 90 degrees with
       small, controlled circles, gradually increasing the size of the
       circle with gains in active control (Fig. 25-5). At the end of
       week 6 to 8, AROM should be within normal limits.
    2. Initiate light, gentle, active internal rotation at 4 to 5 weeks.
    3. Continue to progress shoulder PROM (should be within
       normal limits by week 4 to 6).

D. Weeks 6 to 10
    1. Initiate light isotonic strengthening to shoulder with
       Theraband exercises to be performed at the side or below
       90 degrees (see Fig. 24-4, *A* and *B* in Chapter 24).

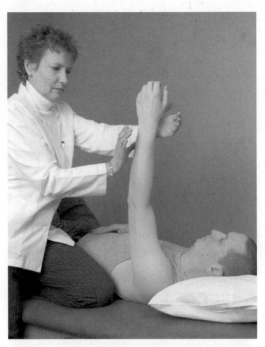

FIG. **25-2** Supine active-assisted place-hold exercise in 90 degrees flexion.

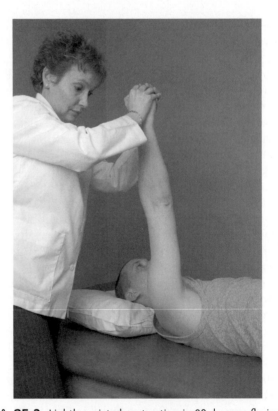

FIG. **25-3** Lightly resisted protraction in 90 degrees flexion.

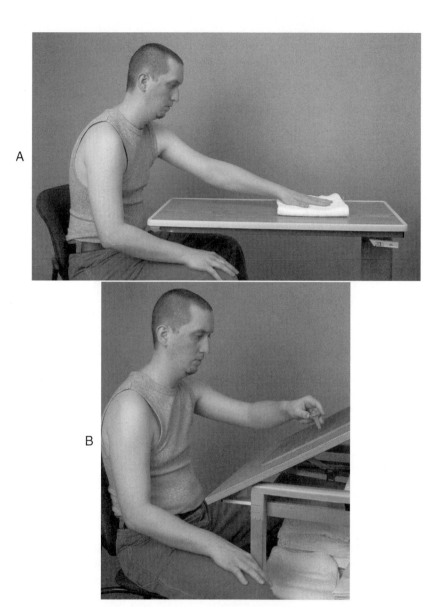

FIG. **25-4** **A,** Supported active range of motion (AROM) on tabletop. **B,** Unsupported AROM.

      2. Continue to progress shoulder strengthening to include resistive exercises in all planes. Gradually work into proprioceptive neuromuscular facilitation (PNF) patterns with Theraband (see Fig. 24-4, *C* through *H* in Chapter 24).

      3. Terminal stretching for full ROM

  II. Open, mini-open with arthroscopic assist, or arthroscopic rotator cuff repair for major tear repairs (1 to 5 cm) and massive tear repairs (greater than 5 cm in healthy tissue with good repair)

    A. Days 1 to 10

      1. Patient education in pain management, positioning of the extremity during sleep and at rest (in approximately 45 degrees scaption with a pillow placed between the sling

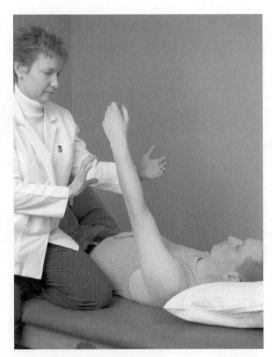

FIG. **25-5** Supine controlled active and active-assisted place-hold exercise with the therapist setting parameters with increasing gravity-resisted planes.

and trunk), and instructions in a home exercise program of pendulum exercises

2. Cold compression and HVG for pain and edema management. The use of TENS, HVG, or an interferential unit with cold is recommended as part of the patient's home program for the control of postsurgical pain and inflammation.

3. Immobilization in a sling with removal for hygiene and exercises. Massive tear repairs, may only be allowed to remove the sling or brace for exercise for the first month.

4. Initiate pendulum exercises on days 3 to 7.

5. Gentle shoulder PROM exercises performed to patient's pain tolerance and restricted to 160 degrees elevation in the plane of the scapula and 60 degrees external rotation in approximately 30 degrees scaption are initiated on days 3 to 7. Massive tear repairs are limited to 100 degrees elevation in the scapular plane and 35 degrees external rotation in approximately 30 degrees scaption.

6. Initiate scapular stabilization exercises with emphasis on serratus anterior and lower trapezius muscle function (see Fig. 24-3, *A* and *F* in Chapter 24).

7. Distal AROM and grasp strengthening, including isometric submaximal biceps strengthening.

8. Instructions in one-handed activities of daily living (ADLs) and the use of adaptive equipment as needed.

B. Day 10 to 4 weeks

1. Continue with exercises described previously.

2. Gradually wean from sling. Wait 4 weeks for major and massive tear repairs.
3. Full PROM in flexion, scaption, and external rotation to tolerance. Wait 4 to 6 weeks for major and massive tear repairs.
4. Initiate AAROM in scapular plane in supine (e.g., practice place-hold, placing the shoulder in a gravity-eliminated position while the therapist directs and supports the shoulder through very controlled patterns of movement) (see Fig. 25-5). Also initiate tabletop AAROM that the patient can perform as part of a home exercise program (e.g., the patient uses uninvolved side to assist involved side in forward flexion with a rolling pin or towel) (Fig. 25-6).
5. Submaximal isometric shoulder exercises to be progressed at the side and advanced to positions throughout the pain-free range (Fig. 25-7, *A* and *B*)
6. Progress scapular stabilization exercises (see Fig. 24-3, *E* and *F* in Chapter 24).

C. Weeks 4 to 6 (wait 6 to 8 weeks for major and massive tear repairs)
1. Continue with the exercises previously described.
2. Initiate gentle passive shoulder internal rotation.

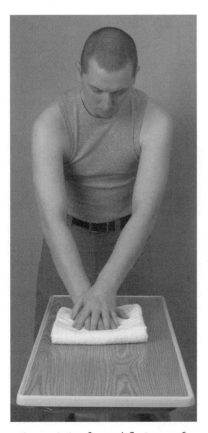

FIG. **25-6** Standing active assistive forward flexion performed using a towel on tabletop.

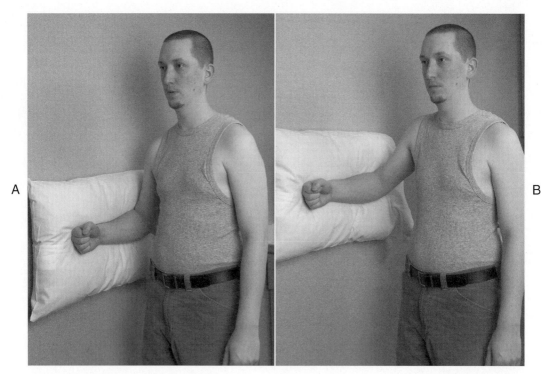

FIG. **25-7** Submaximal isometric shoulder exercises performed at the side; may be advanced to positions away from the side. **A,** Abduction at side. **B,** At 45 degrees.

3. Shoulder AROM. Progress from gravity-eliminated positions in supine with the patient now moving gradually away from 90 degrees shoulder flexion, controlling the arm in wider circles and in short arcs of motion returning to the gravity-eliminated position (see Fig. 25-5). Also, progress to supported tabletop activities, including use of the involved side only, and eventually to nonsupported tabletop activities (e.g., inclined pegboard) (see Fig. 25-4).

4. Initiate light functional ADLs below 90 degrees.

D. Weeks 6 to 8 (wait 3 to 6 months for major and massive tear repairs)

1. Light shoulder isotonic resistive exercises (e.g., light Theraband, rubber tubing, 1 lb weight). Progress from positioning near side to positions throughout the pain-free range (see Fig. 24-4, *A* to *H* in Chapter 24).

2. Progress scapular strengthening exercises (e.g., rowing, push-up plus against wall) (see Fig. 24-3, *A* to *H* in Chapter 24).

3. Stretch tight structures.

E. Weeks 8 to 10

1. Continue to increase isotonic resistive exercises if started at 6 to 8 weeks.

2. Initiate normal use in all light ADLs. Wait 10 to 12 weeks for major and massive tear repairs. It may take 4 to 6 months to return to use in most functional activities and up to 6 to 8 months to return to use in strenuous work or sports activities.

III.   Massive tear limited goal exercise program: This exercise program avoids early overhead AROM exercises and exercises extending into full rotation. The program stresses use of the arm at the side and stability.
  A. Day 2 to 1 month
    1. Proximal immobilization with a sling; an abduction pillow or brace may be used for the first 4 to 8 weeks for protection of the repair.
    2. Passive forward flexion performed on a daily basis; may be limited to 100 degrees depending on the repair and treatment goals
    3. Distal strengthening
    4. Instructions in one-handed ADLs and the use of adaptive equipment as needed.
  B. Months 1 to 3
    1. Continued passive elevation; initiate passive external rotation with the arm at the side (this may be limited to 20 degrees depending on the repair and treatment goals).
    2. Pendulum exercises
    3. Use of the sling between exercise sessions
    4. AAROM, progress to AROM (overhead AROM is delayed until 5½ to 6 months).
  C. Months 2 to 3: Discontinue sling.
  D. Months 3 to 4: submaximal isometric shoulder strengthening
  E. Month 5: progressive resistive exercises
  F. Month 6: activities as tolerated

POSTOPERATIVE COMPLICATIONS

I.   Infection
II. Failed rotator cuff repair with residual impingement
III. Decreased AROM/deltoid weakness
IV. Adhesive capsulitis
V.   Postoperative hematoma
VI. Severe pain

EVALUATION TIMELINE

I.   Incomplete and major tear repairs
  A. Day 3: pain (pain analog scale), posture, distal AROM and grip strength, and ADLs
  B. Day 3 to 3 weeks: PROM of shoulder in scaption, flexion, and external rotation. Wait 4 weeks for passive internal rotation.
  C. Week 6: isometric shoulder strength testing
II. Massive tear repairs
  A. Day 3 to 1 month: pain (pain analog scale), distal ROM and strength, and ADL skills
  B. 1 to 3 months: passive shoulder elevation to 100 degrees and external rotation to 20 degrees
  C. 4 months: isometric shoulder strength testing

OUTCOMES

In a study by Rokito and colleagues,[14] 30 patients (17 with a large tear and 13 with a massive tear) underwent operative rotator cuff repair including an open procedure, anterior-inferior acromioplasty, and partial bursectomy. They were evaluated by isokinetic strength testing and the University of California Los Angeles (UCLA) shoulder score before and after surgery. More than 1 year was needed for strength recovery of a large and massive rotator cuff tear, and the strength achieved was not equal to that of the unaffected shoulder. According to the UCLA shoulder score, improvement in the areas of function, ROM, and pain was significant, with 100% patient satisfaction rating.

In a study by Burkhart and co-workers[15] of 59 shoulders repaired arthroscopically, 95% of the patients had good to excellent results using a modified UCLA scoring system. The authors concluded that results were not dependent on tear size. All patients were able to return to overhead function in an average of 4 months.

A study of 108 patients with massive rotator cuff tears by Vad and associates[16] included 40 patients treated conservatively: 32 who underwent arthroscopic debridement and 36 who underwent primary repair. The authors reported that poor outcomes may be related to the presence of three or more negative prognostic factors. These factors include the presence of glenohumeral arthritis, decreased PROM, superior migration of the humeral head, presence of atrophy, and external rotation and abduction strength less than 3.

Ruotolo and Nottage's[17] review of publications comparing outcome difference for operative versus nonoperative treatment of rotator cuff tears found satisfactory relief of pain in 50% of patients but no improvement in strength at follow-up in nonoperative patients. With operative repair, 85% of patients had a high rate of pain relief with a better return of strength.

Watson and Sonnabend's[18] outcome study included 667 open rotator cuff repairs; patient self-assessment of satisfaction was very high (87.5%).

Hata and associates[19] compared 36 patients subjected to conventional open rotator cuff repair and 22 patients who underwent a mini-open repair; there was no significant difference in UCLA shoulder scores between the two groups at 1 year after repair. The mini-open repair group did significantly better at the 3-month and 6-month assessments, with an earlier return to activities.

Fealy and co-workers[20] reported excellent results with surgical treatment of 75 rotator cuff tears (30 large, 35 moderate, and 10 small) using a mini-open rotator cuff repair and a two-row fixation technique. Patient satisfaction based on primary level of function was 92.6%.

Grondel and colleagues[21] performed retrospective study of 97 rotator cuff tears in 92 patients age 62 years and older. Seven tears were treated arthroscopically, and 85 tears with the mini-open technique. Results based on the UCLA shoulder scoring system were 54% excellent, 33% good, 8% fair, and 5% poor.

REFERENCES

1. Matsen FA, Arntz CT: Rotator cuff tendon failure. In Rockwood CA, Matsen FAL: The Shoulder. Vol. 11. WB Saunders, Philadelphia, 1990, p. 647

2. Neer CS: Cuff tears, biceps lesions and impingement. In Neer CS: Shoulder Rehabilitation. WB Saunders, Philadelphia, 1993, p. 41

3. Breazeale NM, Craig EV: Partial-thickness rotator cuff tears: pathogenesis and treatment. Orthop Clin North Am 28:145, 1997

4. Gartsman GM: Arthroscopic rotator cuff repair. Clin Orthop 390:95, 2001

5. Burkhart SS: Arthroscopic treatment of rotator cuff tears. Clin Orthop 390:107, 2001

6. Brewster C, Moynes Schwab DR: Rehabilitation of the shoulder following rotator cuff injury or surgery. J Sports Phys Ther 18:422, 1993

7. Burke WS, Vangsness CT, Powers CM: Strengthening the supraspinatus: a clinical and biomechanical review. Clin Orthop 402:292, 2002

8. Tempelheh S, Rupp S, Seil R: Age-related prevalence of rotator cuff tears in asymptomatic shoulders. J Shoulder Elbow Surg 8:296, 1999

9. Ruotolo C, Nottage WM: Current concepts: surgical and nonsurgical management of rotator cuff tears. Arthroscopy 18:527, 2002

10. Faryniarz DA, Craig E: Repair technique and mobilization for repair of large cuff defects. Tech Shoulder Elbow Surg 3:124, 2002

11. Lo IK, Burkhart SS: Current concepts in arthroscopic rotator cuff repair. Am J Sports Med 31:308, 2003

12. Yamaguchi K, Levine WN, Marra G, et al.: Transitioning to arthroscopic rotator cuff repair: the pros and cons. Instr Course Lect 52:81, 2003

13. Esch JC: Arthroscopic subacromial decompression and postoperative management. Orthop Clin North Am 24:161, 1993

14. Rokito AS, Cuomo, Gallagher MA, et al.: Long-term functional outcome of repair of large and massive chronic tears of the rotator cuff. J Bone Joint Surg Am 81:991, 1999

15. Burkhart SS, Danaceau SM, Pearce CE Jr: Arthroscopic rotator cuff repair: analysis by tear size and by repair technique—margin convergence versus direct tendon to bone repair. Arthroscopy 17:905, 2001

16. Vad VB, Warren RF, Altchek DW, et al.: Negative prognostic factors in managing massive rotator cuff tears. Clin J Sport Med 12:151-157, 2002

17. Ruotolo C, Nottage WM: Surgical and nonsurgical management of rotator cuff tears. Arthroscopy 18:527, 2002

18. Watson E, Sonnabend DH: Outcome of rotator cuff repair. J Shoulder Elbow Surg 11:201, 2002

19. Hata Y, Saitoh S, Murakami N, et al.: A less invasive surgery for rotator cuff tear: mini open repair. J Shoulder Elbow Surg 10:11, 2001

20. Fealy S, Kingham TP, Altchek DW: Mini-open rotator cuff repair using a two-row fixation technique: outcomes analysis in patients with small, moderate and large rotator cuff tears. Arthroscopy 18:665-670, 2002

21. Grondel RJ, Savoie FH 3rd, Field LD: Rotator cuff repairs in patients 62 years of age or older. J Shoulder Elbow Surg 10:97, 2001

SUGGESTED READINGS

Andrews JR, Harrelson GL: Physical Rehabilitation of the Injured Athlete. WB Saunders, Philadelphia, 1991

Brontzman SB: Clinical Orthopaedic Rehabilitation. Mosby–Year Book, St. Louis, 1996

Burkhart SL, Post WR: A functionally based neuromechanical approach to shoulder rehabilitation. In Hunter JM, Mackin EJ, Callahan AD (eds): Rehabilitation of the Hand: Surgery and Therapy. 4th Ed. Vol. II. Mosby, St. Louis, 1995, p. 1655

Delee C, Drez D: Orthopaedic Sports Medicine: Principles and Practice. Vol. 1. WB Saunders, Philadelphia, 1994

Donatelli RA: Physical Therapy of the Shoulder. 4th Ed. Churchill Livingstone, New York, 2004

Fealy S, Kingham TP, Altchek DW: Mini-open rotator cuff repair using a two-row fixation technique: outcomes analysis in patients with small, moderate, and large rotator cuff tears. Arthroscopy 18:665, 2002

Fenlin JM Jr, Chase JM, Rushton SA, et al.: Tuberoplasty: creation of an acromiohumeral articulation—a treatment option for massive, irreparable rotator cuff tears. J Shoulder Elbow Surg 11:136, 2002

Frieman BG, Albert TJ, Fenlin JM: Rotator cuff disease: a review of diagnosis, pathophysiology and current trends in treatment. Arch Phys Med Rehabil 75:604, 1994

Gartsman GM: Arthroscopic acromioplasty for lesions of the rotator cuff. J Bone Joint Surg Am 72:169, 1990

Goss TP: Rotator cuff injuries. Orthop Rev 15:496, 1990

Jobe FW, Pink M: The athlete's shoulder. J Hand Ther 7:107, 1994

Marks PH, Warner JJP, Irrgang JJ: Rotator cuff disorders of the shoulder. J Hand Ther 7:90, 1994

Miniaci A, Fowler PJ: Impingement in the athlete. Clin Sports Med 12:91, 1993

Nove-Josserand LB, et al.: Coraco-humeral space and rotator cuff tears [French]. Rev Chir Orthop Reparatrice Appar Mot 80:677, 1999 (cited in Lo and Burkhart[11])

Ryu RK, Dunbar WH 5th, Kuhn JE, et al.: Comprehensive evaluation and treatment of the shoulder in the throwing athlete. Arthroscopy 18(Suppl 2):70-89, 2002

Snyder SJ, Pachell AF, Pizza WD: Partial thickness rotator cuff tears: results of arthroscopic treatment. J Arthroscopic Relat Surg 7:1, 1991

Suenagan N, Minami A, Kaneda K: Postoperative subcoracoid impingement syndrome in patients with rotator cuff tear. J Shoulder Elbow Surg 9:275, 2000

Wirth MA, Basamania C, Rockwood CA Jr: Nonoperative management of full-thickness tears of the rotator cuff. Orthop Clin North Am 28:59, 1997

Glenohumeral Instability 26

Gary M. Lynch

The glenohumeral joint trades stability for mobility. The only bony attachment of the shoulder girdle to the trunk is through the sternoclavicular joint; otherwise, the shoulder girdle is stabilized to the thorax through soft tissue connections. The glenohumeral joint in itself is relatively shallow, with a large humeral head sitting in the relatively flat glenoid. Although the joint is concentric, only about 25% of the humeral head is covered[1] by the glenoid without the labrum. The soft tissue labrum does significantly increase this coverage. The primary stabilizer for the glenohumeral joint is positional and is activity dependent. However, the primary stabilizer in most functional activities is the anterior inferior glenohumeral ligament, which is supplemented by the glenoid labrum, the middle and superior glenohumeral ligaments, activity of the rotator cuff, negative pressure inside the glenohumeral joint,[2] and muscular support from a stabile scapular base.

Traditionally, there are two classifications of glenohumeral instabilities: (1) **traumatic unidirectional instability** (TUBS), which often necessitates operative intervention and repair of a bony or soft tissue Bankart lesion; and (2) **atraumatic multidirectional instability** (AMBRII), which is best handled with an intensive rehabilitative program. If surgery is required for AMBRII, then techniques are aimed at decreasing the capsular volume. These procedures include a medial or lateral capsular shift, which may also include closure of the rotator interval. Neer[3] also reported that there may be a third category, **acquired instability**, resulting from repetitive microtrauma related to sport or occupational demands leading to capsular stretching. Pappas and colleagues[4] labeled this a functional instability. It is developed when repetitive microtrauma through sport or activity contributes to capsular stretching.

TRAUMATIC INSTABILITY

Clinical Presentation

TUBS may be related to a single traumatic episode, or it may become episodic or repetitive in nature. The mechanism for this injury is a combination of excessive shoulder abduction, external rotation, and horizontal abduction. If the head of the humerus comes out of place anteriorly, it can shear off the labrum or even a piece of bone, resulting in a soft tissue or bony Bankart lesion. As the humeral head dislocates and the posterior head comes to rest on the anterior glenoid, the head can also sustain a compression fracture called a Hill-Sachs lesion. Passive stabilizers of the anterior capsule are often stretched at the time of dislocation, and in the middle-aged to older patient rotator cuff tears may also occur with anterior dislocation. The dislocation rates after initial dislocation are inversely proportional to age. In athletes and patients with high occupational demands who are younger than 20 years of age, there is an 80% to 90% chance of redislocation after an initial anterior inferior event. In patients age 20 to 40 years the percentage of redislocation is 60%, and in those older than 40 years of age it drops to 10%.[5] In older patients, the more common scenario is gradual development of some osteoarthritis and limited motion after dislocation.

Many surgical procedures have been used over the years to correct anterior instability or to prevent recurrent dislocation. Common early surgeries, such as the Magnuson Stack or the Putti-Platt procedure, significantly limited external rotation, which prevented redislocation but ultimately led to significant loss of external rotation and degenerative arthritic changes at the glenohumeral joint. More anatomically based surgeries are now used that reestablish the labrum and the capsular-labral connections without excessively limiting external rotation. The two most common of these procedures are the Bankart and the Matsen procedures. The Bankart procedure takes the subscapularis in a separate layer from the underlying capsule. The Matsen procedure takes the subscapularis and the capsule as a single layer, peeled medially, followed by repair of the glenoid labrum at the glenoid. Matsen and co-workers[6] have described both procedures in detail.

Surgical Purpose

To restore capsular and labral architecture to as normal a condition as possible, thereby restoring stability to the glenohumeral joint while maintaining normal range of motion (ROM).

Postoperative Rehabilitation Goals

I. Protective phase (0 to 3 weeks)
   A. Reduce soreness.
   B. Prevent stiffness of the distal articulations.
   C. Begin protective ROM.
   D. Begin to use the arm for light activities of daily living (ADLs).
II. Intermediate phase (3 to 6 weeks)
   A. Continue to gain shoulder ROM to near-full flexion and internal rotation.
   B. Promote good proximal control through scapular active movements.
   C. Prevent excessive scar adhesions along the incision site.
   D. Perform personal hygiene tasks and ADLs, within reason, without soreness.

III.   Strengthening phase (6 to 12 weeks)
    A. Full ROM of the shoulder complex.
    B. Increase strength of the shoulder complex.
    C. Increase control of the shoulder complex by introducing plyometric activities.
    D. Obtain manual muscle test scores of 4 to 4+/5 throughout the shoulder complex.

Postoperative Rehabilitation Treatments

  I.   Protective phase (0 to 3 weeks)
    A. While in the sling for 3 weeks, patient begins active motion of the elbow, forearm, wrist, and finger.
    B. Also while in the sling, the patient can begin active-assisted flexion of not greater than 90 degrees, abduction to 60 degrees, and external rotation not beyond neutral.
    C. On or about 2 weeks after surgery, the patient may begin to take off the sling in the home to perform some ADLs and personal hygiene tasks. The patient is to continue to wear the sling in public.
    D. At the discretion of the surgeon, the patient may be instructed on submaximal isometric contractions for abduction and external rotation.
    E. Instruction is given on active scapular and ROM exercises (e.g., circles with emphasis on scapular adduction and depression). This can be done in sitting and sidelying positions during the first week.
 II.   Intermediate phase (3 to 6 weeks)
    A. Use pulleys to obtain passive range of motion (PROM) for flexion to 140 degrees and wand for external rotation to 45 degrees.
    B. Soft tissue mobilization of the subscapularis muscle at the scapula (not near the surgical site) while the patient is in supine position and the arm is abducted to 45 degrees
    C. Instruct patient in scar mobilization techniques to be performed three to four times a day as tolerated (see Chapter 4).
    D. Scapular PROM by the therapist while the patient is in sidelying position
    E. Initiate scapular stabilizations through closed-chain activities. This could begin with wall push-ups and quadruped proprioceptive neuromuscular facilitation (PNF) rhythmic stabilizations.
    F. Initiate glenohumeral closed-chain exercises with use of the upper body ergometer, the Baltimore Therapeutic Equipment (BTE) Work Simulator, or rolling a Swiss ball on the floor, progressing to the wall while standing.
    G. Rotator cuff exercises with light resistance (e.g., bands, hand-held weights)
    H. Rhomboid, levator scapulae, and upper trapezius exercises (i.e., shrugs with and without scapular adduction), using light resistance
     I. Middle trapezius exercises with seated rows, not to break the coronal plane, with light resistance

J. Initiate active-assisted "full can" exercises from 0 to 90 degrees, making sure the arm is maintained in scapular plane.

K. Begin isotonic exercises for the biceps and triceps, using a mirror to reinforce the importance of proper mechanics if appropriate.

L. PROM of the glenohumeral joint, in hooklying position to put the latissimus dorsi muscle on a stretch, working to obtain full external rotation in progressively increasing abduction, using only grade I and II mobilizations

M. Modalities for soreness as needed

III. Strengthening phase (6 to 12 weeks)

A. Continue to progress with all exercises, increasing the weights as long as the patient does not show signs of substitution or soreness.

B. The efficiency of using eccentric exercises in both force production and energy expenditure is well described.[7,8] Exercises should begin with full shoulder elevation in the scapular plane and lowering to the horizontal position. The therapist must provide support of the lowering arm to encourage proper mechanics of the shoulder and to maintain a lumbar neutral position. Once control eccentrically is established, active-assisted concentric elevation may be initiated and progressed. Modified military press, with the arms in more of a sagittal plane, is the goal of this activity.

C. Plyometrics are introduced through bounce passes progressing to chest passes with the therapist, using a basketball. This is progressed to a weighted ball toss into a Plyoback rebounder using both hands, progressing to using only the surgically corrected shoulder, as directed by the surgeon.

D. Increasing weight-bearing on the upper extremity. This is done first in quadruped position by lifting the opposite arm and ipsilateral leg and holding. This is progressed to holding a regular push-up position on toes with only the affected upper extremity.

E. Return to any sport activities is determined by the surgeon based on the type of activity; contact, throwing, and overhead activities are performed at full speed for at least 1 year postoperatively.

Complications

I. Postoperative infection. This has been reduced by the use of prophylactic antibiotics.

II. Postoperative recurrent instability. Special attention needs to be given to the specific surgical procedures and use of appropriate precautions.

III. Neurovascular compromise. Depending on the procedure, injury to the musculocutaneous or axillary nerve may occur. Even with thermal capsulorrhaphy, the axillary nerve[9] could be affected.

IV. Excessive shoulder stiffness.

ATRAUMATIC INSTABILITY

There are a variety of factors that may contribute to the AMBRII type of glenohumeral instability. The glenoid may be small or functionally flat, the capsular volume may be excessive, or there may be weak rotator cuff muscles that allow the shoulder to go beyond its range for stability. Because one or more of these factors could be involved at any time, there is a greater chance of a multidirectional component. This condition typically affects those younger than 30 years of age. There is no one traumatic incident affecting these patients. More likely, they have pain with normal activities and complaints of looseness or a feeling of "slipping out." The instability can be so severe that dislocation occurs during sleep.[10]

Treatment, depending on severity, will most likely begin with a nonoperative approach. Surgical intervention is a medial or lateral inferior capsular shift, performed either openly or arthroscopically,[11] that may be reinforced with a laser-assisted capsular shrinkage procedure.

Nonoperative Treatment Goals

I.   To establish joint compression through exercises.
II. To establish proprioceptive awareness of the affected shoulder.
III. To be able to perform normal daily activities without soreness.

Nonoperative Treatments

This protocol is not as clearcut as most postoperative rehabilitation programs. The therapist must be aware of the direction (or directions) of instability and be able to create an appropriate exercise program. For example, if the instability is in an anterior and inferior direction, then exercises for the rotator cuff in 90 degrees of abduction may be inappropriate early in the rehabilitation process. Morris and colleagues[12] showed that patients with multidirectional instability were stronger than controls for internal rotation in neutral and at 45 degrees abduction. More importantly, they showed the lack of deltoid activity (particularly of the middle and anterior heads) with the arm at 90 degrees while performing internal and external rotation exercises. Uhl and colleagues[13] showed that weight-bearing activities of increasing difficulty also increase the activity of the shoulder stabilizers, including the deltoid. Proprioception has been investigated in patients with anterior shoulder instability[14]; significant preoperative differences for flexion, abduction, and external rotation did not improve until 1 year postoperatively. Swanik and associates[15] showed the usefulness of plyometrics and improvement with proprioception at the shoulder. Because ROM is not the problem with these patients and joint laxity is, there is little reason to do any PROM, other than at the initial evaluation and with reassessments.

Treatments should begin with submaximal isometrics for the glenohumeral stabilizers, including the rotator cuff as appropriate and the deltoid. A stable scapular base needs to be established through scapular stabilization exercises. The lower fibers of the serratus anterior need to be incorporated into the program for smooth scapular upward rotation. As the patient shows proficiency with each level of exercise, he or she can be progressed, working toward the area of difficulty. Activities such as reaching in a variety of positions and pushing and pulling need to be incorporated in the rehabilitation program, because these are some of the activities that affect the patient on a daily basis. This provides a way to monitor progress and to increase the patient's confidence when using the arm. It is important that the patient be monitored for proper mechanics, because poor technique could lead to further problems.

Postoperative Rehabilitation

This program can effectively follow the rehabilitation program for the anterior capsular shift (see discussion of TUBS). There are few modifications. The postoperative delay before initiation of any rehabilitation process could be greater than 1 month with greater instability or with any other systemic conditions that may affect the connective tissue (e.g., Ehlers-Danlos syndrome).[2] If the patient is older than 25 years of age, it may be less than 1 month. ROM is gained through active movements; passive stretching is avoided; and lifting is held to less than 10 lb for 6 months.

ACQUIRED INSTABILITY

Acquired instability is the result of repetitive movements that stress the anterior capsular structures; it is seen most notably in throwing athletes. Burkhart and Morgan[16] believed that this stress, caused by the maximal external rotation at the late cocking phase of the throwing cycle combined with a tight posterior inferior capsule, may cause a torsional peel back of the biceps tendon off the superior glenoid, known as the superior labrum anterior-posterior (SLAP) lesion. This causes a posterior superior instability that leads to undersurface rotator cuff tears. McMahon and co-workers[17] described an increase in translation after a type II SLAP lesion. Surgical techniques use either suture anchors or an absorbable tack to replace the labrum and biceps back onto the glenoid rim. If anterior laxity is detected, an anterior capsulolabral reconstruction, described by Jobe and colleagues,[18] is also performed. The capsulolabral reconstruction follows the traumatic anterior inferior instability rehabilitation program. If the surgery is only to repair the SLAP lesion, the rehabilitation is as follows.

Type II SLAP Lesion Postoperative Therapy after a Biceps Anchor Procedure

Goals

I. Short-term goals (0 to 3 weeks)
   A. Reduce soreness.
   B. Maintain scapular movement, as appropriate.
   C. Maintain normal joint motion with the distal joints of the involved extremity.
   D. Obtain normal scapular posture through appropriate activities and verbal cues.
   E. Obtain full PROM of the glenohumeral joint.
   F. Educate the patient on appropriate level of activity with the involved side.
II. Long-term goals (4 to 12 weeks)
   A. Obtain full active range of motion (AROM) of the shoulder complex.
   B. Return to pain-free ADLs.
   C. Obtain at least equal strength of the involved side compared with the uninvolved side.

   D. Return to previous level of activity.
 III. Sports-related goals (12 to 24 weeks)
   A. Begin interval throwing program.
   B. Begin contact activities with the involved extremity.

Postoperative Precautions

The surgeon determines these precautions. The extent of the injury dictates the aggressive nature of the rehabilitation. If the biceps tendon was not involved, the rehabilitation program may be accelerated as tolerated. If, however, the biceps tendon required stabilization and the inferior glenohumeral ligament needed to be addressed, forearm supination, elbow flexion, and shoulder abduction with external rotation may need to be more slowly progressed. Weight-bearing activities may also need to be graded based on the extent of the structural involvement.[19]

Postoperative Therapy

  I. Days 1 to 7
   A. Sling immobilization
  II. Weeks 2 to 3
   A. Initiate gravity assisted Codman-type activities.
   B. Passive abduction (0 to 90 degrees) and passive external rotation
    while the shoulder is in an adducted position
   C. Initiate scapular active movements while in the sling
    (e.g., scapular clock, manual scapular PNF activities in sitting or
    sidelying position, or non–weight-bearing neurodevelopmental
    treatment (NDT) techniques.
 III. Weeks 3 to 16
   A. Discontinue use of the sling.
   B. Initiate use of the arm for light ADLs.
   C. Passive stretching of the posterior capsule through manual
    techniques; instruct patient on self-mobilization techniques
    (Fig. 26-1).
   D. Patient may begin using a pulley at home.
   E. Initiate submaximal effort isometric abduction to reestablish
    glenohumeral setting.
   F. Begin and progress closed kinetic chain activities for the upper
    extremity.
   G. Quadruped weight shifting and adjusting the level of difficulty
    by lifting the unaffected arm and progressing to lifting the
    contralateral leg.
   H. Standing, quadruped or push-up position (as appropriate) while
    using the Pro Fitter trainer for flexion and extension as well as
    horizontal abduction/adduction.
   I. Swiss ball activities from ROM to wall push-ups.
   J. Initiate active shoulder external rotation in varying abducted
    positions up to 90 degrees.
 IV. Weeks 16 to 24
   A. Continue to progress with passive stretching of the shoulder
    complex, especially the posterior capsule.
   B. Progress with resisted rotator cuff exercises, starting in a neutral

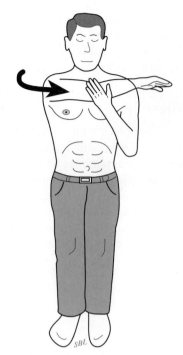

FIG. **26-1** Stretching in cross-body reach with the opposite arm used as the therapist. (From Matsen FA III, Lippitt SB, Sidles JA, et al.: Practical Examination and Management of the Shoulder. WB Saunders, Philadelphia, 1994.)

position, moving to 90 degrees elevation in scapular plane and finally to 90 degrees abduction in frontal plane.

C. Increase difficulty level of closed-chain activities (e.g., by assuming more of a push-up position with the Swiss ball and the Pro Fitter).

D. Begin more isolated biceps curls, including seated rows, latissimus pull-downs.

E. Begin plyometric training with the use of the Plyoball, either into a minitrampoline or ball toss with therapist/trainer.

F. Concentrate on appropriate mechanics for sports activities such as swimming, interval throwing, tennis (no full-speed serving), golf, and volleyball (no smashes), preferably under the watchful eye of a coach.

V.   After 6 months

A. Begin to throw off a mound.

B. Practice tennis serves and volleyball smashes.

C. Begin full level of contact for rugby and football.

OUTCOMES

According to Wahl and colleagues,[20] after any stabilization procedure and depending on the extent of the instability, most patients should regain full ROM at 3 months. Full return to contact sports and overhead activities is delayed until 6 months. Patients who are skeletally immature and diagnosed with recurrent instability, after an open surgical procedure, must go through 6 to 9 months of aggressive rehabilitation and strengthening before they can return to any competitive sports.[21]

REFERENCES

1. Itoi E, et al.: Biomechanics of the shoulder. In Rockwood CA, Matsen FA, Wirth MA, et al. (eds): The Shoulder. 3rd Ed. Elsevier, Philadelphia, 2004

2. McMahon PJ, et al.: Functional anatomy and biomechanics of the shoulder. In Delee JC, Drez D, Miller MD (eds): Delee & Drez's Orthopaedic Sports Medicine. 2nd Ed. WB Saunders, Philadelphia, 2003

3. Neer CS II: Shoulder Reconstruction, WB Saunders, Philadelphia, 1990

4. Pappas AM, et al.: Symptomatic shoulder instability due to lesions of the glenoid labrum. Am J Sports Med 11:279-288, 1983

5. Lintner SA, Speer KP: Traumatic anterior glenohumeral instability: the role of arthroscopy. J Am Acad Orthop Surg 5:233-239, 1997

6. Matsen FA, et al.: Glenohumeral instability. In Rockwood CA, Matsen FA, Wirth MA, et al. (eds): The Shoulder. 3rd Ed. Elsevier, Philadelphia, 2004

7. Komi PV: The stretch–shortening cycle and human power output. In Jones NL, McCartney N, McComas AJ (eds): Human Muscle Power. Human Kinetics Publishers, Champaign, IL, 1986

8. Albert M: Eccentric muscle training in sports and orthopaedics. Churchill Livingstone, New York, 1991

9. Greis PE, et al.: Axillary nerve injury after thermal capsular shrinkage of the shoulder. J Shoulder Elbow Surg 10:231-235, 2001

10. Schenk TJ, Brems JJ: Multidirectional instability of the shoulder: pathophysiology, diagnosis and management. J Am Acad Orthop Surg 6:65-72, 1998

11. Pollock RG, et al.: Operative results of the inferior capsular shift procedure for multidirectional instability of the shoulder. J Bone Joint Surg Am 82:919-928, 2000

12. Morris AD, Kemp GJ, Frostick SP: Shoulder electromyography in multidirectional instability. J Shoulder Elbow Surg 13:24-29, 2004

13. Uhl TL, Carver TJ, Mattacola CG, et al.: Shoulder musculature activation during upper extremity weight-bearing exercises. J Orthop Sports Phys Ther 33:109-117, 2003

14. Zuckerman JD, et al.: The effect of instability and subsequent anterior shoulder repair on proprioception ability. J Shoulder Elbow Surg 12:105-109, 2003

15. Swanik KA, et al.: The effects of shoulder plyometric training on proprioception and selected muscle performance characteristics. J Shoulder Elbow Surg 11:579-586, 2002

16. Burkhart SS, Morgan C: SLAP lesions in the overhead athlete. Orthop Clin North Am 32:431-441, 2001

17. McMahon PJ, et al.: Glenohumeral translations are increased after a type II superior labrum anterior-posterior lesion: a cadaveric study of severity of passive stabilizer injury. J Shoulder Elbow Surg 13:39-44, 2004

18. Jobe FW, et al.: Anterior capsulolabral reconstruction of the shoulder in athletes in overhand sports. Am J Sports Med 19:428-434, 1991

19. Calvert P, et al.: Contribution to the study of pathogenesis of type II superior labrum anterior-posterior lesions: a cadaveric model of a fall on the outstretched hand. J Shoulder Elbow Surg 13:45-50, 2004

20. Wahl CJ, et al.: Shoulder arthroscopy. In Rockwood CA, Matsen FA, Wirth MA, et al. (eds): The Shoulder. 3rd Ed. Elsevier, Philadelphia, 2004

21. Curtis RJ Jr: Glenohumeral instabilities in the child. In Delee JC, Drez D, Miller MD (eds): Delee & Drez's Orthopaedic Sports Medicine. 2nd Ed. WB Saunders, Philadelphia, 2003

SUGGESTED READINGS

Jobe FW, et al.: Rehabilitation of the Shoulder. In Brotzman SB (ed): Clinical Orthopaedic Rehabilitation. Mosby, St. Louis, 1996

Evaluation and Management of Shoulder Injuries in the Athlete [special issue]. J Athletic Training 35(3), 2000

Magee DJ, Reid DC: Shoulder injuries. In Zachazewski JE, Magee DJ, Quillen WS (eds): Athletic Injuries and Rehabilitation. WB Saunders, Philadelphia, 1996

Norkin CC, Levange PK: Joint Structure and Function: A Comprehensive Analysis. 2nd Ed. FA Davis, Philadelphia, 1992

Humeral Fractures 27

Mary Schuler Murphy

PROXIMAL HUMERAL FRACTURES

Proximal humeral fractures are the most common of all humeral fractures (approximately 45%[1-4]) and account for 4% to 5% of all fractures.[1,2,5] In 80% of all proximal humeral fractures, there is no significant displacement of the fracture and the injury can be treated nonsurgically.[1,2,5] The most common mechanism of injury is falling onto outstretched hands from standing height or lower.[1-4,6] Osteoporosis is a major contributing factor in proximal humeral fractures in adults older than 40 years of age.[1,2] In a prospective study of 1027 patients, Court-Brown and colleagues[7] found that 90% of proximal humeral fractures occurred in patients older than 60 years of age. The more complex fractures occurred with osteopenic bone, and the highest incidence was in women between the ages of 80 and 89. Furthermore, they concluded that surgery in the elderly did not improve functional outcomes.[7] The incidence of proximal humeral fractures after 40 years of age increases 76%, with a 2:1 ratio of women to men.[1-4] Proximal humeral fractures in younger age groups are usually secondary to high-velocity injury and typically do not fall into the category of minimally displaced fractures.[1,2] For the purpose of this chapter, a therapeutic treatment protocol has been designed for the treatment of minimally displaced fractures and those fractures stabilized by surgery, permitting early rehabilitation.

Rehabilitation should be initiated early for instruction in control of distal edema and stiffness, as well as increased mobility of the stabilized fractured shoulder. Bertoft and co-workers[8] suggested that the greatest improvement in shoulder range of motion (ROM) after proximal humerus fracture occurs in the initial 3 to 8 weeks. Movement of the fractured shoulder depends on the individual's rate of healing and the stability of the fracture. Clinical unity and clinical union play a paramount role in the physician's decision as to how quickly to move the patient through the rehabilitation program.

Clinical unity occurs when the fracture fragments move in unison. This typically occurs within 1 to 4 weeks and is tested by having the patient stand with the affected arm at the side with the elbow flexed. While the physician places one hand on the humeral head, the humerus is gently rotated by the physician's other hand. If the fracture fragments move in unison, clinical unity has been reached. This may be achieved immediately if internal fixation is used to stabilize the fracture site.[8] If the physician determines that clinical unity is present, the therapy program outlined to initiate movement of the shoulder can begin.

Clinical union is evidence of cancellous healing as seen radiographically. This can occur as early as 6 weeks.[6] Once clinical union is reached, more aggressive movement can be performed safely.

Close communication with the patient's physician provides the therapist with the necessary information to advance the patient's program.

Definition

The **proximal humerus** comprises the humeral head, lesser and greater tuberosities, bicipital groove, and proximal shaft. Proximal humeral fractures may occur between one or all of the four major segments. The **anatomic neck of the humerus** is at the junction of the humeral head and the tuberosities. With anatomic neck fractures, the blood supply to the humeral head is disrupted, increasing the chance of avascular necrosis. The **surgical neck of the humerus** is below the tuberosities. Fractures here are more common and have a better prognosis (Fig. 27-1).

Types of humeral fractures vary greatly, complicating medical management. Proximal humeral fractures are frequently described with the use of Neer's four-segment classification system[3] (Fig. 27-2), which provides a guideline for diagnosis and treatment. This system is based on the number of displaced segments and the amount of their displacement, rather than the number of fracture lines. A one-part fracture has no segments displaced more than 1 cm and no angulation greater than 45 degrees. These fractures are typically treated conservatively with a sling. In a two-part fragment, one segment is displaced in relation to the other three. Depending on the type of two-part fracture, treatment may include either an open or a closed reduction. In a three-part fracture, two segments are displaced in relation to the other segments that are in opposition, and in a four-part fracture, all four segments

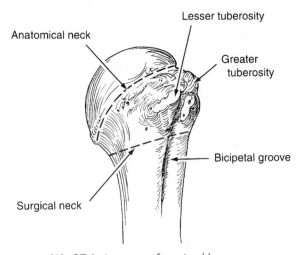

FIG. **27-1** Anatomy of proximal humerus.

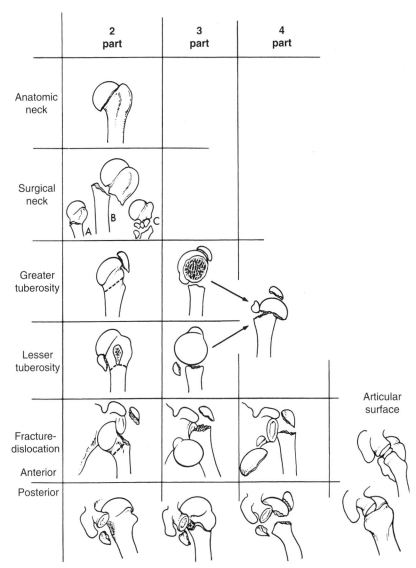

FIG. 27-2 Neer's Classification System. (Redrawn from Neer CS: J Bone Joint Surg Am 52:1077, 1970. From Canale ST: Campbell's Operative Orthopaedics. 10th Ed. Mosby, St. Louis, 2002.)

are displaced. In general, three-part fractures are treated with open reduction and internal fixation. A humeral head prosthesis is frequently the treatment of choice for four-part fractures, especially in the elderly. In a study performed by Bernstein and associates,[9] experts disagreed more than one third of the time using Neer's classification system to identify fracture segments through computed tomography and plain radiography. Sjoden and colleagues[10] reported poor reproducibility with Neer's classification of proximal humeral fractures.

Another classification system, devised by the Orthopedic Trauma Association group, emphasizes the vascular supply to the articular segments (Box 27-1). In a type A fracture, the articular segment is not isolated from its vascular supply. The type B fracture is partially isolated, and the

BOX **27-1** Orthopedic Trauma Association Classification of
         Proximal Humeral Fractures

Type A: extraarticular, unifocal fractures
   A1: avulsion of tuberosity
   A2: impacted metaphysis
   A3: nonimpacted metaphyseal fracture
Type B: extraarticular bifocal fractures
   B1: with metaphyseal impaction
   B2: without metaphyseal impaction
   B3: with glenohumeral dislocation
Type C: articular fractures
   C1: slight displacement, impacted valgus fracture
   C2: marked displacement, impacted
   C3: with glenohumeral dissociation

From Koval KJ, Zuckerman JD: Classification of proximal humeral fractures. In Koval KJ,
Zuckerman JD (eds): Handbook of Fractures. 2nd Ed. Lippincott Williams & Wilkins,
Philadelphia, 2002, p. 81.

type C fracture is totally separated from its blood supply. Decrease in vascular supply to the articular surface directly correlates with fracture prognosis, secondary to the increased possibility of avascular necrosis.[1]

Surgical Purpose

Fractures of the proximal humerus have varying degrees of severity. Those that have a sufficient degree of displacement or comminution may require open reduction and internal fixation (ORIF). The surgical purpose is to restore joint integrity for optimum function after fracture healing. Ideally, fixation of the bone fragments will be constructed with sufficient strength to allow shoulder joint motion during the bone healing phase. In a small percentage of cases, a humeral head prosthesis may be inserted if the humeral head displacement is severe or the vascular integrity of the joint surface is deemed irreparably damaged. Shoulder joint congruity and availability of early motion are the goals.

Treatment Goals

   I.   Promote maximal pain-free shoulder ROM and function.
  II.   Promote normal distal ROM and function.

Nonoperative Indications/Precautions for Therapy

   I.   Indications
      A. Nondisplaced/minimally displaced humeral fractures that are stable.
  II.   Precautions
      A. Greater tuberosity fractures require special consideration secondary to the attachment of the rotator cuff muscles and the potential for displacement of the greater tuberosity fragment.

Other considerations with a greater tuberosity fracture are the possibility of a rotator cuff tear and the potential for impingement of the greater tuberosity against the acromion and posterior glenoid. Greater tuberosity fractures, if not surgically reduced, may be immobilized longer than other nondisplaced or minimally displaced proximal humeral fractures.

B. Associated soft tissue injuries (e.g., ligaments, tendons).

Nonoperative Therapy

I. Day 1
   A. Use of a sling for proximal stabilization. The patient is instructed to wear the sling at all times until the physician gives permission for its removal for hygiene and exercise.
   B. Decrease shoulder pain through the use of modalities. The patient may be instructed in the frequent use of ice at home. Electrical stimulation in the form of transcutaneous electrical nerve stimulation (TENS), high-voltage galvanic stimulation (HVG), or interferential electrical stimulation is recommended for pain not managed by cold compression. Patients in the early stages of proximal humeral fractures frequently sleep in a reclining chair with their injured extremity supported by a pillow, secondary to difficulty lying supine.
   C. Wrist and hand ROM exercise and edema reduction techniques are essential to prevent distal stiffness. Patients with significant distal edema may benefit from an edema glove or kinesiotaping.

II. Days 3 to 7
   A. Initiate weaning from sling: When the patient is sitting, the arm should be supported on a pillow on a stable surface.
   B. Initiate pendulum exercises, typically on day 7 (see Fig. 25-1 in Chapter 25).
   C. Incorporate elbow and forearm ROM with other distal ROM exercises, and continue edema control. Gentle, nonpainful submaximal biceps isometric exercises may be initiated.
   D. Initiate active scapulothoracic stabilization exercises in sitting position (see Fig. 24-3, *A*, in Chapter 24).

III. Days 7 to 3 weeks
   A. Initiate supine shoulder passive range of motion (PROM) and active-assisted range of motion (AAROM) including elevation in the frontal plane, the plane of the scapula, and external rotation. These exercises are performed in supine position with the therapist supporting and protecting the injured shoulder. The patient may be taught to use a dowel to perform these exercises at home after careful instruction by the therapist. As the fracture and surrounding soft tissues heal, the patient may progress to the performance of gravity-eliminated place-hold exercises in supine position in 90 degrees flexion with the therapist's assistance (see Fig. 25-2 in Chapter 25). Encourage active range of motion (AROM) and AAROM at the elbow.
   B. Initiate pulleys for forward elevation. The patient may benefit from the use of pulleys in the home exercise program. Care must be taken to monitor the patient's response to pulley use;

for example, pain with overhead stretching, possibly caused by impingement, should be avoided.

C. Progress from gravity-eliminated position in supine to PROM and AAROM while sitting or standing with the arm supported on a tabletop (see Fig. 25-6 in Chapter 25).

D. Continue to progress scapulothoracic stabilization exercises; may use isometric manual strengthening techniques (see Fig. 24-3, *A*, in Chapter 24). Perform initially in sitting position.

E. Sling discontinued by physician.

IV. $3^1/_2$ weeks: Shoulder PROM, AAROM in extension, and internal rotation

V. 3 to 4 weeks: Rotator cuff, deltoid, and biceps isometric strengthening

VI. 4 to 6 weeks

A. Initiate place and hold AROM in supine position with 90 degrees flexion. Progress from this gravity-eliminated position in supine by having the patient move gradually away from 90 degrees shoulder flexion, controlling the arm in wider circles and in short arcs of motion, then returning to the gravity-eliminated position (see Figs. 25-2 and 25-5 in Chapter 25). Closed-chain exercises may also be incorporated to encourage coordination between shoulder and scapulothoracic musculature (see Fig. 24-3, *F*, in Chapter 24).

B. Progress from tabletop activities, with the arm supported by the table while performing active reaching activities (e.g., placing pegs in a pegboard, dusting), to less support (e.g., using an inclined board) (see Fig. 25-4, *A* and *B*, in Chapter 25).

VII. 6 to 8 weeks

A. Initiate light functional strengthening and endurance-building activities (e.g., copper tooling on an inclined board, sanding, self-care activities of daily living [ADLs]).

B. Continue with PROM, AROM, and AAROM exercises to increase shoulder mobility and function.

C. Initiate shoulder isotonic strengthening using Theraband in proprioceptive neuromuscular facilitation (PNF) patterns; Baltimore Therapeutic Equipment (BTE) Work Simulator may be used for preparation for return to functional tasks. Strengthen through the pain-free range.

VIII. 8 to 12 weeks

A. Continue with stretching ROM exercises to regain end ROM.

B. Progress strengthening exercise; initiate use of free weights (start with 1 lb and progressing to a maximum of 5 lb). Continue to strengthen through the pain-free range.

Nonoperative Complications

I. Unresolved pain

II. Distal edema and stiffness

III. Delayed union

IV. Nonunion

V. Degenerative arthritis

VI. Adhesive capsulitis

VII. Undiagnosed rotator cuff tears

VIII. Shoulder tendonitis/impingement
 IX. Avascular necrosis
  X. Myositis ossificans
 XI. Neurovascular injuries
XII. Reflex sympathetic dystrophy (RSD)

Operative Indications/Precautions for Therapy

  I. Indications: humeral fractures stabilized through surgical reduction
 II. Precautions
    A. Infection
    B. Associated soft tissue injuries or repairs

Postoperative Therapy

The progression of postsurgical repairs (i.e., internal fixation, ORIF) of proximal humeral fractures follows the same treatment guidelines as for nonoperative treatment but may progress at a faster rate because of the stabilization of the fracture provided by the surgery. An example is the tension band wiring supplemented by lag-screw fixation used in two- and three-part fractures, as reported by Cornell.[11] He advocated early aggressive therapy, with PROM initiated on day 1 and AROM and strengthening after postoperative week 4.[8] Hawkins and Angelo[12] also described early AAROM, 5 to 7 days after fixation of a three-part fracture with the wire band principle.

On the other hand, poor fracture stabilization may delay the progression of treatment. If significant pain or crepitation accompanies early motion, ROM should be delayed for 3 to 4 weeks.[12] Secondary to the soft osteogenic bone found frequently in patients with osteoporosis, many ORIFs may be minimally stable. In such cases, patients are frequently treated cautiously with a delayed rehabilitation program. Iannotti and associates[13] reported that, with the use of a proximal pin to secure a greater tuberosity fracture, no motion should be performed until the pins are removed.

Elkowitz and colleagues[14] reported that isolated two-part greater tuberosity fractures are the functional equivalent of a rotator cuff tear. He advocated **ORIF** of these injuries with heavy nonabsorbable sutures placed through the rotator cuff and cortical bone, allowing early postoperative therapy including shoulder PROM. Shoulder AROM is then delayed until 6 weeks after surgery. Park and co-workers[15] demonstrated that 89.3% of their study patients had excellent or satisfactory results with the use of suture fixation of their two- and three-part fractures. The Hughes and Neer[16] three-phrase protocol was initiated during the first postoperative week and progressed according to general time guidelines (Box 27-2).

Therapists' knowledge of the surgical procedure performed and the postsurgical precautions is absolutely necessary for the safe and successful treatment of these fractures. Communication with the surgeon is of paramount importance. The therapist must consult with the surgeon about fracture stabilization and any soft tissue repairs before proceeding with the rehabilitation program.

Postoperative Complications/Considerations

  I. Infection
 II. Hardware failure

BOX **27-2** Three-Phase Protocol Described by Hughes and Neer[16]

Phase I: 4-6 wk
    POD 1-7: pendulums and PROM only (FE in scapular plane 90-100°; ER at side 30°)
    POD 14: Supine ER with stick (start ≤30°)
    Phase II: 6-8 wk (after clinical and radiographical evidence of healing)
    Gentle stretching
    Pulley-assisted elevation
    Isometric strengthening (rotator cuff and deltoid)
Phase III: 8-12 wk
    Rubber band exercises
    Light weights

From Park MC, Murthi AM, Roth NS, et al.: J Orthop Trauma 17:319-325, 2003
ER, External rotation; *FE*, forward elevation; *POD*, postoperative day; *PROM*, passive range of motion.

   III.   Failure to stabilize the fracture
   IV.   Soft tissue repairs
    V.   All nonoperative complications
   VI.   Iatrogenic injuries

Evaluation Timeline

    I.   Nonoperative
       A. Day 1
          1. Wrist and hand AROM and PROM
          2. Distal edema
          3. Sensory screening
          4. Pain assessment
          5. ADL assessment
       B. Days 3 to 7: Elbow and forearm AROM and PROM
       C. Weeks 2 to 3: Passive shoulder flexion and external rotation
       D. Week 4: Passive shoulder extension and internal rotation
       E. Week 6: Shoulder AROM
       F. Week 12: Proximal strength
   II.   Operative: as above, but with variations according to the type of surgical procedure performed (e.g., soft tissue repair)

Outcomes

Court-Brown and colleagues[7] studied 1027 adult proximal humeral fractures, of which 116 were treated surgically and the rest conservatively. They concluded that there was no difference in prefracture level of function. The main determinant of outcome was age. They suggested that proximal fractures in the elderly population are best treated nonoperatively.

De La Hoz Marin and colleagues[17] performed a retrospective study of 29 three-part proximal humerus fractures treated with internal fixation with Kirschner wires. Excellent or satisfactory results were reported in

79.3% of the cases using Neer's criteria. Eighteen patients had no pain or mild pain that did not interfere with function. Twenty-four shoulders had more than 130 degrees active shoulder elevation.

In a study of 104 patients by Koval and co-workers,[18] 86% of the 58 patients who began therapy before 14 days had good to excellent results, compared with 65% of the 46 patients who had delayed therapy (after 14 days).

Hodgson and associates[19] studied conservative treatment in patients with two-part proximal humeral fractures. Those who began therapy within the first week experienced less pain over a 52-week period than did patients who received therapy after 3 weeks.

HUMERAL SHAFT FRACTURES

Humeral shaft fractures comprise approximately 1% of all fractures.[20] These fractures are typically sustained in a fall or caused by a high-energy incident such as a motor vehicle accident. Tytherleigh-Strong[21] reported, in his analysis of 249 patients treated over a 3-year period, that there was a 60% incidence of humeral shaft fractures in patients older than 50 years of age. Eighty percent of these fractures resulted from a simple fall, and 73% occurred in women. Among those younger than 50 years of age, 70% of these fractures were sustained by men, and more than two thirds were the result of moderate to severe trauma. Radial nerve palsy occurs in 20% of closed humeral shaft fractures but spontaneously resolves in 90% of these cases within 4 to 5 months.

Most humeral shaft fractures are treated nonoperatively and respond well to conservative treatment.[22-26] Koval and Zuckerman[22] reported that 90% of all humeral shaft fractures can be treated conservatively. Immediate conservative immobilization management typically includes the application of a hanging cast or a coaptation splint with a collar and cuff or a sling for 1 to 2 weeks. After this period, a custom or prefabricated functional fracture brace may be used. Zagorski and co-workers[27] concluded, in their study of 233 patients with humeral shaft fractures, that the treatment of choice is nonoperative therapy with the use of a fracture brace.

Wallny and associates[28] reported that functional fracture bracing led to significantly better results in terms of ROM, patient comfort, and cost reduction, compared with other conservative treatments (e.g., hanging cast). Fracture bracing compresses the soft tissues surrounding the fracture, providing stabilization and allowing early movement of proximal and distal joints. Fracture bracing also allows micromovement at the fracture site, which promotes fracture healing. The brace is typically applied after the first week, allowing the posttraumatic edema and pain to decrease. Although functional fracture bracing does not restore an anatomic reduction, appearance and function are typically acceptable to the patient. Reports indicate that up to 35 degrees of humeral shaft angulation is acceptable and has been associated with a good functional result.[28] Functional fracture bracing requires that the extremity be positioned in gravity-assisted positions (e.g., sitting, standing) for alignment of the fracture to occur.

A hinged-elbow humeral shaft fracture brace may be indicated for shaft fractures that extend more distally toward the elbow (this is decided by the physician). The expected timeline for clinical union of conservatively treated humeral shaft fractures is typically between 8 to 12 weeks.

Definition

Humeral shaft fractures are those fractures of the diaphysis of the midshaft that do not involve the proximal or distal articular joints. Tytherleigh-Strong[21] defined humeral shaft fractures as those occurring between the border of the insertion of the pectoralis major and the area above the supracondylar ridge. These fractures are frequently classified by Muller's classification system (Fig. 27-3). Type A humeral shaft fractures are most common and are considered to be simple two-fragment fractures. Type B fractures have a wedge, and type C multi-fragment fractures have more complex patterns. These fractures are furthered described in subgroups by location.

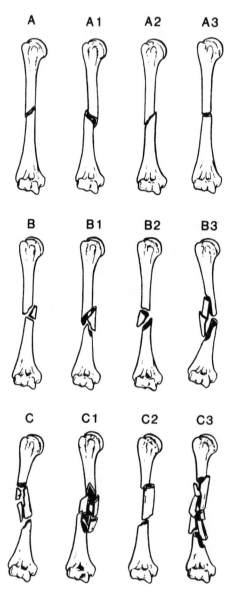

FIG. 27-3 Muller's classification system for humeral shaft fractures. (From Muller ME, Narian S, Koch P, Schatzker J: The Comprehensive Classification of Fractures of Long Bones. Springer-Verlag, Berlin, 1990.)

Treatment Purpose

To return normal shoulder and elbow ROM while protecting and allowing the fracture to heal.

Treatment Goals

I.   Restore full pain-free shoulder and elbow AROM.
II. Restore normal shoulder strength and function.
III. Promote full distal ROM and strength.
IV. Return to all previous ADL function.

Indications

Midshaft fractures that can be managed conservatively with fracture bracing and do not require surgical intervention for stabilization of the fracture. Indications for fracture bracing include closed, spiral, or oblique fractures in the middle or proximal third of the humerus. Patient compliance is essential.

Precautions/Contraindications

I.   Fracture bracing is contraindicated with severe associated soft tissue injuries (e.g., neurological or vascular injuries, open wounds). Fracture bracing is also contraindicated in unreliable patients and in patients who are bedridden and unable to assume gravity-dependent positions of the affected upper extremity that are required for acceptable alignment during healing. Obesity is a relative contraindication secondary to the difficulty of providing enough conformity of the brace for soft tissue compression of the fracture.
II. Weight-bearing and lifting with the affected extremity are commonly contraindicated early in the treatment program unless the fracture was stabilized with an intramedullary rod. Multitrauma patients who require upper extremity use for lower extremity weight-bearing with crutches or a walker may require surgical intervention for early weight-bearing on the injured shoulder. The decision to allow weight-bearing is made by the physician. Tingstad and associates[29] studied the effect of immediate weight-bearing on plated fractures of the humeral shaft (plate and screw fixation with a minimum of six cortices of fixation obtained both proximal and distal to the fracture) and concluded that immediate weight-bearing using a platform walker or crutch is both safe and beneficial, particularly for patients with lower extremity injuries who could be mobilized with upper extremity weight-bearing. Immediate weight-bearing with interlocked intramedullary nails is permitted if the fixation is stable.

Nonoperative Therapy

I.   Days 5 to 7
  A. A custom or prefabricated fracture brace with a collar and cuff or sling is used for fracture stabilization/support. Sarmiento and

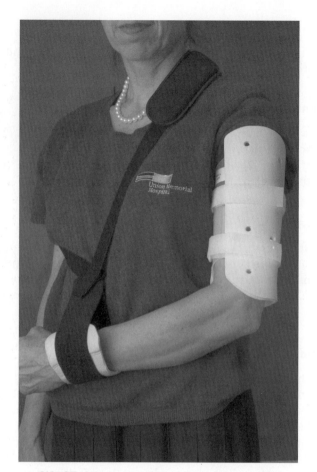

FIG. **27-4** Sarmiento brace with collar and cuff.

colleauges[30] recommended the use of a collar and cuff. Their concern was that, with the use of a sling, there is a greater chance of misalignment of the fracture (Fig. 27-4). The physician determines when the brace may be removed for hygiene, based on the stability of the fracture. This typically occurs after some clinical healing has taken place and the patient's pain has started to subside (at 3 to 4 weeks). If a radial nerve palsy is present, distal neuropathies must be addressed with both protective and functional splinting (Fig. 27-5).

II. Days 7 to 14

A. Instruct the patient in pendulum exercises to be performed at home, in the brace, six to eight times a day for 5 to 10 minutes (see Fig. 25-1 in Chapter 25).

B. Pain management including TENS, HVG, or an interferential unit with cold compression for pain and edema control. Instruct the patient in positioning of the injured extremity during sleep (in approximately 45 degrees scaption with a small pillow placed between the sling and trunk and a pillow support under the entire upper extremity).

C. Initiate AROM and isometric strengthening of the scapulothoracic stabilizers (see Fig. 24-3, *A*, in Chapter 24).

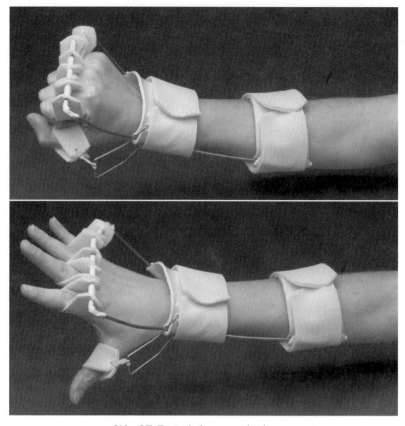

FIG. **27-5** Radial nerve palsy brace.

    D. Instruct the patient in a home program of distal AROM and grasp strengthening using putty. Initiate gentle AAROM at the elbow. Initiate very light submaximal isometric biceps strengthening.

    E. Instruct the patient in one-handed ADLs and the use of adaptive equipment as needed.

III. Weeks 3 to 4

    A. Continue pendulum exercises. Initiate gentle AAROM to the shoulder in standing or sitting position, within the patient's pain tolerance (see Fig. 25-6 in Chapter 25). No shoulder abduction or elevation above 60 degrees should be performed until there is clinical and radiological evidence of clinical unity (this is determined by the physician).

IV. Weeks 4 to 6

    A. Continue with the exercises described previously. Perform shoulder AAROM in supine and sidelying positions. Initiate AROM of the shoulder and elbow. Progress from gravity-eliminated positions in supine (e.g., place-hold performed in 90 degrees shoulder flexion) through gentle movement away from the 90 degrees position with gravity eliminated into gravity-challenged positions by gradually increasing the arc of motion or widening circles (see Figs. 25-2 and 25-5 in Chapter 25).

    B. Progress to isometric strengthening for supination/pronation strength. Progress to gentle active scapular protraction and

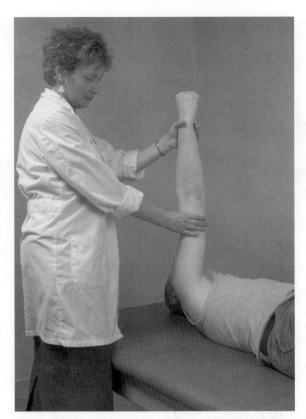

FIG. **27-6** Supine scapular protraction with therapist supporting the shoulder in 90 degrees.

retraction exercises in supine with the therapist supporting the shoulder in approximately 90 degrees flexion (Fig. 27-6).

V. Weeks 6 to 8
  A. Continue with the exercises previously described. Initiate shoulder extension and gentle internal rotation exercises, and progress shoulder abduction/scaption ROM to pain tolerance.
  B. Initiate gentle isotonic exercises to the elbow.
  C. Light weight-bearing is typically permitted at this time
  D. The fracture brace may be discontinued at 8 weeks, depending on fracture healing (decided by the physician).

VI. Weeks 8 to 10
  A. Stretching to the involved shoulder if full PROM is not present and the fracture is stable. Care is taken at the elbow to not become overzealous with PROM of this joint, secondary to problems reported with heterotopic ossification. Elbows may respond well to gentle contraction/relaxation exercises to regain motion.
  B. Light use in self-care ADLs is encouraged.
  C. Initiate gentle submaximal isometric shoulder strengthening.

VII. Weeks 10 to 12
  A. Full weight-bearing and light lifting are permitted.
  B. Isotonic shoulder and elbow strengthening using Theraband, beginning with strengthening at the side and progressing into

PNF patterns and full functional ROM (see Fig. 24-4, *B* to *F,* in Chapter 24).
C. Return to normal upper extremity use in most ADLs. Return to strenuous use or use in sports activities may take longer and should be approved by the physician.

Nonoperative Complications

I. Delayed union or nonunion
II. Unresolved radial nerve palsy

Operative Indications/Precautions for Therapy

I. Indications: humeral shaft fractures stabilized through surgical reduction
II. Precautions
   A. Infection
   B. Associated soft tissue injuries (including neurovascular and nerve injuries)
   C. Radial nerve palsy
III. Specific surgical precautions
   A. Intramedullary nails
      1. Antegrade insertion may result in proximal nail migration into the subacromial space, causing shoulder impingement, damage to the rotator cuff, and/or adhesive capsulitis.
      2. Retrograde insertion may result in distal nail migration, leading to blocked elbow extension, heterotopic ossification, and/or flexion contractures.
   B. External fixation
      1. Shoulder and elbow dysfunction secondary to the tethering of the deltoid and triceps with pin fixation
      2. Pin tract infections
   C. Plating
      1. Iatrogenic nerve palsy
      2. Infection with open fixation

Postoperative Therapy

Once the fracture is stabilized, therapy may follow an advanced nonoperative treatment protocol. Depending on the type of surgical procedure performed, there are some special therapy considerations. Close communication with the surgeon is essential. Interlocked intramedullary nails are frequently used in patients with osteopenic bones. With this type of stabilization, patients are allowed to bear weight and to use the affected extremity for light ADLs as pain permits, provided the fixation is stable. Pendulum, AROM, and AAROM exercises are allowed 1 week after surgery.

External fixation may be the treatment of choice for a comminuted fracture or for an injury in which significant soft tissue has been lost. The therapist should instruct the patient in pin care. At 1 week, pendulum exercises may be performed at the shoulder and elbow AROM and AAROM may be performed. At week 2, AROM and AAROM of the shoulder may be performed in supine position. Light weight-bearing may be initiated at 4 to 6 weeks if approved by the physician.

Stable fixation with plates and screws depends on good bone density. Bone grafting is sometimes used in conjunction with this type of fixation in cases of osteopenic bone. Exercises are the same as for external fixation. Tingstad and associates[29] reported safe immediate weight-bearing with the use of plate and screw fixation with a minimal of six cortices of fixation obtained both proximal and distal to the fracture.

Postoperative Complications/Considerations

I. Same as for nonsurgical management of humeral shaft fractures (e.g., delayed union, nonunion).
II. Possible iatrogenic nerve injuries (e.g., radial nerve palsy may require splint management of distal neuropathies).
III. Failure of surgical hardware to maintain fracture stability. Poor bone quality can contribute to hardware failure. Pins that migrate proximally in intramedullary pinning may interfere with shoulder function and result in pain secondary to rotator cuff impingement or subacromial impingement of the migrating pins. Retrograde insertion of intramedullary nails may block elbow extension. The use of plates may cause elbow stiffness and pain.
IV. Infection
V. Soft tissue resection and repair (e.g., deltoid split for antegrade insertion of an intramedullary nail)
VI. Soft tissue damage (e.g., rotator cuff injury)

Evaluation Guidelines (As Expected with Fracture Brace Protocol)

I. Nonoperative
A. Day 1: wrist and hand ROM, distal edema, sensory screen, pain assessment, and ADLs
B. Days 5 to 7: elbow and forearm ROM
C. Weeks 4 to 6: shoulder AAROM and PROM in flexion within patient's comfort. Full elbow extension is expected at 2 weeks.
D. Weeks 6 to 8: Shoulder AROM. (Secondary to the potential deforming forces across the fracture site, active elevation of the shoulder in flexion, scaption, and abduction is not initiated until there is clinical and radiographical evidence of fracture stability.)
E. Week 12: Isometric proximal strength, return to ADLs
II. Operative
A. Days 2 to 3: wrist and hand ROM, distal edema, sensory screen, pain assessment, ADLs, and surgical incision inspection
B. Week 1: elbow and forearm ROM
C. Week 2: shoulder AAROM supine
D. Weeks 3 to 4: shoulder AROM (if fracture is stable and the patient is relatively pain free)
E. Weeks 4 to 6: isometric shoulder strength

Outcomes

I.   Nonoperative

    A. In a study of 922 patients with a 67% participation rate in follow-up, 90% of humeral shaft fractures healed without surgical intervention. Closed fractures healed in a median time of 9.5 weeks; open fractures, 14 weeks; transverse fractures, 12 weeks; oblique fractures, 10 weeks; comminuted fractures, 10.5 weeks; and segmental fractures, 11.5 weeks. Radial nerve palsy occurred in 67 patients (11%). Full shoulder ROM was achieved in 76% of the patients, and a limitation of 25 degrees or less was found by the time the brace was discontinued.[30]

    B. In a study by Wallny and colleagues,[28] 79 patients with 79 fractures at the proximal and middle third of the humerus were treated with humeral fracture bracing; 86% regained normal elbow and shoulder AROM in comparison with the uninvolved side. Sixty-five percent of the patients had no pain, and 35% had pain with heavy physical exercise.

    C. Radial nerve palsy can occur in up to 17% of cases, with approximately 90% resolving within 3 to 4 months.[31]

    D. In a study by Zagorski and co-workers,[27] 233 patients with humeral shaft fractures were treated with prefabricated braces, including 43 open and 127 closed fractures. All but 3 patients had a good to excellent functional result with near-normal ROM.

II. Postoperative

    A. In a study by Stannard and associates,[26] 42 humeral shaft fractures were surgically treated with intramedullary nailing with a locking flexible nail. Thirty-nine fractures healed, with a mean time of 12 weeks for clinical healing. Thirty-eight patients had no pain, and 36 patients recovered full ROM. Four patients had complications, including 2 nonunions, 2 hardware failures, and 1 wound infection.

    B. In a prospective, randomized study by Chapman and co-workers[24] that compared intramedullary nailing (38 patients) with plating (84 patients), healing occurred in a high percentage of patients in both groups. Antegrade nailing resulted in a higher incidence of shoulder pain and stiffness, whereas plating resulted in a higher incidence of elbow pain and stiffness. Hardware irritation was present in both groups. The authors concluded that either procedure provides a predictable method for fracture stabilization in the subset of patients who require surgical intervention.

REFERENCES

Proximal Humeral Fractures

1. Bigliani LU, Craig EV, Butters KP: Fractures of the proximal humerus. In Rockwood CA Jr, Green DP (ed): Fractures in Adults. 3rd Ed. Vol. 1. Lippincott-Raven, Philadelphia, 1990, p. 871
2. Bigliani LU: Fractures of the proximal humerus. In Rockwood CA, Matsen FA (eds): The Shoulder. Vol. 1. WB Saunders, Philadelphia, 1990, p. 278
3. Basti JJ, Dionysian E, Sherman PW, et al.: Management of proximal humeral fractures. J Hand Ther 7:111, 1994

4. Basti JJ, Dionysian E, Sherman PW, et al.: Management of proximal humeral fractures and fracture dislocations. J Bone Joint Surg Br 72:1050, 1990

5. Neer CS: Fractures. In Neer CS (ed): Shoulder Reconstruction. WB Saunders, Philadelphia, 1990, p. 363

6. Loder RT, Mayhew HE: Common fractures from a fall on an outstretched hand. Am Fam Physician 37:327, 1988

7. Court-Brown CM, Garg A, McQueen MM: The epidemiology of proximal humeral fractures. Acta Orthop Scand 72:365, 2001

8. Bertoft ES, Lundh I, Ringqvist I: Physiotherapy after fracture of the proximal end of the humerus: comparison between two methods. Scand J Rehabil Med 16:11, 1984

9. Bernstein J, Adler LM, Blank JE, et al.: Evaluation of the Neer system of classification of proximal humeral fractures with computerized tomographic scans and plain radiographs. J Bone Joint Surg Am 78:1371-1375, 1996

10. Sjoden GO, Movin T, Guntner P, et al.: Poor reproducibility of classification of proximal humeral fractures. Acta Orthop Scand 68:239, 1997

11. Cornell CN: Tension-band wiring supplemented by lag-screw fixation of proximal humerus fractures: a modified technique. Orthop Rev May (Suppl):19-23, 1994

12. Hawkins RJ, Angelo RL: Displaced proximal humeral fractures. Orthop Clin North Am 18:421, 1987

13. Iannotti JP, Ramsey ML, Williams GR, Warner JJP: Nonprosthetic management of proximal humeral fractures. J Bone Joint Surg 85:1578, 2003

14. Elkowitz SJ, Koval KJ, Zuckerman JD: Decision making for the treatment of proximal humerus fractures. Tech Shoulder Elbow Surg 3:234, 2002

15. Park MC, Murthi AM, Roth NS, et al.: Two part and three part fractures of the proximal humerus treated with fracture fixation. J Orthop Trauma 17:319, 2003

16. Hughes M, Neer CS: Glenohumeral joint replacement and post-operative rehabilitation. Phys Ther 55:850, 1975

17. De La Hoz Marin J, Hernandez Cortes P, Tercedeor Sanchez J: Surgical treatment of three part proximal humeral fractures. Acta Orthop Belg 67:226, 2001

18. Koval KJ, Gallagher MA, Marsicano JG, et al.: Functional outcome after minimally displaced fractures of the proximal part of the humerus. J Bone Joint Surg Am 79: 203-207, 1997

19. Hodgson SA, Mawson SJ, Stanley D: Rehabilitation after two part fractures of the neck of the humerus. J Bone Joint Surg Br 85:419, 2003

Humeral Shaft Fractures

20. Emmett J, Breck LW: A review and analysis of 11,000 fractures seen in private practice of orthopaedic surgery 1937-1956. J Bone Joint Surg Am 40:1169, 1958

21. Tytherleigh-Strong G, Walls N, McQueen MM: The epidemiology of humeral shaft fractures. J Bone Joint Surg Br 80:249, 1998

22. Koval KJ, Zuckerman JD: Humeral shaft upper extremity fractures and dislocations. In Koval KJ, Zuckerman JD (eds): Handbook of Fractures. 2nd Ed. Lippincott Williams & Wilkins, Philadelphia, 2002

23. Georgiadis GM, Behrens FF: Humeral shaft fractures in the elderly. In Koval KJ, Zuckerman JD (eds): Fractures in the Elderly. Lippincott-Raven, New York, 1998, p. 93

24. Chapman JR, Henley MB, Agel J, et al.: Randomized prospective study of humeral shaft fracture fixation: intramedullary nails versus plates. J Orthop Trauma 14:162, 2000

25. Farragos AF: Complications of intramedullary nailing for fractures of the humeral shaft: a review. J Orthop Trauma 13:258, 1999

26. Stannard JP: Intramedullary nailing of humeral shaft fractures with a locking flexible nail. J Bone Joint Surg Am 85:2103, 2003

27. Zagorski JB, Latta LL, Zych GA, et al.: Diaphyseal fractures of the humerus. J Bone Joint Surg Am 70:607, 1988

28. Wallny T, Westermann K, Sagebiel C, et al.: Functional treatment of humeral shaft fractures: indications and results. J Orthop Trauma 11:283, 1997

29. Tingstad EM, Wolinsky PR, Shyr Y, et al.: Effect of immediate weightbearing on plated fractures of the humeral shaft. J Trauma 49:278-280, 2000

30. Sarmiento A, Watson JT : Functional bracing of diaphyseal fractures and operative management of humeral shaft fractures. In Moehring HD, Greenspan A: Fracture Diagnosis and Treatment. McGraw-Hill, Philadelphia, 2000, p. 225

31. Georgiadis GM, Behrens FF: Humeral shaft. In Koval KJ, Zuckerman JD: Fractures in the Elderly. Lippincott-Raven, New York, 1998, p. 93

SUGGESTED READINGS

Proximal Humeral Fractures

Cornell CN, Scheider K: Proximal humerus. In Koval JK, Zuckerman JD (eds): Fractures in the Elderly. Lippincott-Raven, New York, 1998, p. 85

Schlegel TF, Hawkins RJ: Operative treatment of three part proximal humerus fractures. In Craig EV (ed): Master Techniques in Orthopaedic Surgery: The Shoulder (Master Techniques Series). 2nd Ed. Lippincott Williams & Wilkins, Philadelphia, 2003, p. 413

Cornell C: Operative treatment of displaced surgical neck fractures of the proximal humerus. In Crage EV (ed): Master Techniques in Orthopaedic Surgery. 2nd Ed. Lippincott Williams & Wilkins, Philadelphia, 2003, p. 449

Delee JC, Drez D: Orthopaedic Sports Medicine: Principles and Practice. Vol. I. WB Saunders, Philadelphia, 1994

Lin J, Hou SM, Hang YS: Locked nailing for displaced surgical neck fractures of the humerus. J Trauma 45:1051, 1998

Naranja RJ, Iannotti JP: Displaced three and four part proximal humerus fractures: evaluation and management. J Am Acad Orthop Surg 8:373, 2000

Resch H, et al.: Percutaneous fixation of three and four part fractures of the proximal humerus. J Bone Joint Surg Br 79:295, 1997

Wachtl SW, Marti CB, Hoogewoud HM, et al.: Treatment of proximal humerus fractures using multiple intramedullary flexible nails. Arch Orthop Trauma Surg 120:171, 2000

Zyto K, Ahrengart L, Sperber A, et al.: Treatment of displaced proximal humeral fractures in elderly patients. J Bone Joint Surg Br 79:412, 1997

Humeral Shaft Fractures

Brotzman SB, Wilk KE: Clinical Orthopaedic Rehabilitation. 2nd Ed. Mosby, St. Louis, 2003

Gartsman G, Hasan SS: What's new in shoulder and elbow surgery. J Bone Joint Surg Am 86:189, 2004

Hoppenfeld S, Murthy VL: Treatment and Rehabilitation of Fractures. Lippincott Williams & Wilkins, Philadelphia, 2000

Moehring D, Greenspan A: Fractures, Diagnosis and Treatment. McGraw-Hill, New York, 2000

Sarmiento A, et al.: Diaphyseal humeral fractures: treatment options. J Bone Joint Surg Am 83:1566, 2001

Olarte CM, Darowish M, Ziran BH: Radial nerve transposition with humeral fracture fixation. Clin Orthop 413:170, 2003

Shoulder Arthroplasty **28**

Anne Edmonds

The first reported total shoulder arthroplasty was attempted by a French surgeon in 1893.[1] He used a platinum and rubber prosthesis to alleviate shoulder pain in a 37-year-old baker. This prosthesis was removed 2 years later as a result of infection; however, it had been functional for those 2 years. In the 1950s, the constrained prosthesis was introduced, and in 1973 the unconstrained prosthesis was developed.[1]

Shoulder arthroplasty is used to provide a painless range of motion (ROM) by replacing or resurfacing the articulating surface of the humeral head and the glenoid. Patients who present with a history of rheumatoid arthritis, osteoarthritis, avascular necrosis, sickle cell infarction, irradiation necrosis, ochronosis, or gout may benefit from this procedure[2] (Fig. 28-1). Hemiarthroplasty is used for severely displaced and comminuted humeral fractures or dislocations with an interrupted vascular supply. With a properly supervised rehabilitation program, patients undergoing either of these procedures can usually obtain a functional outcome.

DEFINITION

I. **Total shoulder arthroplasty (TSA):** replacement of the humeral head and the glenoid articulating surface with components made of polyethylene or titanium. Three types of replacement components are used
    A. Unconstrained: humeral component that articulates with a scapular component. If musculotendinous units are intact or able to be reconstructed, this implant has the potential for good results.[3] This is the most widely used component (Figs. 28-2 and 28-3).
    B. Constrained: designed for patients who have severe deterioration without a reconstructible rotator cuff but with a functioning deltoid muscle.[1] The glenoid and humeral components are coupled and fixed to bone. The forces acting across the point of coupling cause increasing rates of breakage and loosening.[4]

C. Semiconstrained: monospherical. The humeral head is smaller and spherical, with a head-neck angle of 60 degrees that reportedly permits increased ROM. The glenoid component is matched to the humeral head prosthesis to allow constant surface contact.[1]

II.   **Hemiarthroplasty:** replacement of the humeral head with a stemmed intramedullary implant that articulates with the glenoid, acromion, and distal clavicle[3] (Figs. 28-4 and 28-5).

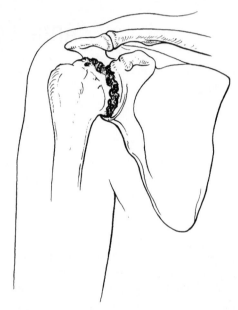

FIG. **28-1** Arthritis of the glenohumeral joint of a shoulder.

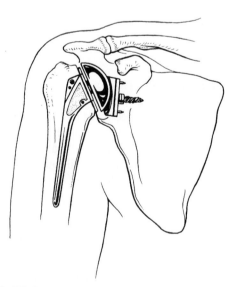

FIG. **28-2** Unconstrained prosthesis of a shoulder.

SURGICAL PURPOSE

To remove painful, irregular, and deformed glenohumeral joint surfaces and replace them with metal or plastic. Restoration approximating normal skeletal alignment and joint stability with an effective pain-free ROM is derived. Avoidance of soft tissue laxity, impingement, and overstuffing of the glenohumeral joint results in the best TSA reconstruction.[5]

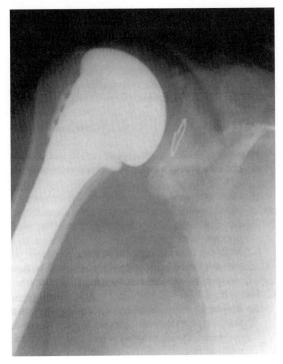

FIG. 28-3   Radiograph of unconstrained shoulder prosthesis.

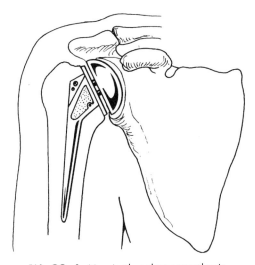

FIG. 28-4   Hemiarthroplasty prosthesis.

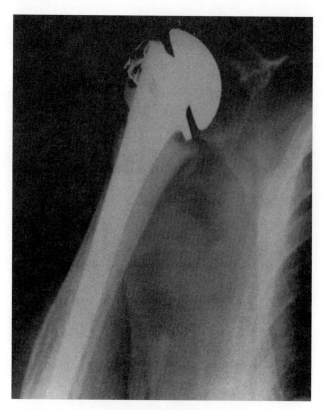

FIG. 28-5   Radiograph of hemiarthroplasty prosthesis.

The shoulder hemiarthroplasty is used to replace a humeral head that has been damaged by a fracture, a vascular necrosis of known or unknown cause, or a destructive tumor. These conditions do not involve the glenoid fossa. Hemiarthroplasty does not disturb the glenoid and is a lesser procedure. It reduces postoperative wound complications, and there are fewer risks of joint component failure compared with a TSA. This facilitates rehabilitation and improves the potential for good shoulder function. Patients may have pain-free shoulders after hemiarthroplasty, but with somewhat reduced motion and strength.[4]

TREATMENT GOALS FOR TOTAL SHOULDER ARTHROPLASTY

I.   To concentrate on rehabilitation of the soft tissues encompassing the implant and to be aware of and monitor the reconstructed structures
II. To restore maximum pain-free ROM
III. To increase function
IV. To maximize strength

OPERATIVE INDICATIONS/PRECAUTIONS FOR THERAPY FOR TOTAL SHOULDER ARTHROPLASTY

I.   Indications
     A. Decreased ROM and function
     B. Decreased strength

II. Precautions
   A. Infection
   B. Integrity of muscle tissue surrounding the implant
   C. Stability of the implant, possible glenoid loosening

POSTOPERATIVE THERAPY FOR TOTAL SHOULDER ARTHROPLASTY

I. Unconstrained prosthesis
   A. ROM
      1. Phase I (0 to 8 days)
         a. Local heat and passive range of motion (PROM) or active-assisted range of motion (AAROM) exercises within the first 2 days. Assess PROM. PROM is restricted to 80 to 90 degrees flexion and 10 to 20 degrees external rotation.
         b. Because of possible displacement of the deltoid tuberosity and pulleys, internal rotation should be avoided.
         c. Pendulum exercises with the body in a forward flexed position, allowing 120 to 130 degrees of flexion for 2 to 3 weeks; the forearm is pronated and supinated while doing circular motion.
         d. External rotation and flexion initiated in supine position. Support is given by towels or a pillow under the humerus. Flexion is limited to ≤140 degrees for the first month postoperative.
         e. Assisted abduction,[6] not past 30 to 40 degrees.[5]
         f. Ipsilateral motion of the hand and elbow to maintain good ROM and function of the distal extremity.
      2. Phase II
         a. 8 to 10 days: Initiate exercise in standing position.
         b. 10 to 14 days: Begin internal rotation exercises, no more than 30 to 40 degrees.
         c. Continue external rotation exercises in standing position until 40 to 60 degrees is obtained.[6]
         d. 17 to 21 days: Begin isometric exercises with elbow flexed to 90 degrees and held close to the body; opposite hand, wall, or door jamb provides resistance.
      3. Phase III
         a. 3 to 6 weeks: assisted shoulder elevation to obtain last 20 degrees of motion.[6] Assess active range of motion (AROM) and PROM.
         b. Assisted external rotation in standing position leaning against wall and stretching axilla
         c. Assisted internal rotation standing with arm behind back and hand resting supine on table
   B. Strengthening
      1. Phase I (6 to 8 weeks): assess strength; gross manual muscle testing (MMT) of upper arm
         a. Exercises done supine without gravity.
         b. Targets primarily supraspinatus and anterior deltoid.
      2. Phase II (8 to 10 weeks)
         a. Targets deltoid and rotator cuff; aggressive stretching[5]

b. Exercises performed against gravity in standing or sitting position.
3. Phase III (10 to 12 weeks)
   a. Isolates anterior, middle, and posterior deltoid and individual rotator cuff muscles
   b. Theraband used for resistance[6]

POSTOPERATIVE COMPLICATIONS FOR TOTAL SHOULDER ARTHROPLASTY

I. Infection
II. Nerve palsy
III. Subluxation/dislocation
IV. Intraoperative fracture
V. Pulmonary embolus
VI. Pneumonia[4]

TREATMENT GOALS FOR HEMIARTHROPLASTY

I. To achieve full PROM gradually rather than quickly
II. To increase function
III. To regain strength

OPERATIVE INDICATIONS/PRECAUTIONS FOR THERAPY FOR HEMIARTHROPLASTY

I. Indications
   A. Decreased ROM and function
   B. Decreased strength
II. Precautions
   A. Stability of implant
   B. Strength of repaired tendons and soft tissues to avoid anterior instability
   C. Infection

POSTOPERATIVE THERAPY FOR HEMIARTHROPLASTY

I. Phase I
   A. 1 to 7 days: Codman exercises, passive flexion within pain-free range
   B. Day 3: passive external rotation to limits defined at surgery[7]
   C. Overhead pulleys and wooden dowel passively
   D. 1 week: Begin isometric exercises if there was good tuberosity fixation at surgery.[7]
II. Phase II
   A. 2 to 3 weeks: gentle active-assisted exercises
   B. 4 to 6 weeks: more aggressive passive stretching; begin AROM
   C. 6 weeks: resistive exercises with rubber tubing
   D. 2 months: should achieve 90-degree active forward flexion[7]

III. Phase III
      A. 4 months: increased resistance using light hand weights
      B. Strengthening to continue for 1 year or longer with
         improvements

POSTOPERATIVE COMPLICATIONS FOR HEMIARTHROPLASTY

I.   Improper positioning of tuberosities, which could cause
     impingement or anterior or posterior subluxation
II. Detachment of subscapularis tendon causing anterior
     instability[7]
III. Disassociation of humeral head component

EVALUATION TIMELINE FOR TOTAL SHOULDER ARTHROPLASTY

I.   ROM
     A. 0 to 8 days: assess PROM and AAROM while supine
     B. 10 to 14 days: assess AROM against gravity
     C. 3 to 6 weeks: assess AROM
II. Strengthening
     A. 6 to 8 weeks: gross MMT upper extremity
     B. 8 to 10 weeks: MMT
     C. 10 to 12 weeks: MMT

EVALUATION TIMELINE FOR HEMIARTHROPLASTY

I.   1 day to 1 week: PROM assessment and initiation of exercises
      (supine progressing to sitting or standing).
II.   2 to 3 weeks: AAROM exercises against gravity.
III. 4 to 6 weeks: AROM.
IV.   6 weeks: Continue exercises; initiate resistance. MMT upper
      extremity.
V.   8 to 10 weeks: Evaluate AROM and MMT.
VI.   4 months to 1 year: Continue strengthening, with
      reevaluation every 3 to 4 weeks.

REFERENCES

1. Sisk TD, Wright PE: Arthroplasty of shoulder and elbow. In Crenshaw AH (ed):
   Campbell's Operative Orthopaedics. Vol. II. Mosby, St. Louis, 1987, p. 1503
2. Alund M, Hoe-Hansen C, Tillander B, et al.: Outcome after cup hemiarthroplasty in
   the rheumatoid shoulder: a retrospective evaluation of 39 patients followed for 2-6 years.
   Acta Orthop Scand 71:180-184, 2000
3. Swanson AB, Cerdo RD, Hynes D, et al.: Bipolar implant shoulder arthroplasty:
   long term results. Clin Orthop 249:227, 1989
4. Johnson RI: Total shoulder arthroplasty. Orthop Nurs 12:1, 1993
5. Owens RA: Total shoulder arthroplasty. AORN J 65:927-932, 1997
6. Brems JJ: Rehabilitation following total shoulder arthroplasty. Clin Orthop 307:70,
   1994
7. Dines DM, Warren RF: Modular shoulder hemiarthroplasty for acute fractures. Clin
   Orthop 301:70, 1994

SUGGESTED READINGS

Clayton ML, Ferlic DC, Jeffers PD: Prosthetic arthroplasties of the shoulder. Clin Orthop
    164:184, 1982

Movin T, Sjoden GO, Ahrengart L: Poor function after shoulder replacement in fracture
    patients: a retrospective evaluation of 29 patients followed for 2-12 years. Acta Orthop
    Scand 69:392-396, 1998

Neer CS, Kirby RM: Revision of humeral head and total shoulder arthroplasties. Clin
    Orthop Relat Res Oct:189-195, 1982

Neer CS, Watson KL, Stanton FJ: Recent experience in total shoulder replacement. J Bone
    Joint Surg Am 64:319, 1982

PART **FIVE**

Elbow

Epicondylitis 29

Jason Leadbetter

Epicondylitis is an extremely common diagnosis given to describe symptoms of pain and weakness occurring over the lateral or medial elbow. The term *epicondylitis* has traditionally implied a state of injury and delayed healing caused primarily by inflammation and commonly referred to as *tendonitis*. Currently, debate exists as to whether this terminology accurately reflects the pathobiology of the condition. Recent histopathological studies of chronically affected elbow tendons have demonstrated varying underlying pathologies, suggesting that the role of inflammation in intratendinous injury may be secondary to a mechanical process of degeneration known as *tendinosis*. The term *angiofibroblastic tendinosis* has been introduced to describe the prevalence of fibroblasts and atypical vascular granulation tissue found microscopically rather than an abundance of inflammatory cells.[1] An inflammatory component may often be evident due to irritation of an affected tendon and surrounding soft tissue or as a primary response to traumatic repair.[2]

DEFINITIONS

Epicondylitis is primarily a degenerative tendinopathy caused by chronic mechanical overloading and failed healing of the involved tendon.

Lateral elbow tendinosis (lateral epicondylitis, or "tennis elbow") primarily involves degeneration of the extensor carpi radialis brevis (ECRB) tendon 1 to 2 cm distal to its origin at the lateral epicondyle.[3] Other structures that may be affected include the extensor digitorum communis (EDC) and extensor carpi radialis longus (ECRL) tendons.[4] Pain and functional weakness are the most overt clinical features associated with microscopic tears within the tendon. Symptoms usually are insidious in nature and relate to changes or faults in training, technique, or equipment. The process by which these factors could affect ECRB tendinopathy in a tennis player is illustrated in Fig. 29-1. Acute pain may also occur from a traumatic tear resulting from a single event of overload on the ECRB tendon (e.g., lifting a heavy toolbox). Biomechanical strain on the tendon can result

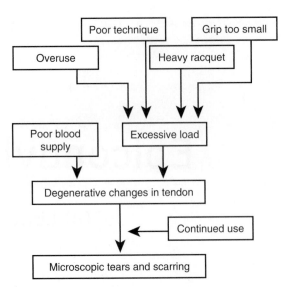

FIG. 29-1 Processes leading to development of extensor carpi radialis brevis (ECRB) tendinopathy. (Redrawn from Bell S: Elbow and forearm pain. In Bruckner P, Khan K [eds]: Clinical Sports Medicine. 2nd Ed. McGraw-Hill, Sydney, 2002, p. 278.)

from either concentrically or eccentrically applied force.[5] Provocative motions typically include repetitive wrist extension under load, forceful gripping, and static wrist extension. These movements are a common part of many sport, occupational, and leisure activities such as tennis, carpentry, bricklaying, clerical tasks, yard work, and sewing.

Medial elbow tendinosis (medial epicondylitis, or "golfer's elbow") usually involves the tendinous origin of the pronator teres, flexor carpi radialis, and palmaris longus at the medial epicondyle, although the flexor carpi ulnaris and flexor digitorum superficialis tendons may also be affected.[6] The process of degenerative tendinopathy that occurs in the flexor/pronator group essentially reflects that of the ECRB tendon at the lateral epicondyle. Upper extremity motions that involve repetitive wrist and finger flexion coupled with active pronation are typically associated with the onset of medial elbow pain and dysfunction. Activities such as overhead throwing, the tennis serve, pull-through swimming strokes, and improper golf technique during the impact phase have been implicated in the development of medial elbow tendinosis.[1,2]

TREATMENT PURPOSE

To reduce pain and restore functional strength and flexibility of the extensor muscle attachments (ECRB) to the lateral epicondyle, or of the flexor pronator origin to the medial epicondyle. Nonoperative management consists of the general principles of treatment of soft tissue injuries. Protection, relative rest, medications, splinting, and the use of modalities are recommended in the acute phase to help relieve pain. A structured rehabilitative program involving graded exercise, control of abusive force loads, modifications of technique or equipment, and counterforce bracing should allow for tendon healing and gradual return to activity.[6] Operative approaches are indicated if conservative management has failed. Persistent pain and dysfunction after

12 months of quality nonoperative care serves as a general guideline for surgery.[2,6] Excision of degenerative tissue within the involved tendon at either the lateral or medial epicondyle typically is the primary surgical purpose. Adjunctive procedures may include release of the ECRB tendon, removal of bony exostosis, and decompression of the ulnar nerve.[1-3]

TREATMENT GOALS

  I. Relief of pain and control of inflammatory mediators
 II. Restoration of flexibility and strength
III. Control of force loads to the affected muscle tendon complex
IV. Prevention of recurrence through improved technique, training, or equipment
 V. Gradual return to sport, work, or recreational activity.

NONOPERATIVE INDICATIONS/PRECAUTIONS FOR THERAPY

  I. Indications
     A. Lateral elbow tendinosis (lateral epicondylitis)
        1. Tenderness to palpation of the extensor muscle group origin—most evident in the ECRB tendon, 1 to 2 cm distal to the lateral epicondyle
        2. Pain on resisted wrist extension or supination
        3. Pain on resisted wrist extension with wrist pronated and radially deviated (Mills' test)[2]
        4. Pain with forceful grip and elbow extended (handshake test)[2,3,7]
        5. Pain with resisted extension of the middle finger
        6. Pain with passive wrist flexion or radial nerve stretch
     B. Medial elbow tendinosis (medial epicondylitis)
        1. Tenderness to palpation of the flexor/pronator group origin at or below the medial epicondyle
        2. Pain on resisted wrist flexion and resisted forearm pronation
        3. Pain with passive wrist extension
 II. Differential diagnosis[1,2]
     A. Lateral elbow pain
        1. Radial tunnel syndrome
        2. Referred pain from cervical radiculopathy or neural tension syndrome
        3. Synovitis of the radiohumeral joint
        4. Radiohumeral bursitis
        5. Osteochondritis dissecans (OCD) of the capitellum or radius (in adolescents)
        6. Humeral or radial head fracture
        7. Degenerative joint disease of the elbow
     B. Medial elbow pain
        1. Medial collateral ligament sprain
        2. Ulnar nerve compression/cubital tunnel syndrome
        3. Referred pain from cervical radiculopathy/thoracic outlet syndrome

      4. Avulsion fracture of the medial epicondyle
      5. Degenerative joint disease of the elbow
III. Precautions
    A. Allergic reactions
      1. Nonsteroidal antiinflammatory drugs (NSAIDs)
      2. Corticosteroid injection
      3. Topical steroid antiinflammatory (iontophoresis/phonophoresis)
    B. Delayed or impaired tissue healing secondary to underlying systemic disease or confounding morbidity (e.g., diabetes)

NONOPERATIVE THERAPY

I.   Acute: protection, rest, ice, compression, elevation, medications, modalities (PRICEMM)
    A. Ice several times a day—ice pack, ice water bath, ice cup massage. Application time may vary from 10 to 25 minutes, and care should be taken to avoid ice-induced neuropraxia.
    B. Promotion of relative rest and termination of the abusive activity. Wrist cock-up splints at 20 degrees extension may be used temporarily (5 to 7 days) to decrease load through the extensor tendons, but complete immobilization should be avoided because of its negative effects on tissue healing.[2,3,7] Splinting may be advisable only at night. Lateral or medial counterforce bracing may be used in conjunction with splinting or independently to control load through the injured tendon. Patients should be given proper instruction on brace use and placement to avoid skin irritation or nerve compression.
    C. Gentle active range of motion (AROM) of the elbow, wrist, and hand. Patients should be encouraged to maintain normal cervical and shoulder ROM, especially if protective posturing caused by pain is observed.
    D. Restrict aggravating motions or postures, such as forceful grasping, pinching, and fine finger movements.
    E. Gentle transverse friction massage or augmented soft tissue mobilization (ASTM)[8]
    F. Electrical stimulation for pain control and edema
    G. Antiinflammatory modalities, iontophoresis, phonophoresis
    H. Submaximal pain-free multiangle isometrics for wrist extensors/flexors
    I. NSAIDs or steroid injections
II. Chronic
    A. Continued control of abusive forces through the forearm. Modification of intensity, frequency, and duration of repetitive gripping and lifting activities involving the wrist extensors and flexors.
    B. Counterforce brace may be used for lateral epicondylitis and medial epicondylitis (Fig. 29-2). Care should be taken not to compress the ulnar nerve.
    C. Modalities: Superficial heat (hot pack) or deep heat (ultrasound) may be considered before stretching or manual therapy, cold therapy (ice pack, ice cup massage) after activity.

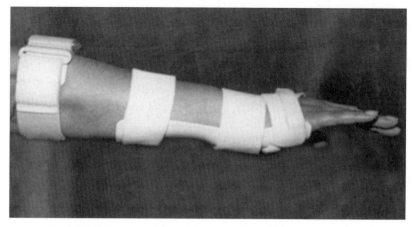

FIG. 29-2 Cock-up splint with tennis elbow counterforce brace.

Electrical stimulation may be used in conjunction with either heat or cold to manage pain.

D. Deep transverse friction massage, manual therapy[8]

E. Stretching
1. Lateral epicondylitis: wrist flexion, pronation; elbow extension.
2. Medial epicondylitis: wrist extension, supination; elbow flexion.
3. General upper extremity and cervical stretches should include upper trapezius, levator scapulae, latissimus dorsi, pectoralis major and minor, sternocleidomastoid, and scalenes.

F. Progressive strengthening program to increase strength and endurance of the entire upper quarter. Initially, the program should focus on the hand, wrist, and elbow complex; then it should be expanded to include muscles of the shoulder and back as well as the scapular stabilizers. Frequency, intensity, and duration of training should be monitored and adjusted in response to pain and fatigue levels. Patients should be given sport-specific or work-specific interval training programs to guide return to activity when appropriate.

G. Education about provocative postures of the hand and wrist during tasks involving lifting, computer work, sports, fine finger motions, and gripping.

H. Modification of equipment or tools. Patients should be provided with instruction in good overall body mechanics and ergonomic workstations to reduce force loads.

I. NSAIDs or steroid injection as appropriate.

III. Prevention
A. Promotion of general health and fitness. The strength, endurance, and flexibility of the wrist extensors and or flexors should be maintained or increased. Overall aerobic and anaerobic conditioning should be encouraged to minimize the opportunity for soft tissue injury.[1,2] Patients should be educated on principles of general stretching and active warm-up before participation in sports or manual work.

B. Ergonomic analysis of worksite conditions and tools
C. Sports equipment modification: proper grip size for tennis racquets and golf clubs. Length, weight, and tension force of equipment should be matched with the physical ability and skills of the individual.
D. Optimal technique through proper posture and positioning during work and sports. Biomechanical analysis and sport-specific coaching may help to reduce the effect of abnormal and chronic compensatory patterns.

NONOPERATIVE COMPLICATIONS

I.   Continued pain and dysfunction.

OPERATIVE INDICATIONS/TECHNIQUES

I.   Operative indication: Failure of a quality rehabilitative program after 12 months.[2,6] This serves a general guideline and may vary by surgeon according to the patient's level of pain and dysfunction and the presence of comorbidities.
II. Operative techniques may vary by surgeon and by type of pathology present. Most surgeries involve excision of pathological tissue and removal of abnormal bone growth if appropriate.[1-3] Ulnar nerve decompression at the medial epicondyle may be performed to alleviate nerve symptoms, and tendon repair may be indicated for acute ruptures.

POSTOPERATIVE INDICATIONS FOR THERAPY

I.   Postoperative therapy initially involves management of the stages of acute inflammation and repair according to the treatment principles for soft tissue injuries. Patients present with severe localized pain, edema, and dysfunction related to surgical trauma. Rehabilitation should progress over a period of 2 to 3 months to address flexibility and strength.

POSTOPERATIVE THERAPY

Postoperative therapy may vary according to type of surgical procedure performed as well as the level of tissue quality existing both preoperatively and postoperatively. It is recommended that the treating therapist communicate with the surgeon regarding progression and intensity of therapeutic activities to promote optimal tissue healing.

I.   Use of ice and antiinflammatory medication. Pain control with appropriate modalities.
II. A removable elbow immobilizer is indicated for a short period after surgery (usually 6 to 10 days). The elbow is usually kept in a 90-degree position with the forearm in a neutral position.[3]
III. AROM of wrist and hand immediately postoperatively. AROM of the elbow should begin within 48 hours and increase as tolerated. Normal shoulder and cervical ROM should be maintained. Light ADL's may be resumed, symptoms permitting.

IV. Progressive resistive exercise should begin at 3 weeks postoperatively with use of a counterforce brace.[3] Use of the brace may be
indicated for 2 months during the strengthening phase. It may be
advisable to begin with isometric strengthening, with progression
to isotonic activity starting with 1 lb. Full active ROM of the hand,
wrist, and elbow should be achieved.

V. Scar management

VI. Functional sport-specific training and eccentric exercise may be
incorporated at 4 to 6 weeks. Upper-extremity closed kinetic chain
activity may also be initiated, with care taken to avoid excessive
loading.

VII. Return to unrestricted activities and light work at 2 months.
Return to competitive athletics or manual work may take
4 to 6 months.[3]

POSTOPERATIVE COMPLICATIONS

I. Infection

II. Recurrent pain and weakness

III. Iatrogenic harm to ligaments or nerves

EVALUATION TIMELINE

I. Initial evaluation

A. Nonoperative
1. AROM and flexibility—hand, wrist, elbow, shoulder and neck
if warranted
2. Pain and related functional impairments
3. Strength of wrist and elbow musculature if pain is low level
and not progressive. Assess proximal muscles in shoulder
and scapula.

B. Operative
1. Pain, edema, bruising, surgical incisions
2. AROM of wrist, hand, shoulder, and neck. Assess elbow
AROM 48 hours postoperatively.

II. Reevaluation

A. Nonoperative: weekly to every other week, depending on
symptoms or progression of strengthening.

B. Operative: biweekly in the initial phase. Passive range of motion
(PROM) and baseline strength may be assessed at 3 weeks.
Patients need functional screening for strength and flexibility
at 2 to 4 months postoperatively for return to work, sports, or
recreational activity.

OUTCOMES

As the rehabilitation sciences evolve through clinical trials, clinicians must
be able to demonstrate the effectiveness of their interventions. Relating
clinical experience to clinical research in today's evidence-based climate has
made treatment of chronic tendinopathy of the elbow more challenging for
the therapist. Numerous conflicting studies have been published regarding
the efficacy of bracing, splinting, therapeutic modalities, therapeutic exercise,

corticosteroid injections, and oral NSAIDs on lateral and or medial elbow tendinosis. Steroid injections and short-term use of either counterforce bracing or splinting appear to have some beneficial effect on pain during the early phases of treatment.[9] The degree to which bracing affects abusive force loads through tendons is the subject of debate, and there are no clear guidelines for use of bracing or splinting beyond the acute phase.[10-16] In addition, the evidence is contradictory and insufficient regarding the effects of manual techniques (transverse friction massage, joint mobilization) and therapeutic modalities (e.g., ultrasound, electrical stimulation, acupuncture, iontophoresis) on tendinopathy.[17-24,27] Strengthening protocols such as the one created by Nirschl and Sobel appear to have the most significant long-term functional impact in chronic cases, although there are many prognostic factors that may affect outcome (e.g., type of work or sport activity).[6,25,26] Until there is a better consensus between clinical experience and clinical research, therapeutic modalities and manual therapies should be used as an adjunct to a progressive rehabilitation program and should not be the primary focus of treatment in the chronic phase.

Surgical outcomes for recalcitrant cases of lateral or medial elbow tendinosis have shown good results regarding both pain and function. Most patients should expect to achieve 80% of their elbow ROM by 3 weeks postoperatively and full AROM by 6 weeks. Premorbid strength should return by 3 to 6 months, but patients who participate in more vigorous activity might expect their power and endurance to return gradually over a period of up to 1 year postoperatively.[3,6,23]

REFERENCES

1. Nirschl RP, Edward SA: Tennis elbow tendinosis (epicondylitis). Instruct Course Lect 53:587-598, 2004
2. Bell S: Elbow and forearm pain. In Bruckner P, Khan K (eds): Clinical Sports Medicine. 2nd Ed. McGraw-Hill, Sydney, 2002, pp. 274-291
3. Nirschl RP: Muscle and tendon trauma: tennis elbow tendinosis. In Morrey BF (ed): The Elbow and Its Disorders. 3rd Ed. WB Saunders, Philadelphia, 2000, pp. 523-535
4. Gabel GT, Morrey BF: Medial epicondylitis. In Morrey BF (ed): The Elbow and Its Disorders. 3rd Ed. WB Saunders, Philadelphia, 2000, pp. 537-542
5. Harrelson GL, Leaver-Dunn D: Elbow rehabilitation. In Andrews JR, Harrelson GL, Wilk KE (eds): Physical Rehabilitation of the Injured Athlete. 2nd Ed. WB Saunders, Philadelphia, 1998, pp. 554-585
6. Johnson B, Nirschl RP: Overuse injuries of the elbow. Orthop Phys Ther Clin North Am 10:617-634, 2001
7. Fedorczyk JM: Therapist's management of elbow tendonitis. In Mackin EJ, Callahan AD, Skirven TM, et al. (eds): Rehabilitation of the Hand and Upper Extremity. 5th Ed. Mosby, St. Louis, 2002, pp. 1271-1281
8. Hammer WI: Friction massage. In Hammer WI (ed): Functional Soft Tissue Examination and Treatment by Manual Methods. 2nd Ed. Aspen, New York, 1999, pp. 463-467
9. Borkholder CD, Hill VA, Fess EE: The efficacy of splinting for lateral epicondylitis: a systematic review. J Hand Ther 17:181-199, 2004
10. Struijs PA, Smidt N, Arola H, et al.: Orthotic devices for the treatment of tennis elbow. Cochrane Database Syst Rev (1):CD001821, 2002
11. Walther M, Kirschner S, Koenig A, et al.: Biomechanical evaluation of braces used for the treatment of epicondylitis. J Shoulder Elbow Surg 11:265-270, 2002
12. Wuori JL, Overend TJ, Kramer JF, et al.: Strength and pain measures associated with lateral epicondylitis bracing. Arch Phys Med Rehabil 79:832-837, 1998
13. Ng GYF, Chan HL: The immediate effects of tension of counterforce forearm brace on neuromuscular performance of wrist extensor muscles in subjects with lateral humeral epicondylosis. J Orthop Sports Phys Ther 34:72-78, 2004

14. Jansen CW, Olson SL, Hasson SM: The effect of use of a wrist orthosis during functional activities on surface electromyography of the wrist extensors in normal subjects. J Hand Ther 10:283-289, 1997

15. Knebel PT, Avery DW, Gebhardt TL, et al.: Effects of the forearm support band on wrist extensor muscle fatigue. J Orthop Sports Phys Ther 29:677-685, 1999

16. Struijs PA, Kerkhoffs GM, Assendelft WJ, et al.: Conservative treatment of lateral epicondylitis: brace versus physical therapy or a combination of both—a randomized clinical trial. Am J Sports Med 32:462-469, 2004

17. Smidt N, Assendelft WJ, Arola H, et al.: Effectiveness of physiotherapy for lateral epicondylitis. Ann Med 35:51-62, 2003

18. Smidt N, Assendelft WJ, van der Windt DA, et al.: Corticosteroid injections for lateral epicondylitis: a systematic review. Pain 96:23-40, 2002

19. Brosseau L, Casimiro L, Milne S, et al.: Deep transverse friction massage for treating tendonitis. Cochrane Database Syst Rev (4):CD003528, 2002

20. Smidt N, van der Windt DA, Assendelft WJ, et al.: Corticosteroid injections, physiotherapy, or a wait and see policy for lateral epicondylitis: a randomized controlled trial. Lancet 359:657-662, 2002

21. Stahl S, Kaufman T: The efficacy of an injection of steroids for medial epicondylitis: a prospective study of sixty elbows. J Bone Surg Am 79:1648-1652, 1997

22. van der Windt DA, van der Heijden GJ, van den Berg SG, et al.: Ultrasound therapy for musculoskeletal disorders: a systematic review. Pain 81:257-271, 1999

23. Roserberg N, Henderson L: Surgical treatment of resistant lateral epicondylitis: follow-up study of 19 patients after excision, release and repair of proximal common extensor tendon origin. Arch Orthop Trauma Surg 122:514-517, 2002

24. Speed CA, Nichols D, Richards C, et al.: Extracorporeal shock wave therapy for lateral epicondylitis: a double blind randomized controlled trial. J Orthop Res 20:895-898, 2002

25. Haahr JP, Andersen JH: Prognostic factors in lateral epicondylitis: a randomized trial with one year follow up in 266 new cases treated with minimal occupational intervention or the usual approach in general practice. Rheumatology (Oxf) 42: 1216-1225, 2003

26. Waugh EJ, Jaglal SB, Davis AM, et al.: Factors associated with prognosis of lateral epicondylitis after 8 weeks of physical therapy. Arch Phys Med Rehabil 85:308-318, 2004

27. Struijs PA, Damen PJ, Bakker EW, et al.: Manipulation of the wrist for management of lateral epicondylitis: a randomized pilot study. Phys Ther 83:608-616, 2003

Elbow Fractures and Dislocations 30

Jane Imle Schmidt

The elbow joint provides an essential link to the forearm, wrist, and hand, allowing the hand to be moved into position for activities of daily living (ADLs) and to transmit heavy loads.[1] The elbow joint allows the motions of flexion, extension, and forearm rotation. Injury to this joint complex can lead to loss of these motions and subsequent loss of upper extremity function.[2] The elbow joint has three articulations. The ulnohumeral joint resembles a hinge joint and allows flexion and extension, and the radio-humeral and proximal radioulnar joint (trochoid joint) allow forearm rotation.[3] Normal range of motion (ROM) is 140 degrees into flexion and 0 degrees into extension, with 75 degrees of supination and 70 degrees of pronation available. Most ADLs can be performed with a ROM of 100 degrees of motion between 30 and 130 degrees flexion and 50 degrees each of pronation and supination[3] (Fig. 30-1). Posttraumatic stiffness and pain can result after both operative and nonoperative treatment of fractures and dislocations of the elbow.[4-6] Soft tissue structures, including the medial and lateral collateral ligaments, the flexor pronator muscle groups, the extensor supinator muscle groups, and the brachialis, are all subject to damage in these injuries. The brachial artery, as well as the median, radial, and ulnar nerve, are also at risk in elbow fractures and dislocations.[7] To restore functional ROM, good communication is required between the physician and therapist. To be able to treat elbow fractures and dislocations safely and effectively, the therapist must know which structures were injured, how they were reduced or repaired, and how stable the reduction or fixation is. To prevent the adverse effects of immobilization, early active range of motion (AROM) to noninjured areas and early protective exercise for injured areas are advocated as soon as the inflammatory process and stability of reduction allow.[7,8]

DEFINITION

I. **Fractures of the distal humerus:** One third of all elbow fractures involve the distal humerus. The mechanism of injury is a fall on an outstretched hand or a direct blow in the case of epicondylar fracture.

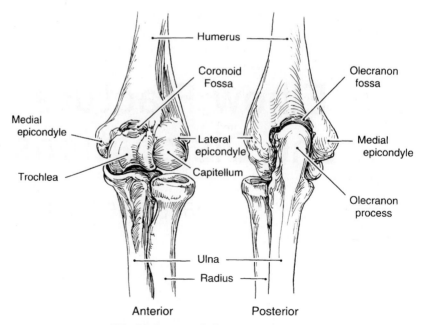

FIG. **30-1** Normal elbow anatomy (left).

Distal humeral fractures may be classified as extraarticular
(supracondylar, transcondylar, or epicondylar) or intraarticular
(T and Y condylar, lateral condylar, medial condylar, or articular
[capitellum, trochlea]). Depending on their severity, these fractures
are treated by closed manipulation or surgical stabilization.
Fractures that extend into the joint usually require open
reduction and internal fixation (ORIF)[9] (Fig. 30-2).

II. **Fractures of the proximal ulna and olecranon:** These fractures
account for one fifth of all elbow injuries in adults and typically occur
indirectly from a fall on the outstretched hand with the elbow in
some flexion, or via a direct blow to the olecranon.[10] These fractures
are classified as nondisplaced, displaced, transverse or oblique,
or comminuted. Nondisplaced fractures are managed with short
immobilization, whereas the other types require surgical
intervention[10-13] (see Fig. 30-2).

III. **Fractures of the proximal radius:** These fractures of the radial
head and neck account for almost half of all fractures about the

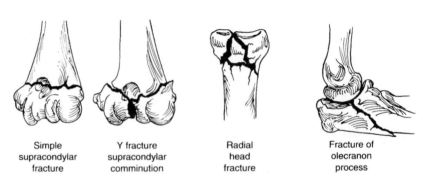

Simple	Y fracture	Radial	Fracture of
supracondylar	supracondylar	head	olecranon
fracture	comminution	fracture	process

FIG. **30-2** Elbow fractures.

elbow in the adult.[10] These fractures occur when an axial load is placed with the forearm in pronation, as in a fall on an outstretched hand. They may be classified as nondisplaced, displaced, and comminuted. Nondisplaced fractures are treated nonoperatively with early AROM. Displaced fractures may be treated nonoperatively, or they may require ORIF or prosthetic replacement. Comminuted fractures of the radial head that are not accompanied by other instabilities are usually treated by complete excision, although there is a trend toward preservation of the radial head if possible after trauma, whereas those radial head fractures that are accompanied by dislocation, ligamentous compromise, and coronoid fracture may require metal prosthetic replacement[14,15] along with medial collateral repair and reconstruction (see Fig. 30-2).

IV.   **Dislocations of the radius and/or ulna:** The elbow joint is the second most commonly dislocated joint in the body.[16] The mechanism of this injury is a fall on an outstretched hand.[16,17] Reduction of these injuries is typically closed unless they have been neglected or fail with closed manipulation, necessitating open reduction to allow sufficient stability for early mobilization.[12,18] Frequently these dislocations are accompanied by a shear fracture of the coronoid[18] (Fig. 30-3). A common pattern of chronic elbow instability is posterolateral rotary instability, which varies in degree of displacement from subluxation to full dislocation with the coronoid behind the humerus.[18] Posterolateral elbow instability and valgus instability usually require reconstruction with a tendon graft. Soft tissue disruption progresses from the lateral side of the elbow, involving the lateral collateral ligament and extensor group, to the medial side, involving the medial collateral ligament and flexor group, with the level of disruption depending on the severity of the disclocation.[18]

V.   **Fractures associated with dislocations**

A. **Monteggia lesions** include all ulnar fractures associated with dislocations of the radiocapitellar articulation. They are divided

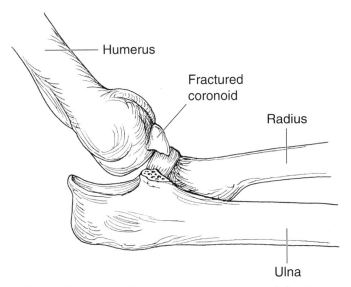

FIG. 30-3 Coronoid fracture with posterior elbow dislocation.

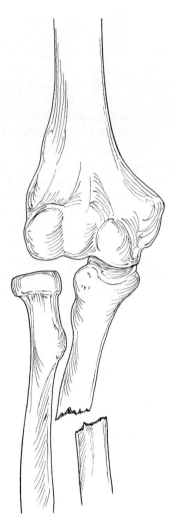

FIG. 30-4 Monteggia fracture.

into four types, with type I (anterior angulation and anterior dislocation of the radial head) being the most common and the only type discussed here[19] (Fig. 30-4). These lesions are relatively uncommon but can cause serious problems. The mechanism of injury may be a direct blow to the ulnar aspect of the forearm or a fall with hyperpronation or hyperextension.[20] Closed methods may be used to treat young patients, but ORIF of the ulna and either closed or open reduction of the radial head is required in adults.[20,21]

B. The **Essex-Lopresti fracture** includes a fracture of the radial head, disruption of the interosseous membrane, and instability of the distal radioulnar joint (DRUJ). In this injury, the brachialis muscle can be torn from its insertion and the brachial artery and the median nerve can also be damaged. The mechanism of injury is a forceful fall onto an outstretched hand, and surgical management is required.[22]

C. **Complex fractures with elbow dislocations** occur when the elbow is protruding from a car window and is struck by an oncoming car or a fixed object. Many different combinations of fractures and soft tissue injuries may be produced, but the most common is an open fracture of the olecranon, anterior dislocation of the head of the radius and the distal fragment of the ulna, and a comminuted fracture of the humerus. Treatment for these injuries is always surgical and involves internal and/or external fixation of the fracture. Other high-energy trauma (e.g., gunshot wounds) can necessitate the use of external fixators to provide stability to the elbow. Either static external fixation or dynamic hinged external fixation, which allows mobilization, can be used.[23,24] Soft tissue coverage is also a component of treatment for these injuries.

SURGICAL PURPOSE

Fractures and dislocations that interrupt the normal elbow anatomy may interfere with effective joint motion and have the potential to cause pain. The elbow joint is complex and allows not only for flexion and extension but also for forearm pronation and supination through the radial head capitellar articulation. Unless normal anatomical relationships are restored after injury, severe limitations of elbow movement will occur. This will impair the individual's ability to carry out ADLs and to hold productive jobs in the workforce.

TREATMENT GOALS

I. Nonoperative
   A. Control edema.
   B. Maintain ROM of uninvolved joints.
   C. Initiate early protective exercise for the injured joints.
   D. Avoid positions of instability.
   E. Return to previous level of function.
II. Operative
   A. Control edema.
   B. Promote wound healing.
   C. Control scar formation.
   D. Maintain ROM of uninvolved joints.
   E. Initiate early protective exercise for the injured joints.
   F. Avoid positions of instability.
   G. Return to previous level of function.

NONOPERATIVE INDICATIONS/PRECAUTIONS FOR THERAPY

I. Indications: Elbow fractures and/or dislocations that have achieved stability through closed techniques
II. Precautions
   A. Associated muscle and/or ligamentous injury
   B. Associated nerve or blood vessel injury
   C. Unresolved hematoma and/or edema
   D. Unstable reduction or history of recurrent dislocations.

NONOPERATIVE THERAPY

Vigorous stretching, whether active or passive, is never permitted in the rehabilitation of elbow fractures and dislocations. These techniques can result in increased periarticular hemorrhage and fibrosis, causing decreased ROM, and can lead to complications of myositis ossificans and the formation of heterotopic bone.[7,8,21,25,26] However, early AROM is advocated to prevent the all too common complication of elbow stiffness. Communication with the physician is necessary to determine when fractures are stable enough to withstand AROM and which ranges constitute the "safe zone" (the ROM that creates no displacement of the fracture or subluxation). This communication allows the therapist to develop the most beneficial therapeutic protocol for each particular patient.[7,8] Continuous passive motion (CPM) machines and hinged elbow splints (commercial or custom-fabricated) allow protected motion while preventing medial and lateral instability.[27,28] Dynamic and static progressive splinting can also be helpful to improve ROM, but timing of the initiation of these devices needs to be determined in collaboration with the physician based on fracture stability, healing, and where the patient is in the inflammatory process.[27-29] Properly used, these devices can be valuable adjuncts to a therapy program. Timelines for strengthening, return to work, and sports/leisure skills need to be determined by the physician based on radiographic union. Fracture union is paramount, because elbow stiffness is easier to manage than loss of skeletal stability and joint alignment.

I. Therapy after distal humeral fractures treated with closed manipulation

    A. Extraarticular supracondylar and transcondylar fractures are immobilized in a posterior splint with the elbow flexed to approximately 90 degrees and the forearm neutral for a period of 2 to 6 weeks, depending on the stability of the fracture. Gentle AROM into flexion can be started at 2 to 3 weeks, with a gradual increase into extension. Strengthening can begin after clearance by the physician has been received.

    B. Medial epicondylar fractures are immobilized in a posterior splint with the elbow flexed to 90 degrees, the forearm in pronation, and the wrist in slight flexion to relax the flexor/pronator muscle group. These fractures are immobilized for 1 to 2 weeks, after which gentle AROM is initiated, with progression to strengthening activities as directed by the physician.

    C. Lateral epicondylar fractures are rare in adults, and treatment consists of immobilization of the elbow in 90 degrees of flexion, with the forearm in supination and the wrist extended to relax the muscles that originate from the fracture surface. Immobilization is for 1 to 2 weeks and is followed by gentle AROM, with progression to strengthening activities as directed by the physician.

    D. Intraarticular T and Y condylar fractures are treated by 3 weeks of immobilization with the elbow in 90 degrees of flexion, followed by splinting with intermittent gentle active mobilization for another 2 to 3 weeks, and progression to strengthening activities as directed by the physician. Displaced fractures of these types require surgical intervention, and their postoperative therapy is described later. Recent practice has changed in that elderly patients may receive surgical treatment, but the so-called "bag of bones" technique is also used. This technique uses compressive manipulation of the distal articular fragments. The elbow is immobilized in as much flexion as possible without compromising circulation for 2 weeks, with AROM into flexion starting at the end of this period. The hand and wrist are mobilized from the day of injury and the shoulder within 2 weeks. At 4 weeks, the elbow should have a 90-degree arc of motion. The patient progresses to a sling, which is adjusted to allow more elbow extension as tolerated, with the sling being discontinued by 6 weeks.

E. Medial and lateral condylar fractures that are undisplaced are splinted or casted for 4 to 5 weeks with the elbow in flexion. These fractures may become displaced, resulting in limitations in motion and arthritis; therefore, communication is needed with the physician to proceed safely with rehabilitation.

F. Capitellar fractures usually are treated with ORIF, as described later.

II. Therapy after fractures of the proximal ulna and olecranon

A. Undisplaced fractures are immobilized in a posterior splint with midflexion of the elbow and neutral forearm rotation. Gentle ROM should begin after 7 to 10 days. Flexion greater than 90 degrees is avoided for 3 to 6 weeks, until bony union is complete. After union is evident, the patient may progress to gentle resistive activities.

B. Displaced fractures usually are treated with surgical management as described later; however, in elderly patients who are not surgical candidates they may be treated with closed methods. The elbow is immobilized in 90 degrees of flexion for a period of 4 weeks, followed by gentle AROM and progression to passive range of motion (PROM) and resistive exercises after healing is evident radiographically.

III. Therapy after fractures of the proximal radius

A. Undisplaced and minimally displaced radial head fractures are managed with immediate AROM or are immobilized in flexion for a period of 5 days to 3 weeks, followed by AROM and progression to strengthening activities as directed by the physician. A loss of full elbow extension may be expected, and displacement can sometimes occur with early motion. Loose bodies can also be problematic with these injuries.

IV. Therapy after dislocations of the radius and/or ulna

A. These dislocations are immobilized in a posterior plaster splint in 90 degrees of elbow flexion and neutral forearm rotation. Circulatory status and neurological status are closely monitored during the first 24 hours for signs of ischemia and compartment syndrome. Motion in the uninvolved joints is begun on the day after reduction, and gentle active flexion from the splint may start during the first week. The physician may be able to indicate a safe zone (i.e., ROM not producing subluxation) for AROM so that a thermoplastic splint, blocking extension at the end of the safe zone, can be fabricated. If no subluxation is evident with extension at week 3, unprotected flexion and extension exercises may be initiated, with progression to strengthening exercises, particularly of the triceps. At 10 to 12 weeks, if an extension loss is still apparent, static progressive splinting may be initiated. Chronic instability is unusual with these injuries.

V. Therapy after fractures associated with dislocation: see Postoperative Therapy.

NONOPERATIVE COMPLICATIONS

I. Loss of motion and need for subsequent surgical procedures to restore motion
II. Nerve injury
III. Malunion
IV. Instability of the fracture and/or recurrent dislocation
V. Vascular injuries and compartment syndrome
VI. Myositis ossificans
VII. Heterotopic ossification
VIII. Nonunion
IX. Residual pain
X. Posttraumatic arthritis
XI. Reflex sympathetic dystrophy

POSTOPERATIVE INDICATIONS/PRECAUTIONS FOR THERAPY

I. Indications: Elbow fractures and/or dislocations that have achieved stability through surgical techniques
II. Precautions
A. Associated muscle and/or ligamentous injury
B. Associated nerve or blood vessel injury
C. Unresolved hematoma and/or edema
D. Unstable reduction or history of recurrent dislocations

POSTOPERATIVE THERAPY

Vigorous stretching, whether active or passive, is never permitted in the rehabilitation of elbow fractures and dislocations. These techniques can result in increased periarticular hemorrhage and fibrosis, causing decreased ROM, and can lead to complications of myositis ossificans and the formation of heterotopic bone.[7,8,21,25,26] However, early AROM is advocated to prevent the all too common complication of postoperative elbow stiffness. In addition, with the newer generation of implants, early ROM can be initiated. Communication with the surgeon is necessary to determine when fractures are stable enough to withstand AROM and which ranges constitute the safe zone (i.e., the range of motion that creates no displacement of the fracture or subluxation). This communication allows the therapist to develop the most beneficial therapeutic protocol for each particular patient.[7,8] CPM machines and hinged elbow splints (commercial or custom-fabricated) allow protected motion while preventing medial and lateral instability.[27,28] Dynamic and static progressive splinting can also be helpful to improve ROM, but timing of the initiation of these devices needs to be determined in collaboration with the physician based on fracture stability,

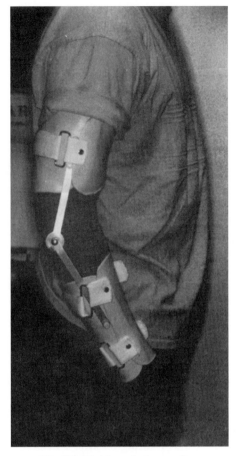

FIG. **30-5** Hinged elbow splint.

healing, and where the patient is in the inflammatory process.[27-29] These devices can be valuable adjuncts to a therapy program (Fig. 30-5). Timelines for strengthening, return to work, and sports/leisure skills need to be determined by the physician based on radiographical union.

I. Therapy after distal humeral fractures treated with surgical stabilization

A. Extraarticular supracondylar and transcondylar fractures that require limited open reduction or percutaneous pinning are immobilized in less elbow flexion than is used with closed methods. The ulnar nerve is usually transposed in these fractures. Gentle AROM into flexion may begin at 2 to 3 weeks, with a gradual increase into elbow extension. Some surgeons prefer earlier AROM or CPM if the fixation is stable. Strengthening may begin after clearance by the surgeon is received.

B. Medial epicondylar fracture: see Nonoperative Therapy.

C. Lateral epicondylar fracture: see Nonoperative Therapy.

D. Intraarticular T and Y condylar fractures that require fixation with screws and Kirschner wires or full exposure with plating of the fracture are splinted in 45 to 90 degrees of elbow flexion postoperatively and are kept elevated. Those fractures requiring full exposure may involve osteotomy of the proximal ulna or release or reflection of the triceps and transposition of the ulnar nerve. Depending on bone quality and stability of the hardware, as indicated by the surgeon, gentle AROM may begin in 3 to 5 days. If bone quality is poor, or if there is question about the stability of the fixation, immobilization will last longer. Once mobilization is allowed, the patient is encouraged to use the extremity in light ADLs, with protective splinting continued between exercise sessions. Patients who have undergone an osteotomy of the proximal ulna and release of the triceps need to avoid active or forceful extension and flexion for 6 weeks because of the stress these actions would place on the extensor mechanism repair. Strengthening is begun at 6 weeks or at the time the fracture demonstrates healing radiographically. Patients whose bone stock is poor, or who have severe destruction of the joint and supporting structures, may be candidates for an elbow arthroplasty. This surgery and rehabilitation is discussed in Chapter 32.

E. Patients with medial and lateral condylar fractures stabilized with screws and/or Kirschner wires may begin AROM 5 to 10 days postoperatively, with the extremity splinted in flexion between exercise sessions for 3 to 5 weeks. If a medial condylar fracture requires plating, the ulnar nerve is usually transposed anteriorly; this possibility should be considered in the rehabilitation.

F. Capitellar fractures treated with surgical reduction and secure fixation (or, rarely, surgical excision) are immobilized in a posterior splint, with AROM into flexion, limited extension, and pronation, begun during the first operative week. Supination exercises are avoided during the first 4 weeks because of the stress they place on the repaired lateral collateral ligament. The patient should also avoid full extension for the first 3 weeks, because this motion generates a shear force across the fracture site. Strengthening is delayed until at least 6 weeks postoperatively.

II. Therapy after fracture of the proximal ulna and olecranon

A. Fracture of the proximal ulna is a common injury, particularly in the elderly patient population. For those fractures that are fixated with Kirschner wires, intramedullary fixation, bicortical screws, plates, or excision of the fracture fragments with reattachment of the extensor mechanism, gentle AROM may be initiated 3 to 5 days postoperatively. Extremes of motion, specifically flexion, are avoided during the first 4 weeks. The elbow may be supported in a protective splint between exercise sessions. Strengthening exercises may be started after the union is firm or at least 8 weeks postoperatively if excision has been performed.

III. Therapy after fracture of the proximal radius

A. Displaced radial head fractures may be treated with ORIF. If the fragment cannot be fixed and in the presence of ligamentous injury or instability, prosthetic replacement is now the treatment of choice over excision of the radial head. Excision of the radial head is still performed if the fracture is severely comminuted. Postoperatively, the patients are immobilized in 90 degrees of elbow flexion and neutral forearm rotation. Gentle AROM is begun at 5 to 10 days, and the patient may be moved from

a splint to a sling. At 3 weeks, the sling is removed. In the case
of a prosthetic replacement, pronation and supination is allowed,
but only with the elbow at 90 degrees of flexion for the first
6 weeks. Strengthening may begin as directed by the physician.

IV. Therapy after dislocation of the radius and/or ulna

    A. As described earlier, most of these injuries are treated by
nonsurgical means unless ligamentous repair is needed for the
elbow to be stable enough to permit early motion. If ligaments
are avulsed, they are repaired to bone with sutures; if torn, they
are reconstructed with a tendon graft. Motion usually begins
within a protective brace during the first week, with care taken
to use a forearm position that protects the repaired structures.
Patients with severe instability or chronic dislocations may be
immobilized for longer periods.[18]

V. Therapy after fractures associated with dislocations

    A. Monteggia fractures can be reduced surgically in a variety of
ways: (1) internal fixation of the ulna with closed reduction of
the radial head, (2) open reduction of the radial head and internal
fixation of the ulna, and, occasionally (3) internal fixation of
the ulna with excision of the radial head. Radial neuropathy,
particularly of the posterior interosseous branch, is frequently seen
in these fractures. Postoperatively, patients with type I fractures
are immobilized in 90 to 120 degrees of elbow flexion with
moderate forearm supination for 4 weeks. AROM is begun at
4 weeks, and gentle pronation and supination are permitted.
The patient may need to be supported in a sling or protective
splint between exercise sessions. Extension of the elbow beyond
90 degrees is not permitted until 4 to 6 weeks after surgery.

    B. Essex-Lopresti fractures can be managed with ORIF of the radial
head in conjunction with reduction of the DRUJ, repair of the
triangular fibrocartilage complex (TFCC), and pinning of the
DRUJ. If there has been severe comminution of the radial head,
a prosthetic replacement must be used with repair and pinning
of the DRUJ. Immobilization is in a Muenster cast, which allows
gentle elbow flexion and extension while preventing forearm
rotation. At 6 weeks, the pin is removed from the DRUJ and
gentle forearm rotation may begin. These patients often develop
chronic problems necessitating future reconstructions.

    C. Complex elbow fractures with dislocations and other high-energy
injuries to the elbow are frequently stabilized with an external
fixator. Initial treatment may include management of skin grafts,
free flaps, and open wounds. Therapeutic treatment depends on
the individual injury and the surgical stabilization performed.
Close communication with the surgeon is imperative for safe
and appropriate progression of these patients to prevent the vast
number of potential complications from these injuries. Nonunion,
infection, and residual pain and stiffness are frequent sequelae.

VI. Therapy after capsular release of the elbow

    A. Because a capsular release is a common secondary procedure
after elbow fracture and dislocation, it is described here. Elbow
contractures are either intrinsic, extrinsic, or mixed in nature.
Extrinsic contractures are caused by thickening of the soft tissues

(capsule, ligaments, muscle) or by heterotopic ossification. Intrinsic contractures are the result of destruction or disruption of the articular surface, including loose bodies and osteophytes.[5] Those patients who after at least 6 months have not obtained a functional ROM via active and passive exercises and a splinting regimen are considered candidates for this procedure.[5]

B. Postoperatively, ROM may begin immediately with CPM, or the surgeon may maintain the elbow splinted in the end range of motion that was lacking, with therapy initiated at 1 week postoperatively. An external fixator may be used if instability of the elbow was present on capsular release. Therapy consists of AROM/PROM exercises as well as intermittent dynamic splinting, with static splinting to maintain gains at nighttime. Modalities for pain and techniques to minimize swelling are crucial in the early stages. Therapy may be continued for up to 3 months after surgery, and splinting may continue after discharge from a formal therapy program.[5]

POSTOPERATIVE COMPLICATIONS

I.   All of the problems listed under Nonoperative Complications
II. The need for hardware removal

EVALUATION TIMELINE

I. Edema measurements are taken on initial evaluation and checked weekly thereafter until resolved or within normal limits (WNL).

II. Pain levels are measured on initial evaluation and checked at each visit during the first 2 weeks, and weekly thereafter, until resolved or WNL.

III. Sensory status is measured on initial evaluation and checked every 4 to 6 weeks, or earlier if the patient indicates a change of status.

IV. Circulatory status is determined on initial evaluation and checked at each visit during the first week.

V. AROM to the uninvolved joints is started on initial evaluation and checked weekly until WNL.

VI. AROM to the involved joints is started as described specifically for each injury and checked weekly thereafter.

VII. Strengthening exercises are started as described specifically for each injury and checked every 3 to 4 weeks thereafter.

VIII. CPM may be initiated after approval by the physician; usually, it is indicated early, with AROM in the safe zone.

IX. Static progressive splinting and dynamic splinting may be initiated after approval by the physician, usually after radiographical union is firm.

OUTCOMES

Outcomes after elbow fractures and dislocations vary widely and depend on many factors, among them the severity of the injury itself, the skill of the physician or surgeon, timely initiation of rehabilitation, patient age, patient compliance, and the skill of the therapist. Outcome tools have been developed in an attempt to predict and quantify results for these injuries.[30,31]

They take into consideration the presence of pain as well as specific daily functional activities. Unfortunately, no one tool is considered standard, and comparisons between tools are difficult and probably not meaningful. However, some generalities are seen with these injuries. The most commonly seen outcome is loss of full elbow extension. This usually is not problematic for the patient if the loss is not greater than 30 degrees. Some patients with specific ROMs needed for vocational or leisure activities require greater extension, and in these cases knowledge of the patient's requirements and mutual goal setting are important. Also common in these patients is loss of full elbow flexion. Keeping in mind that an arc of 100 degrees (between 30 and 130 degrees) is required for many ADLs (e.g., eating, grooming), a therapy program should not sacrifice a functional range of elbow flexion to gain further extension.[3] The best way to avoid or minimize these unfortunate outcomes is through prevention. Good communication with the referring physician allows the therapist to appropriately guide and safely progress each patient through his or her individual rehabilitation program.

REFERENCES

1. Werner FW, An K: Biomechanics of the elbow and forearm. Hand Clin 10:357, 1994
2. Bass RL, Stern PJ: Elbow and forearm anatomy and surgical approaches. Hand Clin 10:343, 1994
3. Morrey BF, An K: Functional evaluation of the elbow. In Morrey BF (ed): The Elbow and Its Disorders. WB Saunders, Philadelphia, 2000, p. 74
4. Weiss AC, Sachar K: Soft tissue contracture about the elbow. Hand Clin 10:439, 1994
5. Vardakas DG, Varitimidis SE, Goebel F, et al.: Evaluating and treating the stiff elbow. Hand Clin 18:77, 2002
6. Morrey BF: Extrinsic contracture: "the column procedure," lateral and medial capsular releases. In Morrey BF (ed): The Elbow and Its Disorders. WB Saunders, Philadelphia, 2000, p. 447
7. Nirschl RP, Morrey BF: Rehabilitation. In Morrey BF (ed): The Elbow and Its Disorders. WB Saunders, Philadelphia, 2000, p. 141
8. Brach P: Reconstruction of the elbow: therapist's commentary. J Hand Ther 12:73, 1999
9. Jupiter JB, Morrey BF: Fractures of the distal humerus in adults. In Morrey BF (ed): The Elbow and Its Disorders. WB Saunders, Philadelphia, 2000, p. 293
10. Nicholson DA, Driscoll PA: The elbow. BMJ 307:1058, 1993
11. McKay PL, Katarincic JA: Fracture of the proximal ulna olecranon and coronoid fractures. Hand Clin 18:43, 2002
12. Bailey CS, MacDermid J, Patterson SD, et al.: Outcome of plate fixation of olecranon fractures. J Orthop Trauma 15:542, 2001
13. Nork SE, Jones CB, Henley MB: Surgical treatment of olecranon fractures. Am J Orthop 30:577, 2001
14. Morrey, BF: Radial head fracture. In Morrey BF (ed): The Elbow and Its Disorders. WB Saunders, Philadelphia, 2000, p. 341
15. Ring D, Jupiter JB, Zilberfarb J: Posterior dislocation of the elbow with fractures of the radial head and coronoid. J Bone J Surg Am 84:547, 2002
16. Royle SG: Posterior dislocation of the elbow. Clin Orthop 269:201, 1991
17. O'Driscoll SW, Morrey BF, Korinek S: Elbow subluxation and dislocation: a spectrum of instability. Clin Orthop 280:186, 1992
18. O'Driscoll SW: Elbow instability. Hand Clin 10:405, 1994
19. Bado JL: The Monteggia lesion. Clin Orthop 50:71, 1967
20. Regan WD, Morrey BF: Coronoid process and Monteggia fractures. In Morrey BF (ed): The Elbow and Its Disorders. WB Saunders, Philadelphia, 2000, p. 396
21. Crenshaw AH: Campbell's Operative Orthopedics. 8th Ed. Mosby, St. Louis, 1992
22. Morgan WJ, Breen TF: Complex fractures of the forearm. Hand Clin 10:375, 1994
23. Morrey BF, Hotchkiss RN: External fixators of the elbow. In Morrey BF (ed): The Elbow and Its Disorders. WB Saunders, Philadelphia, 2000, p. 457

24. Nielsen D, Nowinski RJ, Bamberger HB: Indications, alternatives, and complications of external fixation about the elbow. Hand Clin 18:87, 2002
25. Morrey BF: Ectopic ossification about the elbow. In Morrey BF (ed): The Elbow and Its Disorders. WB Saunders, Philadelphia, 2000, p. 437
26. Ilahi OA, Strausser DW, Gabel, GT: Post-traumatic heterotopic ossification about the elbow. Orthopedics 21:265, 1998
27. O'Driscoll SW: Continuous passive motion. In Morrey BF (ed): The Elbow and Its Disorders. WB Saunders, Philadelphia, 2000, p. 147
28. Morrey BF: Splints and bracing at the elbow. In Morrey BF (ed): The Elbow and Its Disorders. WB Saunders, Philadelphia, 2000, p. 150
29. Lee MJ, LaStayo PC, vonKersburg AE: A supination splint worn distal to the elbow: a radiographic, electromyographic, and retrospective report. J Hand Ther 16:190, 2003
30. Hudak PL, Amadio PC, Bombardier C: Development of an upper extremity outcome measure: the DASH (Disabilities of the Arm, Shoulder, and Hand). The Upper Extremity Collaborative Group (UECG). Am J Indust Med 29:602, 1996
31. Morrey BF: Functional evaluation of the elbow. In Morrey BF (ed): The Elbow and Its Disorders. WB Saunders, Philadelphia, 1993, p. 86

SUGGESTED READINGS

Bell SN, Morrey BF, Bianco AJ Jr: Chronic posterior subluxation and dislocation of the radial head. J Bone J Surg Am 73:392, 1991

Goodwin RC: Pediatric elbow and forearm fractures requiring surgical treatment. Hand Clin 18:135, 2002

Inglis AE: The rehabilitation of the elbow after injury. Instr Course Lect 40:45, 1991

Jupiter JB: Heterotopic ossification about the elbow. Instr Course Lect 40:41, 1991

Lee DH: Treatment options for complex elbow fracture dislocations. Injury 32SD:41, 2001

McKee MD, Jupiter JB: A contemporary approach to the management of complex fractures of the distal humerus and their sequelae. Hand Clin 10:479, 1994

McKee MD, Kim J, Kebaish K, et al.: Functional outcome after open supracondylar fractures of the humerus. J Bone J Surg Br 82:646, 2000

Ring D, Jupiter JB: Fracture-dislocation of the elbow. Hand Clin 18:55, 2002

Rizzo M, Nunley JA: Fractures of the elbow's lateral column radial head and capitellum. Hand Clin 18:21, 2002

Rockwood CA, Green DP, Bucholz RW: Rockwood and Green's Fractures in Adults. 3rd Ed. JB Lippincott, Philadelphia, 1991

Scheckendantz MS: Diagnosis and treatment of elbow disorders in the overhead athlete. Hand Clin 18:65, 2002

Sponseller PD: Problem elbow fractures in children. Hand Clin 10:495, 1994

Zimmerman NB: Clinical application of advances in elbow and forearm anatomy and biomechanics. Hand Clin 18:1, 2002

Elbow Arthroscopy **31**

Frank DiGiovannantonio

Injuries to the elbow can have serious functional consequences in the affected limb. The primary function of the elbow is to place the hand in space, allowing the arm to function as a stabilizer for power and also allowing for fine motor function.[1] The radiohumeral, the ulnohumeral, and the proximal radioulnar joints comprise the three articulations of the elbow which allow flexion/extension and supination/pronation. Even the slightest insult to these joints, including controlled insults such as surgery, can lead to a loss of range of motion (ROM), strength, and function of the affected limb.[1] In an effort to minimize trauma to this very sensitive joint, the concept of arthroscopy has begun to gain popularity in the treatment of some diagnoses that might normally require open surgical technique.

Arthroscopy is being used with increasing frequency to both diagnose and treat many elbow disorders.[2] Some of the proposed advantages of elbow arthroscopy include decreased scarring, decreased postoperative pain, less risk of infection, and, in some cases, better visualization.[2,3] Open surgery often requires extensive dissection and muscle splitting, which may delay rehabilitation.[4] Conversely, arthroscopy causes less surgical morbidity and often allows patients to begin therapy more comfortably immediately after surgery.[4] However, because arthroscopy of the elbow is technically more difficult and poses greater risks than arthroscopy of larger joints, this procedure is not widely used[3] (Figs. 31-1, 31-2 , and 31-3).

The relative complications with arthroscopy of the elbow and the appropriate use of this surgical technique with certain diagnoses have been discussed in the literature.[2-13] This chapter discusses some common pathologies of the elbow that are often treated through the use of arthroscopy.

DEFINITIONS

I. **Diagnostic evaluation:** Arthroscopy can be a useful tool in the evaluation of the chronically painful elbow if a definitive diagnosis is unclear.[6] The minimally invasive nature of arthroscopy makes it a beneficial tool in the evaluation of articular cartilage and may

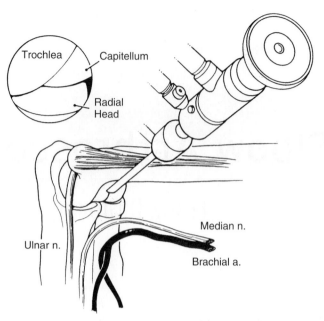

FIG. **31-1** The proximal medial portal view provides a view of the anterior joint. (From Green D: Operative Hand Surgery. 3rd Ed. Churchill-Livingstone, New York, 1993.)

aid the surgeon in determining the most appropriate level of intervention for the patient.[6]

II. **Removal of loose bodies:** The relatively high congruency of the elbow joint, its unique response to joint trauma, and the close interrelationship of the joint capsule with extracapsular muscles predispose the elbow to stiffness.[13] The presence of loose bodies, whether they be bony or soft tissue, can significantly decrease elbow and forearm ROM, causing pain and ultimately limiting an individual's ability to function. The minimally invasive nature of arthroscopy allows removal of these obstructions with less morbidity to the surrounding tissues, often ensuring faster recovery and return to full activity.[4]

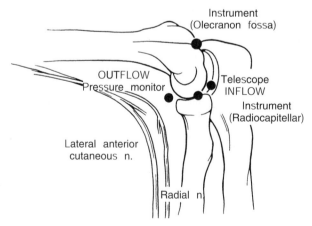

FIG. **31-2** The lateral portal is used to view the olecranon fossa and the posterior radiocapitellar joint. (From Green D: Operative Hand Surgery. 3rd Ed. Churchill-Livingstone, New York, 1993.)

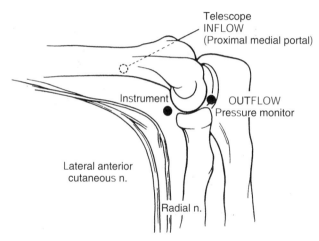

FIG. 31-3 Lateral portals used for anterior joint visualization. (From Green D: Operative Hand Surgery. 3rd Ed. Churchill-Livingstone, New York, 1993.)

III. **Osteochondritis dissecans:** This condition is characterized by damage or lesions to the articular surface of a joint.[14] In the elbow, the capitellum is most often involved.[9,14] Symptoms include elbow pain with activity, a dull aching pain at rest, catching, and locking.[9] This condition is most often seen in adolescents and athletes involved in overhead throwing sports or weight-bearing activities such as gymnastics.[9,12] Conservative treatment typically involves rest and pain management.[9,12] The best prognosis for this condition occurs with early diagnosis and management.[9,12] If left untreated, it can be a potentially disabling condition, leading to a loss of motion, prolonged pain, and an eventual loss of function. Surgical intervention is indicated if conservative treatment fails and is often dictated by the size and location of the lesion, the stability of the fragment, and the preference of the treating physician.[9] Surgical intervention ranges from removal of loose bodies to subchondral drilling, bone grafting, and periosteal transplantation.[9] In the elbow, the most common form of treatment involves the debridement of loose bodies, abrasion chondroplasty, or both.

IV. **Synovectomy:** This procedure is typically performed for patients who have some form of inflammatory disease, such as arthritis. It is often used to delay or postpone the need for total elbow arthroplasty. Either a portion or the entire synovium is removed, to prevent further destruction of the joint and to remove any soft tissue that may block motion because of its bulk.[2]

V. **Capsular release for contractures of the elbow:** The elbow's relatively small capsular volume predisposes the joint to loss of motion with relatively minor effusion, scarring, and thickening.[8] In the contracted elbow, the goal of surgery is to fully resect all pathological tissue and spare the critical ligaments.[8] Surgery is generally indicated for patients whose elbow ROM did not improve with a 3- to 6-month course of physical or occupational therapy and whose lack of motion interferes with activities of daily living (ADLs).[4-6] Morrey[14] described elbow contracture as being caused by intrinsic or extrinsic factors.

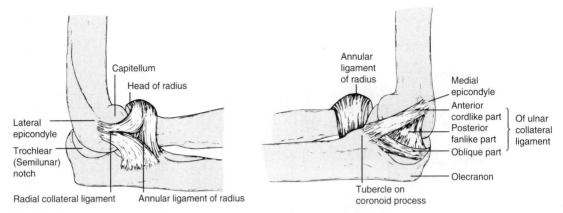

FIG. **31-4** Ligamentous/capsular anatomy of the elbow. (From Mehne DK, Jupiter JB: Fractures of the distal humerus. In Browner BD, Jupiter JM, Levine AM, et al. [eds]: Skeletal Trauma. WB Saunders, Philadelphia, 1992.)

Extrinsic factors include contractures of the joint capsule or collateral ligaments as well as extraarticular malunions. Intrinsic contractures are characterized by irregularity or incongruency of the elbow's bony anatomy. As a general rule, intrinsic contractures frequently have an extrinsic or capsular component[7] (Fig. 31-4).

VI. **Arthroscopic lateral release:** Chronic lateral epicondylitis can also be treated through arthroscopic debridement or release of the lateral epicondyle. (Please refer to the postoperative management section of Chapter 29.)

SURGICAL PURPOSE

Elbow arthroscopy is used to investigate the extent of damage to the cartilage of the elbow without making an extensive incision. Increasingly elbow arthroscopy is used for treatment, including removal of loose bodies, debridement of abnormal synovium, removal of bone spurs, and treatment of lateral epicondylitis. It may also be used to treat infections by irrigation.

TREATMENT GOALS

 I.   Increase/restore ROM to the elbow and forearm.
 II. Decrease pain.
III. Control edema.
 IV. Maintain ROM of the uninvolved joints.
  V. Prevent infection.
 VI. Restore maximum functional capacity.

OPERATIVE INDICATIONS/PRECAUTIONS

  I. Indications
      A. Rheumatoid arthritis[2,4-6]
      B. Degenerative arthritis[2,4-6]
      C. Chronic pain[2,6]

        D. A loss of ROM that interferes with ADLs[4,6]

        E. Disruption of the articular cartilage[5]

        F. Loose bodies[2,4-6]

II.   Precautions

        A. Prior nerve injury, transposition, or repair

        B. Prior elbow fracture or trauma[4-6]

        C. Severe elbow capsular fibrosis

        D. Bridging heterotopic bone[5]

POSTOPERATIVE INDICATIONS/PRECAUTIONS FOR THERAPY

I.   Indications

        A. Edema

        B. Loss of elbow and forearm ROM

        C. Disproportionate pain

        D. Need for static, dynamic, or static progressive splinting

        E. Limited ROM of the uninvolved joints

        F. Nerve paralysis

II.   Precautions

        A. Neurovascular repair

        B. Tendon repair

        C. Muscle lengthening

        D. Collateral ligament repair

        E. Collateral ligament release

        F. Radial head subluxation/instability

        G. Nerve transposition

POSTOPERATIVE THERAPY

I.   Therapy after arthroscopic capsular release, synovectomy, removal of loose bodies, and treatment of osteochondritis dissecans: The goal with all of these procedures is to restore a functional arc of motion and relieve pain. This will allow the patient to perform ADLs and to return to gainful employment or sport activities with limited or no pain in the elbow.

        A. Week 1: During the first postoperative week, the elbow is dressed in a light compressive dressing, and the importance of edema and pain management is stressed. All precautions should be taken to avoid causing excessive pain and edema, which may prevent the patient from performing ROM exercises. The therapist should communicate with surgeon regarding ROM goals. Elbow stability or instability should be determined. Postoperative subluxation is not uncommon with elbow injuries.

           1. Immediately begin full active range of motion (AROM) and passive range of motion (PROM) of all uninvolved joints.

           2. Begin immediate AROM, active-assisted range of motion (AAROM), and gentle PROM of the elbow and forearm. Although increasing ROM is the primary goal at this time, one should exercise caution to avoid increasing edema and inflammation of the joint capsule, which may further decrease ROM.[12]

        3. All therapy sessions should be followed by ice and/or high-voltage galvanic stimulation to assist with minimizing pain, edema, and hemarthrosis, which can lead to joint stiffness.

    B. Weeks 2 and 3: The focus of rehabilitation continues to be increasing the ROM of the elbow and forearm while maintaining full AROM of all uninvolved joints.

        1. PROM via low-load, long-duration stretching should be initiated at this time in the elbow and forearm to address limitations in ROM. Again, care must be taken to minimize pain and edema, which can cause reflexive pain posturing.

        2. Static progressive splinting may be initiated at this time for any patients who present with a hard end feel at either elbow flexion or extension.

    C. Weeks 3 to 6: Strengthening may be initiated, but not at the expense of motion. If strengthening causes disproportionate pain and edema, then this phase of therapy should be delayed.[13]

        1. Isometric strengthening should be used initially; if it is tolerated well, the patient is progressed to isotonic strengthening. Those muscles needed to progress motion are worked.

    D. Weeks 6 to 12: Progress to full activities, return to work, and sports.

        1. Weight-bearing activities can begin at this time.

POSTOPERATIVE COMPLICATIONS

    I. Nerve injuries (both transient and permanent)[2-8,10,11]
    II. Compartment syndrome[2]
    III. Septic arthritis[2]
    IV. Postoperative joint infection[2]
    V. Vascular injury[2]
    VI. Loss of ROM[2-4,6,9]
    VII. Persistent pain
    VIII. Complex regional pain syndrome (CRPS)
    IX. Redislocation of elbow after injury

EVALUATION TIMELINE

    I. Week 1
      A. Wound assessment
      B. AROM/PROM of all uninvolved joints
      C. AROM of the elbow and forearm according to surgeon's instructions
      D. Pain and edema should be closely monitored at all phases of treatment.
    II. Week 2
      A. Evaluate elbow and forearm AROM/PROM (ongoing).
      B. Determine possible need for static progressive splinting.
    III. Week 3
      A. Elbow and forearm strength
      B. Weight-bearing tolerance
      C. AROM/PROM of elbow and forearm
      D. ADL independence

E. Determine possible need for static progressive splinting
F. Grip strength
IV. Weeks 4 to 6
   A. AROM/PROM of the elbow and forearm
   B. Evaluate patient's ability to tolerate throwing and catching activities.
V. Weeks 6 to 12
   A. Continue to assess AROM/PROM and strength.
   B. Determine patient's ability to return to full activity based on pain tolerance.

OUTCOMES

The goal after arthroscopic elbow surgery is to have a pain-free functional arc of motion. Morrey and colleagues[14] reported that the ROM needed to allow independence with ADLs is 30 to 130 degrees in the elbow and 50 degrees of both supination and pronation. The ROM goals after surgery are greatly determined by the intraoperative ROM obtained by the surgeon.[4-6] Communication between therapist and physician is critical to determining ROM goals.

Arthroscopic capsular release of the elbow is typically reserved for those patients whose ROM limitations are greater than 30 degrees into extension or less than 100 degrees of elbow flexion.[4,5] In the literature, reported ROM gains after arthroscopic surgery range from 6 to 25 degrees of extension and 14 to 25 degrees of flexion.[4,6,10,11] Functionally, patients are independent with ADLs and usually able to return to work and sports within 6 to 12 weeks.[4-6,9-11] However, some higher-level athletes treated for osteochondritis dissecans who are involved in throwing sports or weight-bearing activities such as gymnastics are unable to return to their previous level of competition.[11,12,15]

REFERENCES

1. Mackin EJ, Callahan AD, Skirven TM, et al. (eds): Hunter-Mackin-Callahan Rehabilitation of the Hand and Upper Extremity. 5th Ed. Mosby, St. Louis, 2002
2. Kelly EW, Morrey BF, O'Driscoll SW: Complications of elbow arthroscopy. J Bone Joint Surg Am 83:25-34, 2001
3. Kim SJ, Jeong JH: Transarticular approach for elbow arthroscopy. J Arthrosc Rel Surg 19:1-4, 2003
4. Kim SJ, Shin SJ: Arthroscopic treatment for limitation of motion of the elbow. Clin Orthop 375:140-148, 2000
5. Green DP (ed): Operative Hand Surgery. 3rd Ed. Churchill-Livingstone, New York, 1993
6. Bruno RJ, Lee ML, Strauch RJ, Rosenwasser MP: Posttraumatic elbow stiffness: evaluation and management. J Am Acad Orthop Surg 10:106-116, 2002
7. Ball CM, Meunier M, Galatz LM, Calfee R, Yamaguchi K: Arthroscopic treatment of post-traumatic elbow contracture. J Shoulder Elbow Surg 11:624-629, 2002
8. Jupiter JB, O'Driscoll SW, Cohen MS: The assessment and management of the stiff elbow. Instr Course Lect 52:93-111, 2003
7. Hausman M, Gundes H: Treatment of elbow contractures. Curr Opin Orthop 11:310-318, 2000
8. Pill SG, Ganley TJ, Flynn JM, Gregg JR: Osteochondritis dissecans of the capitellum: arthroscopic-assisted treatment of large, full-thickness defects in young patients. J Arthrosc Rel Surg 19:222-225, 2003
9. Menth-Chiari WA, Ruch DS, Poehling GG: Arthroscopic excision of the radial head: clinical outcome in 12 patients with post-traumatic arthritis after fracture of the radial head or rheumatoid arthritis. J Arthrosc Rel Surg 17:918-923, 2001
10. Micheli LJ, Luke AC, Mintzer CM, Walters PM: Elbow arthroscopy in the pediatric and adolescent population. J Arthrosc Rel Surg 17:694-699, 2001

11. Wilk KE, Reinold MM, Andrews JR: Rehabilitation of the throwers elbow. Tech Hand Upper Extremity Surg 7:197-216, 2003
12. Morrey BF: Post-traumatic stiffness: distraction arthroplasty. In Morrey BF (ed): The Elbow and Its Disorders. 2nd Ed. WB Saunders, Philadelphia, 1993, pp. 476-491
13. Yadao MA, Field LD, Savoie FH: Osteochondritis dissecans of the elbow. Instr Course Lect 53:599-606, 2004
14. Morrey BF, Askew LJ, Chao EY: A biomechanical study of functional elbow motion. J Bone Joint Surg Am 63:872-877, 1981
15. Baumgarten TE, Andrews JR, Satterwhite YE: The arthroscopic classification and treatment of osteochondritis dissecans of the capitellum, Am J Sports Med 26: 520-523, 1998

Elbow Arthroplasty 32

Anne Edmonds

In the early 1970s, total elbow arthroplasty came into vogue as a new procedure to eliminate pain, primarily for patients with rheumatoid arthritis (Fig. 32-1). More recently, it was also stated by Graham and Fitzgerald, with reference to Gallay, Richards, and O'Driscoll, that malunions and nonunions of the distal humerus can be treated with total elbow arthroplasty.[1,2]

DEFINITION

Elbow arthroplasty involves the use of prostheses that attempt to duplicate the normal surface anatomy of the distal humerus and proximal ulna. There are three types of total elbow joint (TEJ) prostheses:

I. **Constrained:** constructed with either metal to metal or metal to high-density polyethylene, through a bushing or a separate polyethylene piece.[3] This type of prosthesis is rarely used.

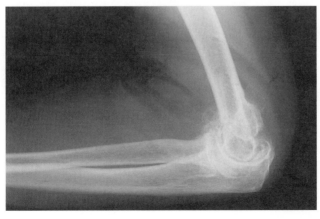

FIG. **32-1** Arthritis of elbow joint.

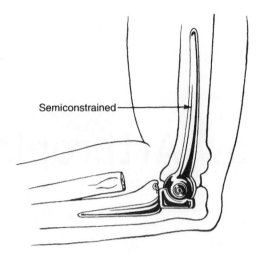

FIG. **32-2**   Semiconstrained elbow prosthesis.

II. **Semiconstrained:** also a sloppy hinge, with stemmed humeral and ulnar components, that allows a few degrees of lateral motion. These may tolerate insufficient soft tissue or loss of metaphyseal bone stock better than the resurfacing implants do[4] (Figs. 32-2 through 32-4). The semiconstrained implants have been accepted for trauma reconstruction. There is no need for the collateral ligaments to be intact to provide stability. If collateral ligaments are intact, then the integrity of the ligaments can prolong the fixation and longevity of the implant. These are cemented implants that allow early mobilization.

III. **Unconstrained:** not hinged, and there is no attachment between the humeral and ulnar components. Sufficient bone stock and soft tissue support is a prerequisite for this type of prosthesis[5] (Figs. 32-5 and 32-6).

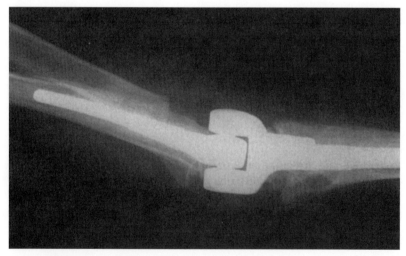

FIG. **32-3**   Anterior/posterior radiograph of semiconstrained prosthesis.

SURGICAL PURPOSE

To remove the irregular and painful ulnohumeral joint and replace these surfaces with new, usually metal or plastic, surfaces. The radial head is excised to improve pronation and supination. Joint stability is restored, and a painless but effective range of motion (ROM) is derived.

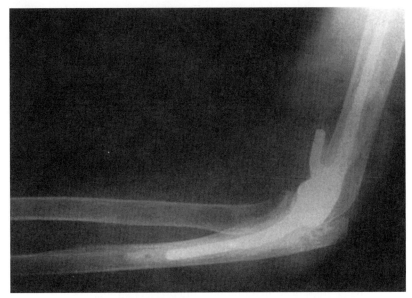

FIG. **32-4** Lateral radiograph of same semiconstrained prosthesis.

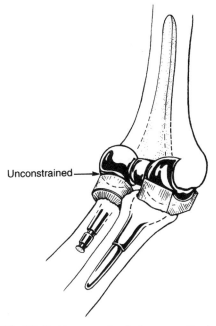

FIG. **32-5** Unconstrained elbow prosthesis.

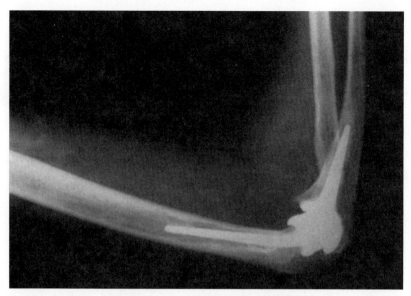

FIG. 32-6 Radiograph of unconstrained capitocondylar elbow prosthesis.

TREATMENT GOALS

I.   Regain maximum elbow ROM to within the limits of the prosthesis.
   A. Constrained: Postoperatively, the patient may expect active extension-flexion to be approximately 44 to 129 degrees, with 68 degrees of pronation and 61 degrees of supination.[6]
   B. Semiconstrained: Postoperatively, the patient may expect active extension-flexion to be approximately 15 to 133 degrees; pronation may increase 10 degrees from 70 to 80 degrees, and supination from 72 to 76 degrees.[7]
   C. Unconstrained: Postoperatively, the patient may expect increases of approximately 16 degrees of flexion, 14 degrees of extension, 19 degrees of pronation, and 26 degrees of supination. Active extension-flexion could be in the range of 47 to 124 degrees.[6]
II. Regain maximum strength.
III. Assess the patient's proficiency of self-care skills.
IV. Assess the patient's home environment for modifications.

OPERATIVE INDICATIONS

I.   Inflammatory arthritis
II. Comminuted fracture of distal humerus/posterior ulna, radius
III. Salvage unconstrained loose bodies
IV. Silicone implant problem
V.   Distal humerus malunion/nonunion

POSTOPERATIVE INDICATIONS/PRECAUTIONS FOR THERAPY

I.   Indications
   A. Immobilization of unconstrained arthroplasty at 90 degrees of flexion for 2 to 3 weeks may be necessary if instability is a

problem. If implant is stable, then immobilization continues for 1 week. Usually, protected motion is initiated at 3 to 5 days if the ligament repair is stable. Bulky dressing is removed after the first week, and a long arm splint is applied.

B. Elbow motion in the rheumatoid patient is usually better after arthroplasty than in a patient with traumatic open reduction and internal fixation.

1. Posttraumatic patients do not achieve the same type of motion, and therapists need to incorporate this knowledge into their treatment and have more realistic goals for the patient.

II. Precautions
   A. Stability of ligamentous repair
   B. Clinical manifestations and selected surgical repair
   C. Avoidance of angular stress or torque on elbow, especially abduction and external rotation.
   D. Eliminating stress on triceps repair
   E. Signs or symptoms of ulnar neuropathy
   F. Infection
   G. Neurovascular status

POSTOPERATIVE THERAPY

Postoperative therapy with triceps sparing must immobilize the elbow in full extension, usually for 8 to 10 days.

I. Immediate active range of motion (AROM) to hand and wrist only.
II. Compressive gloves as needed for edema
III. At 1 week, when bulky dressing is removed, a long arm splint is applied for support. This should be worn at all times when not exercising.
IV. At 3 to 5 days: Begin protected active-assisted elbow flexion/extension.
V. At 5 to 8 days: Begin gentle passive extension and active-assisted supination/pronation.
VI. At 5 to 8 days: Begin simple activities of daily living (ADLs), keep arm adducted, can move shoulder gently. Use long arm splint for up to 6 weeks.
VII. At 12 to 14 days: feeding, buttoning, some grooming
VIII. At 14 to 15 days: If little or no pain is present, begin graded resistive exercise to fingers.
IX. At $3^{1}/_{2}$ to 4 weeks: Maintain adducted position while exercising. May discontinue day splint at 4 weeks; continue at night to 6 weeks.
X. At 5 to 6 weeks: isometrics
XI. At 6 to 7 weeks: Begin resistive activities in the pure planar motions.
XII. Up to 6 months: no lifting, jarring, pounding, pushing, or weight-bearing
XIII. Restrictions
   A. No racquet sports.
   B. No golf or bowling.
   C. No competitive sports activities.
   D. No heavy labor ever.

POSTOPERATIVE COMPLICATIONS

I. Early
    A. Skin/wound problems
    B. Infection
    C. Ulnar neuropathy
II. Late
    A. Triceps weakness
    B. Prosthesis loosening

EVALUATION TIMELINE

I.   AROM of hand and wrist can be measured immediately.
II. Active-assisted range of motion (AAROM) of elbow is measured at 3 to 5 days.
III. At 5 to 8 days, passive extension should be measured. ROM should be measured thereafter every 2 to 3 weeks.
IV. At $3^{1}/_{2}$ to 4 weeks, assess grip and pinch strength, and thereafter every 2 to 3 weeks.

OUTCOMES

Outcomes noted for the different TEJ designs are as follows.

The predominant complication with constrained prostheses is loosening. This is caused by the large torque created by the constrained hinge, which is transmitted to the bone-acrylic bone cement. For this reason, this type of prosthesis is very rarely used.[6] Within a follow-up period of 48.7 months, 63 semiconstrained prostheses showed a 17% increase, 23% decrease, 15% increase, and 48% increase in flexion, extension, pronation, and supination, respectively (compared with preoperative values).[6]

The unconstrained type of TEJ allows extension/flexion of 47 to 124 degrees. It also permits varus/valgus motion at full extension and internal/external rotation at flexion and extension.[6]

Complications for all TEJ designs include staphylococcal infection, ulnar nerve paresthesias transiently; dislocation and loosening may be possible permanent complications.[6]

REFERENCES

1. Gallay SH, Richards RR, O'Driscoll SW: Intra-articular ulnar capacity and compliance of stiff and normal elbows. Arthroscopy 9:9-13, 1993
2. Graham TJ, Fitzgerald MS: The destroyed elbow. Am J Orthop 29(9 Suppl):9-15, 2000
3. Ferlic DC: Rheumatoid arthritis in the elbow. In Green DP (ed): Operative Hand Surgery. 2nd Ed. Vol. 3. Churchill Livingstone, New York, 1988, p. 1767
4. Goldberg VM, Figgie HE, Inglis AE, et al.: Total elbow arthroplasty. J Bone Joint Surg Am 70:778, 1988
5. Dale KG, Orr PM, Harrell PB: Total elbow replacement. Orthop Nurs 2:23, 1992
6. Lewis G: The elbow joint and its total arthroplasty: part I. A state-of-the-art review. Biomed Mater Eng 6:353-365, 1996
7. Hastings H, Theng CS: Total elbow replacement for distal humerus fractures and traumatic deformity: results and complications of semiconstrained implants and design rationale for the Discovery Elbow System. Am J Orthop 32(9 Suppl):20-28, 2003

SUGGESTED READINGS

Ewald FC: Operative Techniques for the Capitello-Condylar Total Elbow Prosthesis. Brigham and Women's Hospital and Harvard University Medical School, Boston

Ewald FC, Jacobs MA: Total elbow arthroplasty. Clin Orthop 182:137, 1984

Kudo H, Iwaro K: Total elbow arthroplasty with a nonconstrained surface-replacement prosthesis in patients who have rheumatoid arthritis. J Bone Joint Surg Am 72:355, 1990

Capitella-Condylar Total Elbow Replacement Protocol. Occupational Therapy Section, Good Samaritan Hospital, Baltimore, MD

Ramsey ML, Adams RA, Morrey BF: Instability of the elbow treated with semiconstrained total elbow arthroplasty. J Bone Joint Surg Am 81:38-47, 1999

Sarris I, Riano FA, Goebel F, Goitz RJ, et al.: Ulnohumeral arthroplasty: results in primary degenerative arthritis of the elbow. Clin Orthop (420):190-193, 2004

Weiland AJ, Weiss AP, Wills RP, Moore JR: Capitellar-condylar total elbow replacement: long term follow-up. J Bone Joint Surg Am 71:217, 1989

PART **SIX**

Wrist and Distal Radial Ulnar Joint

Wrist and Hand Tendinopathies 33

Romina P. Astifidis

The tendons of the normal wrist and hand move freely in their sheaths. Tendinopathies can result if there is swelling or thickening of the tendon, the synovial tissue, or the sheath itself. Pain with movement may inhibit tendon gliding, which is critical for diffusion of fluids. This impaired gliding can compromise blood flow to the tendon and tendon nutrition. Overuse, repetitive tasks, arthritis, diabetes, and pregnancy are the most common predisposing factors to wrist and hand tendinopathy. Vocational or avocational activities that cause tendon stretching, repeated contraction, or direct injury can also lead to tendinopathy.

DEFINITION

Tendinopathies are caused by an inflammation and thickening of the tendon and peritendinous structures. Common symptoms include tenderness, swelling, crepitus with motion, and pain on stretch of involved musculotendinous structure. These pathological conditions can be separated based on the extensor and flexor compartments of the wrist/hand complex, as follows (Fig. 33-1, *A*).

I. Extensors[1]

    A. **De Quervain's tenosynovitis:** stenosing tenosynovitis of the first dorsal compartment of the wrist involving the extensor pollicis brevis (EPB) and abductor pollicis longus (APL) tendons as they pass through the osseoligamentous tunnel of the radial styloid and transverse fibers of the dorsal retinaculum (see Fig. 33-1, *B*).

    B. **Intersection syndrome:** tenosynovitis of the second dorsal compartment involving the tendons of extensor carpi radialis brevis (ECRB) and extensor carpi radialis longus (ECRL) as they pass deep to the muscle bellies of the APL and EPB in the distal forearm. Common to rowers, canoeists, and weightlifters.[1]

    C. **Extensor pollicis longus (EPL) tendonitis** of the third dorsal compartment: common in patients with rheumatoid arthritis or with direct injury and distal radius fracture. Also seen in

Dorsal

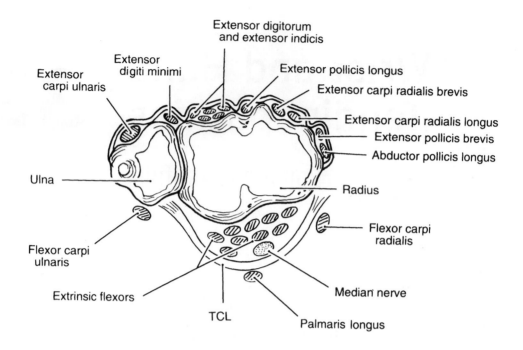

FIG. 33-1 A, Anatomy of wrist tendons.

musicians and writers who position their wrists in dorsiflexion and radial deviation.[2]

D. **Extensor indicis proprius (EIP) syndrome** of the fourth dorsal compartment: stenosis of an abnormally hypertrophic muscle belly within the extensor retinaculum.

E. **Extensor digiti minimi (EDM) tendonitis:** swelling and pain distal to the ulnar head; rarely seen.

F. **Extensor carpi ulnaris (ECU) tendonitis:** tenosynovitis of the sixth dorsal compartment. May be caused by recurrent subluxation of the ECU tendon.

II.   Flexors

A. **Flexor carpi ulnaris (FCU) tendonitis:** pain and swelling proximal to the pisiform and exacerbated by wrist flexion and ulnar deviation. Most common wrist flexor to be involved. Associated with repetitive trauma and racquet sports.

B. **Flexor carpi radialis (FCR) tendonitis:** stenosis in the FCR fibroosseous tunnel with painful radial deviation of the wrist. Commonly coexists with fracture or thumb carpometacarpal joint arthritis.

C. **Trigger digits:** Pathologic thickening of the sheath of the flexor tendons and/or swelling of the tendon itself (especially affecting the flexor digitorum superficialis [FDS]) at the A1 pulley, causing pain and eventually popping as the nodule passes through the pulley (see Fig. 33-1, *C*). Most common in the thumb, ring, and middle finger. [1]

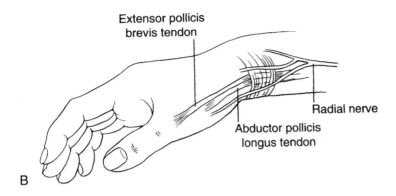

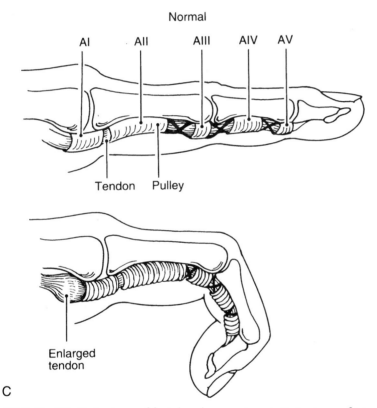

FIG. **33-1, Cont'd B,** Anatomy of first dorsal compartment. **C,** Anatomy of trigger finger.

TREATMENT PURPOSE

Wrist and hand tendinopathy can cause significant pain and limit function. Conservative treatment is indicated to decrease symptoms of pain, swelling, and dysfunction, thereby allowing full use of the hand and upper extremity. If nonoperative methods fail to relieve the inflammation, then surgery may be indicated. The surgical purpose is to release the involved fibrous sheath (release of the compartment), to allow more space for tendon gliding and thus reduce the inflammatory response. Occasionally, the hypertrophied tenosynovium is also excised. It must be recognized, however, that some of the mechanics of pulley function of the involved sheath will be compromised, and this in turn will alter the efficiency of that tendon unit.

TREATMENT GOALS

I.   Restoration of normal, painless use of the involved hand
II.   Resolution of the acute/chronic inflammatory process
III. Prevention of recurrence through education and modification of activities
IV.   Restoration of pain-free tendon glide, full range of motion (ROM), and strength

NONOPERATIVE INDICATIONS/PRECAUTIONS FOR THERAPY

I.   Indications for extensors
   A. De Quervain's tenosynovitis
     1. Pain or localized tenderness on the radial side of the wrist, aggravated by thumb motion
     2. History of chronic overuse of the wrist and hand or pregnancy/postpartum state.
     3. Finkelstein's test: Positive if pain is elicited over the first dorsal compartment when the thumb is held in the palm and the wrist is ulnarly deviated (Fig. 33-2). May also be positive for pain with resisted thumb extension.
     4. Wet leather sign: crepitus with motion of the involved tendons
     5. Palpable ganglions or triggering of the involved tendons
   B. Intersection syndrome
     1. Pain, swelling, and occasionally crepitus are located 4 to 6 cm proximal to Lister's tubercle.[3] In some cases, crepitus is audible.

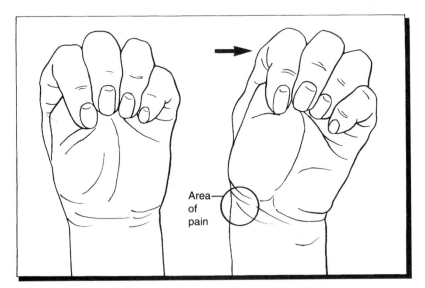

FIG. 33-2 Special test for De Quervain's tenosynovitis (modification of Finkelstein's test).

    2. Weak grip and pinch[1]

    3. History of repetitive wrist/thumb activities

  C. Other extensor wrist tendons (EPL, EIP, EDM, ECU)

    1. Pain with palpation over specific tendon at wrist level

    2. Pain on resisted exercise or passive stretch for the specific muscle/tendon unit

 II. Indications for flexors

  A. Wrist flexors (FCU, FCR)

    1. Pain and often swelling over specific tendon on palpation

    2. Pain on resisted exercise or passive stretch for the specific muscle/tendon unit

  B. Trigger digits

    1. Tenderness or pain over the tendon sheath that increases with active range of motion (AROM) or passive stretch

    2. Tendon nodule and clicking or locking of the digit with finger flexion[4]

    3. Proximal interphalangeal (PIP) joint contracture if tenosynovitis is chronic[4]

III. Precautions

  A. Allergy/intolerance to nonsteroidal antiinflammatory drugs (NSAIDs) or corticosteroids

  B. Contraindications to pertinent modalities

  C. Corticosteroid injections: multiple injections (usually more than two or three) can cause tendon rupture, hypopigmentation of the skin, and subcutaneous fat atrophy.[5]

  D. Rheumatoid arthritis

  E. Immunosuppression: at risk for infection[2]

  F. Diabetes: possible increase in blood sugar after corticosteroid injection (especially with multiple injections), which can be reduced by restricting motion[5]

NONOPERATIVE THERAPY

 I. Extensors

  A. De Quervain's tenosynovitis

    1. Splinting: rigid thumb spica splint (TSS), with thumb immobilized in abduction, wrist in extension (Fig. 33-3, *A*), is used initially to decrease acute symptoms; use of a softer splint is optional after symptoms decrease or if the rigid splint is nonfunctional (Fig. 33-3, *B*).[2]

    2. Local corticosteroid/lidocaine injections[6]

    3. Antiinflammatory modalities, including ultrasound, phonophoresis, iontophoresis with dexamethasone, and electrical stimulation[2]

    4. NSAIDs[6]

    5. Transverse friction massage or soft tissue massage as tolerated

    6. Thermal modalities, including moist heat (chronic) and ice pack or ice massage (acute)

    7. Pain-free AROM of entire wrist/thumb unit. Add tendon gliding/stretching of involved tendons performed actively and without pain into the position of the Finkelestein test. Progress to strengthening oriented toward restoration of function.

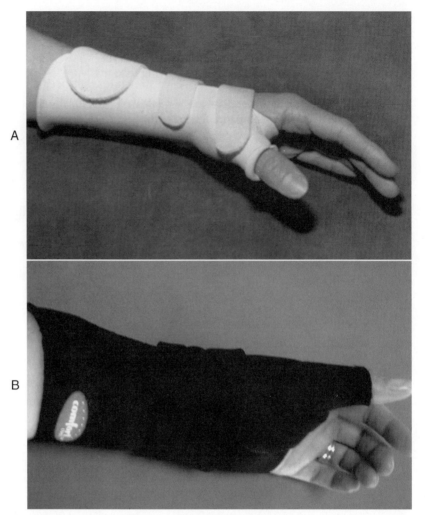

FIG. **33-3 A,** Thermoplastic thumb spica splint. **B,** Neoprene thumb spica splint (Comfort Cool Wrist and Thumb CMC Restriction Splint, North Coast Medical, Inc., Morgan Hill, CA 95037).

8. Modification of activity to avoid combined thumb flexion and ulnar deviation. Examples include split keyboard/modified mouse and handle modifications on tools to encourage neutral positioning.
B. Intersection syndrome
   1. Splint in TSS or wrist splint with slight extension.[1,3]
   2. Other treatment modalities are similar to those used to treat De Quervain's tenosynovitis.[1,3]
   3. Modification/avoidance of inciting activity
C. Other wrist extensors
   1. Splint wrist in neutral position for 4 to 6 weeks with a rigid thermoplastic splint or a prefabricated splint as appropriate to the level of symptoms.
   2. Remove splint frequently for pain-free AROM of entire wrist and hand complex to limit stiffness.

3. Antiinflammatory modalities, including ultrasound, phonophoresis, iontophoresis, and electrical stimulation
4. NSAIDs
5. Corticosteroid injections
6. Deep friction massage or soft tissue massage as tolerated
7. Progress to isometric, isotonic, and eccentric exercises as tolerated after symptoms reduce or resolve. Include work/leisure activity simulation.
8. Educate patient in activity modification to decrease symptoms. Focus on performing activities with wrist neutral. May need to modify workstation or tool use.

II. Wrist and hand flexors
A. Wrist flexors (FCR, FCU)
1. Splint wrist in rigid or prefabricated splint in slight flexion; remove splint frequently for pain-free AROM to prevent stiffness.
2. NSAIDs[2]
3. Corticosteroid injections[2]
4. Educate patients on maintaining wrist neutral with activities; modify tools or use electrically powered tools to limit repetitive wrist flexion activities.

B. Trigger digits
1. Splint involved finger or fingers with metacarpophalangeal (MCP) joint extended (Fig. 33-4, *A*); for thumb trigger, splint with interphalangeal joint extended (Fig. 33-4, *C*).[2,6] Use the least restrictive splint that minimizes triggering.
2. Corticosteroid injections
3. Educate patient in modification of activities to reduce forceful use of hands, including using friction material on tools and utensils, changing size of handle to reduce force required to hold, minimizing direct compression to the A1 pulley, and avoiding forceful pinching, which transmits maximum force to the tendons.[2]
4. Tendon gliding exercises: hook-fisting to promote tendon nutrition (Fig 33-4, *B*)

NONOPERATIVE COMPLICATIONS

I. Continued pain leading to dysfunction
II. Potential tendon rupture and dermatological changes associated with multiple corticosteroid injections[1]
III. Joint stiffness/contracture

OPERATIVE INDICATIONS/PRECAUTIONS

I. Indications
A. Continued/worsening symptoms not relieved by conservative treatment. Typically symptoms have persisted for 3 months or longer.[3]
B. Continued function and limitation due to pain and/or stiffness
C. Fixed flexion contracture in finger due to trigger digit[6]

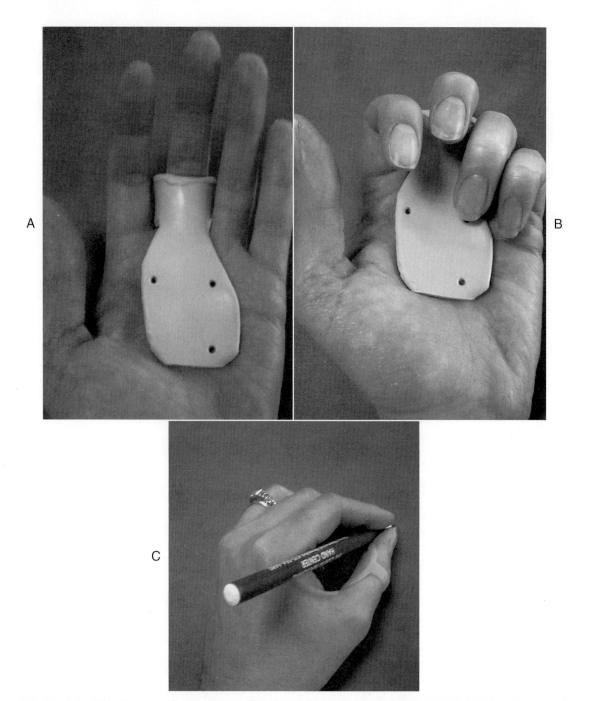

FIG. **33-4 A,** Splint for trigger finger. (From Lindner-Tons S, Ingell K: J Hand Ther 11:206-208, 1998.) **B,** Tendon gliding (hook fist) in trigger finger splint. **C,** Splint for trigger thumb (Oval-8, 3-Point Products, Inc., Annapolis, MD 21401).

II. Precautions
  A. Diabetes mellitus and other immunosuppressive states increase the risk of infection.
  B. Rheumatoid arthritis patients may have progression of MCP-ulnar deviation if the A1 pulley is released for trigger finger management.

POSTOPERATIVE THERAPY

  I. Wrist extensors
  A. De Quervain's tenosynovitis
    1. Immobilize approximately 1 week in TSS. Minimize to prevent extensor tendon adhesion.[5]
    2. ROM as tolerated, with focus on gentle tendon gliding of APL/EPB (in position similar to that for Finklestein's test) with minimal pain.[2]
    3. Scar management, including gel sheets and gentle scar massage. Initiate immediate desensitization program if scar hypersensitivity is observed. Thermal ultrasound may be used over the scar to heat tissue while stretching.
    4. Edema management, including compressive garments such as Isotoner gloves and Tubi-Grip sleeves.
    5. Pain management, including thermal modalities (moist heat and ice) as well as transcutaneous electrical stimulation (TENS)
    6. Gentle strengthening at 2 weeks, progressing as tolerated, with emphasis on work and leisure simulation.[2]
  B. Intersection syndrome[3]
    1. Immobilization in TSS for up to 10 days, followed by initiation of AROM and passive range of motion (PROM) of fingers and wrist
    2. Wrist splint may be worn between exercise sessions and at night for up to 3 to 4 weeks.
    3. Progressive strengthening is begun by 5 to 6 weeks.
  C. Wrist/hand extensor tendinitis
    1. Cast or splint in neutral position for 1 to 2 weeks (this may include the elbow to eliminate supination/pronation). EPL release may not need casting at all.[2]
    2. AROM/PROM after immobilization as tolerated
    3. Strengthening may start at 6 to 8 weeks
  II. Wrist and hand flexors
  A. Trigger finger: Therapy may not be necessary for simple trigger release without complications.[4]
    1. AROM/PROM within first week. Focus on tendon gliding.
    2. Promote wound closure with appropriate dressings and ointments. Initiate scar management after the wound or incision is closed, using gel sheets, elastomer, and scar massage.
    3. Edema management, using compressive garments, elevation, retrograde massage, and frequent gentle motion.
    4. Strengthening after 2 to 3 weeks (avoid if still triggering)[2,3]
    5. Splint PIP joint into extension to correct flexion contracture (usually worn at night).[4] May need to use ultrasound on

shortened tissues to promote lengthening and increase motion.[2]

B. Wrist flexors
1. Initiate motion rapidly.[2]
2. Include edema, scar, and pain management as needed.
3. Progress to strengthening as tolerated.

POSTOPERATIVE COMPLICATIONS

I. Extensors

A. De Quervain's tenosynovitis
1. Neuromas or sensory deficits, usually associated with the superficial radial nerve[5]
2. Scar hypertrophy and adherence to underlying tendons; scar sensitivity[5]
3. Volar subluxation of tendons requiring further surgery.[5] Sometimes prolonged thumb splinting allows this complication to resolve.
4. Recurrent symptoms due to incomplete retinacular release[7]; persistent symptoms if all tendons are not released; specifically, the EPB may be in its own compartmental sheath.
5. Chronic regional pain syndrome (CRPS): previously known as reflex sympathetic dystrophy (RSD).[2]

B. All other wrist extensor compartments
1. Continued pain
2. Scar adherence
3. Loss of motion

II. Wrist and finger flexors

A. Trigger finger
1. PIP joint flexion contracture.
2. Digital nerve/tendon injury[2,6]
3. Sectioning of A2 pulley causing bowstringing.[2]
4. Recurrent trigger[2,6]
5. Scar tenderness[6]
6. Infection[6]

B. Wrist flexors
1. Continued pain
2. Scar adherence
3. Loss of motion

EVALUATION TIMELINE

I. Nonoperative

A. Day 1: Assessment, including history, inciting activities, functional limitations, pain history, provocative testing, sensory testing, and asymptomatic AROM/PROM. Measurements repeated as appropriate every 2 to 4 weeks.

B. Strength measurements at time of painlessness or in nonacute phase.

II. Postoperative

A. Days 1 to 14: Postoperative dressings in place. Assessment as needed to ensure full ROM of uninvolved joints, edema

reduction through elevation and pain management. Assessment, including history, surgical procedure/wound status, pain levels.
B. Days 7 to 14: Sensory testing, edema, and pain-free AROM/PROM. Scar assessment after stitch removal and full wound closure.
C. Days 14 to 21: Strength testing if there is full wound closure, minimal to no pain, and no recurring symptoms (i.e., triggering).
D. 6 to 12 weeks: Assess patient's readiness to return to work or leisure activities based on progress

OUTCOMES

Most research done on wrist and hand tendinopathy is focused on the most common diagnoses, specifically De Quervain's tenosynovitis and trigger finger. Nonoperative treatment of De Quervain's tenosynovitis showed 69% resolution with corticosteroid injection alone, 29% reduction with TSS alone, and 57% resolution with injection and splint combined, questioning the effectiveness of splinting alone.[8] However, some authors still recommend a splinting trial, especially in the acute phase.[2] A retrospective study (1999) examined postoperative satisfaction from De Quervain's release and demonstrated 88% patient satisfaction with surgery and a cure rate of 91%.[7] Those patients with complications after surgery accounted for the rates of dissatisfaction. The duration of symptoms did not correlate with long-term complications, and the patients with the longest duration of symptoms had more postoperative satisfaction.

Conservative treatment of trigger digits demonstrated a 66% to 73% success rate with splinting for trigger digit and lower success with thumb splinting. Results with corticosteroid injection vary from 46% to 92% success, depending on the type of tenosynovitis (nodular versus diffuse) and the type and amount of medication injected.[6] Overall, poorer outcomes were noted with conservative treatment if multiple digits were involved, if duration of symptoms was greater than 4 to 6 months, and if there was diffuse tendon thickening and significant triggering.[2] Generally, authors recommend a trial of splinting and a maximum of two to three steroid injections several weeks to months apart before surgery is considered.[2,6] Operative release of trigger digits has a success rate of 60% to 100%, with most being 85%.[2]

REFERENCES

1. Thorson E, Szabo RM: Common tendinitis problems in the hand and forearm. Orthop Clin North Am 23:65-73, 1992
2. Lee MP, et al.: Surgeon's and therapist's management of tendinopathy in the hand and wrist. In Mackin EJ, Callahan AD, Skirven TM, et al. (eds): Hunter-Mackin-Callahan Rehabilitation of the Hand and Upper Extremity. 5th Ed. Mosby, St. Louis, 2002
3. Kirkpatrick W: Intersection syndrome. Atlas of the Hand Clinics 4(1):55-60, 1999
4. Osterman AL, Sweet S: The treatment of complex trigger finger with proximal interphalangeal joint contracture. Atlas of the Hand Clinics 4(1):9-21, 1999
5. Bednar JM, Santarlasci PR: First extensor compartment release and retinacular sheath reconstruction for deQuervains tenosynovitis. Atlas of the Hand Clinics 4(1):39-54, 1999
6. Taras J, Miskovesky C: Nonoperative management of trigger digits. Atlas of the Hand Clinics 4(1):1-8, 1999
7. Ta KT, et al.: Patient satisfaction and outcomes of surgery for de Quervain's tenosynovitis. J Hand Surg Am 24:1071-1077, 1999
8. Weiss AP, et al.: Treatment of deQuervain's disease. J Hand Surg Am 19:595-598, 1994

SUGGESTED READINGS

Cannon NM (ed): Diagnosis and Treatment Manual for Physicians and Therapists: Upper Extremity Rehabilitation. 4th Ed. The Hand Rehabilitation Center of Indiana, Indianapolis, IN, 2001

Connolly WB: Disorders of tendons and tendon sheaths. In Connolly WB (ed): Atlas of Hand Surgery. Churchill Livingstone, New York, 1997

Lee MP, et al.: Surgeon's and therapist's management of tendinopathy in the hand and wrist. In Mackin EJ, Callahan AD, Skirven TM, et al. (eds): Hunter-Mackin-Callahan Rehabilitation of the Hand and Upper Extremity. 5th Ed. Mosby, St. Louis, 2002

Zelouf DS, Osterman AL (eds): Tendinitis and tenosynovitis. In: Atlas of Hand Clinics. Vol. 1. WB Saunders, Philadelphia, 1999

Wrist Arthroscopy 34

William McKay

Since the introduction of small joint instrumentation in 1985 along with standardized portals, the diagnostic and therapeutic use of arthroscopy in the wrist has expanded.[1-3] The list of indications for arthroscopy of the wrist is increasing.[4-10]

Arthroscopy is conducted through portals on the dorsum of the wrist for most diagnoses (Fig. 34-1); however, for some a volar approach may be preferred.[7] For diagnostic purposes, arthroscopy permits a meticulous study of the anatomy.[11] Arthroscopy provides the best evaluation of the ligaments and joint surfaces.[11] The surgeon may also view the wrist under manipulation, while stressing the surrounding structures.

The advantages of arthroscopy include its utility as both a diagnostic and a therapeutic tool, minimal incisions, low postoperative morbidity, minimal inflammatory response, low hospital cost, and low complication rates.[12] Close communication between the therapist and the surgeon is vital.

DEFINITION

Arthroscopy is a minimally invasive technique that can be used as a diagnostic and therapeutic tool for selected osseous and ligamentous joint pathology, with lower morbidity than for open techniques.[11]

SURGICAL PURPOSE

I. Assess defects/injuries.
II. Diagnose source of pain.
III. Perform therapeutic surgical procedure.

TREATMENT GOALS

I. Maintain/promote maximum range of motion (ROM) in uninvolved joints.
II. When necessary, protect through immobilization.

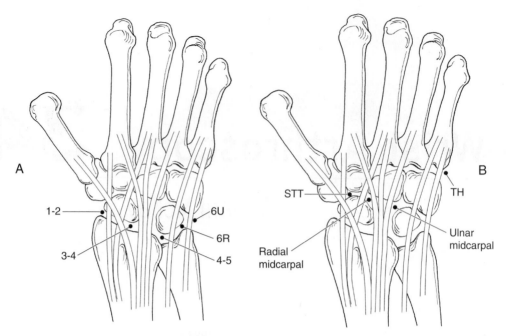

FIG. **34-1** **A,** The standard radiocarpal portals. **B,** The standard midcarpal portals. STT, scaphotrapeziotrapezoid; TH, triquetrohamate. (Modified from Gupta R, Bozentka DJ, Osterman AL: J Am Acad Orthop Surg 3:200, 2001.)

III. Decrease edema.
IV. Decrease pain.
 V. As appropriate, restore active range of motion (AROM) at wrist and forearm.
VI. Prevent infection at portal and pin sites.
VII. Restore patient to maximal functional ability.

OPERATIVE INDICATIONS/PRECAUTIONS

I.   Indications
  A. Diagnostic arthroscopy
    1. Assessment of ligamentous injuries of the wrist
    2. Assessment of chondral defects
    3. Triangular fibrocartilage complex (TFCC) disorders
    4. Assessment of chronic wrist pain of unknown cause
  B. Therapeutic arthroscopy
    1. Arthroscopic reduction and internal fixation (ARIF) of scapholunate tears: see Chapter 35
    2. ARIF of lunotriquetral ligament tears
    3. ARIF of distal radial fractures
    4. ARIF of scaphoid fractures
    5. Removal of loose bodies
    6. Excision of ganglion
    7. Debridement of chondral defects

       8. Synovectomy
       9. Resection arthroplasty
      10. Debridement of and repair of TFCC tears:
          see Chapter 36
      11. Distal ulnar resection: see Chapter 38
II.   Precautions
    A. Associated tendon injuries
    B. Associated bony injuries
    C. Associated nerve injury
    D. Associated vascular injury
    E. Associated ligament injuries
    F. Associated cartilage injuries

POSTOPERATIVE INDICATIONS/PRECAUTIONS FOR THERAPY

  I.   Indications
    A. Ligament repair
    B. Fracture reduction
    C. Painful ROM
    D. Edema
    E. Splinting
  II.   Precautions
    A. Ligament weakness
    B. Fracture instability
    C. Percutaneous Kirschner-wire care
    D. Inflammation
    E. Disproportionate pain
    F. Joint stiffness in uninvolved joints

POSTOPERATIVE THERAPY

   I. Scapholunate tears: see Chapter 35
  II. Lunotriquetral tears
    A. Immediately after surgery to repair the ligaments, the patient is placed in a forearm cast to immobilize the wrist for 6 to 8 weeks, at which time the K-wires are removed. A splint is approved for 3 to 4 weeks of intermittent use.
    B. AROM may begin after the K-wires are removed.
    C. Follow physician's instructions for passive range of motion (PROM).
    D. Strengthening must be performed with great care, because this surgery was performed to return stability to the joint. Begin isometric exercises at 8 weeks after surgery. Free weights are not used until 4 months after surgery, with heavy work performed at 6 months. Monitor for signs of instability, such as carrying angle and clunking.
  III. Intraarticular fractures of the distal radius
    A. Short arm or sugar-tong splint applied in operating room
    B. At 7 to 10 days after surgery, a wrist splint is provided to support the wrist.

C. At 6 to 8 weeks the K-wires are removed; begin AROM/PROM of wrist, and begin gentle strengthening as permitted by the physician.

D. Wrist stiffness may persist for 4 to 6 months.

E. Maximum strength may not return for 6 to 12 months.

IV. Scaphoid fractures fixed with Herbert-Whipple screw

    A. Immobilization for 2 to 4 weeks

    B. Begin AROM at end of immobilization for wrist/thumb

    C. Follow physician restrictions on avoidance of impact loading, torque, and extreme wrist positions.

    D. Possible use of a commercial wrist splint with stops to enforce physician-designated ROM restrictions

    E. Because the scaphoid requires 8 to 10 weeks to heal, strengthening must be delayed until union is accomplished. The purpose in using a compression screw is to permit early mobilization after soft tissue healing. The initial goal for treatment is to regain ROM without disrupting the fracture site.

V. Loose bodies often stem from small to large chondral defects. Immobilization should be minimal, following physician instructions. AROM is usually permitted immediately after surgery. Strengthening as tolerated.

VI. Dorsal ganglion excision

    A. The wrist is immobilized for 7 to 10 days. Digit ROM is begun immediately after surgery to prevent tendon adhesions, especially those dorsally placed.

    B. A light splint is applied for an additional 2 weeks for comfort while active wrist motion is begun.

    C. Light activities for 6 weeks after surgery

    D. Heavy duty at 3 months

VII. Volar ganglion excision

    A. Active wrist movement is begun on day 2.

    B. Address AROM goals to prevent tendon adhesions and prevent tightness of the interossei.

    C. Digit PROM may begin on day 2.

    D. Progressive strengthening as tolerated

VIII. Chondral defects

    A. Treatment involves correction of cause of lesions, which are divided into four types.[4]

       1. Grade I lesion: intact lamina splendens with softer than normal cartilage

       2. Grade II lesion: disruption of lamina splendens, minimal fibrillation

       3. Grade III lesion: deep fissures into articular surface

       4. Grade IV lesion: exposed bone

    B. Variable rehabilitation depending on extent of debridement

    C. Follow physician's instructions for ROM and strengthening.

IX. Rheumatoid wrist synovectomy

    A. Active exercises are started immediately after arthroscopy, and a wrist splint is provided for intermittent use after removal of the bulky dressing.

    B. Some stiffness in the wrist may be desirable to provide stability. Close cooperation with the surgeon is vital, especially in cases

with distal radioulnar joint (DRUJ) involvement. If the DRUJ
was involved, then a sugar tong or Muenster-type splint is
provided immediately after surgery to position the forearm
in supination for 3 weeks.
   C. The length of time the splint is used depends on the amount
   of laxity in the joint.
   X. Proximal row carpectomy
   A. The wrist is immobilized for 4 weeks after surgery; however,
   the patient should be referred for hand therapy within 2 days
   after surgery. AROM/PROM is begun on all noninvolved
   joints as tolerated on the first day of treatment.
   B. Address edema issues with elevation and compressive
   wrapping of digits.
   C. AROM starts along with intermittent splinting during the
   second 4-week interval.[2] Remove splint for increasingly
   greater lengths of time as patient comfort permits.
   D. Begin strengthening at 8 weeks.
   XI. Hemiresection of distal ulna: see Chapter 38
   XII. Radial styloidectomy
   A. AROM at 1 week
   B. Splint the wrist intermittently for 3 weeks
   C. Strengthening at 4 weeks
   XIII. Palmar midcarpal instability: see Chapter 35

POSTOPERATIVE COMPLICATIONS

   I. Traction injury to digital skin[2]
   II. Traction injury to metacarpophalangeal (MCP) joints[2]
   III. Injury to extraarticular structures[2]
   IV. Iatrogenic injury of the chondral surfaces[2]
   V. Forearm compartment syndrome during reduction and
   fixation of distal radius fractures[2]
   VI. Injury to dorsal branch of ulnar nerve during TFCC repair[2]
   VII. Injury to subcutaneous nerves during percutaneous
   pin placement[2]
   VIII. Miscellaneous infection[2]
   IX. Complex regional pain syndrome[2]
   X. Tendon problems[2]
   XI. Edema
   XII. Inflammation
   XIII. Joint stiffness in uninvolved joints

TIMELINE

   I. Edema measurements: at initial evaluation and weekly until
   resolved or within normal limits
   II. Pain measurements: at initial and subsequent visits until resolved
   III. Sensory status: at initial visit and every 4 to 6 weeks as
   necessary if condition warrants
   IV. Circulatory status: at initial and subsequent visits for 1 week
   V. AROM to uninvolved joints: usually begun immediately after
   surgery; checked weekly

VI. AROM to the involved joint: see postoperative care for each diagnosis
VII. Strengthening: see guidelines for each diagnosis in postoperative care
VIII. Joint stability: continuously monitor for carrying angle or clunking sounds after repair of wrist ligaments
IX. Static progressive/dynamic splinting or serial casting may begin with approval of physician.

OUTCOMES

Reported complications from wrist arthroscopy are rare (less than 1%)
I. Lunotriquetral tears: If the ligament is repaired, then some tightness may be accepted as necessary to permit stability in this joint.
II. Wrist fractures usually result in stiffness for 4 to 6 months, with return of full strength requiring 6 to 12 months.[11]
III. Scaphoid fractures fixed with Herbert-Whipple screw: complete bone healing by 12 months.[2]
IV. Dorsal ganglion excision: Average return to work is in 3.5 weeks.[2]
V. Volar ganglion excision: similar to dorsal ganglion excision in that recurrence is the same or better than with traditional methods.[1,8]
VI. Chondral defects: Debridement is likely to reduce pain in types I, II, and III defects; however, long-term benefit in type IV is not assured.
VII. Rheumatoid wrist synovectomy: All patients are expected to experience decreased pain with no loss in motion; however, an increase in level of activity does not always occur.
VIII. Proximal row carpectomy: flexion/extension arc of approximately 80 degrees, with grip strength approximately 75% of that of the unaffected side.

REFERENCES

1. Gupta R, Bozentka DJ, Osterman AL: Wrist arthroscopy: principles and clinical applications. J Am Acad Orthop Surg 3:200, 2001
2. Adler MA, Osterman AL: Arthroscopic surgery of the wrist. In Chapman MW (ed): Chapman's Orthopaedic Surgery. 3rd Ed. Lippincott Williams & Wilkins, Baltimore, 2001, p. 2037
3. Gregory IB, Richards RS, Roth JH: Wrist arthroscopy. In Lichtman DM, Alexander AH (ed): The Wrist and Its Disorders. 2nd Ed. WB Saunders, Philadelphia, 1997, p. 151
4. Poehling GG, Siegel DB, Koman LA, et al: Arthroscopy of the wrist. In Green DP (ed): Operative Hand Surgery, 3rd Ed. Churchill Livingstone, Edinburgh, 1993, p. 189
5. Adolfsson L, Nylander G: Arthroscopic synovectomy of the rheumatoid wrist. J Hand Surg Br 18:92, 1993
6. Shih JT, Hung ST, Lee HM, et al: Dorsal ganglion of the wrist: results of treatment by arthroscopic resection. Hand Surg 7:1, 2002
7. Ho PC, Lo WN, Hung LD: Arthroscopic resection of volar ganglion of the wrist: a new technique. Arthroscopy 19:218, 2003
8. Park MJ, Ahn JH, Kang JS: Arthroscopic synovectomy of the wrist in rheumatoid arthritis. J Bone Joint Surg Br 85:1011, 2003
9. Koh S, Nakamura R, Horii E, et al: Loose body in the wrist: diagnosis and treatment. Arthroscopy 19:820, 2003
10. Ashwood N, Bain GI: Arthroscopically assisted treatment of intraosseous ganglions of the lunate: a new technique. J Hand Surg Am 28:62, 2003

11. Richards RS, James NR: Arthroscopy of the wrist: introduction and indications. McGinty JB (ed): Operative Arthroscopy. 3rd Ed. Lippincott Williams & Wilkins, Baltimore, 2003, p. 721
12. Phillips BB: General principles of arthroscopy. In Canale ST (ed): Campbell's Operative Orthopaedics. 10th Ed. Mosby, Philadelphia, 2003, p. 2507

SUGGESTED READINGS

Hofmeister EP, Dao KD, Glowacki KA, et al: The role of midcarpal arthroscopy in the diagnosis of disorders of the wrist. J Hand Surg Am 26:407, 2001
Whipple TL: The role of arthroscopy in the treatment of wrist injuries in the athlete. Clin Sports Med 3:623, 1998

Carpal Fractures and Instabilities 35

Terri M. Skirven and Lauren M. DeTullio

The wrist is a key joint for upper extremity function. Through its mobility, the wrist allows positioning of the hand for performance of grasp, prehension, and manipulation. Through its stability, the wrist permits transmission of loads involved in lifting, carrying, pushing, pulling, and weight-bearing. The mobility and stability of the wrist are dependent on the integrity of the carpal bones, their articular surfaces, and the carpal ligaments, as well as intact wrist muscle-tendon units. The wrist comprises the radiocarpal, midcarpal, distal radioulnar, carpometacarpal, pisotriquetral, and ulnomeniscotriquetral joints, as well as individual carpal bone articulations. The normal range of motion (ROM) of the wrist averages 70 degrees of wrist extension, 80 degrees of flexion, 20 degrees of radial deviation, and 30 degrees of ulnar deviation.[1] The ROM required for function is less than the normal ROM. For example, Ryu and colleagues,[2] in a study examining the amount of wrist motion required to perform a variety of activities of daily living (ADLs) found that 40 degrees of wrist extension, 40 degrees of flexion, and 40 degrees of combined ulnar and radial deviation were required. A similar study published by Palmer and associates[3] concluded that 5 degrees of wrist flexion, 30 degrees of extension, 10 degrees of radial deviation, and 15 degrees of ulnar deviation were needed for most ADLs.

Fracture of the carpal bones results from traumatic impact loading of the wrist. Carpal fractures may result in stiffness of the wrist, loss of ROM, limited load-bearing capability, and pain. The most commonly fractured carpal bone is the scaphoid, followed by the triquetrum.[4]

Carpal instability results from ligament disruption or ligament laxity. Carpal ligament injuries often occur in combination with carpal fractures. Carpal ligament injuries can cause wrist pain and instability; left untreated, they can lead to carpal collapse with painful degenerative changes and loss of motion. The most common clinical pattern of carpal instability is dorsiflexion instability resulting from ligament disruption between the scaphoid and the lunate.[5]

The approach to rehabilitation of the wrist must take into consideration the specific injury, the stage of healing, the nature of any surgical procedures (whether reparative or salvage), and any resultant alteration in the biomechanics and load-bearing capacity of the wrist. For example, if a surgical procedure is considered salvage, then strenuous efforts to gain wrist ROM at the expense of stability and comfort should be avoided.

DEFINITION

Carpal Fractures

Scaphoid fractures are the most common of carpal bone fractures.[4] The scaphoid connects the distal and proximal carpal rows and acts as a bony block to wrist hyperextension, making it particularly vulnerable to injury from a fall on the outstretched hand. Scaphoid fractures are classified according to location: distal pole, waist, and proximal pole. Approximately 70% to 80% of these fractures involve the waist, 10% to 20% involve the proximal pole, and 10% involve the distal pole.[6] Healing of scaphoid fractures depends on the site and type of fracture. A proximal pole fracture may take 20 or more weeks to heal due to variable blood supply to the proximal pole. There is a high incidence of delayed healing, nonunion, and avascular necrosis of proximal pole fractures. The distal pole has a rich blood supply and requires 8 to 10 weeks for healing. The waist is most commonly fractured and takes up to 12 weeks to heal.[7]

The **triquetrum** is the second most commonly fractured carpal bone.[8] There are two types of triquetral fractures: fractures of the body of the triquetrum and dorsal chip fractures.[9] A triquetral fracture occurs from a dorsiflexion and ulnar deviation force. Clinical presentation includes localized tenderness and swelling. Nondisplaced triquetral fractures typically heal after 4 to 6 weeks of immobilization in a cast.

Trapezial fracture typically results from a direct blow to the abducted thumb or a fall on the hyperextended wrist in radial deviation, which results in impingement of the trapezium against the radial styloid and first metacarpal.[10] There are two main fracture types: trapezial ridge fractures and a split fracture of the trapezium. Trapezial fractures often occur in combination with thumb metacarpal or distal radius fractures. Clinically, ridge fractures are characterized by tenderness at the base of the thumb and pain with resisted wrist flexion; they can be associated with carpal tunnel syndrome or Guyon's canal syndrome. Conservative treatment is a thumb spica cast for 4 to 6 weeks for a nondisplaced fracture.[11]

Hamate fracture involves the body or the hook. Fractures of the hook can occur as a result of impact with the handle of a racquet or club during ball strike or from a fall. The clinical presentation is pain with palpation over the hook and painful grip. Resisted distal interphalangeal (DIP) joint flexion of the ring and small fingers with the wrist in ulnar deviation is painful because the flexor tendons rub against the fractured hamate.[12] Acute fractures of the hook of the hamate are treated with cast immobilization for 6 to 8 weeks or excision.[13] Delayed healing or nonunion of hook fractures can be treated with excision. Complications of hook fracture/nonunion are flexor tendon synovitis, rupture, and ulnar nerve irritation and pain. Body fractures need to be reduced and fixed if unstable; cast immobilization is sufficient if the fracture is stable.

Lunate fractures are usually associated with Kienbock's disease or avascular necrosis of the lunate. The incidence of isolated acute lunate fractures is low.[4] The mechanism of injury with lunate fractures is axial loading by the capitate to the body of the lunate.[14] Treatment for a nondisplaced acute lunate fracture includes cast immobilization for 6 to 8 weeks with repeat radiographs to assess healing.[7] Displacement of lunate fractures greater than 1 mm warrant open reduction and internal fixation (ORIF).[15]

Pisiform fractures usually result from direct trauma over the ulnar volar aspect of the wrist or to the proximal palm over the hypothenar eminence. Pisiform fractures may be associated with triquetrum, hamate, or dorsal radius fractures. Clinical presentation includes pain, swelling, and tenderness of the hypothenar eminence. Ulnar nerve irritation may occur, because the pisiform makes up the ulnar wall of Guyon's canal.[4] Conservative treatment involves 3 to 6 weeks of cast immobilization. Excision is performed in cases of malunion or nonunion.

Capitate fractures may result from direct trauma to the dorsal aspect of the wrist or from extreme dorsiflexion, with radial deviation producing a more complicated fracture-dislocation.[16] The capitate is often associated with transscaphoid, transcapitate, perilunate fracture-dislocation/scaphocapitate syndrome.[17] The isolated nondisplaced capitate fracture can be treated by cast immobilization for 6 weeks.[18] Displaced fractures require surgical intervention with reduction and internal fixation. Postoperative complications include adherence of the extensor tendons, with resultant extensor lag at the metacarpophalangeal joints due to the dorsal surgical approach.

Trapezoid fractures: The protected position of the trapezoid between the base of the second metacarpal, capitate, trapezium, and scaphoid and the strong ligamentous attachments provide much stability, limiting the likelihood of an isolated fracture.[4] Botte and Gelberman[19] reported a 1% incidence of trapezoid fractures in comparison with all carpal bones. The mechanism of injury involves either a crush or a high-energy impact longitudinally along the second metacarpal that indirectly creates a dislocation or fracture-dislocation.[20] Conservative management includes cast immobilization for up to 6 weeks and fusion for late arthritis. Surgical interventions involve closed or open reduction and pin fixation for displaced and unstable fractures. Postoperative complications include edema and dorsal scar adherence of the extensor tendons, which may result in extensor lag or extensor tendon tightness or both.

Carpal Instability

Carpal instability is characterized by malalignment of the carpal bones, inability to bear loads, and disruption of the normal kinematics of the carpal bones during ROM. **Static instability** refers to carpal malalignment that is apparent on standard radiographs. **Dynamic instability** requires provocative maneuvers or stress radiographs to be detected. Carpal instability results from traumatic ligament disruption, from ligament laxity, or from extrinsic factors such as malunion of a distal radius fracture with excessive dorsal tilt. The Mayo classification defines four categories of carpal instability: carpal instability dissociative (CID), carpal instability nondissociative (CIND), carpal instability combined (CIC), and adaptive carpus (AC).[21]

Carpal instability dissociative (CID) refers to instability between carpal bones of the same carpal row. This is caused by partial or complete disruption of the intrinsic interosseous ligaments. Scapholunate instability is an example of CID and is the most frequent form of carpal instability.[5]

Scapholunate instability refers to a spectrum of conditions including the following: subtle instability without overt anatomic disruption but with insufficient load-bearing capacity; dynamic instability that occurs only under load; static instability with full dislocation/rotary subluxation of the scaphoid; and scapholunate advanced collapse (SLAC). Scapholunate ligament injury may result in dorsiflexion instability, with the scaphoid rotating into volar flexion and the lunate and the triquetrum rotating into extension.[5] This pattern is termed dorsal intercalated segment instability (DISI), and it is identified by the dorsiflexed orientation of the lunate with the wrist in neutral position on a lateral radiograph. **Lunotriquetral instability** is the second most frequent form of carpal instability and is another example of CID.[5] Lunotriquetral instability results from disruption of the lunotriquetral interosseous ligament and extrinsic radiocarpal ligaments. Volar rotation of the scaphoid and lunate with extension of the triquetrum can be seen with lunotriquetral instability. This pattern is termed volar intercalated segment instability (VISI). It is identified by the volarflexed orientation of the lunate with the wrist in neutral position on a lateral radiograph.

Carpal instability nondissociative (CIND) refers to instability between carpal rows or between a carpal row and the next adjacent osseous structure. CIND results from injury to the extrinsic or capsular ligaments. Midcarpal instability is an example of CIND and refers to instability between the proximal and distal carpal rows. Palmar midcarpal instability, as described by Lichtman and associates,[22] is an example of CIND and is characterized by a volar sag on the ulnar side of the wrist, a clunk that occurs at the end of the range of ulnar deviation with forearm pronation, tenderness over the triquetral-hamate and capitolunate intervals, and weakness of grip. A lateral radiograph of the wrist in neutral deviation often shows a VISI pattern with slight palmar translation of the distal carpal row.[22]

Carpal instability combined (CIC) refers to instabilities that are combinations of CID and CIND.

Adaptive carpus (AC), adaptive instability (AI), and pseudocarpal instability (PCI) all are terms that refer to carpal instability resulting from an extrinsic cause such as a malunited distal radius fracture. The osseous deformity of the distal radius leads to malalignment of the bones of proximal carpal row, resulting in either midcarpal or radiocarpal instability. Extrinsic midcarpal instability, as described by Lichtman and coworkers,[22] fits in this category.

SURGICAL PURPOSE

Surgical intervention is performed to restore the normal anatomical carpal relationships and to promote healing of carpal fractures and ligament injuries. Unstable and displaced carpal fractures are treated with ORIF with percutaneous pins or compression screws. Bone grafting may be required for comminuted fractures or fracture nonunions. Acute ligament injuries resulting in carpal instability are treated with primary ligament repair or reconstruction and/or augmentation.

If carpal fractures or ligament injuries are not treated primarily and the wrist continues to be subjected to the demands and loads of daily activities, progressive deterioration and collapse of the wrist occurs. In this case, surgery is performed to salvage function and may involve partial or total wrist fusion, replacement arthroplasty, or proximal row carpectomy.

TREATMENT GOALS

I.   Nonoperative
      A. Control edema and pain.
      B. Maintain ROM of uninvolved joints.
      C. Promote functional motion of the wrist after healing permits.
      D. Preserve wrist stability.
      E. Avoid activity and exercise that adversely loads the wrist and undermines recovery of function/healing.
      F. Return to previous level of function after healing permits.
II.   Operative
      A. Control edema.
      B. Promote wound healing.
      C. Control/modulate scar formation.
      D. Maintain ROM of uninvolved joints.
      E. Promote functional motion of the wrist after healing permits.
      F. Monitor response of the wrist to graded exercise and ADLs.
      G. Avoid ADLs and exercises that adversely load the wrist and undermine recovery of function/healing.
      H. Return to previous level of function after healing permits.

NONOPERATIVE INDICATIONS/PRECAUTIONS FOR THERAPY

I.   Indications
      A. Nondisplaced, stable carpal fractures
      B. Ligament injuries with negative radiographic findings that are stable when stressed or under load but symptomatic with palpation
      C. Chronic carpal ligament injuries that are stable with no radiographic findings or are unstable with radiographic findings if not a candidate for surgery
II.   Precautions
      A. Associated nerve injury
      B. Associated tendon injury
      C. Fracture stability, influenced by the type of fracture
      D. Delayed union or nonunion

NONOPERATIVE THERAPY

Carpal Fractures

I.   Therapy for carpal fractures treated nonoperatively with 8 weeks or longer in a short arm cast or splint
      A. During the phase of immobilization, a home program of exercises is provided with instruction in tendon gliding and active range of motion (AROM) exercises for the fingers and other uninvolved joints. Techniques to reduce swelling of the

digits include elevation, retrograde massage, and compressive wrapping.

1. Scaphoid fractures often require long periods of immobilization, resulting in significant stiffness and loss of wrist ROM. The flexible wrist splint[23] (scaphoid mobilization splint) can be used for nondisplaced scaphoid fractures that show evidence of early but incomplete healing after an initial period of cast immobilization. The splint allows limited wrist flexion and extension but prevents radial and ulnar deviation and provides protection and support (Fig. 35-1). The splint is worn full-time and is removed for showers. The intended advantages of the splint include preservation of joint motion, decreased demineralization of bone, and stimulation of fracture healing.[23]

B. After cast removal or discontinuation of continuous splinting, a more formal program of therapy is initiated, including ROM of the wrist and forearm. It is important to have a clear understanding of the extent of carpal bone healing when therapy is initiated and progressed, to prevent overstressing of the bone and undermining of healing due to overaggressive therapy. The focus of therapy after removal of the cast is on resolution of stiffness and recovery of ROM of the wrist. Because of the duration of immobilization, wrist stiffness with limited ROM may be significant. Passive range of motion (PROM) and mobilization techniques are permitted once the fracture is determined by the physician to be completely healed. If goals for wrist ROM are not achieved with ROM and mobilization techniques, static and dynamic splints can be used. These splints are designed to hold the wrist at the end of the available range in the desired direction with either static or dynamic stress applied.

C. Strengthening exercises are begun after healing has been achieved, usually by 3 months. The exact timing of fracture healing depends on the individual patient and the specific fracture and must be verified with the referring physician before a strengthening regimen is begun. Isometric exercises for wrist flexors and extensors are introduced first, with low repetition initially to prevent soft tissue irritation or an inflammatory response. Once the patient demonstrates tolerance, the program is progressed with the introduction of isokinetic and isotonic exercises. The patient should be educated to avoid increasing the weight levels or repetitions too abruptly, which could trigger an adverse symptom response.

Carpal Ligament Injury

Typically, acute wrist ligament injuries are initially immobilized for a range of 3 to 8 weeks, depending on the degree of injury.[24,25] ROM exercises are permitted after this initial period of immobilization. Overaggressive mobilization of the wrist after a ligament injury should be avoided, to prevent exceeding the tensile capability of the healing ligament and possibly undermining the recovery of wrist function. Continuous monitoring of symptom response to therapy is critical to avoid overstress.

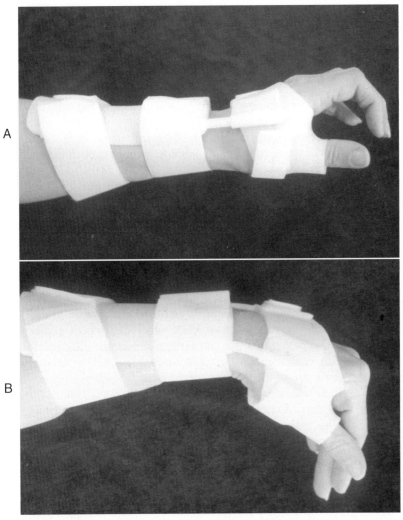

FIG. 35-1 A, Flexible wrist splint used for nondisplaced, incompletely healed scaphoid fractures after an initial period of cast immobilization.[23] B, Splint allows limited wrist flexion and extension but prevents radial and ulnar deviation.

I.   Therapy after acute carpal ligament injuries treated nonsurgically with up to 8 weeks of immobilization
     A. Scapholunate and lunotriquetral ligament injuries
        1. Intermittent, protective splint use after cast removal is usually required for 2 to 4 weeks during the initial stage of rehabilitation to protect against inadvertent stresses to the wrist from ADLs.
        2. AROM exercise to resolve stiffness and promote recovery of motion lost secondary to cast immobilization. Modalities such as hot packs and ultrasound are helpful in increasing tissue extensibility and recovery of ROM. Avoid overzealous mobilization.
        3. Gradual resumption of ADLs and progressive strengthening begins typically 2 to 4 weeks after the initial phase of therapy

and as symptoms permit. The goal is to prepare the wrist to handle the specific demands of ADLs, work, and leisure activities. Isometric exercise is generally tolerated better than isotonic exercise. Continuous monitoring of symptoms is stressed. Persistence of tenderness and swelling over the scapholunate or lunotriquetral intervals with inability to progress to preinjury activity levels indicates the need for reevaluation by the hand surgeon.

II. Chronic carpal ligament injuries: stable with no radiographic findings, or unstable with radiographic findings if not a candidate for surgery

A. Scapholunate and lunotriquetral ligament injuries

1. Symptom management and joint protection through the use of splints and supports and modalities of heat and cold.

2. Job modification and retraining to limit further stress to the wrist from work, sports, and other ADLs and inappropriate exercises. The goal is to discourage the progression of instability and secondary changes.

3. Limited ROM and isometric exercise to maintain functional wrist mobility and strength. Observe caution with exercise: avoid repetitive ROM exercises under load, which are likely to exacerbate symptoms and further undermine the condition of the wrist. Symptom response should routinely be used as an indicator of the tolerance of the wrist to applied stresses.

B. Palmar midcarpal instability

1. Midcarpal stabilization splint (Fig. 35-2) provides dorsally directed pressure on the pisiform to reduce the ulnar volar sag of the carpus and correct the volarflexed position of the proximal carpal row.[22] Midcarpal dynamics are corrected, and the wrist symptoms and the clunk are partially or fully eliminated. The splint allows almost full extension, radial deviation, and ulnar deviation and limits flexion.

2. Avoid standard repetitive grip strengthening and isotonic progressive resistive wrist exercises: The pathomechanics of palmar midcarpal instability are apparent or reproduced with wrist motion under load. Therefore, standard exercise that involves motion under load (wrist curls with free weights) reproduces the pathomechanics of the wrist and usually exacerbates symptoms.

3. Isometric ulnar deviation (extensor carpi ulnaris [ECU] and flexor carpi ulnaris [FCU] strengthening) in supination. The ECU is an important dorsal wrist stabilizer. Contraction of the FCU provides a volar source of ulnar wrist support.[26] Isometric contraction of both ECU and FCU together provides for stabilization of the ulnar carpus. Supination is a more stable position for the wrist because of the tightening effect on the ulnar wrist ligaments with the decrease in ulnar variance that occurs with supination.[27]

4. Lichtman and colleagues[22] described dynamic muscle compression achieved by activation of the ECU and the hypothenar muscles, reproducing the normal joint contact forces in the absence of adequate ligament support.

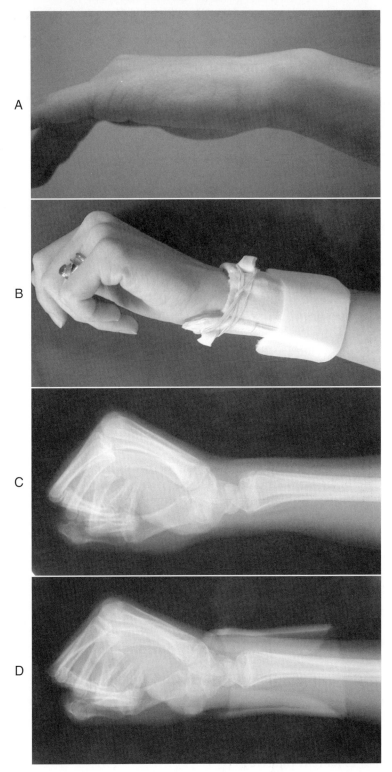

FIG. 35-2 A, Palmar midcarpal instability, as described by Lichtman, is characterized by a volar sag on the ulnar side of the wrist, a clunk that occurs at the end of the range of ulnar deviation with forearm pronation, tenderness over the triquetral-hamate and capitolunate intervals, and weakness of grip.[22] B, Midcarpal stabilization splint provides dorsally directed pressure on the pisiform with counterpressure dorsally over the head of the ulna to reduce the ulnar volar sag of the carpus. C, Volar intercalated segment instability (VISI) pattern with slight palmar translation of the distal carpal row in wrist with palmar midcarpal instability. D, Midcarpal stabilization splint corrects the VISI posture of the wrist.

NONOPERATIVE COMPLICATIONS

I. Nonunion, delayed union
II. Loss of motion and strength
III. Instability of the fracture
IV. Nerve injury
V. Persistent symptoms of pain and tenderness
VI. Carpal collapse
VII. Degenerative changes of the wrist

POSTOPERATIVE INDICATIONS/PRECAUTIONS FOR THERAPY

I. Indications
   A. Carpal fractures and/or ligament injuries that have achieved healing and stability through surgical techniques
II. Precautions
   A. Incomplete healing of bone and/or ligament
   B. Associated nerve and/or tendon injury
   C. Unresolved edema
   D. History of ligament laxity (Ehlers-Danlos syndrome)

POSTOPERATIVE THERAPY

Carpal Fractures

I. Therapy after surgical intervention for carpal fractures
   A. In the early postoperative phase, patients are typically in a bulky postoperative dressing and are encouraged to mobilize the fingers to decrease edema and likelihood of stiffness in uninvolved joints.
   B. At 7 to 14 days postoperatively, AROM may be permitted in all planes. Scar management and desensitization techniques are included at this time to decrease incision scar adherence and hypersensitivity. At 6 weeks, PROM and joint mobilization techniques may be initiated if carpal bone healing permits. In addition, dynamic and static splinting can be used to position the wrist at end range, to enhance the impact on the soft tissues and permit further mobility.
   C. Strengthening begins after healing has been confirmed, as described in the section on nonoperative treatment. The strengthening regimen typically follows, as fractures treated nonoperatively.

Carpal Ligament Injuries

Considerations: vigorous stretching is never indicated after carpal ligament repair or reconstruction. Communication with the referring surgeon concerning the specific procedure and the goals for outcome is imperative; also, timing of the introduction of progressive levels of stress depends on healing as determined by the surgeon through physical examination and radiographic evaluation.

I. Therapy after surgical intervention for scapholunate ligament injury
    A. Arthroscopic stabilization with anatomical reduction and Kirschner-wire placement across the scapholunate interval: After surgery, patients are immobilized in a thumb spica splint or cast for 8 weeks. At 8 weeks, after pin removal, AROM exercises for the wrist are initiated. A removable thermoplastic thumb spica splint is used for intermittent protection and support. Portal site scar massage and desensitization is begun. Light isometric strengthening can begin at 12 weeks. Avoid loading, power grip, weight-bearing, and lifting for 6 months.[28]
    B. Open reduction and pinning with direct scapholunate ligament repair: After surgery, patients are immobilized in a thumb spica splint or cast for 8 weeks. At 8 weeks, after pin removal, AROM exercises for the wrist are initiated. A removable thermoplastic thumb spica splint is used for intermittent protection and support. Scar massage and desensitization is begun. Light isometric strengthening can begin at 12 weeks. Avoid loading, power grip, weight-bearing, and lifting for 6 months.[24]
    C. Blatt dorsal capsulodesis: This operation is described for rotary subluxation of the scaphoid. It involves the use of a proximally based strip of the dorsal wrist capsule attached to the distal pole of the derotated scaphoid to create a dynamic check-rein mechanism that prevents acute flexion of the distal pole of the scaphoid.[29] After surgery, patients are immobilized in a thumb spica splint or cast for 8 weeks. At 8 weeks, after pin removal, AROM exercises for the wrist are initiated. A removable thermoplastic thumb spica splint is used for intermittent protection and support. Scar massage and desensitization are begun. At 12 weeks, light strengthening with isometric exercises can begin; patients are progressed slowly with continuous monitoring of symptoms. No stress loading is permitted for 6 months, and wrist flexion will be limited by 15 to 20 degrees.[29]
    D. Limited intercarpal fusions: These may require wrist immobilization with casting or splinting for up to 12 weeks, until bony consolidation occurs. With more rigid internal fixation, motion may begin earlier. During the phase of immobilization, digital motion and edema control measures are included in a home program. AROM exercises are begun for the wrist after sufficient healing of the fusion has occurred, as determined by the surgeon. ROM of the wrist will be limited, depending on the specific fusion performed, and should not be stressed. Strengthening can begin once there is radiographic confirmation that bony union has been achieved.[30]
II. Therapy after surgical intervention for lunotriquetral ligament injury
    A. Lunotriquetral repair or reconstruction with pinning: Short arm cast or splint for 8 weeks, with digital motion and edema control during the phase of immobilization. Pins are pulled at 8 weeks. A volar splint for the wrist is used for protection for an additional 4 weeks; it is removed for ROM exercises and bathing. AROM exercises for the wrist begin at 8 weeks, after pin removal.

Desensitization, scar massage, and edema management are incorporated as needed. Light strengthening can begin at 12 weeks. Avoid impact loading and forceful rotational motions up to 4 to 6 months.[28]

    B. Lunotriquetral arthrodesis: Short arm cast or splint for 8 weeks, with digital motion and edema control during the phase of immobilization. AROM exercises for the wrist begin at 8 weeks, with a removable volar wrist splint used for protection until healing is complete. Desensitization, scar massage, and edema management are incorporated as needed. Light strengthening can begin at 12 weeks if healing of the arthrodesis is complete.[25]

III. Therapy after surgery for midcarpal instability

    A. Soft tissue repair or reconstruction and pinning: Short arm cast or splint for 8 weeks, with digital motion and edema control during the phase of immobilization. Pins are pulled at 8 to 10 weeks. A volar splint for the wrist is used for protection for an additional 4 weeks; it is removed for AROM exercises and bathing. AROM exercises for the wrist begin at 8 weeks, after pin removal. Passive motion is avoided to prevent reoccurrence of instability. Desensitization, scar massage, and edema management are incorporated as needed. Light isometric strengthening can begin at 12 weeks. Avoid loading, power grip, weight-bearing, and lifting for 6 months.[22]

    B. Limited wrist arthrodesis: wrist immobilization with cast or splint for up to 12 weeks, until bony consolidation occurs. With more rigid internal fixation, motion may begin earlier. During the phase of immobilization, digital motion and edema control measures are included in a home program. AROM exercises are begun for the wrist after sufficient healing of the fusion has occurred, as determined by the surgeon. ROM of the wrist will be limited, depending on the specific fusion performed, and should not be stressed. Strengthening can begin once there is radiographical confirmation that bony union has been achieved.[30]

POSTOPERATIVE COMPLICATIONS

See nonoperative complications.

EVALUATION TIMELINE

   I. AROM of uninvolved joints: at the initial evaluation; weekly reevaluation until ROM is within normal limits.

  II. Edema measurements: at the initial evaluation and then weekly until edema is resolved. Edema measurements can be taken both before and after a therapy session and used as an indicator of tolerance to therapy.

 III. Pain levels: determined at the initial evaluation and at each reevaluation until pain is resolved.

 IV. Symptom response to therapy and to ADLs: assessed at every therapy session.

  V. Sensibility: screened at the initial evaluation. With findings, reassessment is performed every 4 to 6 weeks or if the patient reports a change in status.

VI. ADL function, including self-care, household activities, and work function, is reviewed at the initial evaluation. Reevaluation of goals for function is performed weekly.

VII. AROM of the wrist and forearm is evaluated after casting or continuous splinting has been discontinued and motion is permitted. Reevaluation is performed weekly thereafter. For wrist salvage procedures and carpal instability, wrist ROM measurement in general should not be emphasized and is not the most important indicator of progress.

VIII. Strength measurements of grip and pinch are taken after healing of the involved structures has occurred, as determined by the referring physician. Strength measurements are taken after strengthening exercises are permitted.

IX. Wrist function can be assessed using the Patient Rated Wrist Evaluation (PRWE).[31]

OUTCOMES

Published reports of the outcome after nonoperative and postoperative rehabilitation for carpal fractures and carpal ligament injuries are needed. Outcome measures such as MacDermid's PRWE[31] are appropriate tools that can be used to assess rehabilitation outcomes; this can be administered before and at the conclusion of therapy.

REFERENCES

1. American Academy of Orthopaedic Surgeons: Joint Motion: Method of Measuring and Recording. The American Academy of Orthopaedic Surgeons, Chicago, 1965
2. Ryu J, Cooney WP, Askew LJ, et al.: Functional ranges of motion of the wrist joint. J Hand Surg Am 16:409-419, 1991
3. Palmer AK, Werner FW, Murphy D, Glisson R: Functional wrist motion: a biomechanical study. J Hand Surg Am 10:39-46, 1985
4. Markiewitz AD, Ruby LK, O'Brien ET: Carpal fractures and dislocations. In Lichtman DM, Alexander AH (eds): The Wrist and Its Disorders. 2nd Ed. WB Saunders, Philadelphia, 1997, p. 189
5. Bednar JM, Osterman AL: Carpal instability: evaluation and treatment. J Am Acad Orthop Surg 1:10-17, 1993
6. Kozin S: Incidence, mechanism, and natural history of scaphoid fractures. Hand Clin 17:515-524, 2001
7. Dell PC, Dell RB: Management of carpal fractures and dislocations. In Mackin EJ, Callahan AD, Skirven TM, et al. (eds): Hunter-Mackin-Callahan Rehabilitation of the Hand and Upper Extremity. 5th Ed. Mosby, St. Louis, 2002, p. 1172
8. DeBeer J, Hudson D: Fractures of the triquetrum. J Hand Surg Br 12:52-53, 1987
9. Suzuki T, Nakatsuchi Y, Tateiwa Y, et al.: Osteochondral fracture of the triquetrum: a case report. J Hand Surg Am 27:98-100, 2002
10. Foster RJ, Hastings H 2nd: Treatment of Bennett, Rolando, and vertical intraarticular trapezial fractures. Clin Orthop (214):121-129, 1987
11. Brach P, Goitz R: An update on the management of carpal fractures. J Hand Ther 152-160, 2003
12. Cooney WP, Bishop AT, Linscheid RL: Physical examination of the wrist. In Cooney WP, Linscheid RL, Dobyns JH (eds): The Wrist: Diagnosis and Operative Treatment. Mosby, St. Louis, 1998, p. 254
13. Walsh J, Bishop A: Diagnosis and management of hamate hook fractures. Hand Clin 16:397-403, 2000
14. Cohen M: Fractures of the carpal bones. Hand Clin 13:587-599, 1997
15. Tredget E, Ghahary A: (2004). Hand, Fractures, and Dislocations: Wrist. Available at: http://www.emedicine.com/plastic/topic318.htm (accessed March 30, 2005)

16. Rand JM, Linscheid RL, Dobyns JM: Capitate fractures. Clin Orthop 165:209-216, 1982

17. Vance RM, Gelberman RH, Evans EF: Scaphocapitate fractures: patterns of dislocation, mechanism of injury, and preliminary results of treatment. J Bone Joint Surg Am 62:271, 1980

18. Calandruccio J, Duncan S: Isolated nondisplaced capitate waist fracture diagnosed by magnetic resonance imaging. J Hand Surg Am 24:856-859, 1999

19. Botte MJ, Gelberman RH: Fractures of the carpus, excluding the scaphoid. Hand Clin 3:149-161, 1987

20. Jeong G, Kram D, Lester B: Isolated fracture of the trapezoid. Am J Orthop 30:228-230, 2001

21. Dobyns JH, Cooney WP: Classification of carpal instability. In Cooney WP, Linscheid RL, Dobyns JH (eds): The Wrist: Diagnosis and Operative Treatment. Mosby, St. Louis, 1998, pp. 490-500

22. Lichtman DM, Gaenslen ES, Pollock GR: Midcarpal and proximal carpal instabilities. In Lichtman DM, Alexander AH (eds): The Wrist and Its Disorders. 2nd Ed. WB Saunders, Philadelphia, 1997, pp. 316-328

23. Bora FW, Culp RW, Osterman AL, et al.: A flexible wrist splint. J Hand Surg Am 14:3, 1989

24. Blatt G, Tobias B, Lichtman DM: Scapholunate injuries. In Lichtman DM, Alexander AH (eds): The Wrist and Its Disorders. 2nd Ed. WB Saunders, Philadelphia, 1997, pp. 268-306

25. Alexander CE, Lichtman DM: Triquetrolunate instability. In Lichtman DM, Alexander AH (eds): The Wrist and Its Disorders. 2nd Ed. WB Saunders, Philadelphia, 1997, p. 310

26. Garcia-Elias M: Midcarpal instability: surgical management. Presentation at the Hand Rehabilitation Foundation meeting on Surgery and Rehabilitation of the Hand with Emphasis on the Wrist, Philadelphia, March 8-10, 2003

27. Palmer AK, Glisson RR, Werner FW: Ulnar variance determination. J Hand Surg Am 7:376-379, 1982

28. Whipple TL: Arthroscopic surgery. In Whipple TL (ed): The Wrist. JB Lippincott, Philadelphia, 1992, pp. 119-129

29. Blatt G: Capsulodesis in reconstructive hand surgery: dorsal capsulodesis for unstable scaphoid and volar capsulodesis following excision of the distal ulna. Hand Clin 3:81-102, 1987

30. Feldon PG, Nalebuff EA, Terrono AL: Partial wrist fusions: intercarpal and radiocarpal. In Lichtman DM, Alexander AH (eds): The Wrist and Its Disorders. 2nd Ed. WB Saunders, Philadelphia, 1997, p. 322

31. MacDermid JC, Turgeon T, Richards RS, et al.: Patient rating of wrist pain and disability: a reliable and valid measurement tool. J Orthop Trauma 12:8, 577-586, 1998

Triangular Fibrocartilage Injuries

36

Greg Pitts and Ronald Burgess

DEFINITION

The triangular fibrocartilage complex (TFCC) is the primary stabilizer of the ulnar aspect of the wrist, including both radiocarpal and ulnocarpal relationships. The complex functions as both a load-bearing spacer and a ligament, and the treatment for a pathological lesion of the complex is based on the particular function affected.

ANATOMY

The TFCC is composed of the triangular fibrocartilage and the ulnocarpal ligaments. The triangular fibrocartilage arises from the superior aspect of the radial side of the distal radial-ulnar joint (sigmoid notch) and attaches to the ulna at the fovea at the base of the ulnar styloid. The portions originating at the volar and dorsal aspect of the radius and attaching to the fovea are ligamentous in structure and form stabilizing ligaments for the radioulnar joint. These portions are vascularized and are capable of healing if repaired. The central portion is composed of fibrocartilage and transmits compressive loads from the carpus to the ulnar head. This area is avascular and is not capable of healing if injured.

The ulnocarpal ligaments arise from the fovea of the distal ulna, with the triangular fibrocartilage, and insert on the volar surface of the ulnar carpus; they help stabilize the ulnar side of the carpus. The inner sheath of the extensor carpi ulnaris (ECU) is attached to the dorsal portion of the triangular fibrocartilage and further stabilizes the dorsal portion of the complex (Fig. 36-1).

CLASSIFICATION OF INJURIES

Palmer[1] classified injuries of the TFCC in two main categories based on etiology. The traumatic type occurs with isolated trauma, usually a rotation torque of the distal radioulnar joint. The degenerative type occurs from

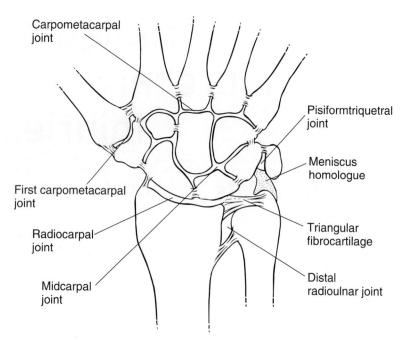

FIG. **36-1** Normal anatomy of the triangular fibrocartilage complex (TFCC). (From Cooney WP, Linscheid RL, Dobyns JH, et al.: The Wrist: Diagnosis and Operative Treatment. Mosby, St. Louis, 1998.)

repetitive compressive forces on the central portion from proximal migration of the lunate toward the ulna with forceful use of the hand. This causes progressive destruction of the central, avascular portion of the cartilage and degenerative changes on either side of the joint.

Traumatic (Type 1) Injuries (Fig. 36-2)

Involved structures may include the following:
    I.   Horizontal tear in the disc adjacent to the sigmoid notch of the radius
   II.   TFCC avulsion from the ulna
  III. Avulsions of the ulnocarpal ligaments from the carpus
  IV. TFCC avulsions from the sigmoid notch of the radius

Degenerative (Type 2) Injuries (Fig. 36-3)

Sequence of degenerative changes:[1]
    I.   Thinning of the TFCC
   II.   Thinning of the TFCC with chondromalacia of the ulna and lunate
  III. Perforation of the TFCC with chondromalacia of the ulna and lunate
  IV. Perforation of the TFCC with chondromalacia of the ulna and lunate and a lunotriquetral ligament tear
   V. Perforation of the TFCC with arthritis of the ulna and lunate and a lunotriquetral ligament tear

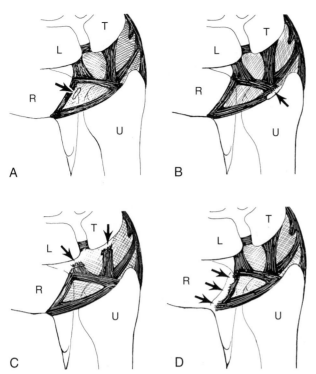

FIG. 36-2 Diagrammatic drawing of traumatic, or class I, abnormalities of the triangular fibrocartilage complex. **A,** Class IA, central perforation *(arrow)*. **B,** Class IB, ulnar avulsion *(arrow)*, with or without distal ulnar fracture. **C,** Class IC, distal avulsion *(arrows)*. **D,** Class ID, radial avulsion *(arrows)*, with or without sigmoid notch fracture. *L,* Lunate; *R,* radius; *T,* triquetrum; *U,* ulna. (Redrawn from Palmer AK: J Hand Surg Am 14:594-606, 1989 with permission from The American Society for Surgery of the Hand.)

TREATMENT INDICATIONS/TECHNIQUE

The indications for treatment of abnormalities of the TFCC are pain and/or instability. The pain may arise from instability of either the ulnocarpal or the radioulnar joints (traumatic injuries), or from the lunotriquetral joint (degenerative injuries), or from progressive degenerative changes between the ulna and lunate.

Traumatic Injuries[2]

I.   The horizontal tear is in the avascular portion of the TFCC and does not involve the ligamentous portions. It is treated by arthroscopic debridement to a stable rim *(debridement treatment program)*.

II. An avulsion of the ligamentous portion of the TFCC off the ulna destabilizes the distal radioulnar joint. The ligament retracts and loses it natural tension when observed arthroscopically (the trampoline effect). It is treated by either direct repair of the ligaments to the ulna or reconstruction of the ligaments with tendon graft *(reconstruction treatment program)*.

III. Although the ulnocarpal ligaments help stabilize the ulnar side of the carpus, injuries to this complex are usually treated by

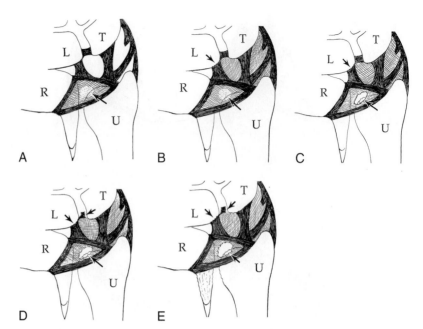

FIG. 36-3 Diagrammatic drawing of degenerative, or class 2, abnormalities of the triangular fibrocartilage complex (TFCC). **A,** Class 2A, TFCC wear *(arrow)*. **B,** Class 2B, TFCC wear with lunate *(small arrow)* and/or ulnar *(large arrow)* chondromalacia. **C,** Class 2C, TFCC perforation with lunate *(small arrow)* and/or ulnar (large arrow) chondromalacia. **D,** Class 2D, TFCC perforation with lunate *(arrow)* and/or ulnar *(large arrow)* chondromalacia and lunotriquetral ligament perforation *(small arrow)*. **E,** Class 2E, TFCC perforation with lunate *(arrow)* and/or ulnar *(large arrow)* chondromalacia, lunotriquetral ligament perforation *(small arrow)*, and ulnocarpal arthritis. *L,* lunate; *R,* radius; *T,* triquetrum; *U,* ulna. (Redrawn from Palmer AK: J Hand Surg Am 14:594-606, 1989 with permission form The American Society for Surgery of the Hand.)

   arthroscopic debridement for pain *(conservative treatment program with wrist gauntlet).*
IV. Avulsions of the TFCC off the sigmoid notch are often seen in conjunction with distal radius fractures, and they are usually initially treated with immobilization *(conservative treatment program with wrist gauntlet splint).* The primary treatment focus should be on the distal radius fracture.

Degenerative Injuries[2]

   I. Thinning of the TFCC from repetitive compressive loads does not require treatment *(conservative treatment program).*
  II. Once the compressive loads are sufficient to cause chondromalacia of the opposing joint surfaces, localized pain develops and can be treated by debridement *(conservative treatment program).*
 III. A central perforation of the TFCC leaves flaps of cartilage that mechanically impinge between the lunate and ulna, making the early degenerative changes of both surfaces more symptomatic. It is treated by debridement of the tears as well as the chondromalacia *(debridement treatment program).*

IV. A degenerative tear of the lunotriquetral ligament adds to the localized pain. Initial treatment consists of debridement of the remaining injured structures *(debridement treatment program)*.

V. If this is insufficient, either lunotriquetral fusion[3] *(reconstruction treatment program)* or ulnar shortening[4] *(debridement treatment program)* may be considered.

VI. Advanced changes are treated with arthroscopic or open ulnar wafer procedure (removal of the distal surface of the ulna down to subchondral bone, typically 3 mm) or ulnar shortening[5] *(debridement treatment program)*.

NONOPERATIVE MANAGEMENT

TFCC injuries to the central avascular articular disk that are confirmed by magnetic resonance imaging often are not amenable to primary repair. Therefore, initial management is aimed at resting the distal radioulnar joint (DRUJ), the ECU, and the TFCC. This is accomplished with a long arm splint or cast to stop forearm rotation and weight-bearing, to facilitate rest. Activity modification and gradual exposure to activities of daily living (ADLs) risk factors is conducted in a controlled manner.

NONOPERATIVE MANAGEMENT TIMELINE[2,6,7]

I. 0 to 6 weeks: Splint is worn 18 hours/day, with no physical activity outside the splint

   A. Long arm cast or long arm splint is fitted with elbow at 70 to 90 degrees flexion, forearm and wrist in neutral[6,8] (Fig. 36-4)

   B. The splint is worn for 6 weeks to rest the TFCC.

   C. Patient education on risk factors with ADL tasks, pathology, and healing timelines

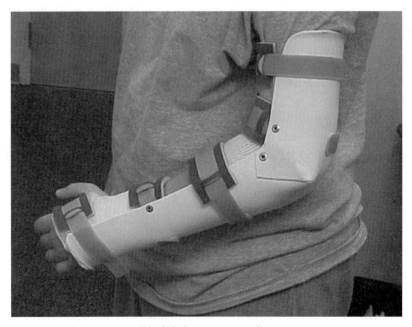

FIG. **36-4** Long arm splint.

D. ADL adaptation is explored, with patient's goals and social roles the major considerations

E. Edema control measures are started with overhead fisting, Coban wraps, and tendon gliding every hour

II. 6 weeks: The focus of rehabilitation in this phase is to restore active range of motion (AROM) of the flexor and extensor compartments and diminish joint stiffness while avoiding an increase in pain.[6]

A. AROM and active-assisted range of motion (AAROM) exercises are performed for the wrist and forearm every hour for 5 to 10 minutes.

B. AROM is conducted for the wrist (linear motion), forearm (in neutral), hand, and digits.

1. Patients can conduct the following:

a. Tendon gliding to restore muscle balance
(1) Basic four hand postures
(2) Joint blocks
(3) Flexor digitorum superficialis (FDS) individual tendon glides

b. Neural gliding to diminish the pain reflex and restore muscle balance
(1) Ulnar nerve gliding
(2) Median nerve gliding (distal)

2. Passive range of motion (PROM) may start with pronation and supination if kept below a pain reflex.

3. ADL training enhances motor control with fine motor and gross motor dexterity tasks (e.g., lacing, buttoning).

a. Basic ADL tasks work well to decrease the pain reflex and restore confidence with basic self-care.

b. *NOTE: Keep wrist in neutral with all tasks.

C. A wrist gauntlet splint (Fig. 36-5) may be appropriate to use after removal of the long arm splint, to increase the patient's tolerance to basic ADL tasks and to rest the wrist complex when not conducting the home exercise program. The splint helps control co-contraction of muscle from joint pain.[8]

III. 8 weeks: Progressive strengthening may be initiated, assuming that there is no increase in pain or discomfort and the patient is totally asymptomatic.

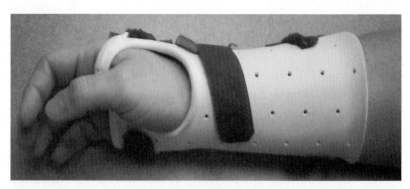

FIG. 36-5 Wrist gauntlet splint.

A. All strengthening is conducted in linear motion patterns while maintaining a neutral forearm position.
   1. Isometric strengthening with grip and hold
   2. Isotonic strengthening with putty
   3. Isotonic wrist flexion and extension with weight
B. Overhead, pronation, supination, torquing and weight-bearing activities are avoided until the patient is asymptomatic with linear-motion, forearm-neutral strengthening tasks.

IV. 10 to 12 weeks: Overhead, torquing, and weight-bearing activities may be initiated if the patient is asymptomatic. These types of tasks place direct biomechanical impingement, soft tissue torsion, and impaction stress on the TFCC. Exposure to these risk factors must be done on a gradual and guarded basis.[9]

A. The Baltimore Therapeutic Equipment (BTE) Work Simulator is recommended as an excellent tool to introduce the risk factors of radial and ulnar deviation, pronation, and supination in a safe and graded manner.
   1. First, introduce the torque motion patterns of ulnar and radial deviation, followed by pronation and supination. Progress slowly until no residual pain is noted the next treatment session. Torque motion with gradual increase in load.
   2. Final stage is torque motion with load and pace.
B. Start gradual exposure to risk factors of overhead activities, torquing tasks, and torquing tasks with load. These tasks have the highest potential for reinjury.
   1. Isometric strengthening with grip and hold (work at 10% or less of maximum voluntary effort [MVE]).
   2. Isotonic strengthening with putty (focus on complete excursion of flexor digitorum profundus [FDP]).
   3. Isotonic wrist flexion and extension with weight
C. Once the patient is asymptomatic with isometric grasp and linear isotonic wrist flexion and extension, exposure to low-load repetitive grasping may be attempted.

V. The patient may consider surgery if the pain continues with torque and weight-bearing tasks.

VI. *NOTE: Conservative management is not always considered if the problem is greater than 6 months in duration.

OPERATIVE INDICATIONS[2,7]

I. Failure of recovery of function with conservative treatment
II. Lunotriquetral ligament injury
III. Distal radioulnar joint instability

DEBRIDEMENT OF THE TFCC

Evaluation and Treatment Timeline

I. Postoperatively in 3 to 5 days[6]
   A. Postoperative dressing is removed, and incision site is inspected for signs and symptoms of infection.

B. Edema control measures are taken with overhead fisting, Coban wraps or edema glove, and tendon gliding every hour.

C. A wrist gauntlet splint is appropriate to use after removal of the dressing to increase the patient's tolerance to basic ADL tasks and to rest the wrist complex when not conducting the home exercise program. The splint helps control co-contraction of muscle from joint pain[8] (see Fig. 36-5).

D. Gentle AROM exercises are initiated at the wrist (linear motion), forearm (in neutral), hand, and digits every hour for 5 to 10 minutes.

   1. Tendon gliding to restore muscle balance

   2. Joint blocking exercises for individual joints

   3. Neural gliding to diminish the pain reflex and restore muscle balance

      a. Ulnar nerve glides

      b. Median nerve glides (distal)

   4. ADL training to enhance motor control with fine motor and gross motor dexterity tasks (e.g., lacing, buttoning)

      a. Basic ADL tasks work well to decrease the pain reflex and restore confidence with basic self-care.

      b. *NOTE: Keep wrist in neutral with all tasks.

II. 7 to 10 days

A. Sutures are removed, and incision site is inspected for signs and symptoms of infection

B. Scar management

   1. Silicone or elastomer applied directly to the scar 1 day after removal of sutures.

   2. Scar pad is worn half of the day and all night to diminish scar pain.

C. Wrist gauntlet is worn part-time for support and comfort as needed for 10 days to 4 weeks.

D. The patient continues to focus on AROM exercises for the digits, hand, and wrist, to create proper muscle lengths to facilitate normal function with ADL tasks.

E. The patient continues self-care ADL tasks to restore motor control.

III. 4 to 6 weeks

A. AAROM and PROM may begin below pain reflex.

B. The patient may start gentle isotonic strengthening with light putty with forearm in neutral position.

C. Treatment focuses on end-range motion below pain reflex to restore full ROM and diminish adaptive shortening of muscles.

D. Patient should continue prior AROM recommendations.

IV. Week 6

A. PROM and static progressive splinting may be considered, assuming that the patient does not have pain with progressive exercises, the scar is mature, and the major limiting factor is extrinsic extensor tightness or joint stiffness.

   1. Static progressive wrist flexion/extension or pronation/supination splinting should be applied with the load tolerable to wear a minimum of 2 hours.

   2. Patient education is critical, with the focus on stretch

versus pain. Directional forces are alternated throughout the day in the exercise program.

3. Emphasis can be placed in a specific direction, but always seek establishment of wrist extension before flexion—this facilitates the grasp reflex, increases function, and diminishes impairment.

B. Progressive strengthening may be initiated.

   1. Isotonic strengthening with putty
   2. Isotonic wrist flexion and extension with weight
   3. Isometric strengthening with grip and hold
      a. Normally, start with a 10-lb gripper—hold 30 seconds, rest 1 minute; do 5 repetitions twice per day. This is increased to hold 1 minute, rest 1 minute with 10-lb gripper 5 times twice per day.
      b. *NOTE: All strengthening is conducted in linear motion patterns while maintaining a neutral forearm position.

C. Overhead tasks, torquing tasks, and weight-bearing tasks are initiated if the patient is asymptomatic with linear-motion, forearm-neutral strengthening tasks. These types of tasks place direct biomechanical impingement, soft tissue torsion, and impaction stress on the TFCC. Exposure to these risk factors must be done on a gradual and guarded basis.[9-11]

   1. First, introduce the torque motion patterns of ulnar and radial deviation; gradual increase in time, with the patient working at his or her own pace.
   2. Ulnar and radial deviation torque motion with load and pace.
   3. Pronation and supination torque motion; gradual increase in time, with the patient working at his or her own pace.
   4. Pronation and supination torque motion with load and pace.

V. The patient may consider vocational change if the pain continues with torque and weight-bearing tasks.

VI. Other treatment considerations

A. Use of minivibrator (padded) for scar pain and adhesions at the incision site

B. Use of transcutaneous electrical nerve stimulation (TENS) unit to diminish pain while conducting exercises after surgery

C. Static progressive splinting (see earlier description) should be used with caution, because it can increase pain and discomfort.

   1. The patient is instructed to set the tension level of the static progressive splint at a point at which the splint can be worn for a minimum of 1 hour without pain; the patient should feel a stretch, but no pain, while using the splint.
   2. The goal is to increase splint wear to 2 hours on, 1 hour off per day. The splint is used until the desired motion is met.

VII. Patient education key points

A. Conduct AROM in a pain-free fashion while not wearing the splint.

B. Avoid overhead activity, torquing tasks (pronation, supination, and radial/ulnar deviation), and weight-bearing tasks.

C. Conduct basic ADL tasks such as laundry, groceries, and meal preparation below pain level with splint until clearance by physician or therapist.

Postoperative Complications with Central Lesion Repair[2,7]

I. Failure of recovery of function
II. Painful neuroma, which can lead to complex regional pain syndrome (CRPS)
III. Infection
IV. Hypersensitive scar
V. DRUJ instability
VI. Extensor tendon injury
VII. Nerve injury

PRIMARY REPAIR OF TFCC PERIPHERAL TEAR

Surgical Indications

Injury to the peripheral TFCC can result in instability of the DRUJ and chronic ulnar carpal pain. Tears to the well-vascularized peripheral area are considered eligible for direct repair. The radial side has poor vascularity but can also be repaired to improve function.[2]

Evaluation and Treatment Timeline[2,6,7]

I. 0 to 10 or 14 days
   A. Immobilization in postoperative splint or cast
II. 7 or 10 days to 8 weeks
   A. The postoperative dressing is removed, and the patient is fitted with a long arm cast or long arm splint with elbow at 90 degrees flexion, forearm in neutral, and wrist in neutral[8] (see Fig. 36-4), or a Muenster-type splint to allow elbow flexion/extension while preventing forearm rotation.
   B. If DRUJ pinned, the patient will conduct pin care with 50% peroxide and 50% sterile water and change of dressings daily or according to the surgeon's preference.
   C. Patient is educated on signs and symptoms of infection with skin care.
   D. AROM exercises are initiated for digits (to prevent or diminish edema, intrinsic tightness, extrinsic tightness, and joint capsule stiffness)
      1. Overhead fisting for edema control
      2. Basic-4 hand postures
      3. Joint blocks for metacarpophalangeal, proximal interphalangeal, and distal interphalangeal joints
III. Weeks 3 to 4
   A. DRUJ pin usually is removed, and gentle wrist flexion and extension is initiated.
   B. PROM with supination to 45 to 60 degrees, depending on the tear, the repair, and the surgeon's preference.
IV. Weeks 6 to 8+
   A. Full AROM for flexion, extension, pronation, and supination should be the treatment goal.
   B. Terminal passive motion to pain tolerance.

V. 8 weeks
   A. AROM/PROM and AAROM are initiated to the forearm, wrist, and hand every hour for 5 to 10 minutes.
   B. PROM (rarely needed) and static progressive wrist splinting may be applied, assuming that the patient does not have pain with progressive exercises.
      1. Static progressive wrist splinting should be applied with the load tolerable to wear a minimum of 2 hours.
      2. Patient education is critical, with the focus on stretch versus pain. Directional forces are alternated throughout the day in the exercise program.
      3. Emphasis can be placed in a specific direction, but always seek to establish wrist extension before flexion; this facilitates the grasp reflex, increases function, and diminishes impairment.
      4. The patient wears a wrist gauntlet to protect the surgical repair while conducting ADL tasks. The splint diminishes pain and allows the wrist joint and muscles to rest while not conducting exercises. ADL training is initiated to restore motor control for self-care, grooming, and fine motor grasp and dexterity (see Fig. 36-5).
VI. 8 to 12 weeks
   A. The patient begins isotonic strengthening with putty, progressing to isometric grip and isotonic wrist flexion and extension.
      1. All strengthening is conducted in linear motion patterns while maintaining a neutral forearm position.
      2. Isometric strengthening with grip and hold (work at 10% or less of MVE)
      3. Isotonic strengthening with putty (focus on complete excursion of FDP)
      4. Isotonic wrist flexion and extension with weight
      5. Focus on speed and control of movement to maximize motor recruitment.
      6. Disallow recruitment of extensor digitorum communis (EDC) for wrist extension, because this will impair the natural grasp reflex.
VII. 12+ weeks
   A. Overhead activities, pronation, and supination torquing tasks and weight-bearing tasks are avoided until the patient is asymptomatic with linear-motion, forearm-neutral strengthening tasks.
   B. Start gradual exposure to overhead activities, torquing tasks, and torquing tasks with load.
      1. Isometric strengthening with grip and hold (work at 10% or less of MVE)
      2. Isotonic strengthening with putty (focus on complete excursion of FDP)
      3. Isotonic wrist flexion and extension with weight
   C. Once the patient is asymptomatic with isometric grasp and linear isotonic wrist flexion and extension, exposure to low-load repetitive grasping may be attempted.

D. If the patient is asymptomatic with repetitive grasping, then progress to overhead, pronation, supination, ulnar and radial deviation, and weight-bearing tasks. These types of tasks place direct biomechanical impingement, soft tissue torsion, and impaction stress on the TFCC. Exposure to these risk factors must be done on a gradual and guarded basis.

    a. First, introduce the torque motion patterns of ulnar and radial deviation, progressing to pronation, and supination. *NOTE: Supination is initiated before pronation, to avoid loading of the TFCC.

    b. Torque motion with gradual increase in load

    c. Final stage is torque motion with load and pace

    d. *NOTE: This progression is critical for predicting a safe return to activity level.

VIII. Other treatment considerations

A. All treatment programs, including splints, should avoid pain reflex and increase in pain, particularly to the ulnar side of the wrist.

B. All exercises, equipment, and strengthening should be performed in a forearm-neutral position, avoiding pronation and supination.

C. These exercises can be gradually progressed to supinated and then pronated postures while strengthening.

D. TENS units may be used and may be found helpful to diminish postoperative joint capsule pain, muscle guarding, and autonomic flare response from the surgical repair.

E. The patient may have to wear a wrist gauntlet splint for heavy instrumental activities of daily living (IADL) tasks such as yard work and manual labor for up to 6 months after surgery to support the TFCC repair.

POSTOPERATIVE COMPLICATIONS WITH PERIPHERAL LESION REPAIR

I. Failure of recovery of function

II. Painful neuroma

III. Infection

IV. Hypersensitive scar

V. Nerve injury (dorsal branch ulnar sensory can lead to CRPS)

VI. Failure to relieve symptoms

OUTCOMES

A radial nerve lesion can be devastating to a patient with the loss of functional dexterity. The functional outcome of radial nerve lesions is dependent on the severity index, location of the injury, age of the patient, and skill levels of the hand surgeon and the hand therapist. The majority of radial nerve lesions when managed by a hand surgeon realize functional recovery and independence with ADL tasks.

The therapist can enhance the functional outcome with detailed evaluations, which will provide the patient with the appropriate custom splints, a graded rehabilitation program, and recommendations on ADL adaptations.

Patient education is a must to diminish fear, provide activity modification, and understand healing timelines.

REFERENCES

1. Palmer AK: Triangular fibrocartilage complex lesions: a classification. J Hand Surg Am 14:594-606, 1989
2. Green DP, Hotchkiss RN, Pederson WP (eds): Green's Operative Hand Surgery. 4th Ed. Churchill Livingstone, St. Louis, 1998
3. Reagan DS, Linscheid RL, Dobyns JH: Lunotriquetral sprains. J Hand Surg Am 9:502-514, 1984
4. Linscheid RL: Ulnar lengthening and shortening. Hand Clin 3:69-79, 1987
5. Feldon P, Belshy MR, Terrono AL: Partial ("wafer") distal ulnar resection for triangular fibrocartilage tears and/or ulnar impaction. J Hand Surg Am 15:826-827, 1990
6. Hunter JM, Schneider LH, Mackin EJ, Callahan AD (eds): Rehabilitation of the Hand and Upper Extremity. 5th Ed. Mosby, St. Louis, 2002
7. Smith P: Lister's The Hand: Diagnosis and Indications. 4th Ed. WB Saunders, St. Louis, 2002
8. Fess EF, Phillips CA: Hand Splinting Principles and Methods. 3rd Ed. Mosby–Year Book, St. Louis, 2001
9. Werner FM, Glisson RR, Murphy DJ, Palmer AK: Force transmission through the distal radioulnar carpal joint: effect of ulnar lengthening and shortening. Handchir Mikrochir Plast Chir 18:304-308, 1986
10. Palmer AK: The distal radial ulnar joint: anatomy, biomechanics, and triangular fibrocartilage complex abnormalities. Hand Clin 3:31-40, 1987
11. Brand PW, Hollister A: Clinical Mechanics of the Hand. 3rd Ed. Mosby, St. Louis, 1999

External and Internal Fixation of Unstable Distal Radius Fractures

37

Georgiann F. Laseter

HISTORY/OVERVIEW

Claude Poteau first described fractures of the distal end of the radius with dorsal displacement of the distal fragment in 1783. However, this dorsally displaced fracture pattern is named for Abraham Colles, who published his now famous article in 1814.[1] Other descriptions of distal radius fracture patterns have been credited to Smith (1838) and Barton (1854).[2]

Distal radius fractures are common and have been estimated to account for approximately one sixth of *all* fractures treated in emergency rooms.[3] The various fracture patterns typically result from a fall on the outstretched hand. Fractures of the distal radius are more common in postmenopausal women and are caused most often by "low-energy" trauma (i.e., falls from level ground). Current evidence[4,5] points out that patients who have a "low-trauma wrist fracture" are at significantly greater risk for development of osteoporosis and hip fractures later in life. Lower bone mineral density (BMD) thresholds have been found in many of these patients, even though they had not yet been diagnosed with osteoporosis. Therefore, the "low-trauma" distal radius fracture should be considered a sentinel event. Orthopedists, hand surgeons, and hand therapists alike can play a proactive role to help reduce the chance of further fractures—and ultimately decrease health care costs—by referring patients back to their internist or family physician for osteoporosis screening.

Epidemiological trends indicate an increase in more complex, unstable distal radius fractures resulting from "high-energy" injuries (i.e., falls from greater than standing height), sports-related activities in younger patients or in a more active elderly population, and motor vehicle accidents.[6,7]

Despite the fact that distal radius fractures were first referenced in the medical literature more than 200 years ago, treatment of these common fractures and their dysfunctional sequelae[8-20] continues to challenge surgeons and therapists. Numerous attempts to establish universal fracture classifications, outcomes reporting, and treatment algorithms are reported in the literature, but there is no consensus.

Reports of distal radius malunions with surprisingly good function can be found in the literature,[21-25] but the more recent literature supports the correlation of anatomical reduction with improved functional outcomes.[26-39] Most surgeons now agree that the best opportunity for an improved outcome with fewer complications is provided by restoration of the distal radius anatomy to as "near normal" as possible.

Numerous techniques for unstable distal radius fracture fixation are outlined in the literature: percutaneous pin fixation, pins and plaster, external fixation, open reduction and internal fixation (ORIF), and arthroscopic reduction. The type of fracture fixation chosen by the surgeon is contingent on a number of variables, which may include the type of fracture displacement, associated injuries, bone "quality" (osteoporosis), patient's age and occupation, and the surgeon's training, preference, and expertise.

TREATMENT AND SURGICAL PURPOSE

Within the past two decades, understanding of the anatomy and biomechanics of the wrist has advanced, and newer imaging techniques are providing better information. The concurrent development and introduction of various fixation techniques and hardware has aided the evolution of distal radius fracture treatment to better restore the distal radius anatomy, improve outcomes, and decrease complications.

Early in treatment, it is important for the surgeon to diagnose fracture patterns that may be the markers of instability. Reduction of unstable fractures can usually be achieved, but a satisfactory reduction may be hard to maintain.[40] This type of fracture does *not* do well in a cast and needs more aggressive treatment.[41] Risk factors for fracture collapse include dorsal comminution, dorsal tilt, radial shortening, and intraarticular involvement. The chance of losing the reduced position of the distal radius increases in proportion to the number of risk factors present.[42]

EXTERNAL FIXATION

Definitions

Various types of percutaneous pinning are used, either alone or in conjunction with casting, external fixation, or arthroscopic reduction.[43,44] External fixation is widely used for treatment of these unstable, displaced distal radius fractures. There are many types of external fixators, each with their own strengths and weaknesses as well as cost differences.[43,45-48] The principle of all external fixation is based on "ligamentotaxis," wherein fracture fragments are aligned by traction across the fracture site through the capsuloligamentous structures.[49,50] External fixation usually does not adequately restore volar tilt in those fractures with excessive dorsal angulation, and supplemental pinning of this fragment is frequently required.[51-54]

The necessary duration of immobilization in an external fixator is still subject to debate among surgeons, but it averages about 6 to 8 weeks, depending on the fracture comminution. If the traction is removed earlier, the fracture may redisplace, because healing times are prolonged with traction.

One of the most common complications seen with external fixation is caused by the pins themselves. Regardless of the method or cleansing agents used, *meticulous* pin tract care is a must! There are other problems inherent with external fixation that can be addressed by the therapist if the

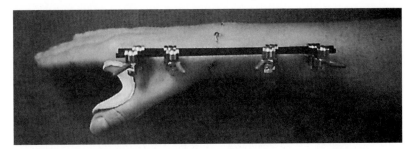

FIG. 37-1 A thermoplastic thumb web spacer splint around an external fixator. Care should be taken to avoid undue stress on the ulnar collateral ligament of the metacarpophalangeal joint (From Laseter GF, Carter PR: J Hand Ther 9:114-128, 1996. Copyright Hanley & Belfus, Philadelphia, used with permission.)

patient is referred for treatment while the external fixator is still in place. Radial abduction and extension of the thumb and flexion of the index finger can be blocked by the position of many external fixators. A thermoplastic web spacer can be fabricated and fit around the external fixator (Fig. 37-1). If the patient has trouble tolerating the hardness of the thermoplastic device, a simple splint can be made from a piece of foam rubber to help stretch the thumb web space (Fig. 37-2). The foam splint can be especially effective if the hand is edematous.[55]

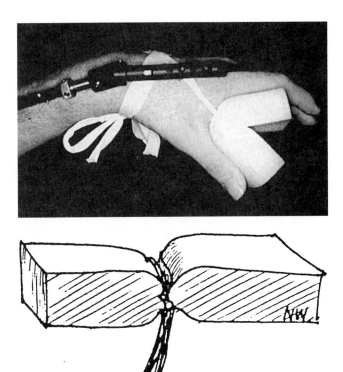

FIG. 37-2 If the hand is edematous or not tolerant of hard thermoplastic, a foam web spacer may be used. A piece of foam 2 × 1 × 2 inches is tied in the center with a length of Surgitube. This is inserted into the web, and the remaining Surgitube is wrapped around the wrist in a figure of 8 and tied in a bow. (From Colditz J: J Hand Ther 4:22, 1991. Copyright Hanley & Belfus, Philadelphia, used with permission.)

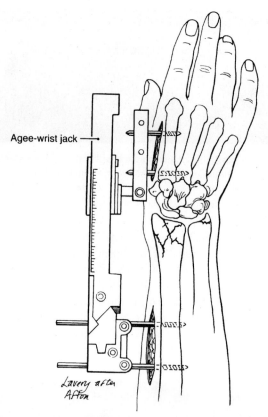

Agee-wrist jack

Lavery after
Afton

FIG. 37-3 Example of external fixation of a distal radius fracture. Note that the percutaneous pins of the fixator transfix the second and third metacarpals and the distal radius.

The second and third metacarpals and the distal radius are transfixed by the percutaneous pins of the external fixator (Fig. 37-3). This supports the longitudinal or fixed arch of the hand, but it does not support the mobile transverse arch. An ulnar gutter splint (Fig. 37-4) that is closely conformed to the palm can support this arch and improve patient comfort. It should be trimmed to allow full finger and thumb motion. It may be short or above-elbow, depending on the need to limit forearm rotation.[56]

Treatment Goals

I. Therapist: while external fixator is in place
   A. Obtain and maintain full range of motion (ROM) of all uninvolved joints by the time the wrist is ready to be mobilized.
   B. Prevent wound and/or pin tract infection.
   C. Resolve pain and edema.
   D. Encourage use of extremity in light functional activities.
II. Therapist: after external fixator is removed
   A. Initiate wrist ROM in a progressive manner, contingent on bony healing and tissue reactivity.
   B. Begin soft tissue and scar mobilization.

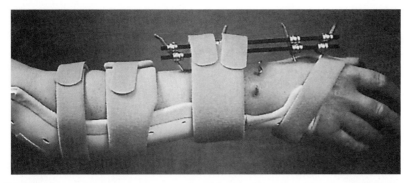

FIG. 37-4 An ulnar gutter support splint fabricated for use with an external fixator. The transverse arch is supported, full motion of the thumb and fingers is allowed, and the length can vary from short to above the elbow, contingent on the need to limit forearm rotation. (From Laseter GF, Carter PR: J Hand Ther 9:122, 1996. Copyright Hanley & Belfus, Philadelphia, used with permission.)

    C. Continue therapeutic interventions for any residual edema, pain, and joint stiffness of uninvolved joints.

    D. Return to previous level of function.

Postoperative Precautions for Therapy

I.   Other associated injuries to tendons, nerves, and soft tissues.

II.   Infections (e.g., open wounds, pin tract infections).

Postoperative Therapy

I.   Week 1 through weeks 6 to 12 (when fixator is usually removed)

    A. Begin the first of many patient education sessions!

      1. Instruction in meticulous pin tract care

      2. Instruction in edema control

    B. Fabricate and fit an ulnar gutter splint to support the mobile transverse arch for patient comfort and support.

    C. Active range of motion (AROM) of shoulder and elbow

    D. AROM, passive range of motion (PROM), and/or combinations of static or dynamic splints to overcome limitations in finger and thumb ROM

    E. Instruction in and emphasis on the importance of being compliant with the home exercise program

    F. Changes in therapy program dictated by patient progress on reevaluation

II.   Weeks 6 to 12 (external fixator is removed by surgeon after radiographical union is demonstrated)

    A. After removal of fixator, fabricate and fit a protective wrist splint (Fig. 37-5) as an interim support between the total immobilization of the fixator and nothing.

    B. Begin soft tissue and scar mobilization.

    C. Begin AROM of wrist in extension and flexion, radial and ulnar deviation, and supination and pronation. Pay particular attention to the patient's ability to extend the wrist *without* using the digital

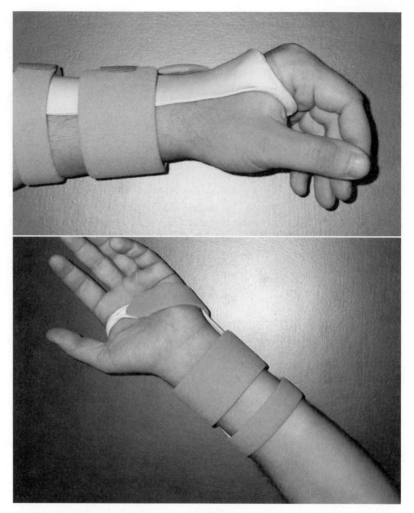

FIG. **37-5** A custom wrist splint is preferable for interim support after the external fixator is removed. This thermoplastic dorsal wrist splint with a slender palmar bar allows full mobility of the fingers and thumb. The open design encourages functional use of the hand while the splint is in use. The dorsal compression provided by the splint is also helpful if dorsal edema is still present. (From Laseter GF: Therapist's management of distal radius fractures. In Mackin EJ, Callahan AD, Skirven TM, et al. [eds]: Hunter-Mackin-Callahan Rehabilitation of the Hand and Upper Extremity. 5th Ed. Mosby, St. Louis, 2002.)

extensor tendons (Fig. 37-6). *Independent* wrist extension is necessary to reestablish power grip.[57,58]

D. Progress to passive stretching (Fig. 37-7) and resistive exercises as tolerated to regain maximum ROM and strength.

E. Continue therapeutic interventions as needed to overcome residual stiffness in shoulder, elbow, fingers, and thumb.

F. Continue emphasis on importance of home exercise program.

Postoperative Complications

I. Loss of reduction, resulting in malunion

II. Problems with hardware

A. Infection

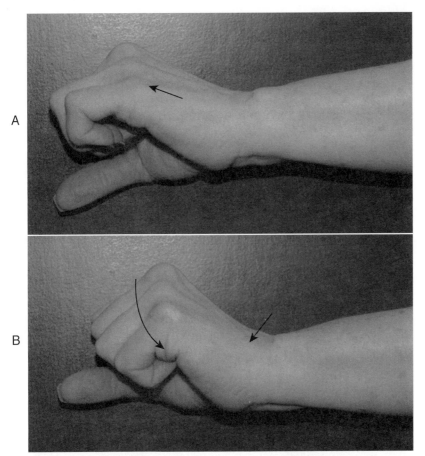

FIG. **37-6 A,** Many distal radius fracture patients have a well-established substitution pattern of using the digital extensors—particularly those in the ring and small fingers—to extend the wrist. **B,** Independent wrist extension is critical to developing the ability to make a fist and in regaining power grip after a distal radius fracture.

     B. Loosening
     C. Fracture of bone at pin site
  III. Complex regional pain syndrome (CRPS); also referred to as reflex sympathetic dystrophy or algodystrophy
  IV. Tendon adherence and/or rupture
   V. Nerve compression/irritation
     A. Median nerve compression can result in carpal tunnel syndrome.
     B. Irritation of dorsal superficial branch of radial nerve can cause "burning" pain along dorsoradial aspect of wrist and thumb.
  VI. Unresolved stiffness of uninvolved joints
 VII. Distal radius malunion
VIII. Refracture or redisplacement of distal radius

Evaluation Timeline

   I. Week 1 through weeks 6 to 12 (when fixator is usually removed)
     A. AROM and PROM measurements of shoulder, elbow, fingers, and thumb of involved extremity

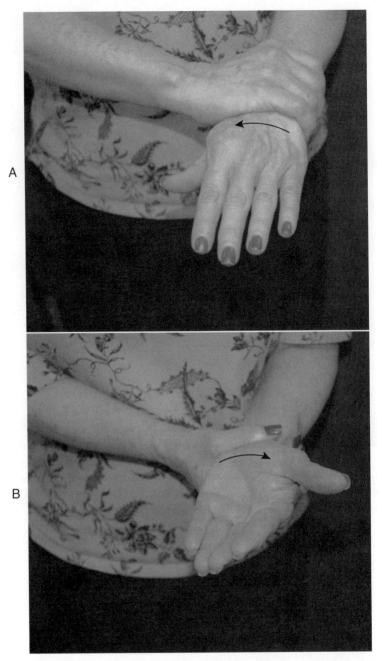

FIG. **37-7** **A,** Passive stretching in pronation is more effective if the opposite hand stretches across the involved distal forearm and "makes a bracelet" around the distal radioulnar joint (DRUJ). Note that the small fingers of both hands are close to each other in the position. **B,** Passive stretching in supination by positioning the thumb of the opposite hand across the distal forearm at about the level of the wrist flexion crease. The fingers of the opposite hand "make a bracelet" on the dorsum of the DRUJ. Note that the thumbs of both hands are close to each other in this position.

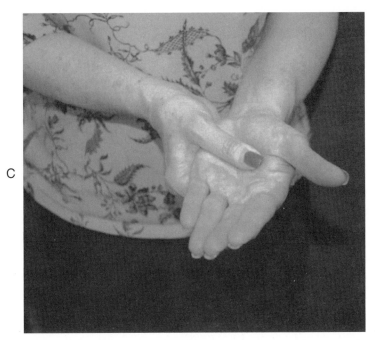

FIG. **37-7, cont'd C,** Incorrect passive stretch in supination. "Twisting the hand on the wrist" does not effectively stretch the DRUJ.

    B. AROM measurements of shoulder, elbow, fingers, and thumb of uninvolved extremity to use as "what's normal" for that patient

    C. Edema assessment

    D. Baseline sensibility assessment using Semmes-Weinstein monofilaments if carpal tunnel syndrome is suspected

II.   Weekly (at least): reassessment of ROM and edema measurements to determine progress and to provide information needed to continue or change the therapeutic program

III. Week 6 to 12 (external fixator is removed by surgeon after radiographic union is demonstrated)

    A. Repeat sensibility assessment if patient continues to report numbness in median nerve distribution.

    B. AROM and PROM measurements of involved wrist in extension/flexion, radial/ulnar deviation, and supination/pronation at first opportunity after removal of external fixator

    C. AROM measurements of uninvolved wrist in extension/flexion, radial/ulnar deviation, and supination/pronation to use as reference for "what's normal" for that patient

    D. Bilateral grip and pinch strength measurements at 2 to 3 weeks after fixator is removed

OPEN REDUCTION AND INTERNAL FIXATION

Definitions

Accurate, stable reduction with rigid fixation and bone grafting, together with an early motion program, has been demonstrated to improve healing and outcomes in other areas of the skeleton. Volar plate fixation of some

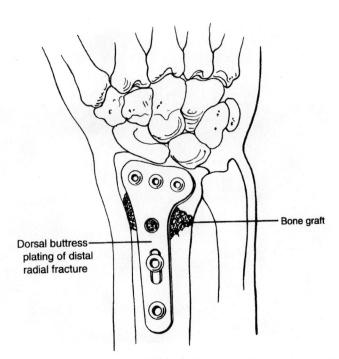

FIG. 37-8 An example of open reduction and internal fixation (ORIF) of a distal radius fracture with dorsal plating and bone graft.

distal radius fractures such as the volar Barton's fracture dislocation has been the standard for more than a decade.[59] ORIF of dorsally displaced distal radius fractures is becoming more predictable with improved techniques and development of low-profile plating systems[60-63] (Fig. 37-8). It may be impossible to reduce and maintain the position of rotated, displaced, and impacted fracture fragments in complex distal radius fractures by traction or other closed means.[56,64,65] Fractures with intraarticular step-off require ORIF.[56,60,64] Significant comminution and/or poor bone stock may require the use of an iliac crest bone graft or synthetic graft material in conjunction with a plate to promote healing of the fracture.

In many cases, stability achieved with this type of fracture fixation is adequate to allow an early motion program of the wrist, starting postoperatively within the first 2 weeks.[60,61,66] The therapeutic management of these fractures continues to evolve. Close communication among surgeon, therapist, and patient, along with careful monitoring of the progress and activity level, is required for at least 8 to 12 weeks postoperatively. Control of edema and pain and restoration of digital motion are priorities during this time, even if an early active motion program for the wrist in flexion/extension, radial/ulnar deviation, and forearm rotation is initiated.

Treatment Goals

I.   Therapist
     A. Reestablish as soon as possible and then maintain full ROM of uninvolved joints.
     B. Prevent wound infection.

C. Eradicate pain and edema as rapidly as possible.

D. Supervise early mobilization program of wrist with a balance of mobilization/immobilization according to surgeon's orders, bony healing, and tissue reactivity.

E. Prevent deep adherence of scar on extensor surface of wrist after dorsal plating.

F. Return patient to previous level of function.

Postoperative Precautions for Therapy

I.   Presence of associated injuries (e.g., ulnar styloid fracture, scapholunate ligament disruption) that might alter postoperative progression of wrist ROM and function

II. Questionable stability of fracture, extreme comminution, poor bone quality, or other "stability-related" issues communicated by surgeon that might delay postoperative progression of wrist ROM and function

III. Infection around incision

Postoperative Therapy

I.   Weeks 1 to 2

A. Begin the first of many patient education sessions!

   1. Instruction in meticulous pin tract and wound care

B. Fabricate and fit a thermoplastic splint to immobilize wrist as directed by surgeon.

   1. Splint should snugly support the wrist and distal radioulnar joint (DRUJ) but should not put any pressure on the distal ulna. It should be trimmed carefully to allow full mobility of the fingers and thumb (Fig. 37-9).

   2. Splint is worn day and night and is removed only for skin care, exercises, and sedentary activities such as watching television.

C. Emphasize importance of edema control and its relationship to improving ROM and decreasing pain

D. Begin active ROM of all uninvolved joints. Early movement of the fingers and thumb takes priority over early movement of the wrist.

E. Gentle active exercises of the wrist in extension/flexion, radial/ulnar deviation, and supination/pronation initiated once or twice per day.

   1. Active ROM of the wrist may be delayed if the patient is having a lot of pain and significant difficulty moving the fingers or seems very apprehensive about moving the wrist.

   2. The ability to extend the wrist without extending the fingers is important in reestablishing the ability to make a fist and in restoration of power grip.

   3. Supination is a key movement in many activities of daily living (ADLs). Most ORIF distal radius fracture patients regain pronation easier and faster than supination.

II. Weeks 3 to 4

A. Remold splint to maintain proper fit if needed.

B. Continue therapeutic intervention to regain full mobility of uninvolved joints if needed. If surgeon indicates that bony

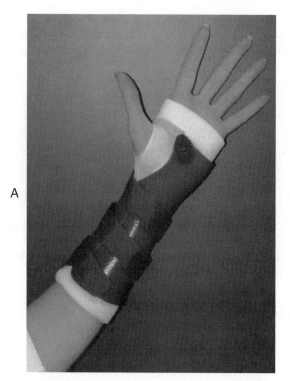

A

FIG. **37-9** An example of a type of wrist splint used postoperatively for patients who have had open reduction and internal fixation (ORIF) for a distal radius fracture. This splint is made of 1/12-inch microperforated plastic. It is lightweight but has a good rigidity because it is circumferential. **A,** Volar view: the splint is trimmed carefully to allow full mobility of the thumb and the fingers—especially on the ulnar half of the hand. Note the overlap of the plastic.

healing is sufficient, gentle passive wrist ROM exercises may be added to the active wrist exercises.
C. Start a more formalized program of soft tissue mobilization and scar massage.
III. Weeks 5 to 8
A. Remold splint to maintain proper fit if necessary.
B. Wean from the splint according to patient's activity level and surgeon's assessment of bony healing.
D. Continue therapeutic intervention to regain full mobility of uninvolved joints if needed.
E. Advance AROM and PROM exercises for the wrist and the soft tissue mobilization contingent on bony healing, tissue reactivity, and progress demonstrated on reevaluation.
IV. Weeks 9 to 12
A. Continue to wean from splint until order to discontinue entirely is received from surgeon.
B. Continue therapeutic interventions as needed to overcome residual stiffness in shoulder, elbow, fingers, and thumb.
C. Continue AROM and PROM exercises and soft tissue mobilization with changes in program reflecting patient's progress.
D. Start strengthening and resistive exercises.

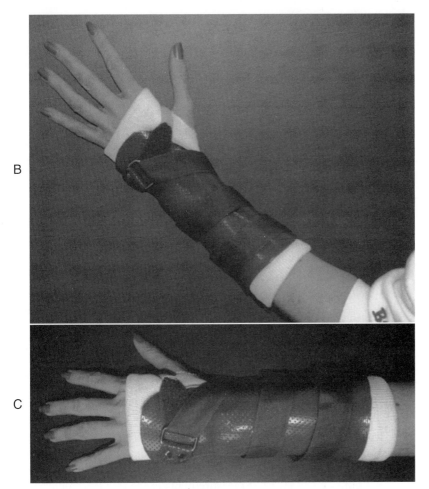

FIG. **37-9, cont'd B,** Dorsal view showing "barber pole" wrap-around strapping arrangement and elevation of the plastic over the distal ulna. **C,** A closer view of the "D-ring" on the dorsum of the splint. This type of strapping arrangement effectively secures the wrist in the splint and helps prevent the tendency of the wrist to fall into flexion, particularly in the early postoperative period.

   E. Continue emphasis on importance of home exercise program.
   F. Resume "normal function" of upper extremity, contingent on what the "normal activity level" is for each patient. Some sports and heavy activities cannot be resumed until 3 to 4 months postoperatively.
   G. Static progressive splinting may be considered if the fracture is healed and AROM has not progressed to functional levels in certain planes of motion.

Postoperative Complications

   I.   Loss of position of fracture, resulting in malunion
   II. "Hardware problems" such as plate breakage or a screw backing out of the bone
   III. CRPS

IV. Compression/irritation of median and/or dorsal superficial branch
     of the radial nerve
V.   Unresolved stiffness of uninvolved joints
VI. Distal radius nonunion

Evaluation Timeline

I.   Weeks 1 to 2
     A. AROM and PROM measurements of shoulder, elbow, fingers,
        and thumb of involved extremity
     B. AROM measurements of involved wrist in extension/flexion,
        radial/ulnar deviation, and supination/pronation
     C. AROM measurements of uninvolved upper extremity for the
        reference of "what's normal" for each patient
     D. Edema assessment
     E. Baseline sensibility assessment using Semmes-Weinstein
        monofilaments if carpal tunnel syndrome is suspected
II. Weeks 3 to 8
     A. Weekly (at least): reassessment of ROM and edema measurements
        to determine progress and to provide information needed to
        continue or change therapeutic program
     B. Repeat sensibility assessment approximately 4 weeks after initial
        assessment if patient continues to report numbness in the
        median nerve distribution
     C. PROM measurements may be made after surgeon gives
        clearance for patient to do PROM exercises.
III. Weeks 9 to 12
     A. Bilateral grip and pinch strength measurements before initiation
        of strengthening
     B. Continue AROM wrist measurements in the six planes of
        motion, and always compare results with ROM of uninvolved
        wrist.

Outcomes

The once well-established belief that deformity from this fracture can be tolerated because there are no long-term functional consequences is no longer
a subject of debate among most surgeons. Restoration of the anatomy is critical to the final radiographical and functional outcome. The development of
imaging techniques beyond radiography and the enhanced understanding of
anatomy and wrist biomechanics within the past two decades have helped
make treatment of these fractures more predictable. Surgeons continue to
develop and refine fixation techniques and hardware to restore distal radius
anatomy with better predictability and fewer complications.

Treatment of unstable distal radius fractures continues to evolve.
Therapists and surgeons must communicate closely, especially during the
early postoperative course of treatment. The functional impact of the
accompanying soft tissue injuries can be just as significant as the fracture
and can lead to finger stiffness and hand dysfunction that remain long
after the fracture has healed.

Maximum improvement in ROM, strength, and function from operative
treatment of unstable distal radius fractures does not occur for many months.

Most patients are discharged from therapy before maximum improvement is reached due to insurance limitations and other "managed care" considerations in the contemporary medical environment. Therapists must become better educators, and distal radius fracture patients must accept responsibility for their rehabilitation to achieve an optimal functional outcome.

REFERENCES

1. Colles A: On the fracture of the carpal extremity of the radius. Edinb Med Surg J 10:182-186, 1814
2. Fernandez DL, Jupiter JB: Fractures of the Distal Radius: A Practical Approach to Management. Springer-Verlag, New York, 1996
3. Owen RA, Melton LJ 3rd, Johnson KA, et al.: Incidence of Colles' fracture in a North American community. Am J Pubic Health 72:605-607, 1982
4. Ashe M, Khan K, Guy P, et al.: Wristwatch–distal radial fracture as a marker for osteoporosis investigation. J Hand Ther 17:324-328, 2004
5. Wigderowitz CA, Rowley DI, Mole PA, et al.: Bone mineral density of the radius in patients with Colles' fracture. J Bone Joint Surg Br 82:87-89, 2000
6. Lawson GM, Hajducka C, McQueen MM: Sports fractures of the distal radius: epidemiology and outcome. Injury 26:33-36, 1995
7. Melton LJ III, Amadio PC, Crowson CS, et al.: Long-term trends in the incidence of distal forearm fractures. Osteoporosis International 8:341-348, 1998
8. Bacorn RW, Kurtzke JF: Colles' fracture: a study of two thousand cases from the New York State Workmen's Compensation Board. J Bone Joint Surg Am 35:643-658, 1953
9. Cooney WP, Dobyns JH, Linscheid RL: Complications of Colles' fractures. J Bone Joint Surg Am 62:613-619, 1980
10. Frykman G: Fractures of the distal end of the radius, including sequelae: shoulder, hand, finger syndrome, disturbance in the distal radioulnar joint and impairment of nerve function. Acta Orthop Scand Suppl 108:1-155, 1967
11. Gartland JJ, Werley CW: Evaluation of healed Colles' fracture. J Bone Joint Surg Am 33:895-907, 1951
12. Green DP: Pins and plaster treatment of comminuted fractures of the distal end of the radius. J Bone Joint Surg Am 57:304-310, 1965
13. Kaempffe FA, Weeler DR, Peimer CA, et al.: Severe fractures of the distal radius: effect of amount and duration of external fixator distraction on outcome. J Hand Surg Am 18:33-41, 1993
14. Kaempffe FA, Walker KM: External fixation for distal radius fractures: effect of distraction on outcome. Clin Orthop 380:220-225, 2000
15. Lidstrom A: Fractures of the distal end of the radius: a clinical and statistical study of end results. Acta Orthop Scand Suppl 41:1-118, 1959
16. Older TM, Stabler EV, Cassebaum WH: Colles fracture: evaluation and selection of therapy. J Trauma 5:469-476, 1965
17. Scheck M: Long term follow up of treatment of comminuted fractures of the distal end of the radius by transfixation with Kirschner wires and cast. J Bone Joint Surg Am 44:337-351, 1962
18. Taleisnik J, Watson HK: Midcarpal instability caused by malunited fractures of the distal radius. J Hand Surg Am 9:350-357, 1984
19. Villar RN, Marsh D, Rushton N, et al.: Three years after Colles' fracture: a prospective review. J Bone Joint Surg Br 69:635-638, 1987
20. Weber SC, Szabo RM: Severely comminuted distal radial fracture as an unsolved problem: complications associated with external fixation and pins and plaster techniques. J Hand Surg Am 11:157-164, 1986
21. Carrozzella J, Stern PJ: Treatment of comminuted distal radius fractures with pins and plaster. Hand Clin 4:391-397, 1988
22. Tsukazaki T, Takagi K, Iwasaki K: Poor correlation between functional results and radiographic findings in Colles' fracture. J Hand Surg Br 18:588-591, 1993
23. Weber ER: A rational approach for the recognition and treatment of Colles' fracture. Hand Clin 3:13-21, 1987
24. Young BT, Rayan GM: Outcome following nonoperative treatment of displaced distal radius fractures in low-demand patients older than 60 years. J Hand Surg Am 25:19-28, 2000

25. Young CF, Nanu AM, Checketts RG: Seven-year outcome following Colles' type distal radial fracture: a comparison of two methods. J Hand Surg Br 28:422-426, 2003

26. Aro HT, Koivunen T: Minor axial shortening of the radius affects outcome of Colles' fracture treatment. J Hand Surg Am 16:392-398, 1991

27. Bass RL, Blair WF, Hubbard P: Results of combined internal and external fixation for the treatment of severe AO-C3 fractures of the distal radius. J Hand Surg Am 20:373- 381, 1995

28. Cooney WP, Berger RA: Treatment of complex fractures of the distal radius. Hand Clin 9:603-612, 1993

29. Kaukonen JP, Karaharju EO, Porras M, et al.: Functional recovery after fractures of the distal forearm: analysis of radiographic and other factors affecting the outcome. Ann Chir Gynaecol 77:27-31, 1988

30. McQueen MM, Caspers J: Colles' fracture: does the anatomical result affect the final function? J Bone Joint Surg Br 70:649-651, 1988

31. McQueen MM, Michie M, Court-Brown CM: Hand and wrist function after external fixation of unstable distal radius fractures. Clin Orthop 285:200-204, 1992

32. Orbay JL: The treatment of unstable distal radius fractures with volar fixation. J Hand Surg Am 5:103-112, 2000

33. Porter M, Stockley I: Fractures of the distal radius: intermediate and end results in relation to radiologic parameters. Clin Orthop 220:241-252, 1987

34. Sanders RA, Keppel FL, Waldrop JI: External fixation of distal radius fractures: results and complications. J Hand Surg Am 16:385-391, 1991

35. Solgaard S: External fixation or a cast for Colles' fracture. Acta Orthop Scand 60:387-391, 1989

36. Steffen T, Eugster T, Jakob RP: Twelve years follow-up of fractures of the distal radius treated with the AO fixator. Injury 25(Suppl 4):S-D44–S-D54, 1994

37. Stewart HD, Innes AR, Burke FD: Functional bracing for Colles' fractures: a comparison between cast bracing and conventional plaster casts. J Bone Joint Surg Br 66:749-753, 1984

38. Strange-Vognsen HH: Intraarticular fractures of the distal end of the radius in young adults: a 16 (2-26) year follow-up of 42 patients. Acta Orthop Scand 62:527-530, 1991

39. Trumble TE, Schmitt SR, Vedder NB: Internal fixation of pilon fractures of the distal radius. Yale Biol Med 66:179-190, 1993

40. Clancey GJ: Percutaneous Kirschner-wire fixation of Colles' fractures. J Bone Joint Surg Am 66:1008-1014, 1984

41. Szabo RM: Comminuted distal radius fractures. Orthop Clin North Am 23:1-5, 1992

42. Lafontaine M, Hardy D, Delince P: Stability assessment of distal radius fractures. Injury 20:208-210, 1989

43. Rodriguez-Mechan EC: Management of comminuted fractures of the distal radius in the adult. Clin Orthop 353:53-62, 1998

44. Ziran BH, Scheel M, Keith MV: Pin reduction and fixation of volar fracture fragments of distal radius fractures via the flexor carpi radialis tendon. J Trauma 49:433-439, 2000

45. Frykman GK, Peckham RH, Willard K, et al.: External fixators for treatment of unstable wrist fractures. Hand Clin 9:555-565, 1993

46. Hertel R, Jakob RP: Static external fixation of the wrist. Hand Clin 9:567-575, 1993

47. Nakata RY, Chand Y, Matiko JD, et al.: External fixators for wrist fractures: a biomechanical and clinical study. J Hand Surg Am 10:845-851, 1985

48. Pennig DW: Dynamic external fixation of distal radius fractures. Hand Clin 9:587-602, 1993

49. Agee J: Distal radius fractures: multiplanar ligamentotaxis. Hand Clin 9:577-585, 1993

50. Vidal J, Buscayret C, Fischbach C, et al.: Une methode originale dans le traitement des fractures comminutives de l'extremite inferieure du radius: "le taxis ligamentaire." Acta Orthop Belg 43:781-789, 1977

51. Bartosh RA, Saldana MJ: Intraarticular fractures of the distal radius: a cadaveric study to determine if ligamentotaxis restores radiopalmar tilt. J Hand Surg Am 15:18-21, 1990

52. Braun RM, Gellman H: Dorsal pin placement and external fixation for correction of dorsal tilt in fractures of the distal radius. J Hand Surg Am 19:653-655, 1994

53. Isani A, Melone CP: Classification and management of intra-articular fractures of the distal radius. Hand Clin 4:349-360, 1988

54. Seitz WH Jr, Froimson AI, Seb R, et al.: Augmented external fixation of unstable distal radius fractures. J Hand Surg Am 16:1010-1016, 1991

55. Colditz J: Practice forum: soft splinting technique for maintaining thumb abduction. J Hand Ther 4:22, 1991

56. Knirk JL, Jupiter JB: Intra-articular fractures of the distal end of the radius in young adults. J Bone Joint Surg Am 68:647-659, 1986

57. ODriscoll SW, Horii E, Ness R, et al.: The relationship between wrist position, grasp size, and grip strength. J Hand Surg Am 17:169-177, 1992

58. Werremeyer MM, Cole KJ: Wrist action affects precision grip force. J Neurophysiol 78:271-280, 1997

59. Frykman G, Kropp W: Fractures and traumatic conditions of the wrist. In Hunter J, Mackin EJ, Callahan AD (eds): Rehabilitation of the Hand: Surgery and Therapy. 4th Ed. Mosby, St. Louis, 1995

60. Carter PR, Frederick HA, Laseter GF: Open reduction and internal fixation of unstable distal radius fractures with a low-profile plate: a multicenter study of 73 fractures. J Hand Surg Am 23:300-307, 1998

61. Hove LM, Nilsen PT, Furnes O, et al.: Open reduction and internal fixation of displaced intraarticular fractures of the distal radius. Acta Orthop Scand 68:59-63, 1997

62. Jakob M, Rikli DA, Regazzoni P: Fractures of the distal radius treated by internal fixation and early function: a prospective study of 73 consecutive patients. J Bone Joint Surg Br 82:340-344, 2000

63. Orbay JL, Fernandez DL: Volar fixation for dorsally displaced fractures of the distal radius: a preliminary report. J Hand Surg Am 27:205-215, 2002

64. Bradway JK, Amadio PC, Cooney WP: Open reduction and internal fixation of displaced, comminuted intra-articular fractures of the distal end of the radius. J Bone Joint Surg Am 71:839-847, 1989

65. Melone CP: Open treatment for displaced articular fractures of the distal radius. Clin Orthop 202:103-111, 1986

66. Smith DW, Brou KE, Henry, MH: Early active rehabilitation for operatively stabilized distal radius fractures. J Hand Ther 17:43-49, 2004

SUGGESTED READINGS

Colditz JC: Therapist's management of the stiff hand in the upper extremity. In Mackin EJ, Callahan AD, Skirven TM, et al. (eds): Hunter-Mackin-Callahan Rehabilitation of the Hand and Upper Extremity. 5th Ed. Mosby, St. Louis, 2002

Collins DC: Management and rehabilitation of distal radius fractures. Orthop Clin North Am 24:365-378, 1993

Fernandez D, Jupiter J (eds): Fractures of the Distal Radius. Springer-Verlag, New York, 1996

Laseter GF: Therapist's management of distal radius fractures. In Mackin EJ, Callahan AD, Skirven TM, et al. (eds): Hunter-Mackin-Callahan Rehabilitation of the Hand and Upper Extremity. 5th Ed. Mosby, St. Louis, 2002

Newport ML (ed): Surgical management of distal radius fractures. In: Techniques in Orthopaedics. Vol. 15, No. 4. Williams & Wilkins, Baltimore, 2000

Saffar P, Cooney WP (eds): Fractures of the Distal Radius. JB Lippincott, Philadelphia, 1995

Ulnar Head Resection

38

Frank DiGiovannantonio

The distal radioulnar joint (DRUJ) is an important and integral part of wrist and hand function. The radius and hand move in relation to and function about the distal ulna.[1] Even the most minor modifications to the relationships among the distal radius, ulna, and ulnar carpus can lead to significant load changes at the distal ulnar and triangular fibrocartilage (TFC).[1] If the DRUJ is unstable, an individual can have decreased range of motion (ROM), and lifting capabilities and grip strength may be diminished or absent.[2]

The current literature describes many variations and modifications to the widely used ulnar head resection, all of which are designed to unload the ulnocarpal articulation.[3] This chapter describes five procedures and their appropriate treatment: (1) Darrach procedure, (2) Bowers' hemiresection-interposition technique (HIT), (3) matched ulna resection, (4) the Sauve–Kapandji procedure, and (5) the ulnar wafer (partial resection) procedure. Communication between therapist and physician is critical because of the variations in surgical technique and purpose for each patient.

Indications for the appropriate surgical procedure to be used during ulnar head resection vary greatly within the literature, as well as among physicians. A review of the literature, however, reveals several diagnoses that are commonly referred for some form of ulnar head resection. They include but are not limited to degenerative arthritis,[2-9] unreconstructable fractures of the ulnar head,[3,4] ulnocarpal impingement,[3,4,6,8-10] chronic painful TFC tears,[3,6,9,11] malunion of a distal radius fracture,[2-6,8,10-12] Madelung's deformity,[3-5,8,10,12] and rheumatoid arthritis.[3,5-11]

DEFINITION

Darrach procedure: Resection of the distal end of the ulna just proximal to the sigmoid notch of the radius[11] (Fig. 38-1).

Hemiresection-interposition technique (HIT): Resection of only the ulnar articular head, leaving the shaft/styloid relationship intact. An interposition

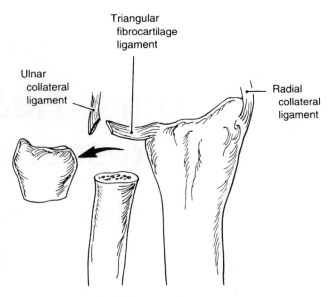

FIG. 38-1 Darrach procedure.

"anchovy" of tendon, capsule, or muscle is placed in the vacant distal radioulnar joint cavity to limit contact of the radial and ulnar shafts. This procedure presupposes an intact or reconstructable triangular fibrocartilage complex (TFCC)[10] (Fig. 38-2).

Matched procedure: The resection of the distal ulna in a smooth, curved, convex fashion to match the contour of the radius throughout forearm rotation[4] (Fig. 38-3).

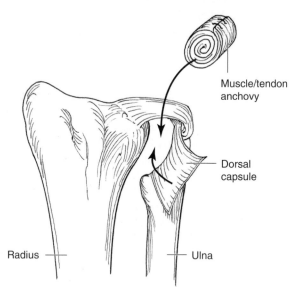

FIG. 38-2 Hemiresection interposition (HIT) technique. (Redrawn from Bowers MS: J Hand Surg Am 10:171, 1985.)

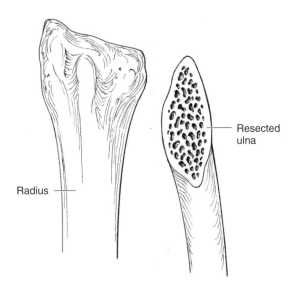

FIG. **38-3** Matched ulna resection. (Redrawn from Watson HK, Gabuzda GM: J Hand Surg Am 17:725, 1992.)

Sauve–Kapandji procedure: A distal radioulnar arthrodesis with the surgical creation of a pseudoarthrosis in the distal ulna[7] (Fig. 38-4). This procedure is often used for the high-demand patient, because the retention of the ulnar head helps to maintain a more normal transmission of loads across the carpus.[13]

Ulnar wafer resection: Open or arthroscopic partial excision of the distal ulna, which retains the ligamentous attachment of the TFCC to the base of the styloid process and preserves the function of the DRUJ.

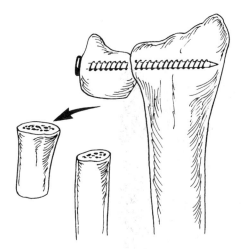

FIG. **38-4** Sauve–Kapandji procedure.

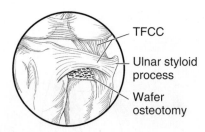

FIG. 38-5 Ulnar wafer resection. (Redrawn from Feldon P, Terrono AL, Belsky MR: J Hand Surg Am 17:735, 1992.)

This procedure is designed to decompress the ulna, TFCC, lunate, and triquetrum[3] (Fig. 38-5).

SURGICAL PURPOSE

Pain at the DRUJ may be caused by a variety of reasons. It is often caused by arthritis between the radius and ulna at that level. This arthritis is often the result of a malalignment of the joint after distal radial fracture, a dislocation, systemic arthritis, or other conditions causing malalignment that brings on cartilage surface changes. The most frequent type of surgery is the resection or reshaping of the distal ulna as it articulates with the radius. These procedures eliminate the joint surfaces and prevent them from rubbing together, thereby decreasing the symptoms of pain.

TREATMENT GOALS

I.   Protect surgical procedure through proper immobilization.
II. Prevent infection at surgical site.
III. Control edema.
IV. Decrease pain.
V.   Maintain/increase ROM of uninvolved joints.
VI. Restore active range of motion (AROM) at wrist and forearm.
VII. Restore patient to maximum functional capacity.

OPERATIVE INDICATIONS/PRECAUTIONS

I. Indications
   A. Rheumatoid arthritis
   B. Degenerative arthritis
   C. Malunited distal radius fracture
   D. TFCC tears
   E. Madelung's deformity
   F. Ulnar head fractures
   G. Ulnocarpal impingement
   H. Chronic dislocation of the DRUJ
II. Precautions
   A. Associated tendon injuries
   B. Associated bony injury
   C. Associated nerve injury
   D. Associated vascular injury

POSTOPERATIVE INDICATIONS/PRECAUTIONS FOR THERAPY

I.   Indications
    A. Distal ulnar resection
    B. Arthrodesis with pseudoarthrosis
    C. Painful ROM
    D. Edema
    E. Splinting
II. Precautions
    A. Ulnar stump instability
    B. Combined tendon interposition or transfer
    C. Painful or nonpainful clicking or popping of the wrist
       during the early stages of AROM
    D. Disproportionate pain

POSTOPERATIVE THERAPY

I.   Therapy after the Darrach procedure, HIT, and the
    matched procedure
    A. Immediately after surgery the patient is immobilized in a
      long arm cast at neutral forearm rotation for 7 to 10 days.
    B. At 7 to 10 days postoperatively, the cast is removed by the
      treating physician and stability is assessed.
      1. If the patient is stable, he or she is placed in a short arm wrist
        splint.
        a. The patient can move safely within 45 to 60 degrees of
          wrist flexion and extension, within the first 2 to 4 weeks
          postoperatively. Forearm supination and pronation can
          begin at 4 weeks postoperatively and be progressed to 45 to
          60 degrees as tolerated. If the patient is relatively pain free
          after 4 weeks, the wrist splint is discontinued and normal
          ROM may be attempted.
        b. Strengthening may begin at 4 to 6 weeks, as tolerated by
          the patient. However, power grasp and excessive lifting
          and carrying should be avoided until 8 to 12 weeks
          postoperatively, to avoid excessive loading of the ulnocarpal
          articulation and impingement of the ulnar stump.
      2. If, after removal of cast, the patient is assessed to be unstable,
        the patient is placed in a long arm splint in neutral forearm
        rotation or as directed by the physician.
        a. AROM to within 45 to 60 degrees of wrist flexion and
          extension and supination and pronation may begin at 7
          to 10 days postoperatively. AROM should be performed
          within pain-free limits and only in the presence of the
          therapist. The patient is to continue to wear the splint at
          all other times. Consult with the physician with regard
          to motion that may promote instability.
        b. At 4 to 6 weeks postoperatively, the long arm splint may be
          discontinued. ROM should continue to be progressed, and
          gradual strengthening may begin.
        c. Avoid power grasp until 8 to 12 weeks postoperatively.

3. If in either of the preceding cases the patient presents with any clicking or popping of the wrist during the early phases of ROM, the physician should be contacted, and consideration should be given to immobilizing the patient in a long arm splint until 6 weeks postoperatively.

II.   Therapy after Sauve–Kapandji procedure

A. The patient is immobilized in a long arm cast for 7 to 10 days postoperatively.

B. If internal fixation was attained using Kirschner wires, the patient is placed in a long arm or Muenster-type splint (Fig. 38-6) at neutral forearm rotation until 3 to 4 weeks postoperatively.[8] In some instances, a short arm cast or splint may be sufficient. This should be discussed with the surgeon.

1. The patient may remove the long arm splint to perform active supination and pronation exercises, within 45 to 60 degrees, again avoiding end-range of motion.

C. If internal fixation is attained through the use of a screw, the patient can be placed in a wrist splint at 7 to 10 days postoperatively, and active forearm supination and pronation within 45 to 60 degrees can begin.

D. In patients with either K-wire or screw fixation, ROM of the wrist may begin at 4 weeks postoperatively.

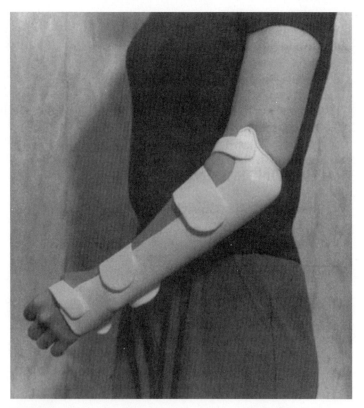

FIG. **38-6** Muenster-type splint. This splint allows elbow flexion and extension while preventing forearm rotation.

E. The wrist splint should be worn between exercise for approximately 6 weeks postoperatively or until fusion between the radius and ulna is achieved. At this point, strengthening may begin.

F. Because this procedure is a pseudoarthrodesis, strengthening may be delayed until fusion between the ulna and radius has taken place. Assuming good bony union, the patient should be able to tolerate moderate resistive use of the involved extremity by 8 to 10 weeks and heavy use by 10 to 12 weeks postoperatively.

III. Therapy after ulnar wafer resection procedure (The protocol for the ulnar wafer procedure assumes that no repair of the TFCC was performed.)

A. The patient is placed in a short arm splint at 0 to 20 degrees wrist extension for 7 to 10 days postoperatively. AROM and passive range of motion (PROM) of all uninvolved joints is initiated.

B. At 1 to 2 weeks postoperatively, the patient begins AROM of the wrist and forearm.

C. At 3 to 4 weeks postoperatively active-assisted range of motion (AAROM) and PROM of the wrist and forearm may begin in order to progress maximum end-range wrist flexion and extension as well as forearm supination and pronation. The use of ice after treatment is encouraged to avoid increased edema and pain. At 5 to 6 weeks postoperatively, begin gentle strengthening of the wrist and forearm.

D. At 6 weeks postoperatively, progress strengthening of the wrist and forearm and begin grip strengthening. Care should be taken and the surgeon notified of any clicking, clunking, or popping about the ulnar wrist.

E. At 8 to 12 weeks postoperatively, plyometric and weight-bearing activities can begin. Resume all activities of daily living (ADLs) and prepare for return to work.

POSTOPERATIVE COMPLICATIONS

I. Stylocarpal impingement[3]
II. Radioulnar impingement[4]
III. Regeneration of the distal ulna[5]
IV. Radial deviation of the wrist[5]
V. Wrist instability[5,6,8,9,11,12]
VI. Tendon rupture[6,11]
VII. Nerve impairment
VIII. Complex regional pain syndrome (CRPS)
IX. Wrist synovitis[7]
X. Instability of the distal ulna
XI. Inadequate bony resection
XII. Extensor carpi ulnaris (ECU) tendonitis

EVALUATION TIMELINE

After Darrach, HIT, matched, Sauve–Kapandji, and ulnar wafer resection procedures

   I. Edema measurement: taken at the initial evaluation and every 3 to 4 weeks thereafter

  II. Pain levels: measured at the initial evaluation and then every week until resolved

 III. Sensation: Tested at the time of the initial evaluation and every 4 weeks thereafter. May be performed more frequently if the patient indicates a change in status.

 IV. AROM of the uninvolved joints: determined at the time of the initial evaluation and every 3 to 4 weeks thereafter.

  V. AROM of the involved joints: started as described earlier, and checked weekly thereafter

 VI. Strength: started as described previously, and checked every 2 to 3 weeks thereafter

VII. Circulation: checked at the time of the initial evaluation and then at each visit during the initial 3 weeks postoperatively

OUTCOMES

The goal after ulnar head resection procedures is to improve the patient's pain-free ROM and maximize functional use of the involved extremity.

   I. Darrach,[11] HIT,[10] and matched procedures[4]: One should strive to attain 40 to 60 degrees of AROM at the wrist within the first 6 weeks postoperatively. The goals for forearm rotation are 60 to 75 degrees within the initial 6 to 8 weeks postoperatively. These patients should be capable of moderate resistive use of the involved extremity by 10 to 12 weeks postoperatively. By 12 to 14 weeks postoperatively, these patients may attempt to resume unrestricted use of the involved extremity.

  II. Ulnar wafer resection procedure[3]: Patients should be capable of attaining 45 to 65 degrees of wrist flexion and extension and 60 to 75 degrees of forearm rotation by 6 to 8 weeks postoperatively. They should be able to tolerate resistive use of the involved extremity by 8 to 10 weeks postoperatively and to return to unrestricted use by 12 weeks postoperatively.

 III. Sauve–Kapandji procedure[13]: These patients should have 40 to 50 degrees of wrist flexion and extension and 60 to 75 degrees of forearm rotation by 8 weeks postoperatively. Restrictions on activity are generally lifted once the fusion between the ulna and radius is confirmed by the physician and the patient is relatively pain free with activity.

REFERENCES

1. Palmer AK, Werner FW: Biomechanics of the distal radioulnar joint. In Leach RE (ed): Clinical Orthopedics and Related Research. Lippincott-Raven, Philadelphia, 1984, p. 26
2. Scheker LR, Babb BA, Killion PE: Distal ulnar prosthetic replacement. Orthop Clin North Am 30:365-376, 2001
3. Wnorowski DC, Palmer AK, Werner FW, et al.: Anatomic and biomechanical analysis of the arthroscopic wafer procedure. J Arthrosc Rel Surg 8:204-212, 1992
4. Sauerbier M, Hahn ME, Fujita M, et al.: Analysis of dynamic distal radioulnar convergence after ulnar head resection and endoprosthesis implantation. J Hand Surg Am 27:425-434, 2002
5. Garcia-Elias M: Failed ulnar head resection: prevention and treatment. J Hand Surg Br 27:470-480, 2002

6. Feldon P, Terrono AL, Belsky MR: Wafer distal ulna resection for triangular fibrocartilage tears and/or ulna impaction syndrome. J Hand Surg Am 17:731-737, 1992

7. Bowers WH: Instability of the distal radioulnar articulation. Hand Clin 7:311-327, 1991

8. Bowers WH: Distal radioulnar joint arthroplasty: the hemiresection-interposition technique. J Hand Surg Am 10:169, 1985

9. Gabuzda GM, Watson HK: Matched distal ulnar resection for posttraumatic disorders of the distal radioulnar joint. J Hand Surg Am 17:724, 1992

10. Dingman PVC: Resection of the distal end of the ulna (Darrach operation). J Bone Joint Surg Am 34:893, 1952

11. Nolan WB, Eaton RG: A Darrach procedure for distal ulnar pathology derangements. Clin Orthop (275):85-89, 1992

12. Vincet KA, Agee JM, Szabo RM: The Sauve-Kapandji procedure for reconstruction of the rheumatoid distal radioulnar joint. J Hand Surg Am 18:978-983, 1993

13. Taleisnik J: The Sauve-Kapandji procedure. Clin Orthop 275:110-123, 1992

SUGGESTED READINGS

Bieber EJ, Linscheid RL, Dobyns JH, et al.: Failed distal ulna resection. J Hand Surg Am 13:193, 1988

Bowers WH: The distal radioulnar joint. In Green DP (ed): Operative Hand Surgery. 3rd Ed. Churchill Livingstone, New York, 1993, p. 973

Darrach W: Anterior dislocation of the head of the ulna. Ann Surg 56:802, 1912

Darrow JC, Linscheid RL, Dobyns JH, et al.: Distal ulnar recession for disorders of the distal radioulnar joint. J Hand Surg Am 10:482, 1985

Frederick HA, Hontas RB, Saunders RA: The Sauve-Kapandji procedure: a salvage operation for distal radioulnar joint. J Hand Surg Am 16:1125, 1991

Gordon L, Levinsohn DG, Moore SV, et al.: The Sauve-Kapandji procedure for the treatment of posttraumatic distal radioulnar joint problems. In Hand Clin 7:397-403, 1991

Hartz CR, Beckenbaugh RD: Long-term results of resection of the distal ulna for post-traumatic conditions. J Trauma 19:219, 1979

Jackson IT, Milward TM, Lee P, et al.: Ulnar head resection in rheumatoid arthritis. Hand 6:172-180, 1974

Noble J, Arafa M: Stabilization of the distal radioulnar joint: anatomy and clues to prompt diagnosis. Clin Orthop 144:154, 1979

Tulipan DJ, Eaton RG, Eberhart RE: The Darrach procedure defended: technique redefined and long-term follow-up. J Hand Surg Am 16:438, 1991

Proximal Row Carpectomy 39

Corie Sullivan

Despite being frequently referred to as a "salvage procedure," proximal row carpectomy (PRC) is actually a reliable and effective surgical procedure that reduces pain and maintains motion at the wrist. When injury to the proximal row of carpals necessitates surgery, PRC has several advantages over other procedures, including a relatively short immobilization period, achievement of functional range of motion (ROM) and grip, and no risk of material failure or prosthetic loosening.[1-3] Unlike wrist arthrodesis, PRC offers the patient a stable yet movable wrist.

DEFINITION

Proximal row carpectomy (PRC) is a surgical procedure whereby the scaphoid, lunate, and triquetrum are excised, allowing the proximal end of the capitate to articulate with the lunate fossa of the radius (Fig. 39-1). Occasionally, a radial styloidectomy may accompany the PRC procedure. The radioscaphocapitate ligament is kept intact so that it can act as a stabilizer, preventing ulnar translation of the capitate out of the lunate fossa.[4]

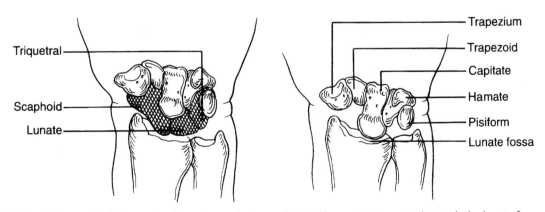

FIG. **39-1** Removal of the proximal row of carpal bones allowing the capitate to articulate with the lunate fossa.

SURGICAL PURPOSE

The primary surgical goal of PRC is pain relief with a stable wrist joint. Other goals include maintaining motion, restoring functional grip strength, and establishing a stable wrist joint. Successful outcomes are dependent on the presence of sufficient articular surfaces of the proximal capitate and the lunate fossa.[4]

TREATMENT GOALS[1,5]

*NOTE: Normal motion is not expected secondary to the kinematic changes at the wrist joint.[6] ROM and strength should not be achieved at the expense of increasing pain. The primary goal of therapy is pain relief with a stable and functional wrist.

  I. Decrease wrist pain.
  II. Minimize edema.
  III. Manage scar formation.
  IV. Maintain/restore wrist motion.
  V. Maintain/restore grip strength.
  VI. Maximize activities of daily living (ADL)/instrumental activities of daily living (IADL) status.
  VII. Normalize any sensory deficits.

POSTOPERATIVE INDICATIONS/PRECAUTIONS FOR THERAPY

  I. Indications [4,6-8]
    A. Chronic perilunate dislocation
    B. Nonreconstructable scaphoid malunion/nonunion
    C. Unsuccessful Silastic implant
    D. Kienböck's disease (avascular necrosis of the lunate) with structured collapse of lunate
    E. Nonreconstructable avascular necrosis of scaphoid or scaphoid nonunion
    F. Preiser's disease
    G. Scapholunate advanced collapse (SLAC) wrist
    H. Scaphoid nonunion advanced collapse (SNAC) wrist
    I. Post-traumatic arthritis
    J. Carpal or ligamentous instabilities
  II. Contraindications [1,2,9,12]
    A. Rheumatoid arthritis
    B. A poor articular surface on the proximal portion of the capitate or on the lunate fossa
  III. Precautions[5]
    A. Overly aggressive ROM or strengthening can lead to synovitis, increased edema, and pain.
    B. Excessive scarring and/or edema can impair rehabilitation.

POSTOPERATIVE THERAPY[1,4,5,9-12]

  I. Days 10 to 14
    A. Remove bulky dressings and fabricate a volar wrist splint.
    B. Encourage edema control and scar management.

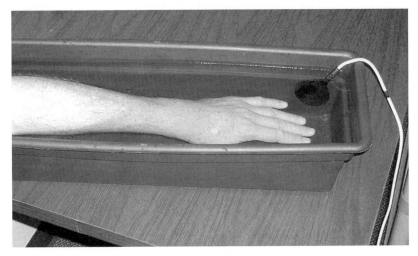

FIG. **39-2** Reducing edema using high-voltage galvanic stimulation.

    C. Reinforce digit and thumb active range of motion (AROM) exercises and instruct patient in tendon gliding exercises.

II.   Weeks 3 to 4 (as early as week 3, no later than week 4)

    A. Begin AROM of the patient's wrist. Exercises should be nonstressful to the tissues, to avoid increasing pain or edema.

    B. The patient may remove the splint for exercises and for short episodes of light, nonstressful activities such as reading, writing, or grooming tasks.

    C. Continue to manage the patient's edema and scarring; high-voltage galvanic stimulation can be especially helpful with chronic edema (Fig. 39-2).

III.   Week 6

    A. Begin gentle isometrics for wrist and grip.

    B. May begin active-assisted range of motion (AAROM).

    C. Avoid simultaneous composite wrist and digit flexion or composite wrist and digit extension; these combined motions may cause excessive stretching of the extrinsic muscles of the forearm.[12]

IV.   Weeks 6 to 8

    A. The patient may begin passive range of motion (PROM) exercises to the wrist as tolerated.

    B. The patient may begin to wean out of the splint for light activities; the goal is to be out of the splint by 3 months after surgery.[1]

V.   Week 8

    A. If the patient is symptom free and wrist motion is within expected/functional ranges, progressive resistive exercises may begin.

    B. Soft wrist supports may be added to supplement the use of the rigid volar splint. Remember, the goal of surgery and therapy is a relatively pain-free and stable wrist.

VI.   Week 12

    A. Composite stretches may be added if needed to increase ROM.

B. Discontinue splint.

C. The patient may return to work if his or her occupation requires minimal lifting and minimal force to the wrist joint. Discuss any needed ergonomic adaptations or modifications with the patient.

VII. 6 months

A. The patient may return to moderate to heavy work.

B. Nonlaborers are more likely to return to their previous occupations than are laborers.[4]

C. Assess the patient's return-to-work needs, including additional wrist supports, ergonomic adaptations or modifications, additional work-conditioning services, or a functional capacity evaluation (FCE).

VIII. Research indicates that it may take up to 12 to 18 months for the patient to realize maximum grip, strength, and ROM levels.[4,6,11]

POSTOPERATIVE COMPLICATIONS

I. Pain

II. Edema

III. Excessive scarring

IV. Sensory impairments: dorsal branch of the radial nerve, posterior interosseous nerve (PIN), or dorsal branch of the ulnar nerve may be affected.[1]

V. Changes to the muscle length-tension relationship can result in decreased digital flexion with subsequent decreased power grip.[1,5]

VI. Arthritic changes in lunate fossa articulation.

EVALUATION TIMELINE

I. Digital ROM/sensation: days 10 to 14 postoperatively

II. Edema/scar: days 10 to 14

III. Wrist AROM: weeks 3 to 4

IV. Wrist PROM: week 6

V. Strength: week 8

VI. Assess return to work status: months 3 to 6

OUTCOMES

I. Approximately half of the motion at the wrist occurs at the midcarpal joint.[5,12] With the removal of that joint, normal wrist motion is not expected, nor should the patient strive to achieve normal motion.[2] The therapist should explain the expectations of therapy and outcomes to the patient at the time of the evaluation.

II. Removal of the proximal row of carpals alters the length-tension relationship of the tendons that cross the joint. Digital flexion can be altered, decreasing grip strength.[1,5]

III. The research findings are mixed regarding return to work for heavy laborers after this procedure.[2,4,6] The therapist should assess the patient for appropriate wrist braces and ergonomic changes, which may facilitate the patient's return to his or her prior occupation.

IV. ROM outcomes vary, but on average the patient can expect a return of 40% to 60% of AROM compared with the unaffected side.[2,4] The average arc of motion is 60% of the unaffected side, or about 80 degrees of combined flexion/extension.[10] Grip strength averages are 60% to 80% of the unaffected side.[3,4,9,13] Radial deviation is the most decreased motion, with flexion next.[2,12] Extension and ulnar deviation are the most important motions for successful ADL function.[1]

V. Maximum ROM and strength can take up to 12 to 18 months to achieve.[4,11]

VI. Long-term studies indicate that there are minimal joint changes at the new articulating joint, so long-term prospects for continued positive outcomes are good.[6,13]

REFERENCES

1. Bednar JM, Von Lersner-Benson C: Wrist reconstruction: salvage procedures. In Mackin EJ, Callahan AD, Skirven TM, et al. (eds): Hunter-Mackin-Callahan Rehabilitation of the Hand and Upper Extremity. 5th Ed. Mosby, St. Louis, 2002, pp. 1195-1202

2. Culp RW, McGuigan FX, Turner MA, et al.: Proximal row carpectomy: a multicenter study. J Hand Surg Am 18:19-25, 1993

3. Imbriglia JE, Broudy AS, Hagberg WC, et al.: Proximal row carpectomy: clinical evaluation. J Hand Surg Am 15:426-430, 1990

4. Culp RW, Williams CS: Proximal row carpectomy for the treatment of scaphoid nonunion. Hand Clin 17:663-669, 2001

5. Kozin SH, Michlovitz SL: Traumatic arthritis and osteoarthritis of the wrist. J Hand Ther 13:124-135, 2000

6. Tomaino MM, Delsignore J, Burton R: Long-term results following proximal row carpectomy. J Hand Surg Am 19:694-703, 1994

7. Rettig ME, Raskin KB: Long-term assessment of proximal row carpectomy for chronic perilunate dislocations. J Hand Surg Am 24:1231-1236, 1999

8. Nakamura R, Horii E, Watanabe K, et al.: Proximal row carpectomy versus limited wrist arthrodesis for advanced Kienbock's disease. J Hand Surg Br 23:741-745, 1998

9. Ferlic DC, Clayton ML, Mills MF: Proximal row carpectomy: review of rheumatoid and nonrheumatoid wrists. J Hand Surg Am 16:420-424, 1991

10. Cohen MS, Kozin SH: Degenerative arthritis of the wrist: proximal row carpectomy versus scaphoid excision and four-corner arthrodesis. J Hand Surg 26:94-104, 2001

11. Wyrick JD: Proximal row carpectomy and intercarpal arthrodesis for the management of wrist arthritis. J Am Acad Orthop Surg 11:227-281, 2003

12. Nagelvoort RW, Kon M, Schuurman AH: Proximal row carpectomy: a worthwhile salvage procedure. Scand J Plast Reconstr Surg Hand Surg 36:289-299, 2002

13. Jebson PJL, Hayes EP, Engber WD: Proximal row carpectomy: a minimum 10-year follow-up study. J Hand Surg Am 28:561-569, 2003

SUGGESTED READINGS

Divelbiss BJ, Baratz ME: The role of arthroplasty and arthrodesis following trauma to the upper extremity. Hand Clin 15:335-345, 1999

Graham B, Detsky AS: The application of decision analysis to the surgical treatment of early osteoarthritis of the wrist. J Bone Joint Surg Br 83:650-654, 2001

Green DP: Proximal row carpectomy. Hand Clin 3:163-168, 1987

Osterman AL, Mikulics M: Scaphoid nonunion. Hand Clin 14:437-455, 1988

Wrist Arthroplasty 40

Brenda A. Kelly

Total wrist arthroplasty was developed in the late 1960s by Swanson.[1] The first wrist replacements were simple one-piece silicone spacers. Several modifications in prosthetic design have occurred, with the most recent consisting of carpal and radial components separated by a polyethylene spacer. Before the development of total wrist arthroplasty, patients were provided with partial or total wrist arthrodesis for pain relief. Patients with rheumatoid arthritis, osteoarthritis, or posttraumatic arthritis may benefit from arthroplasty. The ideal candidate must have intact wrist and digital musculature. Rheumatoid patients with multijoint involvement benefit from the prosthetic joint, which promotes upper extremity motion, function, and independence. Wrist arthroplasty should follow successful completion of any hip, knee, or foot surgeries also required, to avoid unnecessary stress on the upper extremity.

DEFINITION

Design of a wrist prosthesis is challenging due to the complex joint kinematics of the wrist. Multiple designs have been used with limited success and longevity. Before the development of current designs, unacceptable complications arose due to wrist imbalance and implant loosening.[2]

Currently, the most promising prosthetic design, the Universal Total Wrist Prosthesis (KMI, San Diego, CA) provides an unconstrained titanium and polyethylene prosthesis with primary fixation of the carpal component in the capitate and a preserved distal carpal row (not in the third metacarpal), which provides a stable bony support for the carpal component and results in improved longevity.[3] The articular surface of the radial component is inclined 20 degrees, similar to the articular surface of the radius. The carpal component has a titanium surface, which is attached with screws to the carpal bones, and a convex ovoid polyethylene insert, which articulates with the concave radial component.[4] This design has a modified geometry that allows a broader contact area between the radial and carpal components throughout a larger range of motion (ROM).

The prosthesis is designed to allow 35 degrees dorsiflexion, 35 degrees palmar flexion, 10 degrees radial deviation, and 25 degrees ulnar deviation.

SURGICAL PURPOSE

Wrist arthroplasty is performed to replace arthritic joint surfaces (Fig. 40-1) with metal or plastic surfaces (Fig. 40-2), in order to decrease pain and improve hand function.

TREATMENT GOALS

I.   Minimize postoperative pain and swelling.
II. Restore functional digital ROM.
III. Restore wrist ROM within the limits of the prosthesis.
IV. Restore strength sufficient for activities of daily living (ADLs).

POSTOPERATIVE CONSIDERATIONS/PRECAUTIONS FOR THERAPY

I.   Indications
     A. Immobilization of the wrist in a bulky postoperative dressing is needed to allow wound healing.
     B. In the immediate postoperative phase, suction drains and antibiotics are used to prevent hematoma and infection.

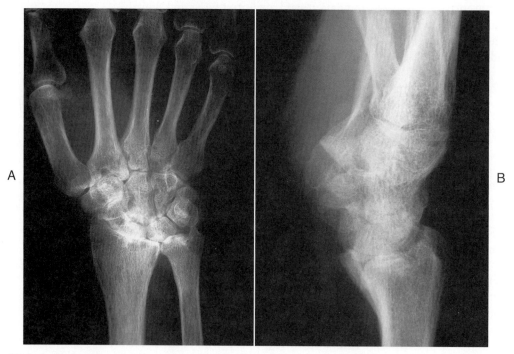

FIG. 40-1 A, Preoperative posterior-anterior radiograph of woman with long-standing rheumatoid disease and symptomatic wrist arthritis. **B,** Preoperative lateral radiograph of woman with long-standing rheumatoid disease and symptomatic wrist arthritis.

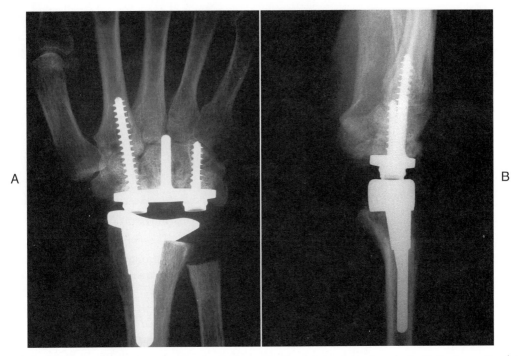

FIG. **40-2 A,** Postoperative posterior-anterior radiograph after total wrist arthroplasty. **B,** Postoperative lateral radiograph after total wrist arthroplasty.

II.   Precautions
   A. Stability of the prosthesis and wrist capsule
   B. Avoidance of excessive movement for flexion and extension and for radial deviation
   C. Infection
   D. Neurovascular status
   E. Protection for tendons that are repaired or lengthened

POSTOPERATIVE THERAPY

   I.   Immediately postoperatively, elevation for edema control
   II.   At 2 days postoperatively, compression garment as needed
   III.   At 2 to 5 days postoperatively, fabricate a removable thermoplastic splint, positioning the wrist in slight extension and permitting unrestricted digital motion (Fig. 40-3).
   IV.   At 2 to 5 days postoperatively, instruct patient in active range of motion (AROM) and gentle active-assisted range of motion (AAROM) of the digits (with compression garment removed) to restore active extension to neutral and active composite digital flexion to the palm. Patients may experience difficulty with activation and glide of the digital extensors because of the operative approach. It is helpful to have patients perform place-and-hold extension exercises in neutral position, as well as bilateral activity to assist with tendon glide.
   V.   At 2 to 5 days postoperatively, with compression garment and splint removed, active wrist flexion and extension via wrist extensors to limits of prosthesis.

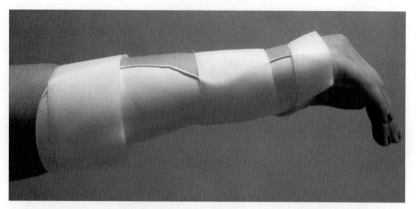

FIG. **40-3** Removable thermoplastic splint.

   VI. At 2 to 5 days postoperatively, active pronation and supination
  VII. At 2 to 5 days postoperatively, initiate instruction in home program to perform exercises described in paragraphs IV, V, and VI several times daily.
 VIII. At 10 to 14 days postoperatively, after suture removal, scar mobilization is initiated. The splint is modified to position the wrist in approximately 20 degrees extension, as ROM allows.
  IX. At 4 weeks postoperatively, initiate passive range of motion (PROM) to assist reaching limits of prosthesis motion
   X. At 8 to 10 weeks postoperatively, gentle resistive exercises may be initiated for wrist and digital musculature if daily activities are limited by weakness.
  XI. Restrictions
    A. Avoid lifting more than 10 lb.
    B. Avoid repetitive lifting of 2 to 10 lb.
    C. Avoid impact loading.
    D. Wear splint during strenuous activities.

POSTOPERATIVE COMPLICATIONS

   I. Infection
  II. Limited soft tissue length, which restricts motion of prosthesis
 III. Prosthetic loosening
 IV. Soft tissue imbalance, which leads to dislocation

EVALUATION TIMELINE

   I. 2 to 5 days: Active shoulder, elbow, wrist, and digital motion may be measured.
  II. 4 weeks: Passive wrist motion may be measured.
 III. Grip and pinch strength may be assessed only after patient is able to maintain the wrist in extended position.

OUTCOMES

Published outcomes are available for the Universal I wrist prosthesis. In the sample of 22 patients, 14 were available for 1-year follow-up and 8 for

2-year follow-up. All patients demonstrated improved ROM postoperatively. Improvements in all arcs of motion (flexion-extension, pronation-supination, and radial-ulnar deviation) as well as Disabilities of the Arm, Shoulder, and Hand (DASH) scores were demonstrated. Motions that were most limited preoperatively (extension, radial deviation, and supination) were most improved postoperatively.

REFERENCES

1. Swanson AB: Flexible implant arthroplasty for arthritic disabilities of the radiocarpal joint: A silicone rubber intramedullary stemmed flexible hinge implant for the wrist joint. Orthop Clin North Am 4:383-394, 1973
2. Adams BD, Khoury JG: Total wrist arthroplasty. In The Wrist. Lippincott Williams & Wilkins, Philadelphia, 2000, pp. 166-176
3. Menon J: Universal total wrist implant: experience with a carpal component fixed with three screws. J Arthroplasty 13:515-523, 1998
4. Divelbiss BJ, Sollerman C, Adams BD: Early results of the Universal total wrist arthroplasty in rheumatoid arthritis. J Hand Surg 27:195-204, 2002

Wrist Arthrodesis 41

Beth Farrell Kozera

Performing functional tasks with the hands would not be possible without a stable wrist to position the hand. Impairment of the wrist leading to instability and pain compromises hand function for activities of daily living (ADLs). Intercarpal, or partial, wrist arthrodesis is useful in treating carpal instability that results from destruction of the carpus, such as in arthritis, advanced Kienböck's or Preiser's disease, and scapholunate instability.[1] This method of treatment restores wrist stability and function while providing pain relief.[2]

Total wrist arthrodesis (fusion) is a reliable method of achieving stability and pain relief. It may be indicated as salvage surgery after failed intercarpal fusion, or for posttraumatic arthritis of the midcarpal and radiocarpal joints.[3] The wrist is usually fused in 10 to 20 degrees extension for optimal hand function. The position of slight ulnar deviation is often used to optimize grip strength.[1] Even with optimal results, however, these patients will have limitations due to loss of wrist motion. Typically these include difficulty with tasks normally requiring wrist extension, use of power or vibratory tools,[4] difficulty with perineal care, and difficulty maneuvering the hand in a tight place.[3]

The immobilization phase after surgery can lead to stiff uninvolved joints of the upper extremity. Therefore, one of the primary goals of therapy is to maintain full range of motion (ROM) of all uninvolved joints. Immobilization can also contribute to upper extremity weakness and decreased endurance. Therefore once fusion is achieved, it is important to begin general conditioning, strengthening, and instruction in compensatory techniques. These techniques enhance the patient's level of functioning for return to work and normal activities.

The therapist plays an important role in the success of wrist arthrodesis. Communication between doctor and therapist regarding the healing process is important in determining the appropriate time to initiate various phases of treatment. The protocol presented here offers only guidelines, which may vary with each patient's particular condition.

DEFINITION

I.   **Total wrist arthrodesis:** the surgical immobilization of the wrist joint. Autogenous or artificial bone graft is inserted with internal fixation to stabilize the wrist in the desired position (Fig. 41-1).

II.   **Intercarpal arthrodesis:** the surgical partial immobilization of the wrist joint. Articular cartilage and subchondral bone is removed[4] from the carpal surfaces being fused. These spaces are filled with autogenous bone graft or allograft and stabilized by pins, screws, or plates (Fig. 41-2).

SURGICAL PURPOSE

The purpose of partial or total wrist fusions is to provide pain relief and wrist stability at the expense of wrist joint motion.

The limited wrist fusion applies to fusing two or more carpal bones together. The most common fusions involve the trapezium, scaphoid, and trapezoid (triscaphe or "STT" fusion); the scaphoid and capitate (SC fusion); and the lunate, triquetrum, hamate, and capitate ("4 corner" or "four-bone" fusion). Other combinations are possible.

The total wrist fusion involves the radius and entire carpus (proximal and distal rows). Internal fixation is frequently used in the form of plates and screws or pins. The distal ulna may be excised if it is arthritic or impinging. Bone grafting from the iliac crest or another source is often required. The average length of time for solid fusion is approximately 12 weeks. Another 12 weeks is usually necessary to reach maximum benefit.

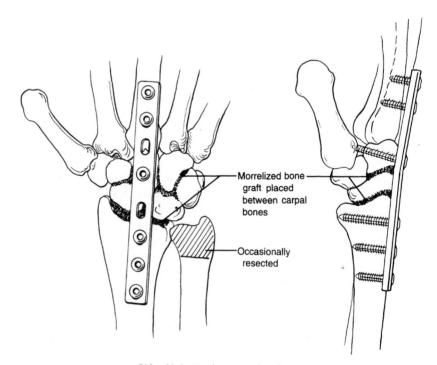

Morrelized bone graft placed between carpal bones

Occasionally resected

FIG. **41-1** Total wrist arthrodesis.

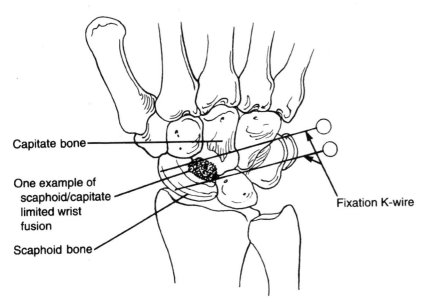

Capitate bone

One example of
scaphoid/capitate
limited wrist
fusion

Scaphoid bone

Fixation K-wire

FIG. 41-2 Intercarpal arthrodesis.

TREATMENT GOALS

   I. Maintain stability of the wrist.
  II. Maximize ROM of wrist (intercarpal arthrodesis).
 III. Protect fusion.
 IV. Control edema.
  V. Minimize pain.
 VI. Minimize adhesions.
VII. Maintain ROM of uninvolved joints.
VIII. Return patient to maximum level of functioning.

OPERATIVE INDICATIONS/PRECAUTIONS
FOR THERAPY

I.   Indications
    A. Intercarpal wrist arthrodesis[1]
      1. Localized arthritis of carpus
      2. Carpal instability
      3. Advanced Kienböck's or Preiser's disease
      4. As salvage surgery for partial carpal bone loss
      5. Sparing of midcarpal joints with destruction limited to
         radiocarpal area
    B. Total wrist arthrodesis
      1. Wrist pain and/or instability resulting from degenerative
         changes
      2. Heavy laborer with advanced radiocarpal joint destruction[2,5]
      3. As salvage surgery for failed procedures[2,5] (e.g., arthroplasties,
         partial wrist fusion)
      4. Paralysis of wrist with the potential for tendon
         reconstruction[2,5]
      5. Reconstruction after tumor resection
      6. Adolescent spastic hemiplegia with wrist flexion deformity[2,5]

       7. Ruptured or nonfunctioning wrist extensors
       8. Rheumatoid arthritis[5]
    C. Precautions for therapy
       1. Vigorous wrist exercise may exacerbate wrist pain[1]
       2. Passive ROM before wrist fusion could lead to a nonunion in partial arthrodesis
       3. Tendon rupture over plate in total wrist fusion
       4. Watch for signs of infection

POSTOPERATIVE THERAPY

The timetable described is only a guideline. It is important to consult with the patient's physician regarding the surgical procedure performed, treatment goals, and healing status of the fused wrist.

  I. Partial wrist arthrodesis
    A. Postoperative day 1 through entire rehabilitation program
       1. Maintain ROM of uninvolved joints
       2. Edema control
       3. Pain control as needed
    B. Cast immobilization for 6 to 8 weeks (for delayed union or nonunion, immobilization time is increased)[7]
    C. Short arm splint or thumb spica splint (depending on procedure) applied for 2 to 3 weeks after cast removal[5,7] (Fig. 41-3)
       1. 6 to 8 weeks: Initiate gentle active range of motion (AROM) of wrist; avoid forced wrist motion.[1]
       2. Initiate scar management and edema control of wrist and digits.
    D. Once the fusion is complete and with the physician's consent, begin passive range of motion (PROM), graded strengthening of the wrist, and work hardening.[1]
  II. Total wrist arthrodesis
    A. A preoperative evaluation is helpful in gathering baseline data on edema, ROM, strength, pain, and function. Patients should be instructed on postoperative functional limitations and the importance of maintaining ROM of uninvolved joints during the immobilization phase. Splinting of the wrist before surgery for a few days to immobilize it in the position of fusion

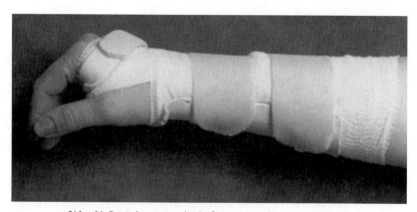

FIG. **41-3** Splint is applied after cast and/or pin removal.

demonstrates to the patient the restrictions that will be encountered.
   B. Postoperative day 1 through entire rehabilitation program
      1. Maintain ROM of uninvolved joints, especially the metacarpophalangeal (MCP) joints. Because the cast usually does not allow for full active MCP flexion, these joints may become stiff. No ROM should be performed on the wrist throughout the entire rehabilitation program.
      2. Tendon gliding exercises for long flexors and extensors[6]
      3. Edema management
      4. Pain management as needed
      5. ADL training/adaptive equipment as needed
      6. Scar management (once the scar is healed)
      7. Home exercise program
      8. Patient education regarding total immobilization of wrist
   C. Postoperative day 7: Check with physician regarding splint versus cast immobilization. Cast immobilization may last up to 6 to 8 weeks,[7] or the patient can be fitted with a short arm wrist or thumb spica splint as early as 1 week postoperatively (with delayed union or nonunion, immobilization time is increased[7]).
   D. Weeks 6 to 12 (if cast was applied for first 6 to 8 weeks): The cast is removed and a short arm splint is applied and worn until fusion is complete (see Fig. 41-3).
      1. Continue with treatment as outlined earlier.[1]
      2. Preparation for return to work once fusion is completely healed. Work hardening and work conditioning programs may be initiated.

POSTOPERATIVE COMPLICATIONS

   I. Pseudoarthroses
   II. Fracture of healed fusion
   III. Nonunion
   IV. Deep wound infection
   V. Superficial skin necrosis
   VI. Hematoma
   VII. Edema
   VIII. Pain
   IX. Transient median nerve or superficial radial nerve compression
   X. Scar adhesions limiting tendon excursion
   XI. Tendon rupture over plate

EVALUATION TIMELINE

   I.   ROM
      A. Intercarpal wrist fusion
         1. Week 1 through entire rehabilitation program
            a. AROM of uninvolved upper extremity joints
            b. Sensory
            c. Pain
            d. Edema

        e. Scar formation

        f. ADL

    2. Weeks 6 to 8 (or once pins are removed) through entire rehabilitation program: AROM of the wrist

    3. Weeks 8 to 12 (or once fusion is complete as confirmed by physician) through entire rehabilitation program

        a. PROM

        b. Grip and pinch strength

        c. Manual muscle testing (MMT) of all upper extremity joints

  B. Total wrist arthrodesis/fusion

    1. Week 1 through entire rehabilitation program

        a. AROM/PROM of uninvolved upper extremity joints

        b. Sensory

        c. Pain

        d. Edema

        e. Scar formation

        f. ADLs

    2. Week 12 (or once fusion is complete as confirmed by physician)

        a. Grip/pinch strength

        b. MMT of all upper extremity joints

OUTCOMES

  I.   Limited wrist fusion

    A. 12 of 15 wrists (4 radiocarpal and 11 intercarpal arthrodeses) showed an average of 32 degrees flexion and 33 degrees extension at 89 months postoperatively.[8]

    B. STT fusion: expected wrist motion is 40 to 60 degrees of flexion and extension, 15 degrees radial deviation, and 25 degrees ulnar deviation.[3]

    C. Four-bone arthrodesis: expect 50% to 60% of wrist motion, compared with the uninvolved side, and 80% of the grip strength of opposite side.[3]

  II.   Total wrist arthrodesis

    A. Weiss and Hastings[9] interviewed 28 patients 2 years after arthrodesis: 13 patients had returned to their same job with no restrictions, and 4 had returned but required weight restrictions; 10 patients had not returned to work but for reasons unrelated to their wrist fusion.

    B. Of the 23 patients studied by Watson and co-workers,[10] 15 returned to their original jobs with modifications required. The tasks reported as most difficult were perineal care and use of the hand in tight spaces.

    C. Weiss and colleagues[11] studied 23 patients over a 7-year period; 15 returned to their same jobs, and 3 were considered permanently impaired. An ADL test was performed. One third of the patients reported no problems with any ADLs, and 50% reported no problems except for personal hygiene. Use of a screwdriver and perineal care received the lowest scores.

REFERENCES

1. Nalebuff EA, Fatti JF, Weil CE: Arthrodesis of the rheumatoid wrist: indications and surgical technique. In Lichtman DM: The Wrist and Its Disorders. WB Saunders, Philadelphia, 1988, p. 365
2. Dick HM: Wrist and intercarpal arthrodesis. In Green DP (ed): Operative Hand Surgery. Vol. 1. Churchill Livingstone, New York, 1982, p. 127
3. Mackin EJ, Callahan AD, Skirven TM, et al. (eds): Hunter-Mackin-Callahan Rehabilitation of the Hand and Upper Extremity. 5th Ed. Mosby, St. Louis, 2002
4. Green DP: Carpal dislocations and instabilities. In Green DP (ed): Operative Hand Surgery. 2nd Ed. Vol. 2. Churchill Livingstone, New York, 1988, p. 925
5. Kozin SH, Michlovitz SL: Traumatic arthritis and osteoarthritis of the wrist. J Hand Ther 13:124-135, 2000
6. Dick HM: Wrist and intercarpal arthrodesis. In Green DP, Hotchkiss RN, Peterson WC (eds): Green's Operative Hand Surgery. 4th Ed. Churchill Livingstone, New York, 1999
7. Feldon P: Wrist fusions: intercarpal and radiocarpal. In Lichtman DM (ed): The Wrist and Its Disorders. WB Saunders, Philadelphia, 1988, p. 446
8. Minami A, Kato H, Iwasaki N, et al.: Limited wrist fusions: comparison of results 22 and 89 months after surgery. J Hand Surg Am 24:133-137, 1999
9. Weiss APC, Hastings H: Wrist arthrodesis for traumatic conditions: a study of plate and local bone graft application. J Hand Surg Am 20:50, 1995
10. Watson HK, Fink JA, Monacelli DM: Use of triscaphe fusion in the treatment of Keinbock's disease. Hand Clin 9:493, 1993
11. Weiss APC, Wiedeman G Jr, Quenzer D, et al.: Upper extremity function after wrist arthrodesis. J Hand Surg Am 20:813, 1995

SUGGESTED READINGS

Clendenin MB, Green DP: Arthrodesis of the wrist: complications and their management. J Hand Surg 6:253, 1981

Cohen MS, Kozin SH: Degenerative arthritis of the wrist: proximal row carpectomy versus scaphoid excision and four corner arthrodesis. J Hand Surg Am 26:94, 2001

Dell PC, Dell RB: Management of rheumatoid arthritis of the wrist. J Hand Ther 9:157-164, 1996

Dick HM: Wrist arthrodesis. In Green DP (ed): Operative Hand Surgery. 3rd. Ed. Vol. 1. Churchill Livingstone, New York, 1993, p. 131

Fisk GR: The wrist: review article. J Bone Joint Surg Br 66:401, 1984

Hastings H II: Wrist (radiocarpal) arthrodesis. In Green DP, Hotchkiss RN, Peterson WC (eds): Green's Operative Hand Surgery. 4th Ed. Churchill Livingstone, New York, 1998

KleinmanWB, Steichen JB, Strickland JW: Management of chronic rotary subluxation of the scaphoid by scapho-trapeqio-trapezoid arthrodesis. J Hand Surg Am 7:125, 1982

Schultz-Johnson K: Splinting the wrist: mobilization and protection. J Hand Ther 9:165-177, 1996

Watson HK, Dhillon HS: Intercarpal arthrodesis. In Green DP (ed): Operative Hand Surgery. 3rd. Ed. Vol. 1. Churchill Livingstone, New York, 1993, p. 113

Watson HK, Weinzweig J: Intercarpal arthrodesis. In Green DP, Hotchkiss RN, Peterson WC (eds): Green's Operative Hand Surgery. 4th Ed. Churchill Livingstone, New York, 1998

PART **SEVEN**

Hand

Dupuytren's Disease **42**

Dale Eckhaus

Dupuytren's disease (DD) is often cited as being of genetic origin.[1,2] Although it is present in various cultural groups,[3] the disease primarily affects individuals of Northern European descent.[4-6] It is often associated with other conditions such as chronic alcoholism, seizure disorders, diabetes mellitus,[2-4] chronic pulmonary disease, hypothyroidism,[4] smoking, and human immunodeficiency virus (HIV) infection.[3,4] The association of seizure disorders with DD can be related to medications.[2,4] The association of hypothyroidism, HIV, diabetes, and smoking can be related to the occurrence of oxygen free radicals.[4] DD in the diabetic is observed to be less progressive and located on the radial aspect of the hand.[4,5] Disease onset is usually in the fifth to seventh decade of life.[4,6] Men are more often affected than women. In most instances, the ulnar side of the hand is affected. The disease can have a slow or rapid progression.[6]

Individuals may sometimes exhibit a Dupuytren's diathesis. In those instances, there is a strong family history, the disease begins at an early age, and there is evidence of fibromatosis in areas other than the volar surface of the hand.[4,6]

The disease is an active cellular process in the fascia of the hand.[4,5] It often manifests initially as a nodule in the pretendinous bands of the ring and small fingers.[4] This is followed by the appearance of tendon-like cords, which are caused by the pathological change in normal fascia. The thickening and shortening of the fascia cause contracture.

Various nonoperative treatments, such as the use of splints, vitamin E, dimethyl sulfoxide (DMSO), and ultrasound, have proved ineffective.[7] Steroid injections have been effective in the treatment of nodules.[8] The use of collagenase offers promising results for nonoperative treatment.[7,9,10] Preoperative use of implanted continuous elongation devices has been effective for minimizing surgical procedures.[7,11-15]

Surgical intervention is recommended according to the progression of the disease and if the contracture becomes a functional problem.[4,16] Surgery is often suggested if the metacarpophalangeal (MCP) joint is contracted to 30 degrees.[2,3] Some surgeons believe that any amount of proximal interphalangeal (PIP) contracture warrants surgery.[3] Others suggest waiting until a PIP is contracted to 30 degrees,[2] or contracted to 30 degrees and accompanied by an MCP contracture.[1]

Many methods of surgical technique have been reported.[3,4] Postoperative management also varies. Common goals of the various methods are to promote wound healing, control scar formation, increase range of motion (ROM), and maximize function.

DEFINITION

Dupuytren's disease is a disease of the fascia of the palm and digits (Figs. 42-1 and 42-2).

SURGICAL PURPOSE

Dupuytren's contractures frequently interfere with normal hand function. The deformities are caused by abnormal thickening and contracture of the palmar fascia and its extensions. Dupuytren's contractures are treated surgically if MCP joint contractures prevent the placement of the hand flat on the table or if PIP joints demonstrate any loss of passive extension. These signs indicate a limitation of hand function and a potential for suboptimal results if left untreated as the disease and deformity progresses.

The fascia is approached with varied palmar skin incisions. These may include planned Z-plasty or skin grafting for wound closure after the contracture is released. The fascia is removed from its dense adhesions to the underlying skin, often leaving thin skin coverage on closure. Digital nerves and arteries may be intimately entrapped in the diseased tissue and risk injury or stretch during the resection. The flexor tendon sheath is not violated, in an attempt to prevent scarring within zone 2. In order to fully release chronically and severely contracted joints, capsulectomies may also be required. After closure of the skin, splinting is employed, and patients are urged to start therapy in the very early postoperative period to maximize improvement in ROM.

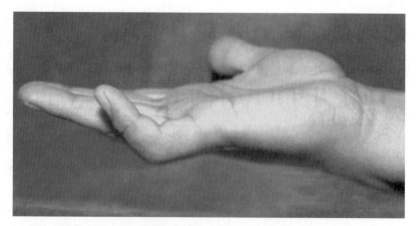

FIG. **42-1** Preoperative positioning of a hand with Dupuytren's disease.

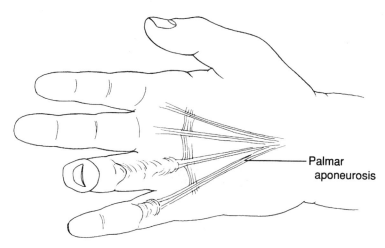

FIG. **42-2**   Dupuytren's disease affects the fascia of the hand.

TREATMENT GOALS

   I. Maintain ROM of uninvolved joints and digits.
  II. Control postoperative edema.
 III. Promote wound healing, especially in open palm techniques.
 IV. Improve active range of motion (AROM) and passive range of motion (PROM) for both extension and flexion.
  V. Control and guide scar formation.
 VI. Monitor and manage postoperative complications.
VII. Recover hand strength and function.

NONOPERATIVE INDICATIONS/PRECAUTIONS FOR THERAPY

Nonoperative therapy, including splinting, has not been effective. There are no therapy applications for nonoperative treatment, but some physicians use nonoperative techniques for the management of some phases of DD.[8,10,11]

POSTOPERATIVE INDICATIONS/PRECAUTIONS FOR THERAPY

  I. Indications: after surgery of the diseased fascia
 II. Precautions
    A. Intraoperative complications involving the neurovascular bundles
    B. Concomitant surgical procedures (e.g., capsulectomy)
    C. Skin grafts
    D. Excessive tissue tension[17]

POSTOPERATIVE THERAPY

  I. During the first week, the postoperative dressing is replaced with a thin, nonadhesive dressing. Depending on extent of surgery and the preference of the surgeon or therapist, a volar or dorsal, hand-based or forearm-based, removable thermoplastic extension splint is applied. Initially, splints are worn during the day except for exercise and hygiene. Splints are worn throughout the night while sleeping. After 2 to 3 weeks, day use is decreased and night use is continued. Regardless of the selected surface application, attention should be given to controlling wound tension through an initial splint design that uses wrist and/or MCP joint flexion (Fig. 42-3).

II. Whirlpool therapy with the extremity positioned horizontally is used early in treatment with an open palm technique or open wounds that result from complications of surgical incisions or grafts.

III. Wound care treatment is used with appropriate wounds, especially with the open techniques.

IV. Edema control methods are instituted.

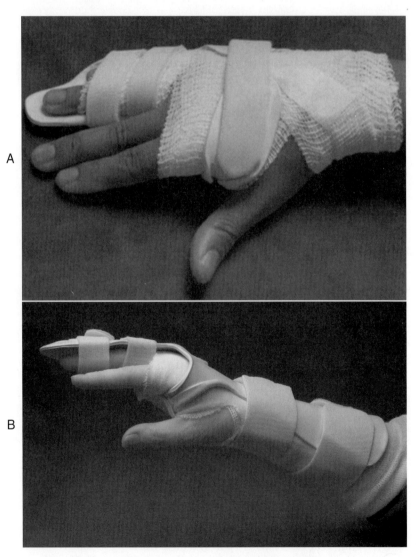

FIG. **42-3** **A** and **B,** Postoperative thermoplastic extension splints.

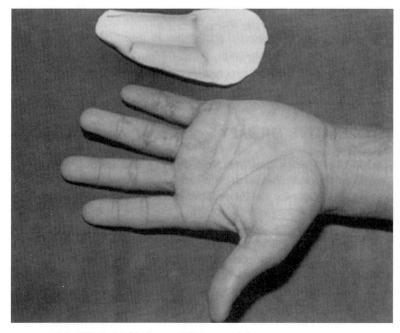

FIG. **42-4** Molded materials are used for scar management.

V. AROM, active-assisted range of motion (AAROM), and PROM exercises are initiated with first treatment session. Within the patient's tolerance, exercises include hook and composite grip, blocked and isolated joint motion, and abduction and adduction. Delay or special care in motion may be necessitated by grafts.

VI. Scar management techniques, including molded materials, are used when wounds are closed and sometimes over nonadherent dressings (Fig. 42-4).

VII. Light activities of daily living (ADLs) are permitted in early postoperative phase.

VIII. Light strengthening exercises, progressing to heavier resistance, are introduced once wounds are healed, edema is controlled, and pressure to the area is well tolerated.

IX. Splints are adjusted and various types are used to achieve full extension and flexion.

X. Splints with scar molds are used for up to 6 months or longer.

POSTOPERATIVE COMPLICATIONS

I. Hematoma

II. Edema

III. Skin necrosis

IV. Infection

V. Stiffness

VI. Pain

VII. Complex regional pain syndrome (CRPS)

VIII. Recurrence of disease

EVALUATION TIMELINE

I.   Initial evaluation at first postoperative visit
     A. Wound and skin condition
     B. Vascular status
     C. Edema
     D. Pain
     E. Sensibility
     F. AROM and PROM
     G. Management of ADLs
II. Reevaluation at 4-week intervals: Assess strength after wounds are closed and palmar surface can tolerate pressure.

OUTCOMES

Various authors have suggested several methods of postoperative splinting, exercise, and treatment programs with satisfactory results.[2,4,16,18,19] One study examined postsurgical management and its effects on patient outcomes[17]; the employment of no tension applied (NTA) in the initial postoperative phase, as related to splinting and exercise, resulted in fewer complications in scar formation and flare reaction when compared with a tension applied (TA) approach. The NTA group wore dorsal postoperative splints that positioned the wrist at 0 degrees extension, the MCP joints at 40 to 45 degrees flexion, and the PIP joints in neutral. The TA group wore splints that applied tension to the palm and digits to achieve an MCP position of 0 to 20 degrees and PIP extension. Both groups performed AROM exercises. The TA group focused on regaining digital extension. Although the final ROM was statistically better in the NTA group, clinical ROM for both groups was similar. The NTA group required fewer treatment sessions.

REFERENCES

1. Burge P: Genetics of Dupuytren's disease. Hand Clin 15:63-71, 1999
2. McFarlane RM, MacDermid JC: Dupuytren's disease. In Mackin EJ, Callahan AD, Skirven TM, et al. (eds): Hunter-Mackin-Callahan Rehabilitation of the Hand and Upper Extremity. 5th Ed. Mosby, St. Louis, 2002
3. Ross DC: Epidemiology of Dupuytren's disease. Hand Clin 15:53-62, 1999
4. Trumble TE: Dupuytren's disease. In Trumble TE (ed): Principles of Hand Surgery and Therapy. WB Saunders, Philadelphia, 2000
5. McGrouther DA: Dupuytren's contracture. In Green DP, Hotchkiss RN, Peterson WC (eds): Green's Operative Hand Surgery. 4th Ed. Churchill Livingstone, New York, 1999
6. Mawhinney I, et al.: Historical, anatomic and clinical aspects of Dupuytren's disease. In Tubiana R (ed): The Hand. Vol. 5. WB Saunders, Philadelphia, 1998
7. Hurst LC, Badalamente MA: Nonoperative treatment of Dupuytren's disease. Hand Clin 15:97-107, 1999
8. Ketchum LD, Donahue TK: The injection of nodules of Dupuytren's disease with triamcinolone acetonide. J Hand Surg Am 25:1157-1162, 2000
9. Starkweather KD, Lattuga S, Hurst LC, et al.: Collagenase in the treatment of Dupuytren's disease: an in vitro study. J Hand Surg Am 21:490-495, 1996
10. Badalamente MA, Hurst LC, Hentz VR: Collagen as a clinical target: nonoperative treatment of Dupuytren's disease. J Hand Surg Am 27:788-798, 2002
11. Messina A, Messina J: The continuous elongation treatment by the TEC device for severe Dupuytren's contracture of the fingers. Plast Reconstr Surg 92:84-90, 1993
12. Brandes G, Messina A, Reale E: The palmar fascia after treatment by the continuous extension technique for Dupuytren's contracture. J Hand Surg Br 19:528-533, 1994
13. Bailey AJ, Tarlton JF, Van der Stappen J, et al.: The continuous elongation technique for severe Dupuytren's disease. J Hand Surg Br 19:522-527, 1994

14. Hodgkinson PD: The use of skeletal traction to correct the flexed PIP joint in Dupuytren's disease. J Hand Surg Br 19:534-537, 1994
15. Citron N, Messina J: The use of skeletal traction in the treatment of severe primary Dupuytren's disease. J Bone Joint Surg Br 80:126-129, 1998
16. Crowley B, Tonkin MA: The proximal interphalangeal joint in Dupuytren's disease. Hand Clin 15:137-147, 1999
17. Evans RB, Dell PC, Fiolkowski P: A clinical report of the effect of mechanical stress on functional results after fasciectomy for Dupuytren's contracture. J Hand Ther 15:331-339, 2002
18. Mullins PA: Postsurgical rehabilitation of Dupuytren's disease. Hand Clin 15:167-174, 1999
19. Abbott K, Denney J, Burke FD, et al.: A review of attitudes to splintage in Dupuytren's contracture. J Hand Surg Br 12:326-328, 1987

SUGGESTED READINGS

Ebskov LB, Boeckstyns ME, Sorensen AI, et al.: Results after surgery for severe Dupuytren's contracture: does a dynamic extension splint influence outcome? Scand J Plast Reconstr Surg Hand Surg 34:155-160, 2000

Jain AS, Mitchell C, Carus DA: A simple inexpensive post-operative management regime following surgery for Dupuytren's contracture. J Hand Surg Br 13:259-261, 1988

McCash CR: The open palm technique in Dupuytren's contracture. Br J Plast Surg 17:271-280, 1964

Prosser R, Conolly WB: Complications following surgical treatment for Dupuytren's contracture. J Hand Ther 9:344-348, 1996

Rayan G, Tubiana R (eds): Dupuytren's disease. In Hand Clinics. Vol. 15. WB Saunders, Philadelphia, 1999

Rivas K, Gelberman R, Smith B, et al.: Severe contractures of the proximal interphalangeal joint in Dupuytren's disease: results of a prospective trial of operative correction and dynamic extension splinting. J Hand Surg Am 17:1153-1159, 1992

Sampson SP, Badalamente MA, Hurst LC, et al.: The use of a passive motion machine in the postoperative rehabilitation of Dupuytren's disease. J Hand Surg Am 17:333-338, 1992

Sinha R, Cresswell TR, Mason R, et al.: Functional benefit of Dupuytren's surgery. J Hand Surg Br 27:378-381, 2002

Smith P, Breed C: Central slip attenuation in Dupuytren's contracture: a cause of persistent flexion of the proximal interphalangeal joint. J Hand Surg Am 19:840-843, 1994

Stiles PJ: Ultrasonic therapy in Dupuytren's contracture. J Bone Joint Surg Br 48:452-454, 1966

Ligament Injuries of the Hand

43

Barbra J. Koczan and Shelby Moore

Functional stability of the hand is provided by the ligamentous structures of the thumb and fingers. Injuries to these structures can affect grasp, prehension, and the overall function of the hand. The primary stabilizers of the small joints of the thumb and fingers include the radial and ulnar collateral ligaments and the volar plate. In general, ligament injuries can be divided into two categories for the purpose of rehabilitation. One category consists of incomplete ligament tears and nondisplaced bony avulsions treated with immobilization. The other category consists of complete tears and displaced bony avulsions treated with surgery and immobilization.

In the thumb, the most commonly injured ligaments are the collateral ligaments of the thumb metacarpophalangeal (MCP) joint. Useful function of the thumb MCP joint depends more on its stability rather than its mobility.[1] Progression through all rehabilitation procedures should be based on continual reassessment of the stability of the ulnar or radial aspect of the joint.

The ulnar collateral ligament (UCL) and radial collateral ligament (RCL) function to provide stability to the MCP joint of the thumb; however, these ligaments vary greatly in their anatomy and their susceptibility to injury. RCL injuries are not as prevalent as UCL injuries, accounting for 10% to 40% of all thumb MCP joint ligamentous injuries.[3] Also, deformity at the MCP joint is more likely to occur with chronic RCL injuries than with chronic UCL injuries. With chronic RCL injuries, deformity is common due to the unopposed action of the strong adductor muscle, which exerts an oblique pull, leading to volar and ulnar subluxation of the MCP joint.[4] With chronic UCL injuries, the unopposed abductor pollicis brevis (APB) and flexor pollicis brevis muscles are aligned in a more vertical orientation, making their pull less destructive to the joint integrity. UCL injuries are also known by names such as gamekeeper's thumb, skier's thumb, and breakdancer's thumb.

The major distinction between partial and complete ligament tears is the likelihood for complete tears to become Stener or Stener-like lesions.[4,5] Unique to UCL injuries, Stener lesions are formed when avulsed ligaments slide out from under the adductor aponeurosis and become entrapped

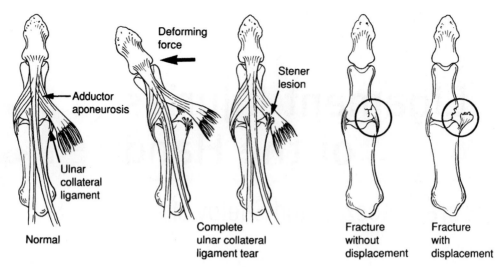

FIG. **43-1** Normal anatomy of thumb metacarpophalangeal joint and associated injuries.

superficial to the adductor aponeurosis (Fig. 43-1). Much less commonly, the APB can displace into the joint space with complete RCL injuries, creating a Stener-like lesion.[4] Both of these lesions require surgical repair to restore medial or lateral stability. Conversely, if the ligament is partially torn and the joint demonstrates minimal instability, the joint can be immobilized in plaster. To ensure stability, the surgeon may position the joint in slight flexion and ulnar deviation for UCL injuries and in slight flexion and radial deviation for RCL injuries.

In contrast to those of the thumb, the ligaments surrounding the MCP joints of the fingers are injured much less commonly than those of the proximal interphalangeal (PIP) joints. The MCP joints are able to absorb more forces because of their ability to move not only into flexion and extension but also into abduction and adduction.

The PIP joint is a hinge joint that allows for good stability of the fingers. Despite its stability, it is the most frequently injured joint in the hand.[6,7] The primary stabilizers of the joint are the soft tissue structures such as the UCL and RCL and the volar plate.[8] The RCL is the most frequently injured PIP joint ligament. RCL injuries occur twice as often as UCL injuries.[7] Injury to the ligaments of the PIP joint are most likely to occur when a torque is applied to an extended joint.

Another commonly injured stabilizing structure in the fingers is the sagittal band (SB). The SBs are part of the extensor retinacular system of the MCP joint, which extends from the volar plate to the extensor digitorum communis (EDC). The purpose of the SB is to provide lateral stability, preventing ulnar or radial subluxation and bowstringing of the EDC.[2] Management of these injuries also is addressed in this chapter.

DEFINITIONS

I.   **Incomplete tears of UCL/RCL:** Partial tears of UCL/RCL with minimal ulnar/radial instability
II. **Nondisplaced bony avulsions:** Injury to bone at attachment of UCL/RCL without displacement

III.   Complete tear of UCL/RCL of the thumb
    A. Complete tear with tendon interposition
       1. **Stener lesions:** Complete UCL tears with UCL entrapment superficial to adductor aponeurosis
       2. **Stener-like lesions:** Complete RCL tears with RCL entrapment superficial to APB tendon
    B. Complete UCL/RCL tears without Stener lesions
    C. Displaced avulsion fracture
IV.   Complete tear of finger (nonthumb) MCP UCL/RCL[9]
    A. Complete tear without SB involvement
    B. Complete tear with SB involvement
 V.   Complete tear of PIP joint UCL/RCL
    A. Complete tear with volar plate involvement
    B. Complete tear without volar plate involvement
    C. Displaced avulsion fracture
VI.   SBs
    A. Type I: incomplete tear of SB without tendonous instability
    B. Type II: incomplete tear of SB with tendon subluxation
    C. Type III: complete tear of SB with tendon subluxation

TREATMENT AND SURGICAL PURPOSE

The UCL of the thumb MCP joint provides stability for that joint against forces applied in a radial direction. The UCL and RCL of the MCP and interphalangeal (IP) joints stabilize the joints against forces applied in a radial or ulnar direction. If ligament integrity is compromised, the ability of the fingers to perform activities such as manipulation, grasp, and pinch can be altered. The SBs act to stabilize the EDC centrally at the MCP joint.

The treatment protocol for ligament injuries depends on the degree of the ligament tear and the amount of instability of the joint. Management ranges from simple splinting to operative repair. The goal is to recognize the extent of the injury early and begin appropriate care. Late reconstruction can seriously compromise the stability and ROM of the joint.

 I.   Collateral ligaments of the thumb MCP joint
    A. Surgical intervention is undertaken in the following settings
       1. A palpable ruptured collateral ligament that is entrapped above the adductor aponeurosis on the ulnar border of the thumb
       2. An unstable joint with greater than 30 degrees of angulation when the injured collateral ligament is stress tested
       3. A displaced avulsion fracture exists at the insertion site of the ligament
       4. Chronic unstable injuries previously unrecognized or failing conservative management
    B. The injuries are approached from a curvilinear dorsolateral incision over the involved side.
    C. The ligament injury is repaired primarily in the setting of an acute injury without bony involvement. This may require the use of bone anchors to fix the ligament to the base of the proximal phalanx.
    D. Fracture avulsions are usually treated with bone anchor, Kirschner wire, or screw fixation.

E. Chronic injuries may require the use of tendon grafts to reconstruct the ligament, or they may be treated by surgical arthrodesis to provide stability.

II. Collateral ligament injuries of the MCP/PIP joints of the fingers
A. Surgical purpose: Collateral ligament injuries at these sites that occur in isolation rarely require surgical intervention.
B. General surgical indications
1. Irreducible MCP or PIP dislocations
2. Displaced fracture dislocations
C. Surgical intervention for irreducible PIP or MCP dislocations focuses on the entrapped soft tissue preventing reduction. In the case of MCP joints, this often is a combination of volar plate, flexor tendons, and intrinsic muscles. In the case of PIP joints, this is often the extensor mechanism, but more rarely it can involve the collateral ligament within the joint. In these cases of severe ligamentous disruption, collateral ligament repair is rarely undertaken, because the long-term functional impairment is usually stiffness rather than instability.
D. Surgical intervention for fracture dislocations involving collateral ligament injuries at these sites focuses on restoration of articular congruity (see Chapter 44).

III. SB injuries
A. Surgical intervention usually is reserved for those instances in which nonoperative treatment has failed to realign and stabilize the extensor mechanism over the MCP joint in digital flexion.
B. The sagittal fibers may be repaired primarily, reinforced with slips of the extensor mechanism or contralateral sagittal fibers, or stabilized with transfers of the lumbrical tendon to the disrupted radial side of the extensor hood.

TREATMENT GOALS

I. Maintain full ROM of all uninvolved joints of the upper extremity.
II. Promote ligament healing.
III. Avoid pin tract and/or pull-out wire tract infection.
IV. Maximize active range of motion (AROM) and passive range of motion (PROM) of involved joint.
V. Maximize ulnar and radial stability of MCP joint during grip and pinch activities.
VI. Return to previous level of function.
VII. Prevent reinjury through patient education.

NONOPERATIVE INDICATIONS/PRECAUTIONS FOR THERAPY

I. Indications
A. Incomplete UCL/RCL tears
B. Nondisplaced bony avulsions at site of UCL/RCL attachment
C. Type I SB injury: minor SB injury without extensor tendon
D. Type II SB injury: moderate SB injury with extensor tendon subluxation

II. Precautions
 A. Avoid directional torque, which would further tear injured ligament.
 B. Extreme pain
 C. Extreme edema
 D. Associated flexor or extensor tendon ruptures
 E. Associated volar plate injuries

NONOPERATIVE THERAPY

 I. Incomplete UCL/RCL tears or nondisplaced avulsion fractures of the thumb
 A. Weeks 1 to 4: thumb spica plaster or thermoplastic splint immobilization for period directed by surgeon.[1,10-12] Consult surgeon as to whether immobilization of the IP and wrist joints is indicated (Fig. 43-2). Maintain AROM of all joints of the upper extremity while in plaster or splint. Concentrate especially on the IP joint to prevent extensor mechanism adhesions.
 B. Week 4: If splint includes the wrist (forearm-based), modify to exclude the wrist (hand-based). Splint use is continued at all times, excluding exercise or hygiene.

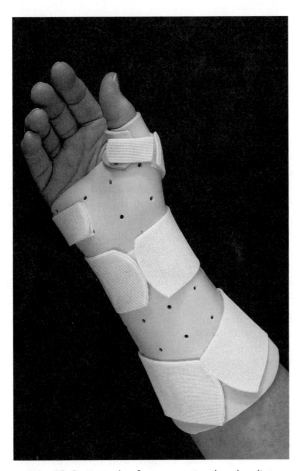

FIG. **43-2** Example of postoperative thumb splint.

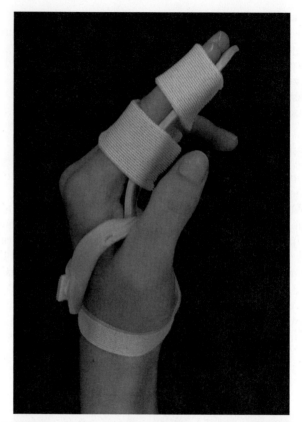

FIG. **43-3** Example of nonoperative or postoperative splint for finger meta-carpophalangeal joint collateral ligament injuries.

    C. Week 5: Begin and progress PROM of the thumb MCP joint.

    D. Week 6: Begin and progress dynamic splinting of the thumb MCP joint as needed. Begin weaning splint use if thumb is stable and asymptomatic.

    E. Week 8: Begin and progress strengthening during grip and pinch, including lateral, tip-to-tip and three-jaw pinch positions. Specifically for UCL injuries, strengthen the locking of the thumb around a 6- to 8-cm-diameter cylinder.[13,14]

    F. Weeks 10 to 16: Begin unrestricted use. May want to tape protectively during sports activities.[15]

  II. Incomplete UCL/RCL tears or nondisplaced avulsion fractures of other digits

    A. Weeks 0 to 3

       1. MCP: hand-based thermoplastic splint with injured and adjacent MCP joints immobilized in 30 to 50 degrees flexion with IP joints free (Fig. 43-3). AROM to all joints not included in splint.

       2. IP: In the daytime, buddy-tape involved digit to adjacent digit on the same side as the injury, using buddy straps at the proximal and middle phalanges and begin AROM (Fig. 43-4). RCL injuries of the index finger and UCL injuries of the small finger should be splinted in an extension gutter splint at all times except during AROM.[6] Concentrate especially on

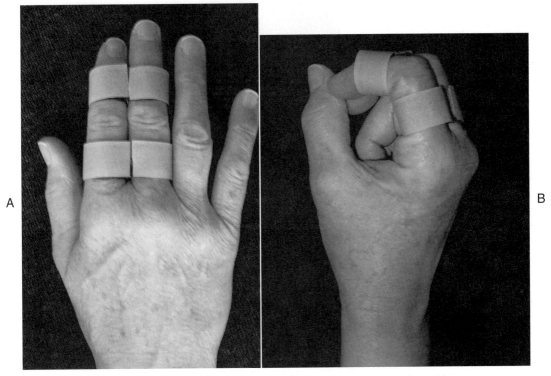

FIG. **43-4** **A** and **B,** Examples of buddy straps for proximal interphalangeal collateral ligament injuries.

   distal interphalangeal (DIP) joint motion to prevent oblique retinacular ligament (ORL) tightness and to encourage tendon gliding.

  3. IP: At nighttime, an extension gutter splint is used on the involved digit. If the joint is extremely painful or the degree of injury high, an extension gutter splint may be used at all times for several days after injury until pain diminishes.

 B. Weeks 3 to 4

  1. MCP: Initiate AROM to the entire digit. Continue with splinting between exercise sessions and at night. A transition may be made to buddy-taping of the injured digit to an adjacent finger on the side of injury, with tape at proximal phalanx, as pain diminishes.

  2. PIP: Discharge splint as pain subsides.

 C. Weeks 6 to 8

  1. MCP: Initiate PROM to entire digit. Begin progressive strengthening. Wean from splint and buddy-tape as pain subsides.

  2. PIP: Discharge buddy tape. Begin progressive strengthening as pain subsides.[6]

 D. Weeks 8 to 12: For both MCP and PIP injuries, progress strengthening and begin unrestricted usage.

III. Type I or II SB injuries

 A. Weeks 0 to 3

  1. Type I: Buddy-tape to adjacent digit on affected side. Initiate AROM to all joints.[16]

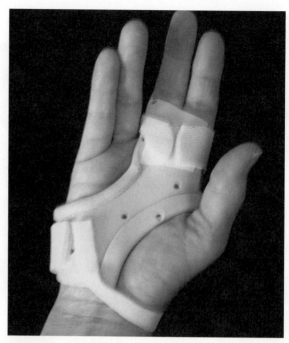

FIG. **43-5** Example of nonoperative splint for sagittal band injuries.

2. Type II: Hand-based splint with MCP of involved and adjacent finger on affected side in full extension with IPs free (Fig. 43-5). Initiate AROM to uninvolved joints.[16]
   B. Weeks 4 to 6
   1. Type I: Add active-assisted range of motion (AAROM) and PROM if needed.[16]
   2. Type II: Initiate AROM to MCP joint.[16]
   C. Weeks 6 to 12
   1. Type I: Discharge buddy straps and add progressive strengthening as tolerated.[16]
   2. Type II: Discharge splint. Change to buddy straps with AROM and AAROM exercises.[16]
   D. Weeks 12 to 16
   1. Type I: Unrestricted usage
   2. Type II: Initiate strengthening, and progress to unrestricted usage.

NONOPERATIVE COMPLICATIONS

   I. Chronic instability and weakness of grip and pinch[10,17]
  II. Persistent pain, stiffness, and arthritis[6-8,11,17]
 III. Decreased ROM of MCP and IP joints[6,17,18]
  IV. Persistent edema[7,16,18]
   V. PIP joint flexion contractures[6]
  VI. Persistent popping of the extensor tendon with MCP flexion
 VII. Visible extensor lag with active extension of the MCP joint
VIII. Decreased MCP joint ROM[18]
  IX. Small finger abduction deformity[2,16]

OPERATIVE INDICATIONS/PRECAUTIONS FOR THERAPY

I.   Indications
     A. Complete UCL/RCL tears
     B. Displaced avulsion fractures at site of UCL/RCL attachment
     C. Complete UCL/RCL tear with associated volar plate rupture
     D. Type III: severe injury to SB with tendon dislocation
     E. Failed conservative treatment of type I or II SB injury
II. Precautions
     A. Avoid directional torque that would further tear involved ligament.
     B. Infection
     C. Extreme pain
     D. Extreme edema
     E. Associated flexor or extensor tendon ruptures
     F. Watch for development of MCP extension lag

POSTOPERATIVE THERAPY

I.   After surgical repair of the thumb MCP joint ligament and removal of K-wires
     A. Day 1 to weeks 2 to 3: Thumb spica plaster cast to immobilize joint for period recommended by surgeon. Mandating AROM for all joints not immobilized, especially the IP joint of the thumb, to prevent extensor tendon adhesions.
     B. Weeks 2 to 3: If surgeon removes cast, K-wire, and pullout wire, apply forearm or hand-based thumb spica splint, according to surgeon's preference. Continue full-time splinting except for supervised ROM of carpometacarpal, IP, and wrist joints.
     C. Week 4: Begin AROM of MCP joint.[19] Protect ulnar/radial stability. Splint use continues at all times excluding exercise and hygiene. The precise duration of immobilization should be determined by the surgeon with his or her knowledge of the actual repair and subsequent expectations.
     D. Weeks 6 to 8: Begin gentle PROM of the MCP joint. Begin and progress dynamic splinting of the MCP joint if indicated. Begin weaning splint use if the joint is stable and asymptomatic.
     E. Weeks 10 to 12: Begin and progress strengthening, during grip and lateral, tip, and three-jaw pinch positions. Specifically for UCL injuries, strengthen the locking of the thumb around a 6- to 8-cm-diameter cylinder.[13,14]
     F. Weeks 12 to 16: Begin unrestricted use.[4] The digit may be taped protectively during sports activities.[12]
II. After surgical repair of other digits and removal of K-wires
     A. Week 2
         1. MCP: If the surgeon removes the plaster cast, proceed with removal of the postoperative bulky dressing. A hand-based thermoplastic splint is fabricated to immobilize the injured digit and an adjacent digit in a safe position with the MCP joint in 30 to 50 degrees flexion with IP joints free (see Fig. 43-3). This position prevents excessive tension on the ligament repair. AROM is applied to all joints not immobilized in splint.[9]

2. PIP: If the surgeon removes the plaster cast, remove the bulky postoperative dressing. Apply hand-based thermoplastic splint to immobilize the injured and an adjacent digit in a safe position with the MCP joints at 45 to 60 degrees flexion with IP joints straight. If there is an associated volar plate injury, the volar plate must be protected by splinting in the safe position with the PIP joint blocked in 20 degrees flexion (see Chapter 44).

B. Weeks 3 to 4: MCP and PIP: Initiate AROM after buddy-taping the injured digit to an adjacent digit. Continue with splint use between exercise sessions and at night.[18]

C. Week 6

1. MCP: Initiate PROM of the MCP joint and gentle strengthening. Splint or buddy-tape as needed for pain relief.

2. PIP: Discharge splint. Buddy-tape for unrestricted AROM and gentle AAROM.

D. Weeks 7 to 8

1. MCP: Discharge splint and buddy tape. Buddy-tape only during sports or heavy activities until weeks 10 to 12. Dynamic flexion splinting may be initiated if ROM deficits persist.[9]

2. PIP: Initiate PROM and dynamic flexion splinting of the PIP joint if needed. Begin gentle strengthening and progress to heavy lifting and repetitive use by 10 to 12 weeks.

III. After surgical repair or reconstruction of the SB with centralization of the extensor tendon

A. Days 3 to 5: If the surgeon removes the plaster cast, proceed with removal of the postoperative bulky dressing. A hand-based thermoplastic splint is fabricated to immobilize the injured digit and an adjacent digit on the affected side with MCP and IP joints in full extension. Initiate AROM to all uninvolved joints, including IP joints of the involved digit.[16]

B. Weeks 3 to 4: Initiate AROM to the MCP joint. Continue splint use between exercise sessions.

C. Week 6: Initiate PROM and dynamic splinting to the MCP joint if needed. Discharge splint use during the day. Warn the patient to monitor for development of extension lag.

D. Weeks 7 to 8: Discharge splint at night.

POSTOPERATIVE COMPLICATIONS

I. Chronic instability and weakness[9]
II. Persistent numbness of ulnar/radial aspect of thumb or digits
III. Persistent pain or arthritis[9,20]
IV. Decreased ROM of MCP and IP joints[20]
V. Infection
VI. Flexion contracture of PIP joint[20]
VII. Persistent edema[18]
VIII. Continuous subluxation/popping of extensor tendon
IX. Extensor lag of MCP joint

EVALUATION TIMELINE

I.   Thumb
  A. Incomplete UCL/RCL tears treated nonoperatively
    1. Week 1: initial AROM and PROM measurements of all upper extremity joints not included in splint
    2. Week 4: initial AROM measurements of entire thumb and wrist joints
    3. Week 5: initial PROM measurements of thumb and wrist joints
    4. Week 8: Assess grip and pinch strength and manual muscle testing (MMT) of the thumb muscles
  B. UCL/RCL tears or nondisplaced avulsion fractures treated operatively
    1. Week 1: same as for incomplete UCL/RCL tears
    2. Weeks 2 to 3: initial AROM measurements of carpometacarpal and IP joints of the thumb and wrist joint
    3. Week 4: Initial AROM measurements of all thumb joints
    4. Weeks 6 to 7: Initial PROM of thumb joints
    5. Week 8: Assess grip and pinch strength and MMT of thumb muscles
II. Finger MCP/IP
  A. Nonoperative
    1. MCP
      a. Weeks 0 to 3: Initial AROM and PROM measurements are taken of all joints not included in splint
      b. Weeks 3 to 4: Initial AROM measurements are taken of entire involved digit
      c. Weeks 6 to 8: Initial PROM measurements of involved digit
      d. Weeks 8 to 12: Assess grip and (if indicated) pinch strength
    2. PIP
      a. Weeks 0 to 3: initial AROM measurements of all joints
      b. Weeks 6 to 8: initial PROM measurements of all joints
      c. Weeks 8 to 12: Assess grip and (if indicated) pinch strength
  B. Operative
    1. MCP
      a. Week 2: initial AROM/PROM measurements of all joints not included in splint
      b. Week 3: initial AROM measurements of the entire involved digit
      c. Week 6: initial PROM measurements of the entire involved digit
      d. Week 8: Assess grip and (if indicated) pinch strength
    2. PIP
      a. Week 2: initial AROM/PROM measurements of all joints not included in splint
      b. Week 3: initial AROM measurements of involved digit
      c. Week 7: initial PROM measurements of involved digit
      d. Week 8: Assess grip and (if indicated) pinch strength

III.   SB injuries
    A. Nonoperative
        1. Type I
            a. Weeks 0 to 3: initial AROM measurements of all joints
            b. Weeks 4 to 6: initial PROM measurements of involved MCP joint
            c. Weeks 8 to 10: Assess grip and (if indicated) pinch strength
        2. Type II
            a. Weeks 0 to 3: initial AROM and PROM measurements of all noninvolved joints
            b. Weeks 4 to 6: initial AROM measurements of involved MCP joint
            c. Weeks 8 to 10: initial PROM measurements of involved MCP joint
            d. Week 12: Assess grip and (if indicated) pinch strength
    B. Operative
        1. Days 3 to 5: initial AROM measurements of all uninvolved joints
        2. Weeks 3 to 4: initial AROM measurements of involved MCP joint
        3. Week 6: initial PROM measurements of involved MCP joint
        4. Week 8: Assess grip and (if indicated) pinch strength

OUTCOMES

After nonoperative or operative management of UCL/RCL injuries of the thumb MCP joint, studies demonstrate that stability and functional ROM is regained. Postoperatively, stability, which was assessed by stress examination, showed an average of 1 to 5 degrees difference between the injured and uninjured sides of the joint.[3,4,21] Results showed that recovery of strength was directly correlated with improved stability. Ninety percent of patients regained near-normal pinch and grip strength postoperatively.[3,4,21] An average of 15 to 20 degrees of thumb MCP joint ROM was lost after operative repair; however, this loss of motion did not impede functional mobility of the hand.[3,4,21] Similar results were found with nonoperative treatment of RCL/UCL thumb MCP joint injuries, with functional mobility regained and a return to premorbid level of activity by 10 to 16 weeks after the injury.[22]

After nonoperative and operative management of UCL/RCL injuries to the finger MCP/PIP joints, the literature shows good results, with most patients regaining full functional strength and stability.[8,9,20] Within 10 to 12 weeks, patients regained full or almost full ROM, with an average loss of 8 to 20 degrees at the involved joint.[9] Subjective complaints of pain, stiffness, and swelling of the involved joint were shown to persist in even minor sprains for up to 6 months after injury.[20]

According to the literature, after type I or II SB injuries treated with immobilization, the best results are achieved with early diagnosis and treatment.[16] Virtually all patients regained full ROM at the MCP joint without residual pain or functional limitations.[16] Similarly to the results with nonoperative treatment, the literature shows the importance of early intervention with operative repair of type III SB injuries. After surgical repair and treatment, patients regained full ROM and strength at the MCP joint and reported a high level of patient satisfaction with return to prior functional level, including competitive sports.[18]

REFERENCES

1. Miller RJ: Dislocations and fracture dislocations of the metacarpophalangeal joint of the thumb. Hand Clin 4:45, 1988
2. Young CM, Rayan GM: The sagittal band: anatomical and biomechanical study. J Hand Surg Am 25:1107-1113, 2000
3. Coyle MP: Grade III radial collateral ligament injuries of the thumb metacarpophalangeal joint. J Hand Surg Am 28:14-20, 2003
4. Melone CP, Beldner S, Basule RS: Thumb collateral ligament injuries: an anatomical basis for treatment. Hand Clin 16:345-357, 2000
5. Stener B: Displacement of the ruptured ulnar collateral ligament of the metacarpophalangeal joint of the thumb: a clinical and anatomical study. J Bone Joint Surg Br 44:869, 1962
6. Chinchalker SJ, Gan BS: Management of proximal interphalangeal joint fractures and dislocations. J Hand Ther 16:117-128, 2003
7. Rhee FY, Reading G, Wray RC: A biomechanic study of the collateral ligaments of the proximal interphalangeal joint. J Hand Surg Am 17:157-163, 1992
8. Kiefhaber TR, Stern PJ, Grood ES: Lateral stability of the proximal interphalangeal joint. J Hand Surg Am 11:661-669, 1986
9. Deleare O, Suttor PM, Degolla R, et al.: Early surgical treatment for collateral ligament rupture of metacarpophalangeal joints of the fingers. J Hand Surg Am 28:309-315, 2003
10. Eaton RG: Injuries of the metacarpophalangeal joint of the thumb. In Tubiana R (ed): The Hand. Vol. 3. WB Saunders, Philadelphia, 1988, p. 887
11. Sandzen SC: The Hand and Wrist. Williams & Wilkins, Baltimore, 1985
12. Green DP (ed): Operative Hand Surgery. 2nd Ed. Churchill Livingstone, New York, 1988
13. Kopandji IA: Biomechanics of the thumb. In Tubiana R (ed): The Hand. Vol. 3. WB Saunders, Philadelphia, 1988, p. 404
14. Aubriot JH: Injuries of the metacarpophalangeal joint of the thumb. In Tubiana R (ed): The Hand. Vol. 3. WB Saunders, Philadelphia, 1988, p. 184
15. Gieck JH, Maxer V: Protective splinting for the hand and wrist. Clin Sports Med 5:795, 1986
16. Rayan GM, Murray D: Classification and treatment of closed sagittal band injuries. J Hand Surg Am 19:590-594, 1994
17. Helm RH: Hand function after injuries to the collateral ligaments of the metacarpophalangeal joint of the thumb. J Hand Surg Br 12:252, 1987
18. Hame SL, Melone CP: Boxer's knuckle: traumatic disruption of the extensor hood. Hand Clin 16:375-379, 2000
19. Adams BD, Muller DL: Assessment of thumb positioning in the treatment of ulnar collateral ligament injuries. Am J Sports Med 24:672-675, 1996
20. Gotoh M, Gotoh H, Shiba Y, et al.: Ulnar deviation after volar subluxation of the proximal interphalangeal joint. Clin Orthop 391:188-191, 2001
21. Fairhurst M, Hansen L: Reconstruction of the ulnar collateral ligament. J Hand Surgery Br 27:542-545, 2002
22. Pichora DR, McMurtry RY, Bell MJ: Gamekeeper's thumb: a prospective study of functional bracing. J Hand Surg Am 14:567-573, 1989

SUGGESTED READINGS

Bowers WH: Sprains and joint injuries in the hand. Hand Clin 2:93, 1986
Eaton RG: Joint Injuries of the Hand. Charles C Thomas, Springfield, MO, 1971
Fess EE, Gettle KS, Strickland JW: Hand splinting principles and methods. Mosby, St. Louis, 1981
Flynn JE: Hand Surgery. 3rd Ed. Williams & Wilkins, Baltimore, 1982

Jupiter JB, Sheppard JE: Tension wire fixation of avulsion fractures of the hand.
   Clin Orthop 214:113, 1987
Milford L: The Hand. Mosby, St. Louis, 1982
Stener B: Acute injuries to the metacarpophalangeal joint of the thumb.
   In Tubiana R (ed): The Hand. Vol. 3. WB Saunders, Philadelphia, 1988, p. 895
Weeks PM: Management of Acute Hand Injuries. 2nd Ed. Mosby, St. Louis, 1978

Digital Fracture Rehabilitation

44

Gregory A. Hritcko

The purpose of this chapter is to provide an overview of fractures of the digits, to review general guidelines, and to present references and resources. There is an inherent danger in presenting protocols, because each case is a unique entity with its own set of issues. A fundamental knowledge base of anatomy and fracture healing, the mechanism of injury, an understanding of the patient and his or her circumstances, and an open line of communication with the treating physician to obtain an appreciation of the treatment option selected are critical to the rehabilitation outcome.

Hand therapy interventions are based on the diagnosis and treatment by the physician. Fig. 44-1 presents an algorithm of healing and the rehabilitation process. Goals of edema reduction, pain control, wound management, maintaining motion of the noninvolved joints, initiating motion of the involved structures, and strengthening should be addressed specifically in each case at the appropriate time relative to tissue healing. The therapist should initiate the treatment, closely monitor the tissue response and the clinical changes, then adapt the treatment as necessary. Swanson, cited by Stern,[1] noted that hand fractures can be complicated by deformity from no treatment, stiffness from overtreatment, and both deformity and stiffness from poor treatment.

DEFINITION

A fracture is defined as a structural break in the integrity of a bone, epiphyseal plate, or cartilaginous surface. Reports of incidence, location, and configuration vary widely in the literature for fractures of the hand. The mechanism of injury, degree of disruption, fracture configuration, and involvement of soft tissue structures are all management considerations. Fig. 44-2 provides an overview of healing based on the physician's treatment methods. A thorough understanding of these methods and techniques will yield a more optimal result.

Meyer and Wilson[2] reported the incidence of fractures in the hand as follows: distal phalanx level, 40% to 50%; middle phalanx, 8% to 12%; proximal phalanx, 15% to 20%; and metacarpal level, 30% to 35%.

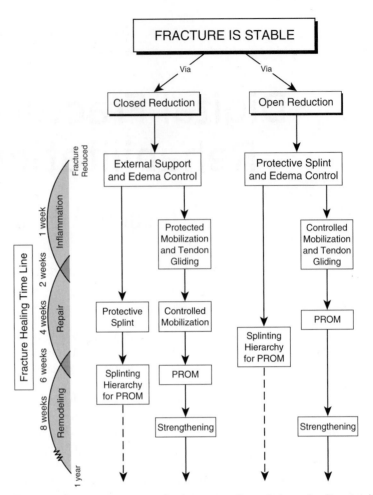

FIG. 44-1 Fracture management and treatment outline relative to healing timeline. Protected mobilization is gentle active and passive range of motion (AROM/PROM) of the nonimmobilized joints to avoid contractures and to glide soft tissue structures. Active motion is emphasized for controlled mobilization and for tendon gliding. (From Lastayo P, Winters K, Hardy M: J Hand Ther 16:90, 2003. Copyright Paul Lastayo, PhD, PT, CHT.)

DISTAL PHALANX FRACTURES

Distal phalanx fractures account for the majority of hand fractures, with incident reports varying. The middle finger and thumb are the most frequently injured digits, owing to their length and use patterns. The mechanism of injury is a crush or blow to the tip of the digit.[3] A modified Schneider classification of distal phalanx fractures, as cited by Stern,[1] includes tuft, shaft, and articular fractures. Tuft fractures often involve a nail bed or pulp injury. Shaft fractures are either longitudinal or transverse; the transverse fracture may be stable or unstable and may require fixation. Articular fractures may be volar, dorsal, or epiphyseal in the child or adolescent. These injuries include avulsion injuries of the distal flexor or extensor tendons and constitute another set of treatment issues that are addressed in Chapters 17 and 21.

Healing Based on Fracture Fixation

Closed Reduction Methods			Open Reduction Methods		
External Immobilization	CREF/CRIF	Co-aptive Fixation	Stable Fixation	Rigid Fixation	
Secondary Healing 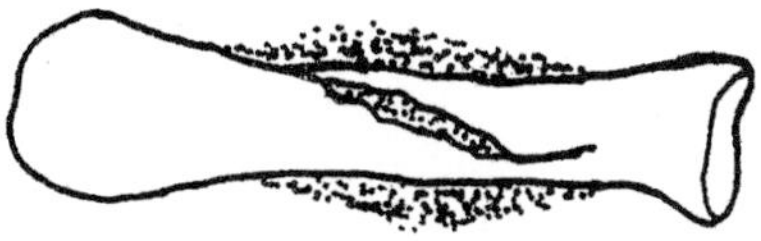			**Primary Healing** 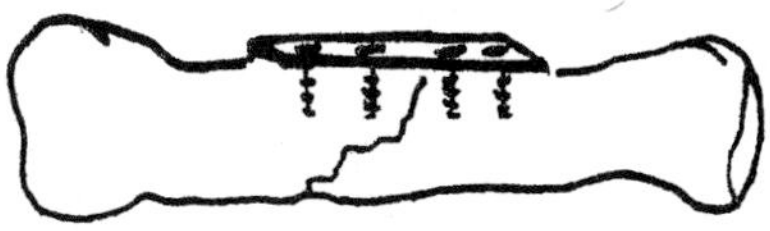		
External Immobilization	CREF/CRIF	Co-aptive Fixation	Stable Fixation	Rigid Fixation	
• Casting	• Percutaneous Pins	• K-Wires	• Inter fragmentary Screw	• Lag Screw	
• Static Splint	• K-Wires	• Interosseous Wiring	• Tension Band Wiring	• Plates	
• Traction Splint (skin, nail)	• Traction Splint (K-wire)	• Intramedullary Pin/Nail	• Tension Band Plating	• 90-90 Wiring	
• Fracture Bracing	• External Fixation				

FIG. 44-2 Healing based on fracture fixation. The method of fixation used relates to the type of fracture healing that will occur. The various methods used to maintain or ensure reduction of the fracture are listed in their appropriate category. (From Lastayo P, Winters K, Hardy M: J Hand Ther 16:87, 2003.)

Treatment Purpose

I.   Promote fracture healing in anatomical alignment in order to achieve pain-free functional range of motion (ROM) and strength.

Treatment Goals

I.   Restore pain-free functional ROM and strength to the involved digit and hand.

Nonoperative Indications/Precautions for Therapy

I.   Indications
     A. Distal tuft fractures that are stable, treated closed with wound care (if indicated) and protective splinting[4]
     B. Distal phalanx fractures (shaft or base) that are stable, treated closed with protective splinting[4]
II. Precaution: unstable reduction

Nonoperative Therapy

I. Distal tuft fractures
    A. Weeks 0 to 3: protective splinting of the distal phalanx[4,5]
       1. Wound care for nail bed injury, if indicated
       2. Coban wrapping for edema control[6]
       3. Early active motion of the noninvolved proximal interphalangeal (PIP)/metacarpophalangeal (MCP) joints[6]
       4. Early active motion of the distal interphalangeal (DIP) joint as indicated/tolerated[6]
       5. Desensitization[4]
    B. Weeks 3 to 4
       1. Protective splinting as needed
       2. Active-assisted range of motion (AAROM) progressing to unrestricted active motion at the DIP level; differential tendon gliding exercises[6,7]
    C. Weeks 6 to 8: Wean from splint.
    D. Weeks 8 to 10: Progress to resistive exercise.
II. Distal phalanx fractures (shaft or base)
    A. Weeks 0 to 4: full-time protective splinting during fracture consolidation phase[3,5]
       1. Coban wrapping
       2. Early active motion of the noninvolved PIP/MCP joints
       3. Desensitization[4]
    B. Weeks 3 to 5: active range of motion (AROM) at the DIP level based on fracture healing.
    C. Weeks 4 to 6: As passive range of motion (PROM) is permitted, taping, PIP/DIP straps, or a form of dynamic flexion device may be initiated.[4,6]
    D. Weeks 8 to 10: Progress to strengthening.

Nonoperative Complications

I.   Loss of reduction
II. Nonunion of fracture[4,6]
III. Infection[8]
IV. Loss of motion
V.   Permanent stiffness
VI. Persistent sensitivity (paresthesias, dysesthesias, or temperature intolerance)[4,6]

Postoperative Indications/Precautions for Therapy

I. Indications
    A. Distal tuft fractures
       1. Nail bed or pulp injury requiring surgical attention
       2. Surgical fracture reduction to address open, unstable fracture, typically Kirschner wire pinning
    B. Distal phalanx fractures (shaft or base)
       1. Nail bed or pulp injury requiring surgical attention
       2. Surgical fracture reduction to address open, unstable fracture. (may include K-wire stabilization or use of screw fixation)

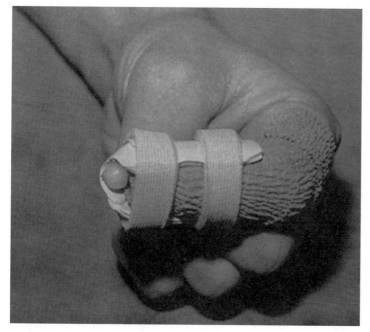

FIG. 44-3 Protective splinting for distal phalanx fracture stabilized with Kirschner wire.

II.   Precautions
      A. Distal tuft fractures
          1. Unstable reduction
          2. Internal/external fixation
          3. Delayed union
          4. Concomitant soft tissue trauma
          5. Limited motion of the noninvolved joints
          6. Distal phalanx fractures

Postoperative Therapy

I.   Distal tuft fractures, transverse or base fracture, nail bed injuries,
     treated with surgical reduction (Fig. 44-3)
     A. 0 to 4 weeks
         1. Fabrication of protective splint for the distal phalanx;
            PIP joint free[5]
         2. Wound care, dressing changes, K-wire pin care as indicated[5,6]
         3. Edema control
         4. AROM of the noninvolved adjacent joints
     B. 4 to 6 weeks
         1. AAROM/AROM of the involved joint (as indicated by
            fracture healing and removal of the fixation)[5,6]
         2. Progress to PROM[5]
         3. Continue with the appropriate therapy interventions
            mentioned previously
         4. Desensitization[6]
     C. 6 to 8 weeks
         1. Unrestricted AROM
         2. Initiation of light resistive exercises

TABLE **44-1** Evaluation Timeline

Treatment and Injury Type	AROM	PROM (wk)	Strength/Endurance (wk)
1. NONOPERATIVE THERAPY			
Distal phalanx			
Tuft fracture	2-4 wk	5-6	7-8
Shaft fracture	3-4 wk	5-7	8
Middle phalanx (nondisplaced)			
Stable	3-5 days	4-5	6-8
Oblique	3 wk	5-6	7-8
Proximal phalanx (nondisplaced)			
Extraarticular	Immediate	4-7	6-8
Intraarticular	2-3 wk	4-5	8-12
2. OPERATIVE THERAPY			
Distal phalanx: shaft fracture PIP	7-10 days (postoperative)	4-6	8
Distal phalanx: (with K-wire fixation) DIP	3-6 wk (at time of K-wire removal)	8	8
Middle phalanx (displaced, ORIF, PIP fracture dislocations)	5-15 days (postoperative)	6-8	7-9
Proximal phalanx (displaced, ORIF)	5-15 days (postoperative)	6-8	8-10

AROM, Active range of motion; *DIP,* distal interphalangeal; *ORIF,* open reduction and internal fixation; *PROM,* passive range of motion.

Postoperative Complications

I. Infection[8]
II. Nonunion/malunion[6]
III. Nail bed deformity[5]
IV. Stiffness/loss of ROM
V. Persistent sensitivity[4,6]

Evaluation Timeline

The evaluation timeline is presented in Table 44-1.

Outcomes

Reports are of a clinical nature and indicate recovery of functional ROM in the vast majority of DIP fractures.[5] At the 6-week postinjury mark, two of every three patients from a total of 110 cases were experiencing sensitivity, numbness, cold sensitivity, restricted motion, and nail growth abnormalities.[1] These findings reinforce the treatment algorithm, which in this time frame indicates that patients are still in the repair stage, moving into remodeling stage (see Fig. 44-1).

MIDDLE PHALANX FRACTURES

Middle phalanx fractures occur at the lowest reported incidence, owing to the hard cortical nature of the bone structure, the short overall length, and the force-absorbing adjacent interphalangeal (IP) joints.[3] It is more likely that a soft tissue component will be compromised before a fracture occurs. PIP collateral ligament tear, avulsion of the central slip, and PIP dislocation are examples of injuries. The mechanism of injury with middle phalanx fractures is usually a direct blow or crush.[3] Given the intimate anatomical relationship of the soft tissue, middle phalanx fractures are likely to develop adhesions or to manifest altered biomechanics as a result of the flexor and extensor tendons.[7,9]

Fracture patterns can be transverse (distal or proximal), short oblique (distal or proximal), or intraarticular.

Those fractures that are closed, nondisplaced, and stable may be simply treated with buddy-taping. Displaced, unstable fractures that are successfully reduced by the surgeon may be casted or splinted during the initial stages of fracture healing.

Displaced and unstable fractures and the treatment required are influenced by the location of the break relative to the insertion of the extrinsic flexor and extensor tendons. Fractures proximal to the insertion of the flexor digitorum superficialis (FDS) angulate apex dorsally. Fractures distal to the FDS insertion tend to angulate apex volarly (Fig. 44-4). Those with greater than a 20 to 30 degree angulation require surgical intervention to attain adequate reduction.[3] This ensures that skeletal length is maintained relative to the relationship of the tendons, leading to optimal function and avoidance of deformity (swan-neck).[9] Distal transverse fractures are reported as being slow to heal (up to 10 to 14 weeks). This time consideration and the mechanism of injury usually result in selection of an operative fixation technique. There appears to be a consensus that there is a tradeoff for placement of rigid fixation and the potential for increased formation of scar adhesions.[7,10] Trumble[7] noted that rigid fixation is not always practical nor necessary. Closed reduction and K-wire stabilization may minimize postoperative

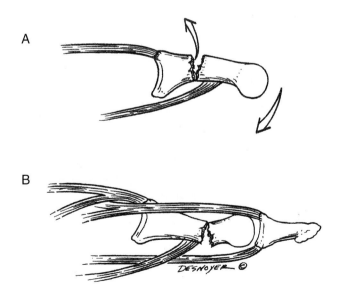

FIG. 44-4 Fracture patterns in transverse middle phalanx fracture. **A,** Fractures proximal to the flexor digitorum superficialis (FDS) insertion angulate dorsally. **B,** Fractures distal to the FDS insertion angulate volarly. (From Hastings H: Management of extraarticular fractures of the phalanges and metacarpals. In Strickland J, Rettig A [eds]: Hand Injuries in Athletes. WB Saunders, Philadelphia, 1992:131.)

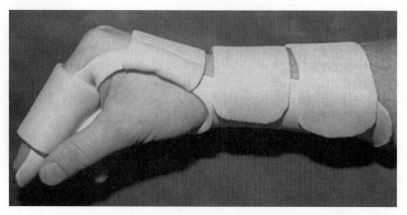

FIG. **44-5** Resting splint in the safe or protected position.

edema and stiffness. The period of immobilization also has been cited as having an impact on functional outcome, with 3 weeks being the cutoff point for immobilization.[1] Many authors cite the need for splinting in the safe or protected position during the course of treatment.[4,5,7,11] The wrist is positioned in slight extension, with MCP joints flexed to 70 to 90 degrees and the IP joints in extension (Fig. 44-5). The soft tissue structures are placed in position to avoid contractures and minimize effects at the fracture site.

Intraarticular middle phalanx fractures are discussed after the outline for short oblique and transverse middle phalanx fractures.

Treatment Purpose

Promote fracture healing in anatomical alignment, so as to achieve pain-free functional ROM and strength.

Treatment Goals

Restore pain-free functional ROM and strength to the involved digit and hand.

Nonoperative Indications/Precautions for Therapy

I.   Indications
     A. Nondisplaced fractures of the middle phalanx, stable and treated closed
     B. Displaced or unstable middle phalanx fractures treated with closed reduction and subsequently stable
II. Precaution: Maintain fracture reduction during initial healing phase.

Nonoperative Therapy

I.   Nondisplaced fractures
     A. Weeks 0 to 3
        1. Buddy-taping to adjacent noninvolved digit[3,8] (Fig. 44-6), or splint immobilization for 1 to 2 weeks and then buddy-taping.
        2. AROM begins, including differential gliding and blocked motion as pain and edema subside.[6,12]

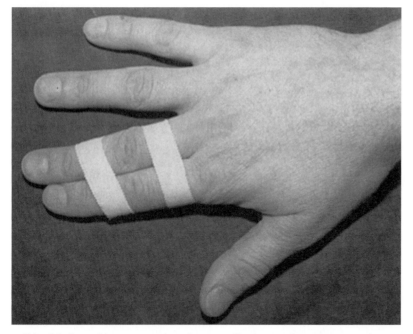

FIG. **44-6** Buddy-taping and application of Coban to the appropriate digit.

       3. Edema control with Coban may be initiated.

       4. Protective splinting may be indicated for contact sports or
         heavy work.[3]

    B. Weeks 4 to 6: PROM exercises and dynamic splinting may begin.[6]

    C. Weeks 6 to 8: Resistive exercises and strengthening begin.

II.   Displaced fractures, closed reduction

    A. Weeks 0 to 3: Continuous splinting in protected, safe splint
      position[3] (see Fig. 44-5)

    B. Weeks 3 to 8

       1. Wean from splint use; additional protective period with
         buddy-taping.[7]

       2. Begin AROM exercises, including tendon gliding and blocked
         motion.[12]

    C. Weeks 4 to 6: Begin PROM.

    D. Weeks 6 to 8: Begin resistive exercise and strengthening.[4]

Nonoperative Complications

  I.   Persistent pain

 II.   Persistent edema

III.   Loss of motion

IV.   Permanent stiffness

  V.   Loss of reduction

Postoperative Indications/Precautions for Therapy

I.   Indications: middle phalanx fractures treated with surgical
   intervention to achieve reduction

   A. K-wire stabilization

B. Interosseous screw/plate or tension band wiring for rigid fixation may be treatment options.

II.   Precautions

A. Less than optimal stabilization

B. K-wire requires pin care, as ordered by the surgeon, to minimize potential for infection.

C. Surgical incisional wound for plate/screw or tension band fixation

Postoperative Therapy

I.   Middle phalanx fracture treated with K-wire stabilization to attain reduction

A. Weeks 0 to 3 or 4

1. Supplemental casting or splinting to ensure adequate reduction[5,7]

2. K-wire pin tract care as ordered by the physician

B. Weeks 2 to 4: AROM begins according to physician recommendation.[5]

C. Weeks 3 to 6

1. K-wire removal may occur and require additional splint protection for 3 to 4 weeks.

D. Weeks 6 to 8: PROM exercises begin.

E. Weeks 8 to 10: Resistive exercise begins.

II.   Middle phalanx fracture treated with plate/screw or tension band rigid fixation

A. Weeks 0 to 4

1. Protective splint in place[13]

2. AROM initiated 3 to 7 days postoperatively[13]

3. Wound care (dressing changes), then scar management on suture removal

4. Edema control: retrograde massage and Coban wrapping

B. Weeks 4 to 6: PROM

C. Weeks 8 to 10: Strengthening begins at the recommendation of the surgeon.

Postoperative Complications

I.   Infection

II.   Loss of reduction

III. Persistent edema

IV.   Stiffness

V.   Scar adhesions limiting active motion

VI.   Decreased functional strength

Evaluation Timeline

The evaluation timeline is shown in Table 44-1.

Outcomes

Factors that affect outcome include patient age, fracture type, wound severity, amount of operative dissection, and factors related to management technique.[4,8]

Immobilization of less than 4 weeks is said to result in a return to 80% of normal AROM. Immobilization for longer than 4 weeks yielded return of 66% of a normal AROM.[1]

INTRAARTICULAR MIDDLE PHALANX FRACTURES

Intraarticular middle phalanx fractures present a clinical challenge to both surgeon and therapist. The optimal treatment allows for adequate reduction and early mobilization. The PIP joint has the largest arc of motion of the digital joints. This implies a complex soft tissue component for stability and tendon interaction for mobility. These injuries are prone to fibrosis and loss of motion with immobilization that lasts longer than 3 weeks.[1,13]

The mechanism of injury is a loading of the middle phalanx with the PIP joint hyperflexing, hyperextending, or an axial loading. These forces more frequently produce a dorsal dislocation and less frequently a volar dislocation (Fig. 44-7). Fracture configurations can include the dorsal lip of the middle phalanx, the palmar lip, or both. Eaton and Littler; Bowers, Hastings, and Carroll; and Schenck[14] have all described classification systems. In general, articular involvement of 30% or less typically is treated by closed reduction methods. If the articular involvement is 30% or greater, the fracture is usually unstable and requires surgical intervention to achieve adequate reduction.

Treatment options include extension block splinting, volar plate arthroplasty, K-wire stabilization, open reduction and internal fixation (ORIF) using screws and/or plates, external fixation, and traction techniques. Dias[15] reviewed two variations of the Agee technique, the Suzuki and the Push traction techniques (Fig. 44-8). There are also several variations and refinements of the Schenck protocol[14,16,17] (Fig. 44-9). The therapist must be familiar with the specific details of the method selected by the surgeon. The time frames and interventions are similar because they are based on the same fundamental foundations relative to the healing stages.

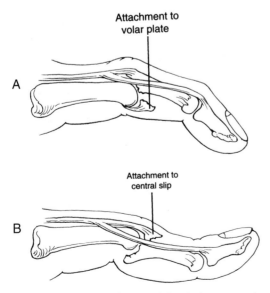

FIG. 44-7 Intraarticular fractures of the middle phalanx. **A,** Volar fragment with dorsal dislocation. **B,** Dorsal fragment with volar dislocation.

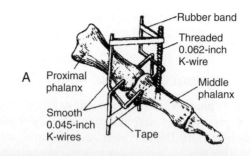

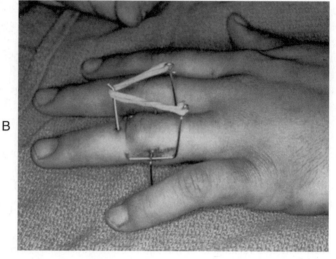

FIG. **44-8** **A,** Representation of the Agee force-couple. **B,** Use of the Agee force-couple in treatment of a fracture dislocation. (**A,** From Blazar P, Steinberg D: J Am Acad Orthop Surg 8:388, 2000.)

Definition

Volar dislocation: middle phalanx moves volar in relation to proximal phalanx (see Fig. 44-5)

  Dorsal dislocation: middle phalanx moves dorsally in relation to proximal phalanx (see Fig. 44-5)

Treatment Purpose

Promote fracture healing in optimally reduced alignment, in order to restore maximum active motion to the involved joint. This may or may not involve surgical intervention, based on the physician's assessment and treatment selection. Surgery may require a period of immobilization or mandate a mobilization protocol. There are several intervention procedures that require the therapist to be involved soon after surgery. The therapist must have a thorough understanding of the problem, procedure, and protocol, as well as close communication with the surgeon, for an optimal outcome. There are traction/distraction protocols with specific parameters[11,14-18] that may be changed by input from the surgeon on radiographical follow-up.

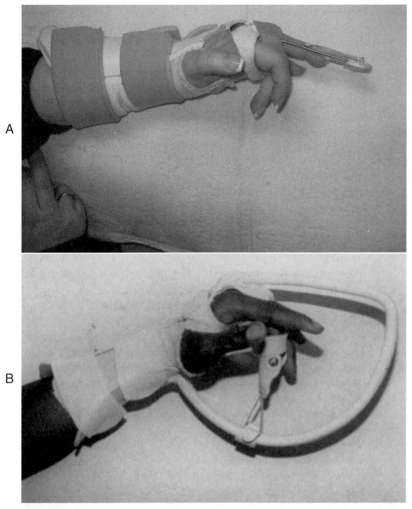

FIG. 44-9 A, Example of the modified Schenck dynamic traction splint. B, Dynamic traction splint modified by Dennys.

Treatment Goals

   I.   Maintain reduction for adequate fracture healing.
  II.   Early mobilization to minimize scarring and adhesions.
 III.   Prevent recurrence of dislocation.
 IV.   Maximize the return of AROM.

Nonoperative Indications/Precautions for Therapy

   I.   Indications: intraarticular fracture dislocation of the PIP joint treated with closed reduction, buddy-taping, and/or extension block splinting
  II.   Precautions: unstable reduction

Nonoperative Therapy

I. Stable closed reduction: volar-based fragment
    A. Weeks 1 to 3: Extension block splint to reduce a volar-based
       fragment (Fig. 44-10). This can be achieved with the use of
       a hand-based thermoplastic splint or an Alumafoam splint.
       The flexion angle may be decreased according to the surgeon's
       instructions after interpretation of the radiographical results.
       1. A combination of buddy-taping and extension block splinting
          may be required to yield optimal early AAROM.[13,15]
       2. AROM flexion to full and extension limit of the splint.
    B. Week 3
       1. Extension block splint may be removed and buddy-taping
          initiated.
       2. Continue with AROM flexion.
       3. May begin to wean from extension block splint, depending on
          the integrity of the central slip.[19]
       4. Initiate AROM exercises to the involved joint and to the DIP
          level of the involved digit.
    C. Week 4: May begin dynamic extension splint to PIP level if
       necessary.
    D. Week 6: PROM initiated
    E. Weeks 8 to 10: Resistive exercises begin during this time frame.
II. Stable closed reduction: dorsal-based fragment
    A. Weeks 1 to 3
       1. For a dorsal-based fragment up to 3 weeks of immobilization
          of the PIP joint may be necessary.
       2. AROM to noninvolved joints and to the DIP level of the
          involved finger.

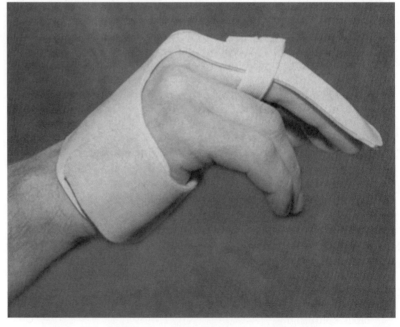

FIG. **44-10** Dorsal-based extension block splint.

B. Weeks 3 to 4: Initiate AROM to involved joint with surgeon's recommendation.
C. Weeks 4 to 6
1. Initiate PROM.
2. Wean from splint.
3. Dynamic splinting to assist return of flexion or extension.
D. Weeks 8 to 10: Initiate resistive exercise.

Nonoperative Complications

I. Loss of reduction or subluxation
II. Restricted PIP joint motion
III. Permanent stiffness

Postoperative Indications/Precautions for Therapy

I. Indications: PIP joint fracture-dislocations treated with closed reduction, percutaneous K-wire pinning, ORIF, volar plate arthroplasty, the Agee force-couple traction splint, or the Schenck dynamic traction/mobilization procedure
II. Precautions
A. Unstable reduction
B. Internal or external fixation components
C. Surgical wound or pin tract site
D. Epiphyseal plate fracture

Postoperative Therapy

I. Volar plate arthroplasty or percutaneous pinning
A. Weeks 0 to 2: immobilization with K-wire; protective splint in safe position may be indicated.[15]
B. Weeks 2 to 3: K-wire removed by the surgeon
1. Begin extension block splinting to −25 degrees of full extension.
2. Begin AROM with unrestricted flexion, total arc, and blocked isolated joint motion for the involved digit. Initiate full active extension for all digital joints to the limits of the extension block splint. Full active unrestricted extension of the digital joints blocked individually to tolerance.
C. Week 3: Volar plate arthroplasty, pull-out wire may be removed by surgeon if appropriate. Another fixation technique is a suture loop, which eliminates the need for a pull-out wire.[7] At this time, it may be appropriate to initiate active extension.
D. Week 4: Begin progressive extension splinting after surgeon approval and light functional tasks while buddy-taped.
II. Unstable acute fracture dislocations managed with the force-couple traction (see Fig. 44-8)
A. Days 0 to 2: postoperative dressing in place[18]
B. Days 3 to 5
1. Dressing removal and pin care initiated according to the surgeon's instructions. Apply hydrogen peroxide, isopropyl alcohol, and/or antibiotic ointment to pin tract.
2. AROM flexion is initiated.[18]

C. Weeks 3 to 6: On removal of the force-couple splint, follow the "unstable closed reduction or volar plate arthroplasty" as reviewed above.

III. Unstable fracture dislocations managed with dynamic traction splinting and early PROM (see Fig. 44-9).[14,16,17] On completion of the traction splint, radiographical review by the surgeon should confirm adequacy of traction for reduction.

A. Weeks 0 to 6
1. Wear dynamic traction splint continuously; rubber band traction should be checked and replaced as needed. Radiographical review by surgeon to ensure alignment should occur weekly.
2. AAROM/PROM exercises consist of moving the digit through a full, stable arc of motion, with 5 to 10 repetitions every 1 to 2 hours.[17]
3. AROM exercises consist of blocked DIP motion.
4. Coban wrapping for edema control
5. Pin tract care according to the surgeon's instructions[17]

B. Week 3: Remove splint, begin wrist AROM, replace splint and continue with exercises outlined in weeks 0 to 3.

C. Week 6
1. Pin is usually removed by the surgeon by this time frame.
2. Protective hand-based splint for an additional 1 to 2 weeks[17]
3. AROM blocked and total active arc flexion and extension to the PIP joint.

D. Weeks 8 to 12
1. Progress to PROM and dynamic splinting to achieve end-range motion in all planes.
2. Progress to resistive exercises by weeks 10 to 12[17]

Postoperative Complications

I. Recurrent subluxations
II. Pin tract infections
III. Loss of motion secondary to tendon adhesions (flexors and extensors)
IV. Permanent joint stiffness
V. Traumatic arthritis

Evaluation Timeline

The evaluation timeline is presented in Table 44-1.

Outcomes

Dias[15] presented an excellent overview of outcomes of the techniques used for PIP fracture dislocations. All techniques appeared to render a functional ROM with a total arc of 60 to 90 degrees. Most authors reported that extension lag was an issue.[9,10,16,17] Dennys and colleagues[17] reported a total arc for AROM of 81 degrees in their dynamic traction series. Active extension was −8 degrees, and flexion was 89 degrees. Schenck[16] observed active extension at a mean average of −5 degrees and flexion to 92 degrees.

PROXIMAL PHALANX FRACTURES

Proximal phalanx fractures prove to be clinically challenging in the same mechanical and anatomical manner as do middle phalanx fractures. The proximal phalanx is less protected than the other phalanges, and it is exposed to a variety of forces, which produce varying fracture patterns. The extensor and flexor mechanisms essentially encase the proximal phalanx. Trumble[7] noted an arc of 270 degrees of the extensor hood covering the proximal phalanx. The potential for developing adhesions limiting motion is great as a result of the close interface and interaction of the soft tissue.[7,9,12,13] Proximal phalanx shaft fractures typically manifest with an apex volar angulation as a result of the volar force of the intrinsics and the dorsal force of the extensor mechanism and central slip.[4,7] For closed fractures of the proximal phalanx, there are two basic classifications: nondisplaced and displaced. K-wire fixation or ORIF is frequently required to achieve adequate reduction. Methods and techniques are as varied as the fracture patterns seen, and close communication with the surgeon is required.[4,8,12,17]

Treatment Purpose

Provide fracture stabilization, minimal soft tissue disruption, and early active mobilization.[4,7]

Treatment Goals

  I.   Maintain reduction for adequate fracture healing.
 II.   Early mobilization to minimize scarring and adhesions[4,7]
III.   Maximize the return of AROM.

Nonoperative Indications/Precautions for Therapy

  I.   Indications
      A. Nondisplaced proximal phalanx fractures
      B. Displaced proximal phalanx fractures managed with closed reduction
 II.   Precaution: unstable closed reduction of displaced fracture

Nonoperative Therapy

  I.   Weeks 0 to 3.5
      A. Minimally displaced and stable fractures may be treated with buddy-taping and immediate AROM.[4,12]
      B. Splinting in the safe position may be required for others needing additional protection.[4,12]
 II.   Weeks 3.5 to 4
      A. Splint is removed and AROM initiated; buddy-taping may be required.[4,12]
      B. AROM is initiated, including differential tendon gliding and blocked motion.[8,12]
III.   Weeks 4 to 6
      A. Splints are discontinued.[4]

B. PROM and dynamic splinting may be indicated.

C. Light resistive exercises[4]

IV. Weeks 6 to 8: Heavy resistance and strengthening exercises are initiated.[4]

Nonoperative Complications

I. Loss of reduction

II. Restricted PIP joint motion[4]

III. Permanent stiffness[4]

Postoperative Indications/Precautions for Therapy

I. Indications: closed, displaced, unstable proximal phalanx fractures

A. Treated with Kirschner wire stabilization

B. Treated with ORIF (screw or plate) rigid stabilizing fixation

II. Precautions

A. Unstable reduction[7]

B. Internal or external fixation components

C. Surgical wound or pin tract site[4]

Postoperative Therapy

I. Days 2 to 3 postoperatively

A. Postoperative dressing removed and wound/pin care initiated[4,8]

B. Gentle AROM is initiated for the stable fracture, with differential tendon gliding and blocked motion to avoid adhesions.[7,12]

C. Edema control using Coban is begun.[12]

D. Safe position splint is indicated.[7,12]

II. Days 3 to 10

A. Gentle AROM may be ordered by the physician for those fractures that are less than optimal with fixation.[7,8]

B. Scar management begins on suture removal.

C. PROM may be ordered by the physician.[8]

III. Week 3

A. AROM may be more vigorous for fractures with less than optimal fixation.[7]

B. PROM begins for these fractures, with physician approval.

C. Dynamic splinting may be used in all cases with the surgeon's approval.

IV. Weeks 4 to 6

A. Protective splint may be discontinued for day use; use is continued at night to maintain extension, and buddy-taping is initiated.[7]

B. Light resistive exercises are begun.[7,8]

C. Dynamic splinting is used to regain end-range motion.[7]

V. Weeks 6 to 8: Heavy resistance and strengthening exercises are initiated.

Postoperative Complications

I. Loss of reduction

II. Pin tract infections[8]

III.   Nonunion or malunion[7,8]
IV.   Permanent joint stiffness[7,8,12]
V.   Loss of motion secondary to tendon adhesions (flexors and extensors).[12]

Evaluation Timeline

Appropriate baseline measures should be taken at initiation of specific exercises and repeated at 4- to 6-week intervals for documentation of progress (see Table 44-1).

Outcomes

A universal tenet would appear to be that of early motion with differential tendon gliding and blocked motion to minimize adhesion formation.[4,7,8,12,15,19] Feehan and Bassett[20] concluded that further investigation is indicated for early mobilization in extraarticular hand fractures. Their findings suggested that early mobilization results in earlier recovery of mobility and strength, facilitates an earlier return to work, and does not affect fracture alignment. Blazar and Steinberg[13] reported a study with a mean average 3-year follow-up on condylar fractures treated by ORIF with a mean active range of 71 degrees. A second review of condylar ORIF found a mean range of −8 to +95 degrees for five cases after 1 year.[13]

REFERENCES

1. Stern P: Fractures of the metacarpals and phalanges. In Green D (ed): Operative Hand Surgery. 3rd Ed. Churchill Livingstone, New York, 1993
2. Meyer FN, Wilson RL: Management of nonarticular fractures of the hand. In Hunter JM, Mackin EJ, Callahan AD (eds): Rehabilitation of the Hand: Surgery and Therapy. 4th Ed. Mosby, St. Louis, 1995
3. Hastings H: Management of extra-articular fractures of the phalanges and metacarpals. In Strickland J, Rettig A (eds): Hand Injuries in Athletes. WB Saunders, Philadelphia, 1992
4. Purdy PA, Wilson RL: Management of nonarticular fractures of the hand. In Mackin EJ, Callahan AD, Skirven TM, et al. (eds): Hunter-Mackin-Callahan Rehabilitation of the Hand and Upper Extremity. 5th Ed. Vol. 1. Mosby, St. Louis, 2002
5. Cannon N: Rehabilitation approaches for distal and middle phalanx fractures of the hand. J Hand Ther 16:105-128, 2003
6. Mannarino SL: Skeletal injuries. In Stanley, BG (ed): Concepts in Hand Rehabilitation. FA Davis, Philadelphia, 1992
7. Trumble TE: Hand fractures. In: Trumble TE (ed): Principles of Hand Surgery and Therapy. WB Saunders, Philadelphia, 2004
8. Freeland AE, Torres JE: Extraarticular fractures of the phalanges. In Berger RA, Weiss A-PC (eds): Hand Surgery. Lippincott Williams & Wilkins, Philadelphia, 2004
9. Agee J: Common hand problems: treatment principles for proximal and middle phalangeal fractures. Orthop Clin North Am 23:35-40, 1992
10. Klien D, Belsoe R: Percutaneous treatment of carpal, metacarpal and phalangeal injuries. Clin Orthop 375:116-309, 2000
11. Kearney LM, Brown KK: The therapist's management of intra-articular fractures. Hand Clin 10:199-209, 1994
12. Freeland AE, Hardy MA, Singletary S: Rehabilitation for proximal phalanx fractures. J Hand Ther 16:129-142, 2003
13. Blazar P, Steinberg D: Fractures of the proximal interphalangeal joint. J Am Acad Orthop Surg 8:383-390, 2000
14. Chinchalkar SJ, Gan BS: Management of proximal interphalangeal joint fractures and dislocations. J Hand Ther 16:117-129, 2003

15. Dias JJ: Intraarticular injuries of the distal and proximal interphalangeal joints. In Berger RA, Weiss A-PC (eds): Hand Surgery. Lippincott Williams & Wilkins, Philadelphia, 2004
16. Schenck RR: The dynamic traction method: combining movement and traction for intra-articular fractures of the phalanges. Hand Clin 10:187-198, 1994
17. Dennys LJ, Hurst LN, Cox J: Management of proximal interphalangeal joint fractures using a new dynamic traction splint and early active movement. J Hand Ther 5:16-24, 1992
18. Agee JM: Unstable fracture dislocations of the proximal interphalangeal joint treatment with a force couple splint. Clin Orthop 214:101-112, 1987
19. Campbell PJ, Wilson RL: Management on joint injuries and intra-articular fractures. In Mackin EJ, Callahan AD, Skirven TM, et al. (eds): Hunter-Mackin-Callahan Rehabilitation of the Hand and Upper Extremity. 5th Ed. Vol. 1. Mosby, St. Louis, 2002
20. Feehan LM, Bassett K: Is there evidence for early mobilization following an extraarticular hand fracture. J Hand Ther 17:300-308, 2004

SUGGESTED READINGS

Breenwald J: Fracture healing in the hand. Clin Orthop 327:9-11, 1996
Bryan BK, Kohnke EN: Therapy after skeletal fixation in the hand and wrist. Hand Clin 13:761-776, 1997
Flowers KR: A hierarchy of splinting for joint stiffness. J Hand Ther 15:58-62, 2002
Groner J, Weeks P: Healing of hand and soft tissues in the hand. In Strickland J, Rettig A (eds): Hand Injuries in Athletes. WB Saunders, Philadelphia, 1992
Lastayo P, Winters K, Hardy M: Bone healing, fracture management, and current concepts related to the hand. J Hand Ther 16:81-93, 2003

Replantation 45

J. Martin Walsh

Experiments on limb replantation were reported in the late 1800s, but it was not until the operating microscope allowed repair of small vessels in the 1960s that microvascular surgery began. More and more reports of successful replantations occurred after improvements in instrumentation, surgical techniques, suture materials, patient selection, and preoperative and postoperative management were introduced. With the success of replantation, greater focus is now placed on functional recovery of the replanted digits.

Replantation is defined as "the reattachment of a body part that has been totally severed from the body without any attachments. This term differs from revascularization, which is defined as the reattachment of an incompletely amputated part, in which vessel reconstruction is necessary to assure viability."[1]

After amputation occurs, recovery of function depends on the preservation of cellular structure, as well as on the restoration of blood flow. Cellular damage may develop as an immediate result of ischemia. Extreme or irreversible ischemic tissue damage before replantation is often seen and can be prevented by proper cooling.[1-3] The amputated part should be wrapped in a slightly moistened, sterile gauze with saline solution (it should not be soaked). It should then be enclosed in a container or sealed in a plastic bag and placed on ice. The amputated part should not be submerged in the ice, because this can cause cold injury to the part. A compressive dressing is placed on the stump.[4,5]

For digital and hand replantation, the surgical sequence to follow varies but is generally as follows. Surgical debridement is performed first, followed by bone shortening and bone fixation. Bone nonunion rates for digital replantations range from 10% to 30%, and interosseous wiring has been shown to have the lowest nonunion and complication rates. In general, bone problems are present in almost 50% of all replantations.[6] After bony fixation, the tendons are repaired. If possible, both the flexor digitorum superficialis (FDS) and the flexor digitorum profundus (FDP) are repaired. The extensor tendons are also repaired, either at this point or later on, when the dorsum of the hand is surgically addressed. Both digital arteries are repaired, if possible; if there is substantial vessel damage, interpositional vein grafts can be used. Nerves are then repaired, and again both nerves are repaired, if possible, for overall improved functional use of the hand postoperatively. Because the bone has been shortened, end-to-end nerve repairs are usually possible; however, if the length is not sufficient for an end-to-end repair, nerve grafting may be necessary. Once the arteries have been repaired, the veins may be addressed. The general rule is to anastomose two veins for every artery repaired. Finally, the skin is closed without tension. With major limb replantations, circulation is established as soon as possible, and the arteries are repaired earlier than in the above sequence[5,7,8]

Postoperatively, the patient is placed in a bulky dressing and plaster splint, and the replanted extremity is elevated and kept warm to promote perfusion.[7] The postoperative dressing is not changed for the first 3 to 7 days unless it has become restrictive due to dried blood. Color, pulp, turgor, surface Doppler, capillary refill, and warmth are monitored routinely. If the skin temperature of the replanted part falls below 30°C, vascular insufficiency is certain and the cause must be corrected.[8] Other monitoring techniques include transcutaneous oxygen measurements; laser, surface, and internal Doppler fluorometry; and fluorescein perfusion.[7,8] In most instances, patients are given anticoagulant therapy for up to 7 days and are restricted to bedrest. Smoking is prohibited postoperatively, because it causes severe vasoconstriction and increases the failure rate after replantation. The limb must be kept free from drafts, because cold can cause vasospasm as well.[8] Dressing changes therefore must be performed in a warm, draft-free environment. Hand therapy is initiated after the patient has been discontinued from the anticoagulant medication.

DEFINITION

Replantation is the reattachment of a body part that has been totally severed from the body without any attachments[1,9] (Fig. 45-1).

Revascularization is the repair of a body part that has been incompletely amputated from the body and requires vascular repair.[8]

SURGICAL PURPOSE

Under many circumstances, totally amputated parts of the upper limb can be reattached using current surgical techniques. Amputation causes damage to every anatomical structure. Restoration of the critical components, such as bone, tendons, arteries, nerves, veins, and skin, is essential for the survival of the amputated segment or segments. Not all of these segments will be suitable for replantation, nor will they all survive replantation. The purpose is to restore those parts necessary for good arm and hand function.

TREATMENT GOALS

I. Protect all repaired structures: vessels, nerves, tendons, fractures.
II. Promote/monitor wound healing and care.
III. Decrease adhesions and encourage tendon gliding.
IV. Promote intrinsic healing and increase tensile strength of healing tissues.

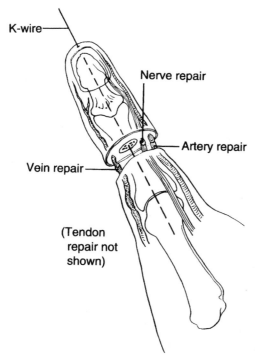

FIG. **45-1** Replantation is the reattachment of a totally severed body part.

V. Prevent joint contractures.
VI. Maintain range of motion (ROM) of all proximal uninvolved joints of the upper extremity.
VII. Reduce edema, taking into consideration vein repairs over repaired parts.
VIII. Splint hand and fingers in as functional a position as possible.
IX. Minimize complaints of pain.
X. Educate patient and family in the care of the replanted part and treatment.
XI. Promote independence in activities of daily living (ADL) for the patient, with assists as needed.
XII. Evaluate the need for psychological intervention and provide support as needed.

OPERATIVE INDICATIONS/PRECAUTIONS

I. Indications: In general, the following are strong indications for replantation.[2,5,8,10,11]
   A. Thumb amputation
   B. Partial hand amputation through the palm
   C. All digits in children are replanted, if possible.
   D. Individual digits are replanted if all fingers are required for professional or social purposes (e.g., musicians).
   E. Incomplete amputations of digits that are devascularized, especially if the flexor tendon and/or digital nerves are intact
   F. Finger replantations distal to the FDS insertion
   G. Replantations at the distal forearm and wrist levels
   H. Sharp injuries

II.   Precautions: The following are considered contraindications for replantation.[2,5,8,10,11]

    A. Avulsion injuries generally are not advised except for the thumb.

    B. Multiple-level and severe crush injuries

    C. Amputations in patients who have poor general health, systemic illness, or a surgical history precluding replantation

    D. Amputations with a warm ischemia time greater than 6 hours. (Digit replantation may be tried in this circumstance.)

    E. Amputations proximal to the midforearm

    F. Self-mutilation, psychotic patients

IMMEDIATE POSTOPERATIVE COMPLICATIONS

I.   Vasospasm: A finger turns pale due to decreased blood supply. This can result from manipulation of the finger, especially during dressing changes.[4]

II.   Venous insufficiency: A finger turns blue and feels tense to the touch. This is the most common source of replantation failure. Time is critical, because prolonged venous obstruction can lead to arterial obstruction and eventually to loss of the replanted part.[4]

III.   Arterial insufficiency: A finger turns white or pale in color. If arterial insufficiency is suspected and does not resolve, then surgery must be performed immediately and the anastomosis must be redone.[2]

IV.   Infection: Daily wound checks are performed.

POSTOPERATIVE INDICATIONS/PRECAUTIONS FOR THERAPY

I.   Indications: The replanted digit or part has been cleared by the surgeon for viability after the initial postoperative dressing is removed and replaced with a lighter dressing by the surgeon and the patient's anticoagulant medications have been discontinued.[4,10,12]

II.   Precautions

    A. Avoid exposing the replanted part to cold, because it is a vasoconstrictor. Hand therapy treatment and dressing changes must be performed in a warm, draft-free environment. Cold modalities are not to be used on a replanted part during the acute phase of rehabilitation.[10]

    B. Pressure on the replanted part by straps, tight dressings, and compressive wraps should be avoided.

    C. The hand or replanted part should be elevated above the heart at all times. Dependent positions are to be avoided, because they can overburden the circulatory system, causing venous congestion.[10]

    D. Whirlpool treatments should be avoided, because they place the extremity in a dependent position.[13]

    E. Heat modalities should be avoided until 8 weeks postoperatively because of the lack of sensation and the fact that the lymphatic system is unable to dissipate heat effectively, making the replanted part highly susceptible to burns.[14]

F. Smoking is not allowed, nor is any exposure to secondary smoke, because nicotine is a vasoconstrictor.[15]

G. Any changes in the circulation or condition of the wounds is a precaution.

POSTOPERATIVE THERAPY

Digital Replantation

I.   Days 0 to 5

A. The patient receives anticoagulant treatment for the first 5 to 7 days and must remain in bed. Therapy is not appropriate at this time because of the risk of compromising the newly repaired vessels.[4,10]

B. Elevate the hand on pillows above the level of the heart; care must be taken so that the involved digits are not in a dependent position.[10]

C. Keep the replanted part warm.[4,10]

D. If the postoperative dressing and cast are taken down because of excessive drainage, occlusive dressing, or poor positioning, a volar resting splint is fabricated. A volar splint is used at this time to promote rest and for ease in monitoring of the replanted digit. The splint should maintain the wrist in neutral extension, with the digits supported in the postoperative position, encouraging metacarpophalangeal (MCP) flexion and interphalangeal (IP) extension. Care must be taken to move the digits as little as possible at this time.[16] Velcro straps usually are not used during this time frame; instead, the splint is secured using a bias or gauze wrap.

E. Patient/family education is initiated regarding precautions as well as discharge planning.

II. Days 5 to 10 (depending on the discontinuation of anticoagulant medication and the vascular stability of the digit)[4]

A. Splinting: A dorsal protective splint is fabricated (Fig. 45-2). If a volar splint was fabricated during the first 5 days postoperatively, it should be replaced with a dorsal protective splint.[4,17] Dorsal splints are preferred because volar splints may migrate distally, thus positioning the hand into an intrinsic minus position. Straps should not interfere with blood supply and should not be placed over sites of anastomosis. The straps should be wide and well padded. Internal Doppler devices are helpful for monitoring blood supply after application of the splints. The splint should position the wrist in a neutral position, with the MCP joints in 45 to 50 degrees flexion and the IP joints in extension. The splint may need serial adjustments to obtain an optimal position.[4,14]

B. Wound care: Perform daily wound care and dressing changes after the first postoperative dressing change is performed by the physician. The dressing changes should be performed gently, with the extremity elevated, and in a warm, draft-free room to avoid vasospasm of the involved vessels.[10] Dressings should be nonadherent and nonrestrictive. Whirlpool therapy is

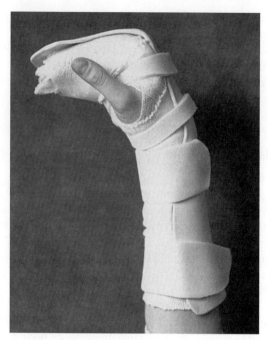

FIG. **45-2** Postoperative splint that may be fabricated on doctor referral.

not recommended, because it places the digit in a dependent position.[13]

C. Early protective motion I (EPM I) is begun[10,14]: Active wrist flexion to tension, allowing the tenodesis effect to extend the MCP and IP joints (Fig. 45-3). This is followed by active wrist extension to neutral with simultaneous gentle passive MCP joint flexion (Fig. 45-4). (The ratio of wrist to MCP motion must be proportional; if MCP ROM is severely restricted, the corresponding wrist ROM should be adjusted accordingly.)[10,14,18]

D. Active range of motion (AROM) and passive range of motion (PROM) of the uninvolved digits, unless there is a direct effect on the replanted digits and repaired tendons

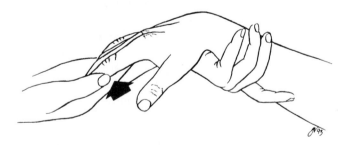

EPM I A.

FIG.**45-3** Early protective motion I (EPM I): Active wrist flexion to tension, allowing the tenodesis effect to extend the metacarpophalangeal and interphalangeal joints. (From Hunter JM, Mackin EJ, Callahan AD [eds]: Rehabilitation of the Hand: Surgery and Therapy. 4th Ed. Mosby, St. Louis, 1995.)

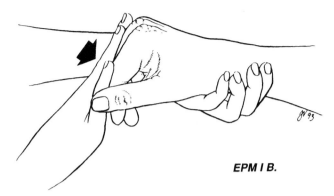

EPM I B.

FIG. 45-4 Early protective motion I (EPM I): This is followed by active wrist extension to neutral with simultaneous gentle passive metacarpophalangeal joint flexion. (From Hunter JM, Mackin EJ, Callahan AD [eds]: Rehabilitation of the Hand: Surgery and Therapy. 4th Ed. Mosby, St. Louis, 1995.)

    E. Edema control, consisting of elevation only, with the elbow and hand positioned at the level of the heart. Compressive dressings and other edema-reducing techniques are contraindicated at this time.

III. Days 10 to 14
    A. Continue with EPM I.
    B. Passive early protective motion II (EPM II)[10,14] is initiated if the IP joints are free of fixation. EPM II consists of the intrinsic-minus position (hook position), with neutral wrist, MCP joints extended to neutral, PIP joints flexed up to 60 degrees, and minimal DIP flexion (Fig. 45-5). This is followed by the intrinsic-plus position (tabletop position), with neutral wrist, MCP joints flexed, and IP joints extended (Fig. 45-6).[10,14]
    C. Progress to gentle place-and-hold exercises in these positions.[19]

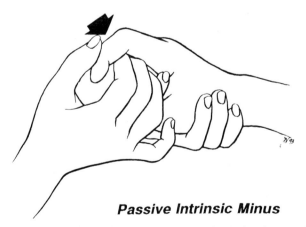

Passive Intrinsic Minus

FIG. 45-5 Passive early protective motion II (EPM II): Intrinsic-minus position (hook position): neutral wrist, metacarpophalangeal (MCP) joints extended to neutral and proximal interphalangeal (PIP) joints flexed up to 60 degrees with minimal distal interphalangeal (DIP) joint flexion. (From Hunter JM, Mackin EJ, Callahan AD [eds]: Rehabilitation of the Hand: Surgery and Therapy. 4th Ed. Mosby, St. Louis, 1995.)

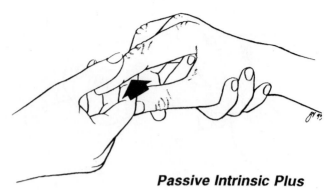

Passive Intrinsic Plus

FIG. **45-6** Passive early protective motion II (EMP II): This is followed by the intrinsic-plus position (tabletop position) with neutral wrist, metacarpophalangeal (MCP) joints flexed, and interphalangeal (IP) joints extended. (From Hunter JM, Mackin EJ, Callahan AD [eds]: Rehabilitation of the Hand: Surgery and Therapy. 4th Ed. Mosby, St. Louis, 1995.)

IV.   Days 14 to 21
    A. Begin active EPM II as described previously[4,14]
       (Figs. 45-7 and 45-8).
 V.   Weeks 3 to 4
    A. Continue with EPM I and EPM II through 5 weeks.[4,14]
    B. Begin scar massage after the wound has healed.
    C. Begin light Coban wrapping and/or retrograde massage
       if edema is extreme and if cleared by the physician.
VI.   Weeks 4 to 5
    A. Gradual active and passive wrist extension past neutral is
       initiated as tolerated.[14]
    B. Simultaneous MCP and IP flexion and extension (composite
       digit motion) is initiated with the wrist in neutral position.[10]
    C. Neuromuscular electrical stimulation (NMES) may be used
       if needed.
    D. May begin light Coban wrapping and retrograde massage.[20]

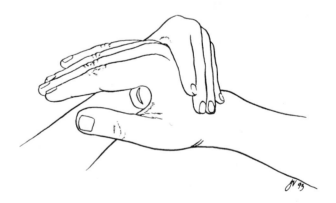

Active Intrinsic Plus

FIG. **45-7** Active early protective motion II (EPM II): With the wrist in neutral, the patient is asked to gently assume the intrinsic-plus position. (From Hunter JM, Mackin EJ, Callahan AD [eds]: Rehabilitation of the Hand: Surgery and Therapy. 4th Ed. Mosby, St. Louis, 1995.)

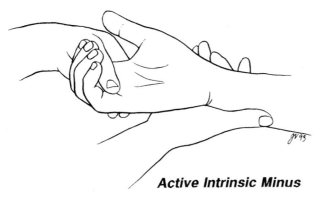

Active Intrinsic Minus

FIG. **45-8** Active early protective motion II (EPM II): With the wrist in neutral and the metacarpophalangeal (MCP) joints supported in extension, the patient is asked to gently assume the intrinsic-minus position. (From Hunter JM, Mackin EJ, Callahan AD [eds]: Rehabilitation of the Hand: Surgery and Therapy. 4th Ed. Mosby, St. Louis, 1995.)

VII. Weeks 5 to 6
   A. Begin composite wrist and finger flexion and extension, passive and active.[14]
   B. Begin gentle blocking exercises to isolate joint motion.[14]
   C. Begin differential tendon gliding exercises.[14]
   D. Dynamic splinting as indicated. Patients may be insensate, and extreme care must be taken with dynamic splinting. Splint should be monitored closely for decreased circulation and pressure areas.[14]
   E. Static volar extension pan splinting at night, as indicated for flexor tightness.[14]
   F. Light functional activities are incorporated (sponges, pegs).[14,16]

VIII. Weeks 6 to 8
   A. Discontinue use of protective splints, although gutter splints may be needed to protect unhealed fractures.[10]
   B. Continue with light functional activities.

IX. Week 8 and later
   A. Begin light resistive activities and progressive strengthening exercises as tolerated.
   B. Begin sensory reeducation after patient perceives protective sensation.
   C. Formal sensory evaluation, if not performed already, should be done to provide a baseline for monitoring of future nerve growth and regeneration.
   D. Progress toward work simulation by 12 weeks.

Thumb Replantation[10,17]

   I. Days 5 to 10 (depending on discontinuation of anticoagulant medication and vascular stability of the digit)
   A. A dorsal protective thumb splint is fabricated with neutral wrist and digits free. The thumb is positioned in abduction with no tension placed on the repaired structures. If both flexor and extensor tendons were repaired, the thumb should be positioned with less tension placed on the flexor tendons.[14]

B. Gentle passive carpometacarpal (CMC) ROM is begun, as well as gentle passive wrist flexion to tension and extension to neutral.[2,14]

C. Active CMC ROM should be added if PROM is well tolerated.[10]

D. Begin AROM and PROM of the uninvolved digits.[10]

E. Wound care, as described for digital replantation.

II. Days 10 to 14: Begin gentle isolated passive MCP and IP ROM if free from fixation. The wrist should remain in a neutral position. Avoid full composite flexion or extension until 5 weeks postoperatively.[4]

III. Days 14 to 21: Begin isolated active MCP and IP ROM in protective position.[4]

IV. Weeks 3 to 4: Begin scar massage.[4]

V. Weeks 4 to 5

A. Begin gradual active and passive wrist extension past neutral.[4]

B. Begin Coban wrapping for edema.[4]

C. May begin NMES if needed.[4]

VI. Weeks 5 to 6

A. Active and passive composite thumb and wrist motions are allowed.[4]

B. Blocking exercises are performed, and a blocking splint may be fabricated to improve isolated joint motion.[4]

C. Begin dynamic splinting if fractures are stable.[4]

D. Initiate light functional activities.[4]

VII. Weeks 6 to 8

A. Discontinue the use of the dorsal protective splint.[4]

B. A thumb web space splint may be necessary at this point. The web space splint may be fabricated once the vascular status has been stabilized, wounds are healed, and fractures are stable and can tolerate stress.[4,10]

C. Progress as described for digital replantation.[4]

Hand Replantation[10,17]

I. Days 2 to 7

A. A protective positioning splint is often constructed earlier postoperatively due to the need for improved wrist and hand positioning. The vascular status tends to stabilize earlier with hand replantations, and positioning becomes more of a priority.[4,10] The wrist is positioned in neutral, and the digits are placed in an intrinsic-plus position (MCP joints in 50 to 60 degrees flexion and IP joints in extension). Depending on the structures repaired and the amount of tension on the repaired structures, more or less MCP flexion may be required.[4,10]

B. Wound care as for digital replantation.

C. Passive EPM II (as described for digital replantation) is initiated to the thumb and finger MCP and IP joints after anticoagulation therapy has been discontinued.

II. Days 7 to 14

A. Begin retrograde massage to the digits and hand if edema is a problem.

B. Elbow and shoulder ROM are evaluated and included in therapy as indicated. Wrist and forearm motions are contraindicated.[4]

III. Days 14 to 21: Begin active and active-assisted EMP II. Because the intrinsic muscles are denervated, MCP flexion is assisted while the patient tries to extend the IP joints.[4]

IV. Weeks 3 to 4: Begin scar management and edema control techniques, as for digital replantation.[4]

V. Weeks 4 to 5
   A. Begin gentle AROM and PROM to the wrist if there is no bony fixation or if it has been removed from the wrist.[4]
   B. May initiate NMES.[4]
   C. Initiate dynamic finger splinting as needed.[4]

VI. Weeks 5 to 6
   A. Begin composite active and passive wrist and finger motions.[4]
   B. Blocking exercises may be initiated, and a blocking splint may be fabricated as needed.[4]
   C. Begin static volar extension splinting at night if indicated.[4]
   D. Light functional activities are incorporated.[4]

VII. Weeks 6 to 8: Discontinue use of protective splints, although the patient may require the use of splints to position the MCP joints in flexion and the thumb in opposition due to the loss of intrinsic function ("nerve-palsy" type splints).[4,12]

VIII. Week 8 and later
   A. Begin dynamic wrist splinting with physician approval.
   B. Progress as described for digital replantation.

Arm Replantation[10,17]

I. Days 2 to 7
   A. A protective splint is fabricated early due to a need for improved positioning. The elbow is usually splinted in the postoperative position. A second, detachable hand splint is made with the wrist in 0 to 30 degrees extension, MCP joints in 45 to 65 degrees flexion, the IP joints in extension, and the thumb in abduction.[4]
   B. Wound care and dressing changes are performed by the therapist, as described for digital replantation, after anticoagulation therapy has been discontinued.[4]

II. Days 7 to 14: PROM to the wrist, fingers, and thumb is begun after vascular status is stabilized and anticoagulant therapy is discontinued.[4]

III. Days 14 to 21: Begin AROM and PROM to the shoulder. Stress to wounds or repair sites should be avoided. Shoulder motion should be cleared by the physician secondary to differences in type, level, and severity of the repaired structures.[4]

IV. Week 3
   A. Continue with PROM and begin AROM to the wrist, fingers, and thumb as indicated. Depending on the level of replantation and whether the replantation was total or subtotal, AROM may be possible.
   B. Begin elbow PROM and AROM if the joint is free from fixation. All motion should be cleared by the physician. Gains in motion

should be gradual, to prevent stress on repairs that cross the elbow joint.[4]

C. Initiate edema reduction techniques such as Coban wrapping and retrograde massage.[4]

D. A sling or other arm support should be provided to keep the arm from being in a dependent position during ambulation.[4]

V.   Weeks 4 to 6

A. Begin dynamic splinting and splinting to prevent deformity. Because of the loss of intrinsic function, "nerve-palsy" type splints may be used, as described for hand replantation.[4]

B. Once the vascular status of the forearm is stabilized, Coban wrapping of the forearm may be initiated when approved by the surgeon.

VI.   Weeks 6 to 8

A. Discontinue the use of protective splints; continue to use the "nerve-palsy" splints until intrinsic function has returned.[4,12]

B. Maintain PROM of affected joints until muscle function returns.

C. Maintain and increase strength of existing musculature as nerve regeneration occurs.

D. Sensation is evaluated and sensory education and muscle reeducation are performed as the nerve regenerates.

POSTOPERATIVE COMPLICATIONS

If any of the following changes occurs, contact the patient's physician immediately.

I.   Change in temperature of replanted part
II.   Change in color of replanted part
III.   Replanted part begins to bleed profusely
IV.   Increase in necrotic tissue noted over repaired sites
V.   Any pus discharge or any other signs of infection
VI.   Any sudden increase in edema of the hand and/or replanted part
VII.   Any sudden increase in pain of the hand and/or replanted part

EVALUATION TIMELINE

I.   0 to 5 days: Surgeon and nurses monitor for any changes in temperature and/or color of replanted part through observation and Doppler checks. A volar resting splint may be fabricated at this time if ordered by the surgeon. During this time, the therapist can begin to gather information regarding the patient's surgery/injury and begin the treatment planning process.

II.   5 to 21 days: A dorsal protective thermoplastic splint is made. If a volar splint was fabricated earlier, it is remolded to a dorsal splint. Patient and therapist monitor and check temperature, color, and viability of the replanted part. No ROM measurements are taken at this time. Note and document the position of the fingers in the splint. The wound is evaluated and recorded, as is pain.

III.   3 to 4 weeks: Active protected ROM measurements can be recorded. Evaluate and record wound viability, scar adhesions, and edema.

IV.   4 to 6 weeks: Record AROM and PROM measurements in a protected position. Evaluate the splint and adjust to increase the functional position. Continue with wound evaluation and scar mobilization, and begin more vigorous edema-reducing techniques such as compressive wraps, if approved by physician.

V. 6 to 9 weeks: Record AROM and gentle PROM measurements. Evaluate joint stiffness and begin, with physician's approval, dynamic flexion and/or extension splinting. Continue with edema reduction and scar mobilization techniques.

VI. 9 to 12 weeks: AROM and PROM measurements are taken, as well as early grip and pinch measurements (if bone fixation is good). Sensory evaluation and record of progressing Tinel's sign. Prework hardening activities can begin with evaluation of patient's ability for return-to-work activities. Desensitization may be initiated.

VII. 12 weeks: Return-to-work goals are assessed, as well as the need for any secondary surgical procedures. If the patient does not need additional surgery, work conditioning is implemented. If the patient requires a secondary procedure, therapy needs are addressed in preparation for this surgery.

OUTCOMES

Replantation surgery has been successfully performed for more than 30 years, with overall average survival rates of the replanted parts being 80%.[8] "When comparing patients with replantations to those with revision amputations at similar levels, satisfactory results were reported in 60% to nearly 80%."[21] The type of injury is an important factor influencing late functional outcomes for replantations. Sharp injuries produce the best overall results, and crush and avulsion amputations produce the poorest outcomes.[22] Prolonged ischemia time also influences the overall functional outcomes. More distal injuries have a better result in terms of function, and multilevel injuries do not do as well as single-level injuries. Recovery is better in children than in adults.

Sensibility recovery is comparable to that of a severed peripheral nerve repair.[8] Two-point discrimination for replanted thumbs is on average 11 mm, and for replanted fingers it is 8 mm.[8] In general, therefore, diminished protective sensibility can be expected for replanted digits.

AROM, again, depends on the level and type of injury. PIP range of motion can be expected to be 35 degrees if the injury is between the wrist and the insertion of the FDS, and 82 degrees if it is distal to the FDS insertion.[8,22] Intrinsic muscle function is weak or absent with replantations at or distal to the wrist, and pinch and grip strengths can be reduced by 10% to 60% at this level of replantation.[22]

Cold intolerance is present in almost all replantations and may not resolve for more than 2 years after the injury.[8] The appearance of the replanted part is generally preferable to that of a prosthesis, and, when compared with a prosthesis, the replantation most often produces superior functional results.[23]

REFERENCES

1. Urbaniak JR: Microsurgery for Major Limb Reconstruction. Mosby, St. Louis, 1987, pp. 2-37, 56-66
2. Morrison WA, O'Brien BMcC, MacLeod AM: Digital replantation and revascularizations: a long term review of one hundred cases. Hand 10:125, 1978

3. Smith AR, van Alphen B, Faithfull NS, et al.: Limb preservation in replantation surgery. Plast Reconstr Surg 75:227, 1985

4. Buncke HJ (ed): Microsurgery: Transplantation Replantation, An Atlas-Text. Lea & Febiger, Philadelphia, 1991

5. Trumble TE: Replantation. In Trumble TE (ed): Principles of Hand Surgery and Therapy. Saunders, St. Louis, 2000

6. Whitney TM, Lineawearver WC, Buncke HJ, et al.: Clinical results of bony fixation methods in digital replantation. J Hand Surg Am 15:328-334, 1990

7. Lim BH, Tan BK, Peng YP: Digital replantations including fingertip and ring avulsions. Hand Clin 17:419-431, 2001

8. Goderner RD, Urbaniak JR: Replantation. In Green DP, Hotchkiss RN, Peterson WC, et al. (eds): Green's Operative Hand Surgery. 5th Ed. Churchill Livingstone, Philadelphia, 2005

10. Buncke H, Jackson R, Buncke G, et al.: The surgical and rehabilitative aspects of replantation and revascularization of the hand. In Hunter JM, Mackin EJ, Callahan AD (eds): Rehabilitation of the Hand: Surgery and Therapy. 4th Ed. Mosby, St. Louis, 1995

11. Chen ZV, Meyer UE, Kleinart HE: Present indications and contraindications for replantation as reflected by long term functional results. Orthop Clin North Am 3:849-870, 1981

12. Scheker LR, Hodges A: Brace and rehabilitation after replantation and revascularization. Hand Clin 17:473-480, 2001

13. Michlovitz SL: Thermal agents in rehabilitation. In Michlovitz SL (ed): Contemporary Perspectives in Rehabilitation. 2nd Ed. Vol. 6. FA Davis, Philadelphia, 1990

14. Silverman P, Mac N, Willette GV: Early protective motion in digital revascularization and replantation. J Hand Ther 2:84, 1989

15. van Adrichem LN, Hovius SE, van Strik R, et al.: The acute effect of cigarette smoking on the microcirculation of a replanted digit. J Hand Surg Am 17:230-233, 1992

16. Chan SW, Jaglowski JM, Kaplan R: Rehabilitation of hand injuries. In Cohen M (ed): Mastery of Plastic and Reconstructive Surgery. Little, Brown, Boston, 1994

17. Jones N, Chang J, Kashani P: The surgical and rehabilitative aspects of replantation and revascularization of the hand. In Mackin EJ, Callahan AD, Skirven TM, et al. (eds): Hunter-Mackin-Callahan Rehabilitation of the Hand and Upper Extremity. 5th Ed. Mosby, St. Louis, 2002

18. Chan SW, LaStayo P: Hand therapy management following mutilating hand injuries. Hand Clin 19:133-148, 2003

19. Kader PB: Therapist's management of the replanted hand. Hand Clin 2:179, 1986

20. Michlovitz SL, Segal LR: Physical agents and electrotherapy techniques in hand rehabilitation. In Stanley BG, Tribuzi SM (eds): Concepts in Hand Rehabilitation. FA Davis, Philadelphia, 1992

21. Kitay GS, Steinberg B: Upper Extremity Replantation. Jacksonville Medicine, May 1998

22. Bolton M, Bajaj AK, Gupta S: Reassessing the Indications for Digit Replantation: A Meta-Analysis of Functional Outcomes. American Society of Plastic Surgery 2003 Annual Meeting. Hand/Upper Extremity Papers, San Diego, October 29, 2003

23. Graham B, Adkins P, Tsai TM, et al.: Major replantation versus revision amputation and prosthetic fitting in the upper extremity: a late functional outcomes study. J Hand Surg Am 23:783-791, 1998

SUGGESTED READINGS

Amadio PC, Lin GT, An KN: Anatomy and pathomechanics of the flexor pulley system. J Hand Ther 2:138, 1989

Axelrod TS, Buchler U: Severe complex injuries to the upper extremity: revascularization and replantation. J Hand Surg Am 16:574, 1991

Baker GL, Kleinert JM: Digit replantation in infants and young children: determinants of survival. Plast Reconstr Surg 94:139, 1994

Browne EZ, Ribik CA: Early dynamic splinting for extensor tendon injuries. J Hand Surg Am 14:72, 1989

Dellon AL: Sensory recovery in replanted digits and transplanted toes: a review. J Reconstr Microsurg 2:123, 1986

Doyle JR: Anatomy of the flexor tendon sheath and pulley system: a current review. J Hand Surg Am 14:349, 1989

Duran RJ, Houser RG: Controlled passive motion following flexor tendon repair in zones 2 and 3. AAOS Symposium of Tendon Surgery in the Hand. Mosby, St. Louis, 1975, p. 105

Evans RB: Therapeutic management of extensor tendon injuries. Hand Clin 2:157, 1986

Evans RB, Burkhalter WE: A study of the dynamic anatomy of extensor tendons and implications for treatment. J Hand Surg Am 11:774, 1986

Glickman LT, MacKinnon SE: Sensory recovery following digital replantation. Microsurgery 11:236, 1990

Goldner RD, Stevanovic MV, Nunley JA, et al.: Digital replantation at the level of the distal interphalangeal joint and distal phalanx. J Hand Surg Am 14:214, 1989

Jupiter JB, Pess GM, Bour CJ: Results of flexor tendon tenolysis after replantation in the hand. J Hand Surg Am 14:35, 1989

Kleinert HE, Kutz JE, Cohen MJ: Primary repair of zone 2 flexor tendon lacerations. AAOS Symposium on Tendon Surgery in the Hand. Mosby, St. Louis, 1975, p. 91

Milford L: The Hand. 2nd Ed. Mosby, St. Louis, 1982

O'Brien BMcC: Reconstructive microsurgery of the upper extremity. J Hand Surg Am 15:316, 1990

Strickland JW: Biologic rationale, clinical application and results of early motion following flexor tendon repair. J Hand Ther 2:71, 1989

Tark KC, Kim YW, Lee YH, et al.: Replantation and revascularization of hands: clinical analysis and functional results of 261 cases. J Hand Surg Am 14:17, 1989

Werntz JR, Chester SP, Breidenbach WC, et al.: A new dynamic splint for postoperative treatment of flexor tendon injury. J Hand Surg Am 14:559, 1989

Whitney TM, Lineaweaver WC, Buncke HJ, et al.: Clinical results of bony fixation methods in digital replantation. J Hand Surg Am 15:328, 1990

Tsau TM: Upper extremity amputations and management of acute microsurgical treatment prostheses and rehabilitation. Hand Clin 17(3):343-510, 2001

Digital Amputation and Ray Resection

46

Linda Coll Ware

Partial digit amputations are the most common type of amputation seen in the upper extremity.[1] Various ways to treat these injuries include split-thickness skin grafts, bone shortening with primary closure, healing by secondary intention, V-Y advancement flap, volar advancement Moberg flap, cross-finger flap, thenar flap, and hypothenar flap.[1-4] Regardless of surgical technique, the goals of surgery are (1) wound closure, (2) preservation of functional length, (3) preservation of useful sensibility, (4) prevention of symptomatic neuromas, and (5) quick return to work or play.[1]

Partial digit amputations can occur at various levels. The level of the amputation can affect the amount of recoverable movement. If the amputation is distal to the sublimis insertion, the middle phalanx segment will be able to participate effectively in grasping activities. If the amputation occurs proximal to the insertion, however, there will be no active flexion of the remaining middle phalanx. Once an amputation has occurred proximal to the proximal interphalangeal (PIP) joint, the remaining proximal segment is controlled by the intrinsic muscles and the extensor digitorum communis. This may allow only 45 degrees of active flexion of the metacarpophalangeal (MCP) joint. If the amputation occurs at the MCP level, the patient is left with a space that makes it difficult to keep small objects in the palm. At this point a ray resection may be considered.

A ray resection with or without digital transposition is often performed electively after consideration is given to this option. Before making this decision, the patient may regain maximum function with the initial surgical treatment and adapt to using the altered hand. Considerations should include the possible loss of power grip with ray resection and the decreased breadth of the palm. Conversely, the cosmesis and symmetry of the hand are improved after ray resection.

Loss of a digit can be devastating for the patient. Emotional support and referral to a social worker or psychiatrist may be necessary.

DEFINITION

A **partial digit amputation** is a digital amputation at or distal to the MCP joint (Fig. 46-1). A **ray resection** is a digital amputation through the

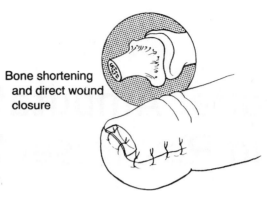

Bone shortening
and direct wound
closure

FIG. **46-1** Digital amputation.

metacarpal bone. Ray resection with a transposition additionally involves an osteotomy of an adjacent border metacarpal and its fixation to the remaining metacarpal bone of the resected digit (Figs. 46-2 and 46-3).

SURGICAL PURPOSE

Traumatized fingers may require digital amputation if the distal tissue is nonsalvageable or nonreplantable. In some cases, replantation may be possible but digital amputation offers a superior result. A properly performed amputation should have adequate bulk of soft tissue at the volar pad, with a tension-free closure to avoid delayed wound healing or bony prominence. Tendons are resected away from the skin closure to prevent postoperative tendon imbalance or quadrigia. Nerves are resected back from the closure site to make neuroma formation or tip hypersensitivity less likely. It is important to maintain the integrity and mobility of the proximal joints to optimize hand function.

Ray resection may be performed with two essential goals in mind: function and cosmesis. For the long and ring fingers, patients may prefer the less noticeable appearance of the ray-resected digit to the visible gap in

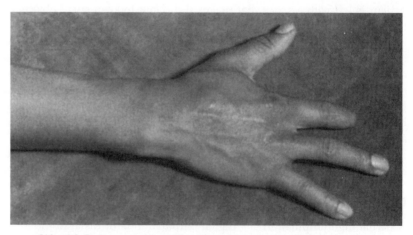

FIG. **46-2** Ray resection with transposition and partial amputation.

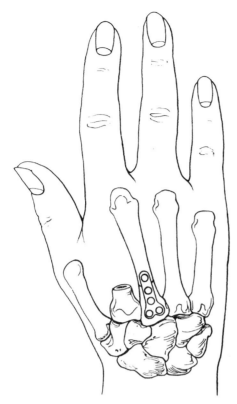

FIG. **46-3** Ray resection with transposition.

the hand created by a digital amputation. Patients also report that ray resections of these digits better enable them to hold smaller objects (e.g., coins) with the digits adducted and hand supinated. Without transposition, the gap is closed by firm repair of the intermetacarpal ligaments at the level of the metacarpal neck. Ray amputations of the index finger are often performed to deepen the first web space in the traumatized hand. The resection is typically performed at the metacarpal metaphyseal base, preserving the carpometacarpal articulation and wrist extensor insertions. Care is taken to preserve glabrous volar skin and to place incisions dorsally. Nerves are resected back and buried in muscle to prevent neuroma formation.

TREATMENT GOALS

   I.   Promote wound closure and optimal scar formation.
  II.   Maintain full range of motion (ROM) of all uninvolved joints.
III.   Maximize ROM of all involved joints.
 IV.   Desensitization/sensory reeducation of injured tip.
  V.   Return patient to previous level of function.

NONOPERATIVE INDICATIONS/PRECAUTIONS
FOR THERAPY

   I.   Indications: digit amputations allowed to heal by secondary intention

II.   Precautions
       A. Exposed bone
       B. Associated nail bed injury
       C. Associated fractures
       D. Associated nerve lacerations
       E. Associated tendon lacerations

NONOPERATIVE THERAPY

   I. Wound care (see Chapter 1)
  II. Protective splinting
 III. ROM
  IV. Edema control
   V. Desensitization/sensory reeducation
  VI. Scar management after wound is healed
 VII. Strengthening
VIII. Fine motor and functional activities
  IX. Fitting of cosmetic prosthesis

NONOPERATIVE COMPLICATIONS

   I. Infection
  II. Prolonged open wound
 III. Hypersensitivity
  IV. Diminished sensation
   V. Neuroma
  VI. Poorly shaped tip
 VII. Adherent scar
VIII. Limited ROM
  IX. Alienation of digit
   X. Quadrigia syndrome
  XI. Empty space when fisting

POSTOPERATIVE INDICATIONS/PRECAUTIONS FOR THERAPY

   I. Indications
       A. Partial digit amputations closed by sutures, skin grafts, or flaps
       B. Ray amputations with or without digital transposition
  II. Precautions
       A. Presence of graft or flap
       B. Associated nail bed injuries
       C. Associated fractures
       D. Associated nerve lacerations
       E. Associated tendon lacerations

POSTOPERATIVE THERAPY

   I. Wound care, including donor site
  II. Protective splinting
       A. If the third or fourth ray has been surgically resected, it is
          important to apply firm circumferential support to the palmar
          arch to prevent the metacarpals from spreading apart. This can

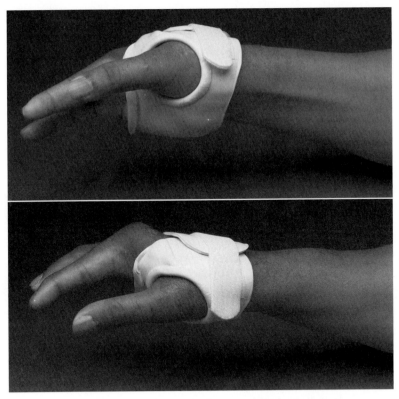

FIG. **46-4** Circumferential splint supporting palmar arch.

be achieved by a palmar bar splint, which supports the
transverse and longitudinal arches of the palm. The splint may
be discontinued at 6 to 8 weeks postoperatively[5] (Fig. 46-4).
- B. With a ray resection of the second metacarpal and a transfer
  of the first dorsal interossei, an index proximal phalanx block
  should be added to the palmar bar to prevent motion at the
  MCP joint and stretching of the transfer.[5]

III. Edema control

IV. ROM
- A. Active range of motion (AROM) may begin immediately with
  partial tip amputations and most ray resections.
- B. If a ray resection of the index finger with a first dorsal interossei
  transfer has been performed, AROM is started 3 to 4 weeks
  postoperatively and passive range of motion (PROM) is started
  6 weeks postoperatively in the middle finger MCP joint.
- C. The type of fixation determines when to begin AROM of a ray
  resection with digital transposition. Rigid fixation with plates
  and screws allows motion early.[5] Consult with the physician.

V. Desensitization/sensory reeducation

VI. Scar management after wound is closed

VII. Strengthening
- A. Strengthening can begin after the amputation wound is healed.
- B. Strengthening can begin 6 to 8 weeks after a ray resection.
- C. Strengthening can begin after the osteotomy has healed with
  a ray resection and digital transposition.

VIII. Fine motor control, functional activities, and work hardening
IX. Fitting of cosmetic prosthesis

POSTOPERATIVE COMPLICATIONS

  I. Graft or flap infection, hematoma, necrosis
  II. Donor site infection
  III. Hypersensitivity in fingertip and/or donor site
  IV. Diminished sensation in fingertip and/or donor site
  V. Neuroma
  VI. Poorly shaped tip
  VII. Adherent scar
  VIII. Limited ROM
  IX. Alienation of digit
  X. Spreading of metacarpals
  XI. Scissoring of digits

EVALUATION TIMELINE

I. Nonoperative
  A. Immediately
    1. Wound assessment
    2. AROM and PROM measurements of all joints
  B. After wound is healed
    1. Scar assessment
    2. AROM and PROM measurements of all joints
    3. Strength measurements
    4. Sensory evaluation
    5. Fine motor and functional assessments
II. Operative
  A. Immediately
    1. Wound assessment including donor site
    2. AROM and PROM of uninvolved joints
    3. ROM of involved joints may be delayed until graft or flap, first dorsal interossei transfer, or osteotomy has fixation. Consult physician.
  B. After graft or flap is well established
    1. Scar assessment
    2. AROM and PROM of all joints
      a. AROM at 3 to 4 weeks of the middle finger MCP if first dorsal interosseous is transferred; PROM at 6 weeks
      b. AROM and PROM for ray resection with digital transposition depends on type of fixation used.
    3. Strength measurements: 6 to 8 weeks for ray resection/transposition
    4. Sensory evaluation
    5. Fine motor and functional assessments

OUTCOMES

I. Nuzumlali and colleagues[7] compared ring finger ray resections and ring finger partial digital amputations. Ray resections demonstrated decreased grip strength, key pinch strength, three-jaw pinch strength, hand circumference, and palmar volume. Partial ring finger amputations displayed only grip strength and pulp pinch strength loss. The authors suggested that ray resection should be avoided in patients with occupations that require strong pinch functions.

II. Melikyan and associates[6] reported the results of 20 ray amputations and showed an average of 27% less grip and 22% less three-point pinch strength in the operated hand. The Disability Shoulder, Arm, and Hand (DASH) questionnaire function score was 29.2 (on a scale of 0 to 100, with 0 indicating no disability).

III. Karle and coworkers,[8] in the article, "Functional Outcome and Quality of Life after Ray Amputation versus Amputation Through the Proximal Phalanx of the Index Finger," showed no significant loss of strength between the two. Patients with amputations through the proximal phalanx demonstrated a better functional outcome, whereas aesthetic appearance was rated higher after ray amputation.[8]

REFERENCES

1. Jebson PJ, Graham TJ: Amputations. In Green DP, Hotchkiss RN, Peterson WC (eds): Green's Operative Hand Surgery. 4th ed. Churchill Livingstone, New York, 1999, p. 48

2. Levin LS, Moorman GJ, Heller L: Management of skin grafts and flaps. In Mackin EJ, Callahan AD, Skirven TM, et al. (eds): Hunter-Mackin-Callahan Rehabilitation of the Hand and Upper Extremity. 5th Ed. Mosby, St. Louis, 2002, p. 347

3. Schenck RR, Cheema TA: Hypothenar skin grafts for fingertip reconstruction. J Hand Surg Am 9:750, 1984

4. Tupper J, Miller G: Sensitivity following volar V-Y plasty for fingertip amputations. J Hand Surg Br 10:183, 1985

5. Cannon NM (ed): Diagnosis and Treatment Manual for Physicians and Therapists. The Hand Rehabilitation Center of Indiana, Indianapolis, IN, 1991

6. Melikyan EY, Beg MS, Woodbridge S, et al.: The functional results of ray amputation. Hand Surg 8:47-51, 2003

7. Nuzumlali E, Orhun E, Ozturk K, et al.: Results of ray resection and amputation for ring avulsion injuries at the proximal interphalangeal joint. J Hand Surg Br 28:578-581, 2003

8. Karle B, Wittemann M, Germann G: Functional outcome and quality of life after ray amputation versus amputation through the proximal phalanx of the index finger. Handchir Mikrochir Plast Chir 34:30-35, 2002

SUGGESTED READINGS

Arata J, Ishikawa K, Soeda H, et al.: The palmar pocket method: an adjunct to the management of zone I and II fingertip amputations. J Hand Surg Am 26:945-950, 2001

Chow SP: Hand function after digital amputation. J Hand Surg Br 18:125, 1993

Lister GD, Pederson WC: Skin flaps. In Green DP, Hotchkiss RN, Peterson WC (eds): Green's Operative Hand Surgery. 4th Ed. Churchill Livingstone, New York, 1999, p. 1783

Pillet J, Mackin EJ: Aesthetic hand prosthesis: its psychologic and functional potential. In Mackin EJ, Callahan AD, Skirven TM, et al. (eds): Hunter-Mackin-Callahan Rehabilitation of the Hand and Upper Extremity. 5th Ed. Mosby, St. Louis, 2002, p. 1461

Sagiv P, Shabat S, Mann M, et al.: Rehabilitation process and functional results of patients with amputated fingers. Plast Reconstr Surg 110:497-503; discussion 504-505, 2002

Metacarpal and Proximal Interphalangeal Joint Capsulectomy

47

Rebecca J. Saunders

Capsulectomies of the metacarpophalangeal (MCP) and proximal interphalangeal (PIP) joints are performed to improve motion and functional use of stiff joints with normal articular surfaces. Some of the common diagnoses that may result in capsulectomy are metacarpal and phalangeal fractures, crush injuries, nerve injuries, burns, and Volkmann's contracture.[1] Capsulectomies are necessary if stiff joints fail to respond to a conservative treatment program that includes splinting and exercise. Surgery is usually performed 4 to 6 months after the initial injury or most recent surgery, to ensure that the remodeling stage of wound healing has been reached and the patient has had a substantial trial of therapy.[2]

Most capsulectomies are performed on an outpatient basis. The use of local anesthesia with sedation is advocated by Idler[3] and Schneider.[4] This allows the patient to actively move the involved joint and can aid in assessing whether the release is effective. It can also aid in identifying other structures limiting motion (e.g., tendon adhesions).

Many anatomic structures within the finger may limit joint motion[5]:
I. Limited flexion (extension contracture)
   A. Scar contracture of skin over the dorsum of the finger
   B. Contracted long extensor muscle or adherent extensor tendon
   C. Contracted interosseus muscle or adherent interosseus tendon
   D. Contracted capsular ligament, particularly the collateral ligaments
   E. Bony block or exostosis
   F. Flexor tendon adherence
II. Limited extension
   A. Scar of skin on the volar surface of the finger
   B. Contraction of the superficial fascia in the finger, as in Dupuytren's contracture
   C. Contraction of the flexor-tendon sheath within the finger
   D. Contracted flexor muscle or adherent flexor tendon
   E. Contraction of the volar plate of the capsular ligament

F. Adherence of the collateral ligaments with the finger in the flexed position

G. Bony block or exostosis

These multiple factors need to be evaluated clinically and at the time of surgery. Capsulectomies are frequently performed concurrently with other surgical procedures, such as intrinsic releases or flexor and/or extensor tenolysis. To facilitate effective postoperative management, the therapist should obtain a copy of the operative report. If possible, the therapist should speak to the surgeon directly before seeing the patient. It is important to know which structures were involved, the status of the articular surfaces, the quality of the tendons involved, and the range of motion (ROM) that was obtained intraoperatively.[1,3] Patients who have undergone an extensive tenolysis may require a frayed tendon program. As Curtis[5] stated, "the results seem to indicate that the more anatomical structures are involved in the limitation of motion, the poorer is the end result."

The therapist's role in postoperative management of capsulectomies begins before surgery. Patient education should emphasize what will be expected of the patient postoperatively and why the patient's postoperative performance is critical to obtaining the maximum functional benefit from the surgery.[6] According to Curtis,[5] "one should not expect to restore function completely by this procedure, but one can expect to improve it."

Successful management after capsulectomy requires skillful observation, constant reassessment, and adaptation on the part of the therapist as well as a motivated and compliant patient. Maximum gains in ROM are usually obtained 3 to 5 months postoperatively. However, patients requiring fewer surgical maneuvers may continue to gain ROM for up to 6 to 8 months.[7]

DEFINITION

I.   **MCP capsulectomy:** surgical release of the dorsal and/or volar joint capsule and collateral ligaments

II. **PIP capsulectomy:** surgical release of the dorsal and/or volar joint capsule and collateral ligaments.

SURGICAL PURPOSE

I.   MCP capsulectomy: to restore MCP joint motion where either a flexion or extension contracture exists. The capsular structures have contracted or are locally adherent to other surrounding elements (Fig. 47-1). These structures are surgically released and partially excised. Joint stability must be maintained. The passive range of motion (PROM) obtained at the time of surgery is approximately the active range of motion (AROM) that can be expected with postoperative wound healing.

II. PIP capsulectomy: to restore motion to a joint that has less than a 45-degree range. The tissues surrounding the PIP joint must be considered as contributing to the contracture (e.g., skin, tendons, joint capsule, joint surfaces) (Fig. 47-2). Tissue equilibrium (scar maturity) must be present before surgery. Offending scar and capsule are released or excised, but joint stability is maintained. The PROM achieved at the time of surgery approximates the expected AROM with healing.

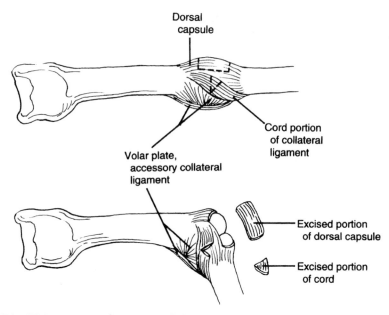

FIG. **47-1** Anatomy of metacarpophalangeal joint structures and capsulectomy.

TREATMENT GOALS

I.   MCP capsulectomy: Increase PROM and AROM of the MCP to approximately 60 to 70 degrees flexion, and increase functional use of the hand.

II. PIP capsulectomy: Restore AROM and PROM of PIP joint flexion and extension.

III. Functional goal postoperatively for both procedures: Achieve AROM equal to the PROM present after the surgical release.

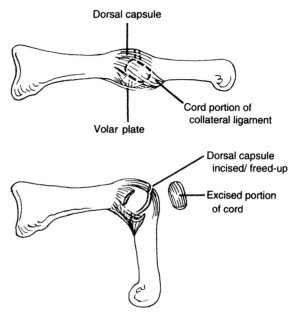

FIG. **47-2** Anatomy of proximal interphalangeal joint structures and capsulectomy.

POSTOPERATIVE INDICATIONS/PRECAUTIONS FOR THERAPY

I.   Indications
   A. MCP capsulectomy: If tendons are adherent and also limiting flexion, a concurrent tenolysis may have been performed. (Review the operative note.)
   B. PIP capsulectomy: This procedure is often performed in combination with other surgical procedures (e.g., tenotomy of contracted interossei, flexor and/or extensor tenolysis). The operative report should be reviewed to ensure adequate protection and treatment of the involved anatomic structures.
II. Precautions
   A. Intrinsic releases: Splinting should include an intrinsic stretch splint and instruction in stretching exercises.
   B. Extensor tenolysis with volar capsulectomy secondary to flexion contracture requires dynamic extension splinting to protect the weakened and frequently stretched extensor tendon while promoting active flexion; static extension splinting is required at night.

POSTOPERATIVE THERAPY

I.   General treatment principles for capsulectomies secondary to limitations of flexion and/or extension
   A. Edema control: As with acute hand injuries, effective management of edema is critical to a successful outcome. Postoperative edema needs to be monitored closely. Edema control includes elevation of the hand above the level of the heart to reduce limb dependency, use of light compressive dressings, and exercise. Cold packs applied with the extremity in elevation for 15- to 20-minute periods may be used as long as the dressing is kept dry and sterile and there is no vascular compromise. Postoperative edema should gradually subside over 2 to 3 weeks.
   B. Pain management: Patients' experiences of pain postoperatively vary widely. Some patients require narcotic relief for a short period. Pain, if present, needs to be managed effectively so that the patient can participate in therapy and the home exercise program. Transcutaneous electrical nerve stimulation (TENS), high-voltage galvanic stimulation (HVG), and other types of electrical stimulation can be helpful in reducing postoperative discomfort.
   C. Wound care: Universal precautions should be used when performing dressing changes and exercises.
   D. Initiation of AROM according to the physician's orders (usually within 24 to 48 hours after surgery).
   E. PROM: instruction in gentle, passive stretching.
   F. Scar management
   G. Splinting
      1. An appointment for postoperative therapy should be made when the surgery is scheduled.

2. Dynamic splints are used during the day as an adjunct to the patient's active exercise program and to protect weakened structures.

3. Static progressive splints are used at night to maintain gains in ROM and to provide a prolonged gentle stretch to the involved soft tissues.

4. All splints need to be monitored and adjusted frequently as the soft tissues respond to the stresses applied through active and passive exercise. The patient should be provided with detailed wearing instructions and precautions.

5. Splinting is continued until the patient is able to maintain the ROM present postoperatively with AROM and PROM (approximately 3 to 5 months).

6. If passive motion exceeds active motion, the emphasis on active exercise should be increased to overcome tendon weakness or adherence.

H. Functional activities and light use of the hand should be incorporated early to promote use of available ROM and to increase strength. Pain and edema need to be monitored closely as activities are incorporated.

I. Grip strengthening may be initiated at 6 weeks postoperatively; however, if a concurrent tenolysis was performed, it is deferred until 8 to 10 weeks postoperatively.

II. Postoperative management of MCP capsulectomy

A. Begin AROM 1 to 3 days postoperatively according to the physician's orders. Active exercises should include blocked and full-excursion flexion and extension.

B. PROM: instruction in *gentle* passive stretching.

C. Splinting

1. Instruction in skin care and routine checking for pressure areas to prevent skin breakdown

2. Static splint: MCPs are placed near the limit of obtainable flexion with the wrist in extension. The static splint is to be used at night and during the day when the patient is not exercising; it needs to be monitored closely and adjusted frequently as flexion increases. Continue night splinting until ROM goals are met and maintained for a few weeks (Fig. 47-3).

3. Dynamic splinting to increase MCP flexion should be used intermittently during the day. Splint use should be followed by active exercise to help maintain gains in PROM achieved by splinting (Fig. 47-4).

4. If an extension lag is present, dynamic flexion splinting should be alternated with dynamic extension splinting (Fig. 47-5).

D. Functional activities should be promoted to utilize gains in ROM and to increase strength.

E. Muscle reeducation of wrist extensors may be necessary, because patients may have been substituting their digital extensors for wrist extension; this pattern can contribute to stiffness in extension of MCPs and also can interfere with grip strength.[6]

F. Continuous passive motion (CPM) can be a useful adjunct to help decrease postoperative pain and edema while increasing PROM.[1]

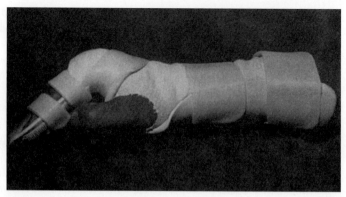

FIG. **47-3** Postoperative night positioning for metacarpophalangeal capsulectomy.

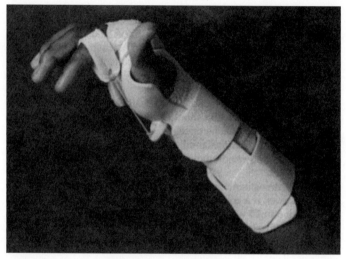

FIG. **47-4** Dynamic metacarpophalangeal flexion splint used intermittently during the day.

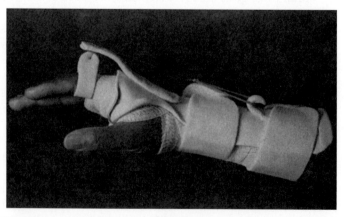

FIG. **47-5** Dynamic extension splint should be used during the day if an extension lag is present.

III. Postoperative management of PIP capsulectomy
    A. PIP capsulectomy secondary to extension contracture
        1. Dynamic flexion and extension splinting are alternated during the day (ratio of flexion versus extension splinting is determined by the available ROM and postoperative ROM goals).
        2. AROM should emphasize blocked active flexion and extension exercises.
        3. Static night splint position is determined by the available ROM and the anatomic structures involved.
    B. PIP capsulectomy secondary to flexion contracture
        1. Depending on the severity of the contracture and the surgeon's preferred method, the PIP joint may be pinned in extension postoperatively, with initiation of exercise and splinting deferred until pin removal at 1 to 2 weeks postoperatively.
        2. The static splint maintains PIP joint extension at night and between active exercise sessions (Fig. 47-6).
        3. Alternate dynamic extension and flexion splinting may be used during the day (as indicated by ROM) (Figs. 47-7 and 47-8).
        4. An active exercise program should include blocked PIP flexion and extension (Figs. 47-9 and 47-10). If an extension lag is present it is important to protect it, via splinting, and to prevent further loss of extension as ROM into flexion improves. Failure to monitor PIP joint extension closely can result in recurrence of the flexion contracture.
        5. The oblique retinacular ligament may have become tight secondary to the flexion contracture, and stretching exercises should be initiated (Fig. 47-11).

POSTOPERATIVE COMPLICATIONS

    I. Hematoma: Notify physician immediately, because this condition may require treatment by the physician.
   II. Infection: Notify physician immediately.
  III. Limitations in ROM secondary to edema and/or pain.
  IV. Weakness of previously adherent tendons
    V. Joint subluxation secondary to excessive ligament excision.
  VI. Complex regional pain syndrome

EVALUATION TIMELINE

    I. Preoperative evaluation 1 to 2 weeks before surgery
        A. AROM/PROM
        B. Grip and pinch strength.
        C. Sensation
        D. Functional assessment of activities of daily living, vocational and avocational activities
   II. Postoperative evaluation
        A. Initial AROM postoperatively; AROM should be reassessed at every treatment session for the first few weeks.
        B. Weekly reevaluation of AROM/PROM

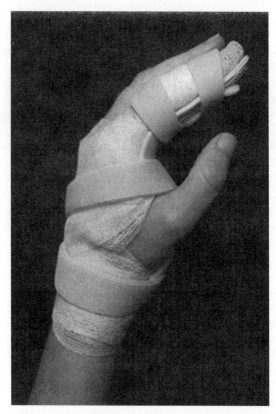

FIG. **47-6** Static proximal interphalangeal extension splint used at night and between active exercises.

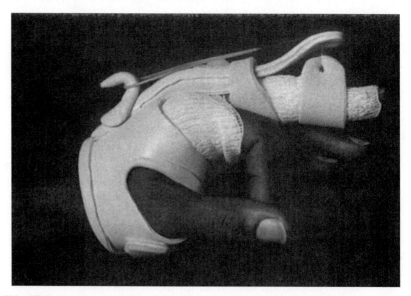

FIG. **47-7** Dynamic extension splint can be used during the day to increase extension.

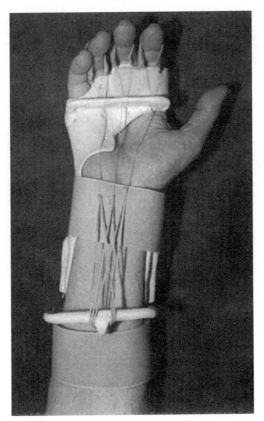

FIG. 47-8 Dynamic flexion splint can be used during day to increase flexion.

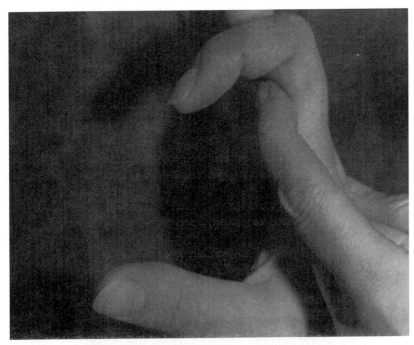

FIG. 47-9 Blocked range-of-motion exercises should be included in the exercise program.

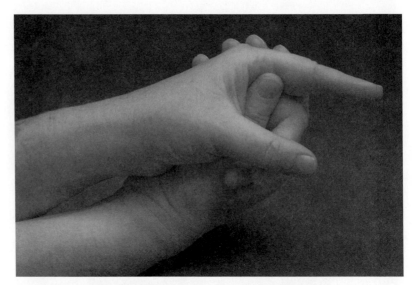

FIG. **47-10** Proximal interphalangeal extension with metacarpophalangeal joint blocked in flexion.

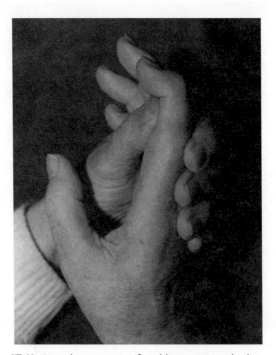

FIG. **47-11** Stretching exercise for oblique retinacular ligament.

C. At 6 to 8 weeks: evaluation of ROM, sensation, and strength.
If a concurrent tenolysis was performed, evaluation of strength
is deferred until 8 to 10 weeks postoperatively.

OUTCOMES

The results of surgery are inversely related to the number of structures
involved in the procedure. The goal of capsulectomy is to increase ROM
and improve function. Restoration of normal AROM is rare.

REFERENCES

1. Cannon NM: Postoperative management of metacarpophalangeal joint capsulectomies.
   In Mackin EJ, Callahan AD, Skirven TM, et al. (ed): Hunter-Mackin-Callahan
   Rehabilitation of the Hand and Upper Extremity. 5th Ed. Vol.1. Mosby, St. Louis, 2002
2. Jabaley ME, Freeland AE: Capsulectomy of the proximal interphalangeal joint.
   In Blair WE (ed): Techniques in Hand Surgery. Williams & Wilkins, Baltimore, 1996
3. Idler RS: Capsulectomies of the metacarpophalangeal and proximal interphalangeal
   joints. In Strickland JW (ed): Master Techniques in Orthopaedic Surgery: The Hand.
   Lippincott-Raven, Philadelphia, 1998
4. Schneider LH: Tenolysis and capsulectomy after hand fractures. Clin Orthop (327):
   72-78, 1996
5. Curtis RM: Capsulectomy of the interphalangeal joints of the fingers. J Bone Joint
   Surg Am 36:1219, 1954
6. Laseter G: Postoperative management of capsulectomies. In Hunter JM, Schneider LH,
   Mackin EJ, et al. (eds): Rehabilitation of the Hand: Surgery and Therapy. 3rd Ed.
   Mosby, St. Louis, 1990, p. 364
7. Gould JS, Nicholson BG: Capsulectomy of the metacarpophalangeal and proximal
   interphalangeal joints. J Hand Surg Am 4:482, 1979

SUGGESTED READINGS

Canale ST (ed): Campbell's Operative Orthopaedics. 10th Ed. Mosby, St. Louis, 2002
Cannon N: Postoperative management of metacarpophalangeal joint capsulectomies.
    In Hunter JM, Mackin EJ, Callahan AD (eds): Rehabilitation of the Hand: Surgery
    and Therapy. 4th Ed. Mosby, St. Louis, 1995, p. 1173
Diao E, Eaton G: Total collateral ligament excision for contractures of the proximal
    interphalangeal joint. J Hand Surg Am 18:395, 1993
Flowers KR: Edema: differential management based on stages of wound healing. In Hunter JM,
    Mackin EJ, Callahan AD (eds): Rehabilitation of the Hand: Surgery and Therapy.
    4th Ed. Mosby, St. Louis, 1995, p. 87
Flynn MD: Hand Surgery. 3rd Ed. Williams & Wilkins, Baltimore, 1982
Green DP (ed): Operative Hand Surgery. 2nd Ed. Churchill Livingstone, New York, 1988
Innis PC, Clark GL, Curtis RM: Management of the stiff hand. In Hunter JM, Mackin EJ,
    Callahan AD (eds): Rehabilitation of the Hand: Surgery and Therapy. 4th Ed. Mosby,
    St. Louis, 1995, p. 1129
McEntee P: Therapists management of the stiff hand. In Hunter JM, Schneider LH,
    Mackin EJ, et al. (eds): Rehabilitation of the Hand. 3rd Ed. Mosby, St. Louis, 1990,
    p. 328
Minaamikawa Y, Hori E, Amadio PC, et al.: Stability and constraint of the proximal
    interphalangeal joint. J Hand Surg Am 18:198, 1993
Smith RJ: Nonischemic contractures of the intrinsic muscles of the hand. J Bone Joint Surg
    Am 53:1313-1331, 1971
Young VL, Wray RC Jr, Weeks PM: The surgical management of stiff joints in the hand.
    Plast Reconstr Surg 62:835, 1978

Thumb Carpometacarpal Joint Arthroplasty

48

Rebecca J. Saunders

The basal joint complex consists of the trapeziometacarpal joint and the articulations of the trapezium with the scaphoid, trapezoid, and second metacarpal. The unique saddle shape of the trapeziometacarpal or first CMC (carpometacarpal) joint accounts for the mobility of the thumb. It is frequently described as the basal joint and is the major source of thumb pain. Pellegrini[1-3] stated that there is concurrent involvement of the scaphotrapezial joint in 50% of the cases.

Basal joint arthroplasty is indicated when there is significant arthritis of the trapeziometacarpal joint, or of the adjacent joints of the thumb, that results in disabling pain and loss of hand function (Fig. 48-1). Surgical intervention may be necessary if there is no response to a conservative management regimen of splinting, nonsteroidal antiinflammatory drugs (NSAIDs), and/or steroid injection. Patient education is also an important factor in conservative management and should include joint protection techniques and activity modification. Building up handles on tools, utensils, and sports equipment can decrease pain with activities. Some authors advocate strengthening exercises for the muscles of the thenar cone, as well as the extrinsic abductor, long extensor, and long flexor.[2,4,5] Arthritic changes can be degenerative, traumatic, or caused by systemic disease (e.g., rheumatoid arthritis). Disease of the thumb CMC joint occurs more frequently in women than in men. In published series of basal joint reconstructions, the female-to-male ratio ranges from 10:1 to 15:1.[3] CMC arthritis is thought to be related to hormonal changes, ligamentous laxity, and activities that require continuous tone in the thenar musculature during thumb flexion-adduction.[6]

The surgical options in basal joint arthroplasty are implant insertion and soft tissue reconstruction. Implant arthroplasty usually is reserved for the relatively low-demand rheumatoid hand, because of the potential complications of silicone synovitis or subluxation or both. Many different types of soft tissue reconstructions are performed. The following protocol is based on the Burton-Pellegrini procedure of ligament reconstruction and tendon interposition (LRTI) after resection of the trapezium.[7] Range of motion (ROM) after this procedure is approximately the same as it was

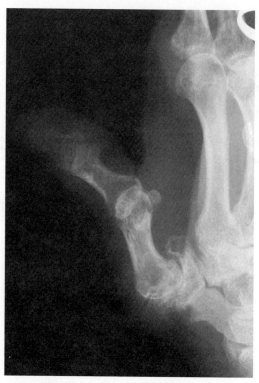

FIG. **48-1** Advanced CMC arthritis with osteophyte formation, MCP hyperextension, and adduction deformity.

before surgery. Functionally, a slight decrease in grip and pinch strength is to be expected initially, because of the slight shortening of the first ray, although these functions are less painful after this procedure.[8] Patients with advanced disease may require concomitant surgical procedures (e.g., hemi-trapezoidectomy due to scaphotrapezial arthritis). Patients who have metacarpophalangeal (MCP) joint hyperextension of greater than 30 degrees frequently require MCP fusion or capsulodesis of the MCP joint to prevent attenuation of the reconstructed ligament.[9-11] The prevalence of carpal tunnel syndrome in patients undergoing basal joint reconstruction has been reported to be 26% to 29%.[12] As with any surgical procedure involving the hand, close communication with the surgeon is necessary to facilitate complete patient care.

DEFINITION

During thumb CMC joint arthroplasty, the trapezium may be trimmed, but more often it is excised and the base of the first metacarpal is resected. A soft tissue spacer is constructed from part of the flexor carpi radialis (FCR) or from the whole tendon and is inserted in the trapezial space; then the joint capsule is closed. Ligamentous stability is often augmented by taking part of the FCR through a drill hole in the first metacarpal and then suturing it back on itself. The abductor pollicis longus tendon is also sometimes imbricated to increase stability (Fig. 48-2).

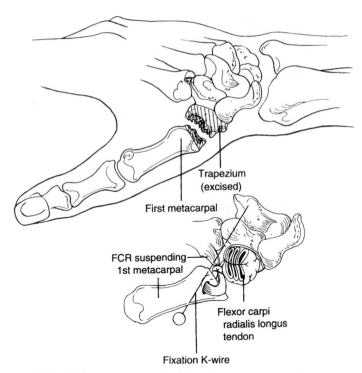

Trapezium
(excised)

First metacarpal

FCR suspending
1st metacarpal

Flexor carpi
radialis longus
tendon

Fixation K-wire

FIG. 48-2   Reconstruction of thumb carpometacarpal joint.

SURGICAL PURPOSE

Surgical correction of arthritis of the CMC joint of the thumb is designed mainly to relieve pain. Secondary gains are the improved positioning of the thumb with greater active range of motion (AROM) as a result of decreased pain. This provides better thumb function and appearance. If there is secondary deformity of the MCP joint, it may also have to be surgically corrected.

TREATMENT GOALS

   I.   Edema control
  II.   Pain control
 III.   Promotion of a stable, pain-free and mobile joint.
 IV.   Increase ROM, strength, and functional use of the hand.

POSTOPERATIVE INDICATIONS/PRECAUTIONS FOR THERAPY

MCP joint hyperextension can be a concurrent problem, and this may necessitate additional surgical procedures such as MCP fusion or capsulodesis. The operative note should be consulted if possible.

POSTOPERATIVE THERAPY

   I.   0 to 2 weeks: The patient is immobilized in a thumb spica cast.
  II.   2 to 4 weeks
      A. The bulky, postoperative dressing and sutures are removed, and the use of elastic stockinette or Coban can be initiated for edema control.

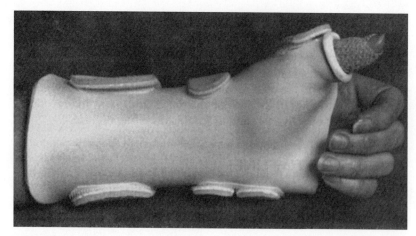

FIG. **48-3** Coban used for edema control may be worn with a thumb spica splint.

      B. The patient is fitted with a thumb spica cast or splint with the interphalangeal (IP) joint left free for ROM (Fig. 48-3).

      C. The cast or splint is used continuously until the initiation of AROM of the CMC at 4 to 6 weeks postoperatively.

  III. 4 to 6 weeks

      A. Active-assisted range of motion (AAROM) and AROM are initiated to the thumb and wrist.

      B. Exercises should emphasize CMC abduction, radial extension, and opposition to each fingertip. Isometric thenar abduction strengthening may be initiated at this time.[3,5] Pinch and grip strengthening are not initiated until 8 to 10 weeks postoperatively.

      C. Early metacarpal flexion and adduction puts undue stress on the reconstructed ligament and should be minimized at this time.

      D. Complete flexion across the palm to the base of the fifth metacarpal should not be attempted until the thumb can oppose each fingertip with ease and gradually be worked down to the base of the small finger actively.[6]

      E. Splinting is continued after exercise and at night, primarily for patient comfort. Patients may resume use of the hand for light activities of daily living (ADLs) with the splint on, as long as they are asymptomatic during performance of the activity.

  IV. 7 weeks: Dynamic splinting to increase MCP and IP joint motion may be initiated if the CMC joint is well stabilized.

   V. 8 to 10 weeks

      A. Static splint use may be discontinued if the joint is stable and the patient is asymptomatic.

      B. Gentle strengthening including grip and pinch strengthening may be initiated if the joint is stable and relatively pain free.[13] Cooney and Chao[14] found that the compressive force generated at the CMC joint is 12 times the force generated at the thumb and index finger (IF) tip with lateral pinch. This factor should be kept in mind as use of the hand and strengthening activities are progressed. No attempt should be made to pinch to the ring and small fingers, because this risks stretching out the ligament reconstruction.[11]

VI.   10 to 12 weeks: Normal use of the hand may be resumed without restrictions if the joint is stable and the patient is asymptomatic.

POSTOPERATIVE COMPLICATIONS

I.   The carpal tunnel is in close proximity to the basal joint, and postoperative edema can exacerbate an underlying median nerve problem or cause an acute carpal tunnel. This responds well to conservative management. If a concurrent carpal tunnel release was performed, the patient may take longer to regain strength.

II.   De Quervain's syndrome may become symptomatic during therapy. If recognized, it responds well to conservative treatment, including splinting, NSAIDs, and/or injection.[8]

III.   Hypersensitivity of the thenar region and incisional area is not an uncommon complication. If present, it needs to be treated with desensitization and pain control techniques. The therapist should be on the alert for signs and symptoms of complex regional pain syndrome (CRPS), because prompt diagnosis and early intervention are the most effective treatments for this disabling disease.

EVALUATION TIMELINE

I.   Preoperative evaluation should include:
A. ROM
B. Grip and pinch strength
C. Sensation
D. ADL function

II.   Postoperative evaluation
A. 2 weeks: Blocked active and passive MCP and IP ROM
B. 4 weeks
  1. MCP and IP ROM
  2. CMC abduction and extension
  3. Opposition, active only
  4. Wrist ROM
C. 8 weeks
  1. Thumb ROM (CMC, MCP, IP)
  2. Wrist ROM
  3. Grip and pinch strength (provided that the CMC joint is stable and the patient is asymptomatic)[13]
  4. Sensation
D. Functional assessment of ADLs, vocational and avocational activities.

OUTCOMES

Tomaino and colleagues[15] reported on the long-term follow up after LRTI as described by Burton and Pellegrini.[7] Twenty-two patients (24 joints) were evaluated at follow-up examinations after 2, 6, and 9 years. All but two patients had complete relief of pain and were satisfied with their thumb at each follow-up interval. Key pinch and grip strength continued to improve at the 2- and 6-year follow-up intervals. At the 9-year follow up, there was an average 93% improvement in grip strength and 34% improvement in pinch strength, compared with preoperative levels. Twenty-one (95%) of the patients reported excellent pain relief and were satisfied with the outcome.

Nylen and associates[16] reported on a prospective study of 100 basal joint arthroplasties performed as described by Burton and Pellegrini. Their average follow-up time was 36 months. Eighty-eight percent of patients were satisfied with the procedure and four of the dissatisfied patients stated they would have had the procedure done with hindsight. Grip strength improved in 44% and pinch strength in 72% of the patients.

Varitimidis and co-workers[17] reported on 58 patients (62 joints) who underwent LRTI using the entire FCR tendon. Their average follow-up interval was 42.5 months. Fifty percent of their patients also underwent a partial trapezoidectomy due to scaphotrapezial arthritis. Key pinch improved by 86% and grip strength improved by 69%. Excellent pain relief was reported by 95% of the patients. The authors stated that no morbidity was observed with use of the entire FCR tendon.

Tomaino and Coleman[18] reported on the effect of use of the entire FCR tendon on wrist function. Nine patients were tested preoperatively and postoperatively. The findings indicated no impairment in wrist motion or strength at 1 year follow-up by either subjective or objective measures. At 6 months postoperatively, wrist flexion strength had returned to near-baseline levels.

REFERENCES

1. Pellegrini VD: Osteoarthritis of the trapezio-metacarpal joint: the pathophysiology of articular cartilage degeneration: I. Anatomy and pathology of the aging joint. J Hand Surg Am 16:967, 1991

2. Poole JU, Pellegrini VD: Arthritis of the thumb basal joint complex. J Hand Ther 13:91-107, 2000

3. Pellegrini VD: The basal articulations of the thumb: pain, instability and osteoarthritis. In Peimer CA (ed): Surgery of the Hand and Upper Extremity. Vol. 1. McGraw-Hill, New York, 1996, pp. 1019-1042

4. Burton R: Basal joint implant arthroplasty in osteoarthritis. Hand Clin 3:473, 1987

5. Burton R: Resection/suspension arthroplasty of the basal joint of the thumb for osteoarthritis. In Strickland J (ed): Master Techniques in Orthopaedic Surgery: The Hand. Lippincott-Raven, Philadelphia, 1998

6. Burton R: Complications following surgery on the basal joint of the thumb. Hand Clin 2:265, 1986

7. Burton R, Pellegrini V: Surgical management of basal joint arthritis of the thumb: part II. Ligament reconstruction with tendon interposition arthroplasty. J Hand Surg Am 11:324, 1986

8. Eaton R: Trapezometacarpal osteoarthritis staging as a rationale for treatment. Hand Clin 3:455, 1987

9. Lourie GM: The role and implementation of metacarpophalangeal joint fusion and capsulodesis: indications and treatment alternatives. Hand Clin 17:255-260, 2001

10. Tomaino MM: Ligament reconstruction tendon interposition arthroplasty for basal joint arthritis: rationale, current technique and clinical outcome. Hand Clin 17:671-686, 2001

11. Burton R: Ligament reconstruction tendon interposition arthroplasty. In Osterman AL: Atlas of the Hand Clinics. Vol. 2, No. 2, 1997, pp. 77-99

12. Florack TM, Miller RJ, Pellegrini VD, et al.: The prevalence of carpal tunnel syndrome in patients with basal joint arthritis of the thumb. J Hand Surg Am 17:624, 1992

13. Cannon NM, Eaton R, Glickel S (eds): Soft tissue reconstructions: CMC joint. In Diagnosis and Treatment Manual for Physicians and Therapists. 3rd Ed. Hand Rehabilitation Center of Indiana PC, Indianapolis, IN, 1991

14. Cooney WP, Chao EY: Biomechanical analysis of static forces in the thumb during hand function. J Bone Joint Surg Am 59:27-36, 1977

15. Tomaino MM, Pellegrini VD, Burton RI: Arthroplasty of the basal joint of the thumb: long-term follow-up after ligament reconstruction with tendon interposition. J Bone Joint Surg Am 77:346, 1995

16. Nylen S, Johnson A, Rosenquist AM: Trapeziectomy and ligament reconstruction for osteoarthrosis of the base of the thumb: a prospective study of 100 operations. J Hand Surg Br 18:616-619, 1993

17. Varitimidis SE, Fox RJ, King JA, et al.: Trapeziometacarpal arthroplasty using the entire flexor carpi radialis tendon. Clin Orthop (370):164-170, 2000

18. Tomaino MM, Coleman K: Use of the entire width of the flexor carpi radialis tendon for the ligament reconstruction tendon interposition arthroplasty does not impair wrist function. Am J Orthop 29:283-284, 2000

SUGGESTED READINGS

Amadio P, Millender L, Smith R: Silicone spacer or tendon spacer for trapezium, resection arthroplasty: comparison of results. J Hand Surg Am 7:237, 1982

Colditz J: Anatomic considerations for splinting the thumb: In Hunter JM, Mackin EJ, Callahan AD (eds): Rehabilitation of the Hand: Surgery and Therapy. 4th Ed. Mosby, St. Louis, 1995, pp. 1161-1172

Colditz JC: The biomechanics of a thumb carpometacarpal immobilization splint: design and fitting. J Hand Ther 13:228-235, 2000

Eaton R, Glickel S, Littler W: Tendon interposition arthroplasty for degenerative arthritis of the trapeziometacarpal joint of the thumb. J Hand Surg Am 10:645, 1985

Le Viet DT, Kerboull L, Lantieri L, et al.: Stabilized resection arthroplasty by an anterior approach in trapeziometacarpal arthritis: results and surgical technique. J Hand Surg Am 21:194, 1996

Lins RE, Gelberman RH, McKeown L, et al.: Basal joint arthritis: trapeziectomy with ligament reconstruction and tendon interposition arthroplasty. J Hand Surg Am 21:202-209, 1996

Mureau MA, Rademaker PC, Verhaar JA, et al.: Tendon interposition arthroplasty versus arthrodesis for the treatment of trapeziometacarpal arthritis: a retrospective comparative follow-up study. J Hand Surg Am 26:869-876, 2001

Roberts RA, Jabaley ME, Nick TG: Results following trapeziometacarpal arthroplasty of the thumb. J Hand Ther 14:202-207, 2001

Swigart CR, Eaton RG, Glickel SZ, et al.: Splinting in the treatment of arthritis of the first carpometacarpal joint. J Hand Surg Am 24:86-91, 1999

Weiss S, LaStayo P, Mills A, et al.: Prospective analysis of splinting the first carpometacarpal joint: an objective, subjective and radiographic assessment. J Hand Ther 13:218-226, 2000

Wolock BS, Moore JR, Weiland AJ: Arthritis of the basal joint of the thumb: a critical analysis of treatment options. J Arthroplasty 4:65, 1989

Metacarpophalangeal Joint Arthroplasty 49

Lorie Theisen

Flexible implant arthroplasty is frequently indicated for patients with rheumatoid arthritis who have pain, joint instability, and deformities of the metacarpophalangeal (MCP) joints. Typically, in rheumatoid arthritis, ulnar drift of the fingers and subluxation of the MCP joint occur. Radial deviation of the metacarpals secondary to wrist malalignment is thought to cause the ulnar drift deformity. Other causes include posture, gravitational forces, and dynamic flexion forces.[1-3]

In flexible implant arthroplasty, the term *implant* refers to a flexible Silastic spacer rather than a joint. One of the main functions of the spacer is to maintain alignment and spacing during the early stages of healing and rehabilitation. Early motion is important in promoting the development of a fibrous joint capsule. The process whereby the implant acts as a spacer to support the newly forming fibrous capsule is the encapsulation process.[4-7] Early protected motion ensures a greater range of motion (ROM), assists in decreasing edema, promotes an organized arrangement of collagen fibers, and prevents malalignment. Alternative splinting and rehabilitation programs have emerged whereby patients use static splints and perform ROM exercises without the use of a dynamic splint.[8]

There is increasing research and development of the new implants such as pyrolytic carbon metacarpophalangeal implants.[9] Operative and postoperative management of patients with rheumatoid arthritis is clearly evolving.

DEFINITION

Metacarpophalangeal joint arthroplasty is a surgical formation or reformation of the MCP joints, typically using a flexible implant (Fig. 49-1).

SURGICAL PURPOSE

To restore skeletal alignment and tendon repositioning for more effective and efficient finger function. Flexible implant arthroplasty is most commonly

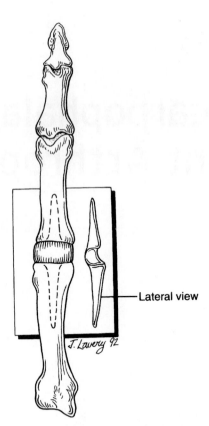

FIG. **49-1** Views of implant.

used for patients with rheumatoid arthritis. The surgery is also performed in cases of other types of arthritic conditions resulting from trauma, infection, or systemic diseases. The silicone implant acts primarily as a bone spacer. Soft tissue reconstruction around the joint may include collateral ligament repair and extensor tendon realignment. Postoperative therapy and monitoring are integral parts of the treatment to ensure a satisfactory result. Greatly improved appearance of the hand is also achieved and has been shown to influence the patient's postprocedure satisfaction.[10] Also, as patients with rheumatoid arthritis have more pharmacological interventions available to them and therefore are remaining more functional, the expectation of the implants is increasing.[11]

TREATMENT GOALS

    I.   Monitor wound healing.
   II.   Decrease edema.
 III.   Prevent scar adherence.
 IV.   Obtain active MCP flexion to 70 degrees and extension to neutral.
  V.   Obtain neutral alignment of each digit with the corresponding metacarpal.
 VI.   Prevent rotational deformities.

POSTOPERATIVE INDICATIONS/PRECAUTIONS FOR THERAPY

I.   Indications: MCP arthroplasty with flexible implant
II. Precautions
    A. Extensive reconstruction of soft tissues, limited bone stock, or arthrodesis of adjacent joints may require a delay in initiating postoperative rehabilitation and may require additional protective splinting during the postoperative rehabilitation.
    B. Delay in wound healing that may be caused by medical conditions and/or use of nonsteroidal antiinflammatory drugs (NSAIDs) or steroids
    C. Presence of osteoporosis
    D. Greater than expected postoperative pain may indicate a flare-up of rheumatoid arthritis or infection
    E. Additional deformities of the hand and wrist that are common in patients with rheumatoid arthritis may effect MCP ROM and position. For example, radial deviation of the wrist is considered a contributing factor to the ulnar deformity of the digits. Proximal interphalangeal (PIP) joint deformities may reduce the effectiveness of the digital flexors or extensors and subsequently effect MCP ROM.

POSTOPERATIVE THERAPY

I.   2 to 6 days postoperatively: The bulky dressing is removed and a static splint is fabricated. The surgeon should be consulted if there is any question about the timing of the first visit. Immobilization for longer periods is practiced, so communication with the physician is considered essential. At the first or a subsequent visit, a dynamic MCP extension splint is applied over a lightly padded dressing (Fig. 49-2). The splint design must consider the patient's ability to apply it correctly, because the contralateral hand may have functional limitations as well. A low-profile splint, in which the outrigger is no more than 2 inches from the dorsum of the metacarpals, seems to be more accepted by patients yet requires careful design and fabrication to meet splinting goals of MCP positioning and allow desired motion. The pull of the slings is full MCP extension when at rest and appropriate tension to allow active MCP flexion. Keep in mind that the final goal is 70 degrees MCP flexion and full MCP extension. The slings should also pull the MCP joints in a radial direction to prevent ulnar forces. Interphalangeal (IP) extension blocks or troughs to prevent PIP joint flexion during active MCP flexion exercises may be applied. If the troughs are applied volarly, care should be taken that the digits are not positioned in an ulnar direction. Dorsally applied troughs may be easier to apply correctly. The dynamic splint is worn continuously, with a static splint for night use (Fig. 49-3). Active MCP flexion exercises are performed intermittently throughout the waking hours. Initiate edema control via elevation and retrograde massage, with careful attention to avoid any lateral forces and meticulous wound care techniques.

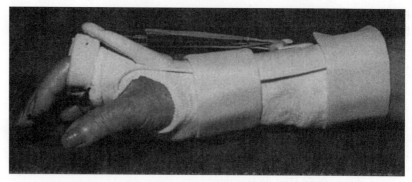

FIG. **49-2** Dynamic extension splint for postoperative treatment.

II.   2 to 3 weeks postoperatively: MCP flexion assists (e.g., dynamic flexion splinting) may be initiated for intermittent use throughout the day. The MCP flexion splint should not pull the fingers in an ulnar direction. It is important to work diligently to obtain MCP extension and flexion goals in the first 3 weeks.[6,12] Initiate scar management once the surgical wound has healed, with massage and or a compressive gel-type sheet.

III. 6 weeks postoperatively: Dynamic MCP extension splinting is gradually tapered to night splinting only, except in the presence of MCP extension lag or MCP flexion contracture. In these cases, continue splinting for the existing deformities. Initiate appropriate activities of daily living (ADLs) and education on joint protection techniques (see Chapter 52).

IV.   8 to 10 weeks: Mild isometric resistive exercises may be initiated, if ulnar forces are avoided. Isometric exercises may be useful in preventing ulnar forces. Assess for hand-based splinting to minimize ulnar forces.

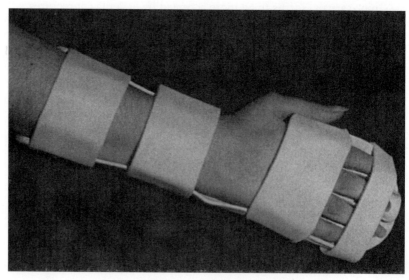

FIG. **49-3** Static positioning splint.

POSTOPERATIVE COMPLICATIONS

I. Pronation deformity or medial rotation may occur, especially in the index finger. To resolve this deformity, additional outriggers to provide a rotational force at the MCP joint may be necessary. The combined pull of a force couple may be necessary. (A force couple consists of two equal and opposite forces that act along parallel lines.[12]) The force couple is obtained by applying another outrigger to the digit with a pronation tendency. The combined forces produce a force in the supination direction of the digit and allow MCP extension and flexion.[13]

II. Extension contracture at the fifth digit may occur. Therefore, carefully monitor and provide verbal or visual cueing to the patient regarding active MCP flexion of the small finger. Tension on the dynamic MCP extension splint may need to be reduced for the fifth digit. If joint tightness is noted, dynamic splinting may be helpful. Dynamic splinting and ROM programs should be carefully monitored.

III. Dislocation or fracture of implant may occur.

IV. Slow healing with steroid medication may occur; use wound care precautions.

EVALUATION TIMELINE

I. 2 to 7 days postoperatively: initial assessment including active ROM measurement of the MCP joints

II. Reassessment of ROM every week thereafter

III. 8 to 10 weeks: Grip strength using a modified blood pressure cuff may be initiated.[14]

OUTCOMES

Recent strides in rheumatology and pharmacology have led to better overall health for patients with rheumatoid arthritis. It has been suggested that such patients therefore have a longer and more active life expectancy. The long-term results of metacarpophalangeal arthroplasty are gaining attention, and there are growing numbers of publications regarding metacarpophalangeal joint arthroplasty. Researchers and health care providers are challenged with first identifying the goals and desirable outcomes of this surgical procedure.

Providers and researchers are investigating the patients' and health care providers' perspectives. Mandi and colleagues[15] studied the varying opinions about what constitutes a good result. They found that patients' satisfaction after MCP implant arthroplasty was primarily related to postoperative appearance and secondarily to reduction in pain. Massey-Westropp and associates[11] examined patients after implant arthroplasty and found that, when assessing hand function, one must consider many factors (e.g., speed, ease of completing the task, pain). By using accurate methods of assessing function, particularly the quality of function, changes in patients' status will be noted. Therefore, the emerging research focusing on patients' expectations will ultimately lead to improved outcomes and satisfaction.

A recent study by Goldfarb and Stern[10] showed a deterioration of initially good results over time. This shows the importance of studying the long-term results after these procedures.

REFERENCES

1. Flatt A: Care of the Rheumatoid Hand. 4th Ed. Mosby, St. Louis, 1983
2. Smith RR, Kaplan E: Rheumatoid deformities at the MCP joints. J Bone Joint Surg Am 49:31, 1967
3. Hakstan R, Tubiana R: Ulnar deviation of the fingers: the role of joint structure and function. J Bone Joint Surg Am 49:299, 1967
4. Flatt AS: Restoration of rheumatoid finger joint function. J Bone Joint Surg Am 45:753, 1961
5. Swanson A: Flexible implant arthroplasty for arthritis finger joints. J Bone Joint Surg Am 54:435, 1972
6. Swanson A, Swanson G, Leonard J: Postoperative rehabilitation programs in flexible implant arthroplasty of the digits. In Hunter J, Schneider LH, Mackin EJ, et al. (ed): Rehabilitation of the Hand: Surgery and Therapy. 3rd Ed. Mosby, St. Louis, 1990, p. 912
7. Leonard J, Swanson A, Swanson G: Post-operative Care for Patients with Silastic Finger Joint Implants. 4th Ed. Dow Corning Corporation, Midland, MI, 1985
8. Burr N, Pratt A, Smith P: An alternative splinting and rehabilitation protocol for metacarpophalangeal joint arthroplasty in patients with rheumatoid arthritis. J Hand Ther 15:41-47, 2002
9. Cook S, Beckenbaugh R, Redondo J, et al.: Long term follow up of pyrolytic carbon metacarpophalangeal implants. J Bone Joint Surg Am 81:635, 1999
10. Goldfarb C, Stern P: Metacarpophalangeal joint arthroplasty in rheumatoid arthritis. J Bone Joint Surg Am 85:1869-1878, 2003
11. Massey-Westropp N, Massey-Westropp M, Rankin W, et al.: Metacarpophalangeal arthroplasty from the patient's perspective. J Hand Ther 6:315-319, 2003
12. Madden JW, Devore G, Arem AJ: A rational post-operative management program for metacarpophalangeal joint implant arthroplasty. J Hand Surg Am 2:358, 1977
13. Devore G, Muhleman C, Sasarita S: Management of pronation deformity in metacarpophalangeal joint implant arthroplasty. J Hand Surg Am 11:859, 1986
14. Melvin J: Evaluation of muscle strength. In Melvin J (ed): Rheumatic Disease Occupational Therapy and Rehabilitation. 2nd Ed. FA Davis, Philadelphia, 1982, p. 291
15. Mandi L, Galvin D, Bosch J, et al.: Metacarpophalangeal arthroplasty in rheumatoid arthritis: what determines satisfaction with surgery? J Rheumatol 29:2488-2491, 2002

SUGGESTED READINGS

Aren A, Madden J: Effects of stress on healing wounds: intermittent noncyclical tension. J Surg Res 20:93, 1976

Beckenbaugh R, Dobyns J, Linscheid R: Review and analysis of silicone-rubber metacarpophalangeal implants. J Bone Joint Surg Am 58:483, 1976

Bieber E, Weiland A, Volenec-Dowling S: Silicone rubber implant arthroplasty of the metacarpophalangeal joints for rheumatoid arthritis. J Bone Joint Surg Am 68:206, 1986

Bryant M: Wound healing. Clin Symp 29:2, 1977

Ehrlich G: Rehabilitation Management of Rheumatic Conditions. 2nd Ed. Williams & Wilkins, Baltimore, 1986

El-Gammal TA, Blair W: Motion after metacarpophalangeal joint reconstruction in rheumatoid disease. J Hand Surg Am 18:504, 1993

Gardner R, Mowat A: Wound healing after operations on patients with rheumatoid arthritis. J Bone Joint Surg Br 55:134, 1973

Kirschenbaum D, Schneider LH, Adams DC, et al.: Arthroplasty of the metacarpophalangeal joints with use of silicone-rubber implants in patients who have rheumatoid arthritis. J Bone Joint Surg Am 75:3, 1993

Kloth L, McCulloch J, Feedar J: Wound Healing: Alternatives in Management. FA Davis, Philadelphia, 1990

Lundborg G, Branemark PI, Carlsson I: Metacarpophalangeal joint arthroplasty based on the osseointegration concept. J Hand Surg Br 18:693, 1993

Melvin J: Rheumatic Disease in the Adult and Child. 3rd Ed. FA Davis, Philadelphia, 1982

Peimer CA, Medige J, Eckert BS, et al.: Reactive synovitis after silicone arthroplasty. J Hand Surg Am 11:624, 1986

Stephens J, Pratt N, Parks B: The reliability and validity of the Tekdyne hand dynamometer: part I. J Hand Ther 9:10, 1996

Stephens J, Pratt N, Michlovitz S: The reliability and validity of the Tekdyne hand
dynamometer: part II. J Hand Ther 9:18, 1996

Stothard J, Thompson AE, Sherris D: Correction of ulnar drift during Silastic metacarpophalangeal joint arthroplasty. J Hand Surg Br 16:61, 1991

Swanson AB, Swanson GG, Leonard JB: Postoperative rehabilitation programs in flexible
implant arthroplasty of the digits. In Hunter JM, Mackin EJ, Callahan AD (eds):
Rehabilitation of the Hand: Surgery and Therapy. 4th Ed. Mosby, St. Louis, 1995

Swanson AB, Swanson GG, Winfield DC: The pronated index finger deformity in the
rheumatoid hand. Bull Hosp J Dis Orthop Inst 44:498, 1989

Utsinger P, Zuaifler N, Ehrlich G: Rheumatoid Arthritis Etiology, Diagnosis, and
Management. JB Lippincott, Philadelphia, 1989

Vahuanen V, Viljakka T: Silicone rubber implant arthroplasty of the metacarpophalangeal
joint in rheumatoid arthritis: a follow-up study of 32 patients. J Hand Surg Am 11:333,
1986

Proximal and Distal Interphalangeal Joint Arthroplasty

50

Lorie Theisen

Flexible implant arthroplasty may be indicated for the proximal interphalangeal (PIP) or the distal interphalangeal (DIP) joints of the digits. PIP or DIP joint arthroplasty is indicated in the presence of pain, stiffness, deformities, instability about a joint, and loss of cartilage. These findings may be sequelae of osteoarthritis, rheumatoid arthritis, or trauma (Fig. 50-1).

An acceptable alternative procedure to flexible implant arthroplasty of the distal joints is arthrodesis. The advantages and disadvantages of each procedure are weighed carefully by the surgeon. Because hand function is significantly limited by a decrease in range of motion (ROM) at the PIP joints, particularly of the ulnar fingers, arthroplasty of the PIP joint is often preferred over arthrodesis. Hand function is only minimally limited by a decrease in DIP joint ROM; therefore, arthrodesis is often preferred at the DIP joint. Arthroplasty of the DIP joint is indicated if ROM as well as pain relief is necessary. Surgical methods typically use a dorsal approach, although an anterior approach has also been described.[1]

DEFINITION

PIP or DIP arthroplasty is a surgical formation or reformation of the PIP or DIP joints with the use of Silastic or a soft tissue spacer.

SURGICAL PURPOSE

The surgical management of acquired or posttraumatic arthritis of the PIP or DIP joints can improve function and joint alignment. Two basic types of arthroplasty may be used: Silastic joint spacers or a soft tissue interpositional

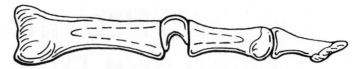

FIG. **50-1** Flexible implant arthroplasty of a proximal interphalangeal joint.

joint spacer. Relief of pain and improvement of joint motion is of primary importance in undertaking these operations.

TREATMENT GOALS

The usual postoperative treatment goals regarding wound healing, edema control, scar management, and activities of daily living (ADLs) function apply. The encapsulation process and associated rehabilitation principles described in postoperative guidelines for metacarpophalangeal (MCP) joint arthroplasty also apply (see Chapter 49). Specifically, after PIP arthroplasty of the ring and small fingers, the goal is pain-free active range of motion (AROM) to 70 degrees flexion and neutral extension. For the index and middle fingers, less flexion is acceptable. After DIP arthroplasty, the goal is 30 degrees flexion and neutral extension. Tendencies toward deformities (e.g., boutonniere, swan-neck) should be addressed. Finally, the surgeon should be contacted if there is any question regarding joint stability or progression of the mobilization phase of rehabilitation.

POSTOPERATIVE INDICATIONS/PRECAUTIONS FOR THERAPY

I.   Indications
    A. Rehabilitation is indicated after surgical reformation of a joint and surgical implant of a flexible Silastic spacer.
II. Precautions
    A. The initiation of the remobilization program depends on the stability of the joint. Consult the physician about the timing of the ROM exercise program.
    B. Additional surgical procedures, such as ligament repair, tendon repositioning or reconstruction, tenolysis, or volar plate release, may require adherence to additional rehabilitation principles and precautions.

POSTOPERATIVE THERAPY

I.   PIP arthroplasty
    A. For a preoperative stiff PIP joint requiring joint release procedures.
      1. 3 to 5 days postoperatively: Begin AROM of the PIP joint, avoiding any lateral deviation.
      2. Continuous static extension splinting (Fig. 50-2), except during exercise, is applied for 6 weeks postoperatively. Alternatively, dynamic PIP extension splinting with intermittent active flexion in the splint may be used.

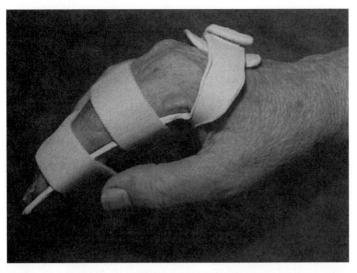

FIG. **50-2** A static proximal interphalangeal (PIP) extension splint may be used after arthroplasty for a stiff PIP joint.

> The dynamic splint should be designed to control lateral forces (Fig. 50-3).

3. Dynamic flexion splinting, to gain 70 degrees, may be initiated after consultation with the physician depending on joint stability. Care must be taken to avoid lateral forces from the splint (Fig. 50-4).

B. For a boutonniere deformity, the main goal is to maintain PIP extension and DIP flexion.

1. Maintain static protective splinting with the PIP joint in full extension and continue for 3 to 6 weeks postoperatively.

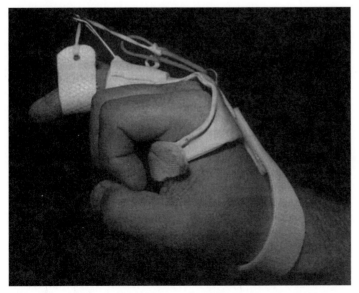

FIG. **50-3** Dynamic proximal interphalangeal (PIP) extension splint may be used after arthroplasty for a stiff PIP joint.

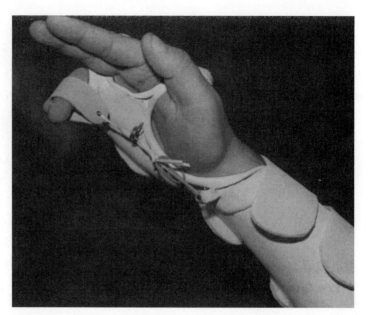

FIG. **50-4** Dynamic flexion splinting may be used to improve proximal interphalangeal flexion.

Active DIP flexion exercises with the PIP joint extended are indicated to maintain the oblique retinacular ligament length.

2. 10 to 14 days postoperatively: Active flexion and extension exercises of the PIP joint are initiated with the MCP joint in extension. Static extension splinting continues with intermittent AROM exercises up to 10 weeks postoperatively.

3. Buddy taping may be indicated to protect against lateral forces (Fig. 50-5).

C. For a swan-neck deformity, the main goal during the postoperative rehabilitation process is to maintain PIP flexion and DIP extension.

1. 0 to 10 days postoperatively: Continue digital static extension splinting with the PIP in 10 to 20 degrees flexion and DIP in full extension.

2. 10 to 14 days postoperatively: Initiate AROM. During exercise, maintain 10 degrees of flexion at the PIP joint and avoid extreme flexion at the DIP joint.

3. 14 days postoperatively: Initiate gentle passive exercises in flexion and extension.[1]

II. DIP arthroplasty

A. Without Kirschner wire fixation

1. PIP and DIP joints are in extension for 2 weeks.

2. The DIP joint is held in extension for an additional 2 weeks, and PIP joint AROM is initiated.

3. Gentle active flexion is initiated after this immobilization period. Flexion should be performed gradually, progressing to 30 degrees flexion. Night extension splinting continues for an additional 6 weeks.

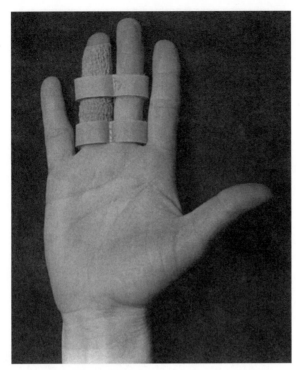

FIG. 50-5 Buddy tapes may be used after arthroplasty for a boutonniere deformity.

      B. With K-wire fixation
          1. 3 to 4 weeks of fixation is followed by an additional 4 weeks of DIP extension splinting (Fig. 50-6).
          2. Gradual AROM to 30 degrees of DIP flexion may be initiated after removal of fixation.
          3. Night DIP extension splinting continues for another 2 months.
III. Function: When orthopedic condition allows, address ADL function. In particular, address those activities that involve grasping of objects smaller than 2 inches in diameter (e.g., toothbrush, kitchen utensils, screwdriver) and those requiring fine motor tasks (e.g., buttoning, zippering). Strength testing and treatment is initiated after restrictions from the surgeon have been lifted.

POSTOPERATIVE COMPLICATIONS

  I.   PIP arthroplasty
      A. Flexor tendon adherence
      B. Malalignment
      C. Extension lag
      D. Fracture of the prosthesis
      E. Synovitis/injection
  II.   DIP arthroplasty
      A. Malalignment
      B. Mallet finger
      C. Fracture of the prosthesis
      D. Synovitis/injection

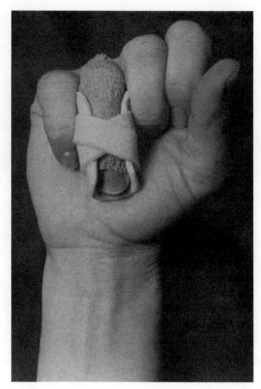

FIG. 50-6 Distal interphalangeal (DIP) extension splinting after K-wire immobilization for a DIP arthroplasty.

EVALUATION TIMELINE

I. PIP arthroplasty
    A. 3 to 5 days postoperatively: initial AROM measurements
    B. Reevaluation every 2 weeks thereafter
    C. Strength measurements after joint stability is well established and with physician approval. A modified blood pressure cuff may be indicated for strength testing.[2]
II. DIP arthroplasty
    A. 4 weeks postoperatively: initial AROM measurements
    B. Reevaluation every 2 weeks thereafter
    C. Strength measurements after joint stability is well established and with physician approval. A modified blood pressure cuff for testing may be indicated.

OUTCOMES

Research on outcomes after interphalangeal arthroplasty is limited. The few long-term follow-up research articles state that the overall goals are to relieve pain as well as to provide ROM, stability, flexibility, and function. Takigawa and associates[3] reviewed postoperative results of 48 patients an average of 6.5 years after PIP implant arthroplasty. They discovered that the joint replacement did provide pain relief but did not improve motion or correct deformities. Early results of osseointegrated endoprosthesis PIP joint arthroplasty suggest significant improvement in ROM along with good pain relief.[4] Moller and co-workers[4] report an average of 56 degrees PIP joint flexion and an 11-degree extensor lag at 27 months after the procedure. Further investigation of this prosthesis is needed, particularly regarding the durability of the implant. Researchers noted the incidence of both fracture and deformation of the implant. Outcome research in this area should lead toward development of an implant that provides durability, ROM, and pain relief for optimal hand function in those patients with PIP dysfunction.

REFERENCES

1. Lin H, Wyrick J, Stern P: Proximal interphalangeal joint silicone replacement arthroplasty: clinical results using an anterior approach. J Hand Surg Am 20:123-132, 1995
2. Swanson AB, Swanson-deGroot G, Leonard J: Post-operative rehabilitation programs in flexible implant arthroplasty of the digits. In Hunter J: Rehabilitation of the Hand. 2nd Ed. Mosby, St. Louis, 1984, pp. 133, 142
3. Takigawa S, Meletiou S, Sauerbier M, et al.: Long-term assessment of Swanson implant arthroplasty in the proximal interphalangeal joint of the hand. J Hand Surg Am 29:785-795, 2004
4. Moller K, Sollerman C, Geijer M, et al.: Early results with osseointegrated proximal interphalangeal joint prosthesis. J Hand Surg Am 24:267-274, 1999

SUGGESTED READINGS

Adamson GJ, Gellman H, Brumfield RH, et al.: Flexible implant resection arthroplasty of the proximal interphalangeal joint in patients with systemic inflammatory arthritis. J Hand Surg Am 19:3, 1994

Beckenbaugh RD, Linscheid RL: Arthroplasty in the hand and wrist. In Green DP (ed): Operative Hand Surgery. 2nd Ed. Vol. 1. Churchill Livingstone, New York, 1988, p. 167

Hage J, Yoe E: Proximal interphalangeal joint silicone arthroplasty for posttramatic arthritis. J Hand Surg 24:73-77, 1999

Melvin JL: Evaluation of muscle strength. In Melvin JL (ed): Rheumatic Disease: Occupational Therapy and Rehabilitation. 2nd Ed. FA Davis, Philadelphia, 1982, p. 291

Milford L: Reconstruction after injury. In Crenshaw AH (ed): Campbell's Operative Orthopaedics. 6th Ed. Vol. 1. Mosby, St. Louis, 1987, p. 283

Pellegrini D, Burton R: Osteoarthritis of the proximal interphalangeal joint of the hand: arthroplasty or fusion? J Hand Surg Am 15:194, 1990

Smith RJ: Balance of kinetics of the fingers under normal pathological conditions. Clin Orthop 104:92, 1974

Stanly JK, Evans RA: What are the long term follow up results of Silastic metacarpophalangeal and proximal interphalangeal joint replacements. Br J Rheumatol 31:839, 1992

Stephens J, Pratt N, Parks B: The reliability and validity of the Tekdyne hand dynamometer: part I. J Hand Ther 9:10, 1996

Stephens J, Pratt N, Michlovitz S: The reliability and validity of the Tekdyne hand dynamometer: part II. J Hand Ther 9:18, 1996

Swanson AB, Maupin BK, Gajjar NV: Flexible implant arthroplasty in the proximal interphalangeal joint of the hand. J Hand Surg Am 10:796, 1985

Swanson AB, Swanson-deGroot G: Treatment considerations and resource materials for flexible (silicone) implant arthroplasty. Orthopedic Research Dept., Blodgett Memorial Medical Center, Grand Rapids, MI, 1987

Swanson AB, Swanson-deGroot G: Postoperative Care for Patients with Silastic Finger Joint Implants (Swanson Design). 4th Ed. Orthopaedic Reconstructive Surgeons P.C., Grand Rapids, MI, 1985

Swanson AB, Swanson-deGroot G, Leonard JB: Postoperative rehabilitation programs in flexible implant arthroplasty of the digits. In Hunter JM, Macklin EJ, Callahan AD (eds): Rehabilitation of the Hand: Surgery and Therapy. 4th Ed. Mosby, St. Louis, 1995, p. 1351

Zimmerman NB, Shuhey PV, Clark GL, et al.: Silicone interpositional arthroplasty of the distal interphalangeal joint. J Hand Surg Am 14:882, 1989

Small Joint Arthrodesis of the Hand

51

Lauren Adelsberger

The goal of any arthrodesis is to achieve painless solid fusion in the proper position in reasonable time. Pain, instability, and joint deformity are possible indications for arthrodesis.[1] Conditions such as acute trauma, posttraumatic arthrosis, primary osteoarthrosis, rheumatoid or psoriatic arthritis, chronic deep infections, and fixed contractures may require arthrodesis.[2,3]

The position of the fused joint is important for functional results. There is no desirable position in which to fuse the finger metacarpophalangeal (MCP) joint secondary to the loss of grasp function or the ability to flatten the hand. The index finger MCP joint is most commonly considered for fusion to restore the stability needed for lateral pinch. Recommended positions for MCP fusion are at 25, 30, 35, and 40 degrees of flexion (for the index finger through small finger, respectively).[4] The proximal interphalangeal (PIP) joints commonly are fused at 40, 45, 50, and 55 degrees of flexion (index finger through small finger, respectively).[4] The distal interphalangeal (DIP) joint is fused for the benefit of pinch and grasp at 0 to 20 degrees of flexion.[4,5]

The thumb interphalangeal (IP) and MCP joints are fused at 10 to 30 degrees of flexion for the benefit of pinch. The position of thumb carpometacarpal (CMC) joint fusion varies. Ideally, moderate abduction and opposition are needed to allow pinch with the index and middle fingers. Typically, the first metacarpal is fused at 20 to 40 degrees flexion and 35 to 45 degrees palmar abduction, and the thumb is pronated.[4,6]

Potential surgical techniques include Kirschner wires, intraosseous wiring, mini-plate fixation, tension bands, Herbert screws, and A-O compression screws (Figs. 51-1 through 51-3). Each technique has its own advantages and disadvantages (Table 51-1).

DEFINITION

Joint fusion is surgical immobilization of a joint in a functional/optimal position.

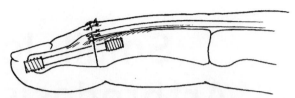

FIG. 51-1 Screw fixation of distal interphalangeal joint. (From Trumble TE: Principles of Hand Surgery and Therapy. WB Saunders, St. Louis, 2000, p. 424.)

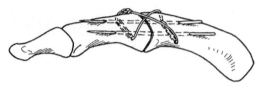

FIG. 51-2 Tension band arthrodesis of the proximal interphalangeal joint. (From Trumble TE: Principles of Hand Surgery and Therapy. WB Saunders, St. Louis, 2000, p. 425.)

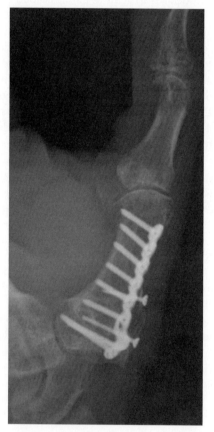

FIG. 51-3 Carpometacarpal arthrodesis using a vascularized node graft for the radius and a mini-condylar plate. (From Trumble TE: Principles of Hand Surgery and Therapy. WB Saunders, St. Louis, 2000, p. 432.)

TABLE **51-1** Options for Fixation Methods for Small Joint Arthrodesis

Type	Advantages	Disadvantages
Kirschner wires	Technically easy	Crossed wires may distract
		Pin tract infections
Herbert screw	Rigid fixation	Technically demanding
Tension band	Rigid fixation	Increased soft tissue disruption
Intraosseous band	Rigid fixation	Increased soft tissue disruption
External fixation		Pin tract infections
		Devices interfere with adjacent fingers
Plate fixation	Rigid fixation	Increased soft tissue disruption
Intramedullary bone peg	Increased bony apposition	Technically demanding

From Divelbiss BJ, Baratz ME: Hand Clin 15:335-345, 1999.

TREATMENT AND SURGICAL PURPOSE

Small joint arthrodeses of the hand vary in indication and goals, depending on the joint involved and the goals of the patient. The range of motion (ROM) of a joint in its fully functional state is proportional to the loss of function the patient will sustain after fusion of that joint. In the four ulnarmost digits, the CMC and DIP joints can readily be fused with little negative impact on the function of the hand. Conversely, PIP and MP joint fusions result in significant morbidity and are undertaken as a salvage option if restoration or arthroplasty is impossible.

Thumb MCP and IP joint fusions result in minimal functional disability, whereas CMC fusions limit thumb motion significantly.

The joints are surgically approached dorsally to limit the impact on flexor tendons. Positions are selected to minimize the morbidity of motion loss (discussed earlier). The joints are prepared by removing cartilage and subchondral bone to reach soft medullary bone on both ends. The bone fusion angle is obtained either by making sharp-angled cuts with a saw or by fashioning the opposing ends into a "cup and cone" configuration. Great care is taken to prevent rotation or angulation of the digit. The most common fixation methods are K-wires alone, wires with tension banding, and screw fixation. The more rigid the fixation, the more likely it is that a successful fusion will be achieved. Rigid fixation also permits the patient and therapist to pursue active range of motion (AROM) at adjacent joints sooner.

TREATMENT GOALS

   I.   Protect fusion.
  II.   Control edema.
 III.   Minimize pain.
  IV.   Maintain uninvolved joint ROM.
   V.   Reach maximal level of function.

POSTOPERATIVE INDICATIONS/PRECAUTIONS FOR THERAPY

   I.   Indications for therapy
        A. Uninvolved joint stiffness
        B. Education needs: uninvolved joint ROM, strengthening, edema control

C. Edema management

D. Protective splinting

II.   Precautions for therapy

A. Solid arthrodesis needs to be achieved before splint discharge and strengthening are undertaken.

B. Special care is required with DIP ROM after PIP joint arthrodesis. PIP splint axial loading and torque across the PIP joint during DIP ROM may delay DIP ROM.[7]

POSTOPERATIVE COMPLICATIONS

I.   Nonunion

II.   Infections

III. Hardware failure

IV.   Cold intolerance

POSTOPERATIVE THERAPY

I.   Finger MCP, PIP, DIP; thumb IP and MCP: Usually one to three visits are needed.

A. Therapy day 1: Educate the patient on the following.

1. Edema management

2. Application of the appropriate splint. A gutter splint is used for finger DIP and PIP fusion (Fig. 51-4). A static hand-based splint that includes the MCP joint is used only for finger MCP fusion. Thumb spica is used for thumb MCP fusion. A protective splint is used for thumb IP fusion.

3. Scar management with elastomer, gel sheeting, and/or scar massage

4. Uninvolved joint AROM and passive range of motion (PROM). Special care must be taken with DIP joint ROM after PIP arthrodesis; discuss this with the physician.

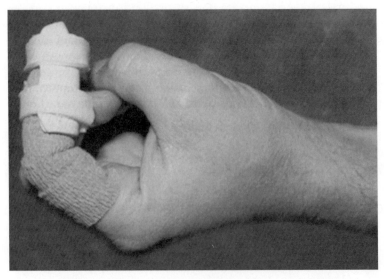

FIG. **51-4** Protective splint for distal interphalangeal arthrodesis.

B. 6 to 8 weeks postoperatively: consult physician
  1. Discontinue splinting when healing permits.
  2. Educate patient on progressive strengthening.
II.   Thumb CMC: The number of visits varies.
  A. Therapy day 1: Educate the patient on the following.
    1. Edema management
    2. Application of thumb spica splint
    3. Scar management with elastomer, gel sheeting, and/or scar massage
    4. Uninvolved joint AROM and PROM
  B. 6 to 8 weeks postoperatively: consult physician
    1. Discontinue splinting.
    2. Initiate strengthening after fusion is achieved.

EVALUATION TIMELINE

I.   Finger MCP, PIP, DIP; thumb IP and MCP: Usually one to three visits are needed.
  A. Visit 1
    1. Evaluate edema.
    2. Evaluate splinting needs.
    3. Evaluate AROM and PROM of uninvolved joints.
    4. Evaluate scar.
II.   Thumb CMC: Number of visits varies.
  A. Visit 1
    1. Evaluate edema.
    2. Evaluate splinting needs.
    3. Evaluate AROM and PROM of uninvolved joints.
    4. Evaluate scar management needs.
  B. 6 to 8 weeks postoperatively, with physician approval
    1. Evaluate grip and pinch strength.

OUTCOMES

I.   Finger fusions: outcomes vary according to the technique used (Table 51-2).
  A. Union is achieved typically at 7 to 12 weeks.
  B. Union rates typically are 90% to 100%.

TABLE **51-2** Outcomes

Procedure and Joints	Fusion Rate (%)	Time to Union (wk)	Reference
Herbert screw (DIP and thumb IP)	93	10	El-Hadidi and Al-Kdah[1]
Tension band (PIP, thumb IP, and MCP)	100	7-8 for trauma, 12-14 for rheumatoid or psoriatic arthritis	Stahl and Rozen[3]
Kirschner wires and intraosseous wires, "pepper-pot" technique (PIP, DIP, MCP, and thumb IP)	90	7	Shanker et al.[2]
Plate and screw (CMC)	92	Not stated	Forseth and Stern[8]
Cannulated screw (thumb MCP)	100	7 clinically, 10 radiologically	Messer et al.[9]
Power staple (CMC)	93	8	Lisanti et al.[10]
K-wires and bone graft (CMC)	100	7	Ishida and Ikuta[5]

CMC, Carpometacarpal; *DIP,* distal interphalangeal; *IP,* interphalangeal; *MCP,* metacarpophalangeal; *PIP,* proximal interphalangeal.

II.   Thumb fusions: outcomes vary according to the technique used (see Table 51-2).
A. Union is achieved typically at 8 to 12 weeks.
B. Union rates are 90% to 100%.
C. Grip strength after CMC fusion is 97% compared with the uninvolved side.
D. Pinch strength after CMC fusion is 79% of the uninvolved side.

REFERENCES

1. El-Hadidi S, Al-Kdah H: Distal interphalangeal joint arthrodesis with Herbert screw. Hand Surg 8:21-24, 2003
2. Shanker HK, Johnstone AJ, Rizzo L, et al.: "Pepper-pot" arthrodesis of the small joints of the hand: our experience in 68 cases. J Hand Surg Br 27:430-432, 2002
3. Stahl S, Rozen N: Tension-band arthrodesis of the small joints of the hand. Orthopedics 24:981-983, 2001
4. Divelbiss BJ, Baratz ME: The role of arthroplasty and arthrodesis following trauma to the upper extremity. Hand Clin 15:335-345, 1999
5. Ishida O, Ikuta Y: Trapeziometacarpal joint arthrodesis for the treatment of arthrosis. Scand J Plast Reconstr Hand Surg 34:245-248, 2000
6. Klimo GM, Verma RB, Baratz ME: The treatment of trapeziometacarpal arthritis with arthrodesis. Hand Clin 17:261-270, 2001
7. Estes JP, Bochenek C, Fasler P: Osteoarthritis of the fingers. J Hand Ther 13:108-123, 2000
8. Forseth MJ, Stern PJ: Complications of trapeziometacarpal arthrodesis using plate and screw fixation. J Hand Surg Am 28:342-345, 2003
9. Messer TM, Nagle DJ, Martinez AG: Thumb metacarpophalangeal joint arthrodesis using the AO 3.0-mm cannulated screw: surgical technique. J Hand Surg Am 27:910-912, 2002
10. Lisanti M, Rosati M, Spagnolli G, et al.: Trapeziometacarpal joint arthrodesis for osteoarthritis. J Hand Surg Br 22:576-579, 1997

SUGGESTED READINGS

Damen A, Dijkstra T, van der Lei B, et al.: Long-term results of arthrodesis of the carpometacarpal joint of the thumb. Scand J Plast Reconstr Surg Hand Surg 35:407-413, 2001

Lamas GC, Proubasta I, Escriba I, et al.: Distal interphalangeal joint arthrodesis: treatment with Herbert screw. J South Orthop Assoc 12:154-159, 2003

Lourie G: The role and implementation of metacarpophalangeal joint fusion and capsulodesis: indications and treatment alternatives. Hand Clin 17:255-260, 2001

Mackin EJ, Callahan AD, Skirven TM, et al. (eds): Hunter-Mackin-Callahan Rehabilitation of the Hand and Upper Extremity. 5th Ed. Mosby, St. Louis, 2002

Mader K, Gausepohl T, Wolfgarten B, et al.: Percutaneous arthrodesis of small joints in the hand. J Bone Joint Surg Br 85:1016-1018, 2003

Trumble T: Principles of Hand Surgery and Therapy. WB Saunders, St. Louis, 2000

PART **EIGHT**

Special Topics

Conservative Management of Arthritis

52

Paige E. Kurtz

Therapists can offer nonoperative treatment of arthritis that can be beneficial for patients in both earlier and more advanced stages, to decrease pain and inflammation while increasing range of motion (ROM), joint stability, and functional use of the hand and upper extremity. A comprehensive program may include education in disease process and joint protection, use of adaptive equipment and techniques, energy conservation, ROM/exercise program, pain-reducing modalities, and splinting. Nonoperative (or conservative) management of arthritis may give patients enhanced control over their disease and symptoms, decreasing the incidence of deforming and destabilizing forces on joints and increasing functional use of the hands when incorporated into activities of daily living (ADLs).

DEFINITION

Arthritis is characterized by destruction of joint surfaces that results in pain, stiffness, and inflammation in the joints. This is most commonly caused by inflammatory processes, as seen in rheumatoid arthritis (RA), or by degenerative changes from overuse or trauma, as seen in osteoarthritis (OA). Systemic lupus erythematosus, scleroderma, and psoriatic arthritis are three less common forms of arthritis that share some characteristics with RA. Most of the treatment principles outlined in this chapter may be applied to these forms as well.

TREATMENT GOALS

A conservative arthritis management program should achieve the following.
  I.   Decrease pain and inflammation.
 II.   Decrease destabilizing and destructive forces on joints.
III.   Increase or preserve ROM as appropriate. Avoid fixed contractures and deformities.
 IV.   Increase function.
  V.   Slow the progression of the disease.

TREATMENT PURPOSE

To provide a nonsurgical option in treatment to decrease pain and other symptoms while increasing functional use of the involved extremity.

NONOPERATIVE INDICATIONS/PRECAUTIONS FOR THERAPY

I. Indications
    A. RA, OA, or other forms of arthritis affecting/limiting lifestyle
    B. Early- or later-stage arthritis
    C. Principles of conservative management may also be applied postoperatively to maximize benefits of surgery and to protect joints after surgery.
II. Precautions
    A. Patient compliance and motivation are necessary, with an understanding of the rationale for treatment and an ability to follow through with the home program.
    B. Some interventions should be limited if an active inflammatory process is present.
    C. The benefits of nonoperative treatment are limited if the disease has progressed to joint destruction, severe imbalance, or dislocation.

CONSERVATIVE MANAGEMENT AND TREATMENT OF ARTHRITIS

I. Evaluation: a variety of evaluations are available to the therapist. A thorough evaluation should include the following.
    A. History of problem, including onset, history of flares and remissions, medications, and other past treatment interventions
    B. Joints affected, considering the entire body, with emphasis on the hands, pain levels, and fluctuations
    C. Relevant ROM measurements, strength, sensibility, and dexterity. Intrinsic tightness should be evaluated in the patient with RA. Look for and note laxity or hypermobility, stiffness or ankylosis, subluxation, deviation, or crepitus at wrist and finger joints.
        1. Common deformities seen in RA include laxity of the volar plate at the metacarpophalangeal (MCP) joint and at the proximal interphalangeal (PIP) joint. The latter often leads to swan-neck deformity, seen as PIP hyperextension with distal interphalangeal (DIP) flexion. The MCP joint in the rheumatoid hand is also subject to subluxation and ulnar deviation, which may be measured or noted on evaluation.
        2. Patients with OA or RA may present with boutonniere deformity, in which the PIP joint maintains a flexion contracture and the DIP joint hyperextends. In the patient with OA, osteophytes may limit PIP extension, resulting in PIP flexion resembling a boutonniere deformity, or they may create lateral deviation at the PIP.

3. Nerve compression may be present due to structural and neurovascular changes in the extremities. Evaluate via Semmes-Weinstein monofilaments.

D. ADL/functional evaluation: It is important to identify areas in which function is limited due to arthritis, because functional improvement is one of the primary goals of conservative management.

1. Consider common bilateral and daily activities, including the following.
   a. Cooking and eating (e.g., cutting food and serving; stirring; opening jars, boxes, and cans)
   b. Dressing (e.g., buttoning, tying shoes, managing zippers, pulling up pants)
   c. Self-care (e.g., grooming, brushing teeth, hair care, applying makeup, toileting, bathing)
   d. Other ADLs (e.g., writing, driving, opening doors, using a key, fastening seatbelt)
   e. Leisure activities (e.g., sewing, reading, gardening, golfing, playing cards)

2. Consider whether the individual is modifying the way in which an activity is performed (awkwardly, or with abnormal motions, or using incorrect postures). It may be helpful to use a functional test to observe the hands in use, observing any substitution patterns, awkward positions, or other problems.

3. Consider whether an increase in pain accompanies or immediately follows performance of an activity.

4. Consider whether it takes longer than normal to complete an activity.

5. Use observation of the patient or an evaluation tool such as the Disability of the Arm, Shoulder, and Hand (DASH) questionnaire, the Arthritis Hand Function Test (AHFT), or the Patient-Rated Wrist/Hand Evaluation (PRWHE).[1-4]

II. Splinting: Appropriate splints can help to immobilize and rest a joint to decrease pain and inflammation. Splints protect against destabilizing forces on joints and promote proper positioning and alignment. The therapist should consider the patient's needs with regard to splinting, as well as probable use and wear circumstances. This may affect the choice of materials used and whether a prefabricated or a custom-molded splint is more appropriate. Often, the patient with RA can tolerate soft splints better than thermoplastic ones, due to medication-related skin conditions. Functional use and potential compliance should also be considered, because splints are helpful only if they are used. Several examples are noted here for reference; however, there are many different splinting options and approaches that may be used.

A. RA
   1. Antideviation (Fig. 52-1)
   2. Swan-neck, figure of 8 (Fig. 52-2)
   3. Resting (Fig. 52-3)
   4. Finger gutter splint
   5. Wrist support

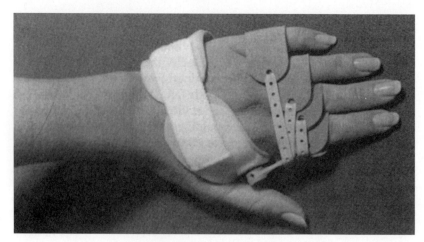

FIG. **52-1** Rolyan hand-based arthritis splint.

B. OA
 1. Carpometacarpal (CMC) support (Figs. 52-4 through 52-6)
 2. Thumb spica
 3. Finger splint for DIP or PIP
III. Patient education: Patients are often more compliant with home
 programs if education is provided in lay terms about their arthritis,
 including disease process, effect on joints, and how it progresses.
 A variety of publications are available for patient education from
 sources such as the American Occupational Therapy Association
 and the Arthritis Foundation. Other resources are noted at the end
 of this chapter.
IV. Joint protection: Principles of joint protection should be taught
 as part of a comprehensive nonoperative arthritis management
 program. Activity and ADL analysis can help to tailor specific

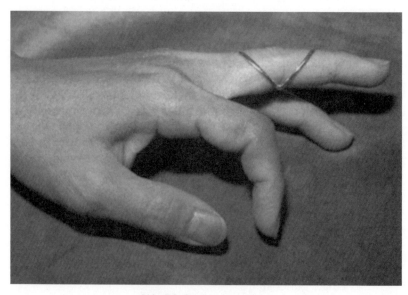

FIG. **52-2** Tripoint splint.

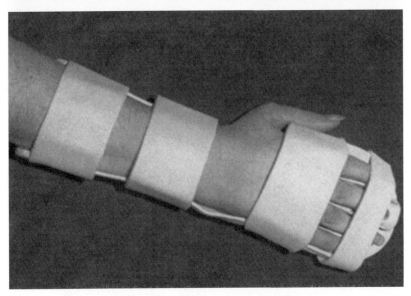

FIG. **52-3** Static positioning splint.

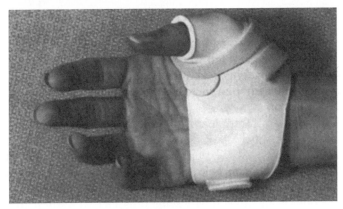

FIG. **52-4** Thumb carpometacarpal splint.

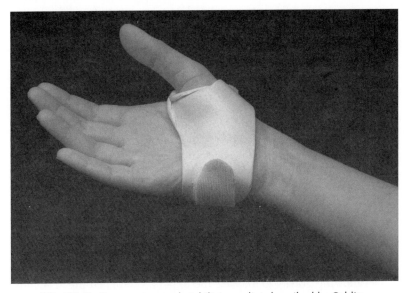

FIG. **52-5** Carpometacarpal stabilizing splint described by Colditz.

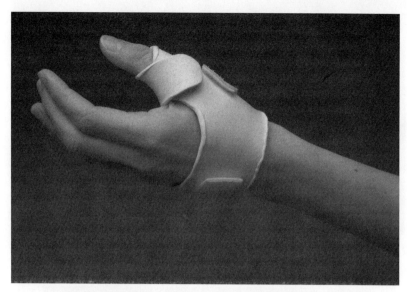

FIG. **52-6** Dorsal carpometacarpal splint.

modifications to the patient's uses and lifestyle. General considerations are as follows.

A. Respect pain: Pain is not always observed during an activity; therefore, it is important to develop an awareness of pain with consideration of any activities completed during the previous 12 to 24 hours. Any pain that lingers more than 2 hours after completion of an activity should also be considered a warning that the activity should be modified or eliminated. Exercises should be modified if flare symptoms such as warmth and redness are noted around the joints.[5]

B. Use larger/stronger joints and muscles if possible: Protect the more delicate joints of the hands by using larger, more proximal muscles and joints to perform ADLs. For example, using the forearm or shoulder to push open a door protects the fingers. Groceries should be carried in paper bags, with the hip and arm supporting the bag's weight, rather than stressing finger joints by carrying plastic bags with a hook grasp.

C. Avoid tight or prolonged grasp: Build up or purchase utensils, tools, and pens with enlarged handles. Modify door handles with levers. Use adaptive equipment for assistance in opening jars, turning knobs, turning keys, and so forth. Change grasp as often as able to avoid static positioning.

D. Avoid positions of deformity: Help the patient understand which movements and positions contribute to his or her pain and instability patterns, and then help find ways to avoid or modify these while remaining functional. In RA, this often means activities that push the fingers ulnarly, such as wringing a washcloth, pinching against the index finger, opening jar lids, or lifting objects such as a pot of coffee with the forearm in neutral, allowing gravity to displace the fingers. Prolonged intrinsic-plus positioning, as in needlework, may lead to tightening of the intrinsic musculature. With OA, stress to the unstable CMC joint is often a problem, and static lateral/key pinch should be avoided. Tripod or three-point pinches stress the PIP and DIP joints. Good body mechanics should be taught and encouraged for all joints.

    E. Avoid remaining in one position for a long period. This can increase joint pain, strain, and instability. Stop, take a break, and move around as often as possible, preferably every 20 minutes.

    F. Balance rest and activity: Plan ahead so that rest breaks can be scheduled. Do not start activities that cannot be stopped if needed. Use energy conservation techniques and labor-saving devices (see later discussion). Use stress management and relaxation techniques. Stress, rest, and sleep can have a significant effect on symptoms.

V. Pain management: Modalities should be used in the clinical setting and incorporated into a home program.

    A. Heat increases circulation and decreases joint stiffness and soreness, which makes it useful in decreasing morning stiffness and as a passive "warm-up" before exercise. It may include application of paraffin, moist heat packs, fluidotherapy, or warm water soaks. Caution: inflammation may be exacerbated by heat if used inappropriately. Make certain that clear parameters are explained with regard to appropriate temperatures and application times before adding this modality to a home program. Heat should be discontinued or used cautiously if significant inflammation or swelling is present.

    B. Cold is best used for reducing pain when there is acute inflammation—for example, during a "flare" or after "overdoing it," particularly if the joints feel warm to the touch. Although cold is good at reducing pain and edema, it may lead to increased stiffness in the joints of the hand. Soaking the hands in cool or cold water may be more comfortable than using ice packs.

    C. Contrast baths help to "pump" out swelling and pain and are soothing to joints. Techniques and protocols vary, but all methods alternate between warm and cold water soaks.

VI. ROM and exercise: The goals of a program for ROM and strength in the arthritis patient center on maximizing pain-free *functional* ROM, rather than normal ROM, and increasing functional strength and cardiovascular wellness. Studies have shown that weight-bearing and ROM exercises have beneficial nutritional effects on articular cartilage, but this has not been well studied in the hands and upper extremities. Daily use of the hands generally provides more than enough "exercise" to the joints themselves.

    A. ROM exercises are prescribed to maximize the pain-free arc of active and active-assisted ROM in joints without overstressing them. Often this means limiting exercises to the midrange of available motion, or going just to the end range. Appropriate ROM and strengthening exercises should be taught, practiced in the clinical setting, and included in a home program. Aggressive stretching should be avoided. Leonard[5] described a series of stretches that she has found successful for maximizing ROM in patients with inflammatory disorders.

        1. Intrinsic stretching: One of the hallmark deformities in the rheumatoid hand is intrinsic tightness, coupled with MCP joint ulnar deviation. Gentle stretching of the ulnar

intrinsic muscles of the hand may help to reduce these problems.

B. Strengthening: The status and stability of affected and surrounding joints should be taken into consideration when prescribing resistive exercises for the patient with upper extremity arthritis. Consider the effect of joint compressive forces and joint biomechanics. "Dosing" of exercise with the arthritic patient should be done with care to offer enough resistance to increase strength but not too much resistance, which could increase joint stress and instability. Strengthening may be less traumatic to joints if isometric contractions are used in different positions, avoiding close-packed and compressive positions at end range. Description of all the specifics of strengthening considerations and protocols are beyond the scope of this chapter. The reader is referred to Lockard's article in the *Journal of Hand Therapy* for specific considerations that apply to patients with OA and RA.[6]

1. A CMC protocol for degenerative joint disease, described by Poole and Pellegrini in the *Journal of Hand Therapy*,[7] involves strengthening of the thenar musculature, abductor pollicis longus, and extensor pollicis longus and may help to minimize the deforming forces that lead to the adduction deformity commonly seen with degenerative joint disease at this joint.

C. Aerobic exercise: Low- to moderate-impact exercise benefits the entire body by increasing general health and well-being, as well as increasing cardiovascular fitness, strengthening muscles, and helping to stabilize joints. Water or pool-based therapeutic exercise is a good option because of its non–weight-bearing nature, and heated pools are available in many areas.

VII. Energy conservation: Basic principles should be incorporated into patient education. These include sitting when able, planning ahead (e.g., gathering needed items together before starting an activity), organizing work and storage spaces for accessibility, keeping most commonly used items within easy access, resting during activities as able, and using timesavers such as prepared foods.

VIII. Adaptive equipment and techniques go "hand in hand" with joint protection techniques. Many different catalogs offer equipment, and many stores now carry items such as modified cooking, writing, or cutting utensils. Problem ADLs identified during evaluation should be discussed. Changes in techniques may be suggested and tried out, and use of modified equipment should be practiced in the clinical setting whenever possible. Patients are often resistant to use of adaptive devices, seeing them as crutches rather than as enablers that increase independence. Sometimes trial use of an item helps an individual see its positive side. Examples of commonly available adaptive equipment include zipper pulls, enlarged handle knives and other utensils, large grip pens, jar openers, and key holder/turners. A number of hand therapy vendors offer these items through their catalogs, and an increasing number of retailers also offer specialty equipment.

FURTHER INFORMATION

I. Arthritis Foundation: PO Box 7669, Atlanta, GA 30357-0669. 1-800-283-7800. http://www.arthritis.org (accessed April 4, 2005). Offers educational information, programs, and publications.

II. American Occupational Therapy Association: 4720 Montgomery Lane, P.O. Box 31220, Bethesda, MD 20824-1220. http://www.AOTA.org (accessed April 4, 2005).

III. Useful web sites

A. American Society for Surgery of the Hand: http://www.ASSH.org (accessed April 4, 2005).

B. Arthritis Foundation: http://www.arthritis.org (accessed April 4, 2005).

C. American Occupational Therapy Association: http://www.AOTA.org (accessed April 4, 2005).

D. Medline Plus, a service of the National Institutes of Health: http://www.nlm.nih.gov/medlineplus/arthritis.html

REFERENCES

1. MacDermid JC, Richards RS, Donner A, et al.: Responsiveness of the Short Form-36, Disability of the Arm, Shoulder, and Hand Questionnaire, Patient-Rated Wrist Evaluation, and physical impairment measurements in evaluating recovery after a distal radius fracture. J Hand Surg Am 25:330-340, 2000

2. MacDermid JC, Tottenham V: Responsiveness of the Disability of the Arm, Shoulder, and Hand (DASH) and Patient-Rated Wrist/Hand Evaluation (PRWHE) in evaluating change after therapy. J Hand Ther 17:18-23, 2004

3. Backman C, Mackie H, Harris J: Arthritis hand function test: development of a standardized assessment tool. Occup J Res 11:245-256, 1997

4. Hudak PL, Amadio PC, Bombardier C, for the Upper Extremity Collaborative Group (UECG): Development of an upper extremity outcome measure: the DASH (Disabilities of the Arm, Shoulder and Hand). Am J Ind Med 29:602-608, 1996

5. Leonard JB: Joint protection for inflammatory disorders. In Hunter JM, Mackin EJ, Callahan AD (eds): Rehabilitation of the Hand: Surgery and Therapy. 4th Ed. Mosby, St. Louis, 1995, p. 1377

6. Lockard MA: Exercise for the patient with upper quadrant osteoarthritis. J Hand Ther 2:175-183, 2000

7. Poole JA, Pellegrini VD: Arthritis of the thumb basal joint complex. J Hand Ther 2:91-107, 2000

SUGGESTED READINGS

Fries J: Arthritis: A Complete Guide to Understanding Your Arthritis. 3rd Ed. Addison-Wesley, Reading, MA, 1990

Journal of Hand Therapy. Special edition on Osteoarthritis and Traumatic Arthritis of the Upper Quadrant. 2:77-192, 2000

Leonard JB: Joint protection for inflammatory disorders. In Hunter JM, Mackin EJ, Callahan AD (eds): Rehabilitation of the Hand: Surgery and Therapy. 4th Ed. Mosby, St. Louis, 1995, p. 1377

Lorig K, Fries J: The Arthritis Helpbook. 3rd Ed. Addison-Wesley, Reading, MA, 1990

Meenan RF, Mason JH, Anderson JJ, et al.: AIMS2: the content and properties of the revised and expanded Arthritis Impact Measurement Scales health status questionnaire. Arthritis Rheum 35:1, 1992

Melvin JL: Osteoarthritis: Caring for Your Hands. The American Occupational Therapy Association, Bethesda, MD, 1995

Moskowitz R: Osteoarthritis. Arthritis Foundation, Atlanta, 1990

Ouellette EA: The rheumatoid hand: orthotics as preventative. Semin Arthritis Rheum 21:65, 1991

Palmieri TJ, Grand FM, Hay EL, et al.: Treatment of osteoarthritis in the hand and wrist: nonoperative treatment. Hand Clin 3:371, 1987

Philips CA: Therapist's management of patients with rheumatoid arthritis. In Hunter JM, Mackin EJ, Callahan AD (eds): Rehabilitation of the Hand: Surgery and Therapy. 4th Ed. Mosby, St. Louis, 1995, p. 1345

Pinals R, Zvaifler N: Rheumatoid Arthritis. Arthritis Foundation, Atlanta, 1990

Semble EL: Rheumatoid arthritis: new approaches for its evaluation and management. Arch Phys Med Rehabil 76:190, 1995

Slonaker D, Feinberg J, Holsten D: Taking Care: Protecting Your Joints and Saving Energy. Arthritis Foundation, Atlanta, 1986

Sutej PG, Handler NM: Current principles of rehabilitation for patients with rheumatoid arthritis. Clin Orthop 265:116, 1991

Congenital Differences in the Hand and Upper Extremity

53

Cheryl S. Lutz and Scott H. Kozin

Congenital differences are challenging for the physician and therapist. Many conditions require coordinated care to maximize hand use, function, and independence. Ample time is required to explain to the family the "congenital difference" and proposed treatment plan. Certain conditions are associated with other systemic or musculoskeletal problems. These differences require accurate diagnosis and appropriate referral to pediatric specialists and geneticists.

This chapter covers numerous congenital differences that require coordinated care by physician and therapist. Treatment goals are highlighted for each entity to ensure realistic expectations. Indications, guidelines, and techniques for nonoperative, operative, and postoperative management are detailed. Classification schemes are selected that provide guidelines for nonoperative and operative treatment.

GENERAL GUIDELINES FOR THERAPY EVALUATION

I. History
II. Physical examination
   A. Detailed active range of motion (AROM) and passive range of motion (PROM) evaluation of entire upper extremity
   B. Upper extremity manual muscle testing
   C. Strength assessment: pinch and grip measurements
   D. Observation of prehensile patterns
   E. Sensory evaluation
      1. Threshold and functional two-point discrimination for older patients

2. O'Riain wrinkle test or ninhydrin test for younger children.
*Note: For younger children, assessment may be limited to observation of prehensile patterns and preferences during play activities and PROM evaluation

III.   Functional assessment
   A. Achievement of developmental milestones (may be affected by upper extremity anomalies, such as decreased ability for rolling, crawling, or using arms to transition from supine to sitting to standing position)
   B. Observation of upper extremity positioning during functional activities (e.g., use of compensatory patterns for hand-to-mouth activities or perineal activities)
   C. Detailed description of adaptive techniques or equipment used
   D. WeeFIM, Functional Independence Measure, or other age-appropriate measure of independence level[1,2]

IV.   Client/family goals for therapy (e.g., Canadian Occupational Performance Measure[3,4])

TRANSVERSE DEFICIENCY

Definition

Transverse deficiency, also known as **congenital amputation,** is defined by the last remaining bone segment. Transverse deficiencies are usually unilateral and sporadic in occurrence. Amputation through the proximal third of the forearm (short below-elbow) is the most common level of upper extremity transverse deficiency (Fig. 53-1). The diagnosis should not be

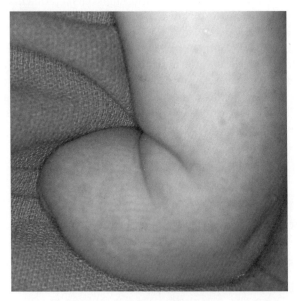

FIG. **53-1** A 1-year-old child with short below-elbow transverse deficiency. (Courtesy Shriners Hospital for Children, Philadelphia, Penn.)

confused with amniotic band or constriction band syndrome, which is a result of entrapment of developing embryonic tissue by fetal lining. This syndrome can manifest as amputation of a part and most commonly affects the digits of the hands or feet. The diagnosis of constriction band syndrome requires the presence of a constriction band either in the involved extremity or elsewhere.[5]

Clinical Presentation

The anatomy of the affected limb is normal up to the level of the amputation. The end of the residual limb usually is well padded, and in individuals with transverse deficiency below the elbow it may possess rudimentary nubbins or dimples.

Classification

Transverse deficiencies are classified by the last remaining bone segment (Fig. 53-2).

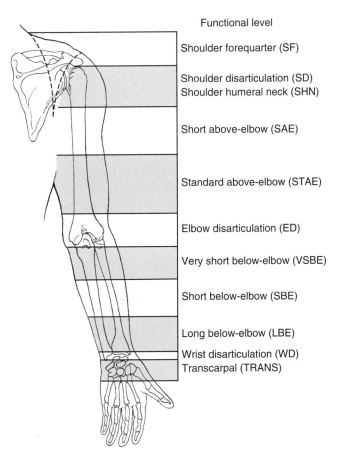

Functional level

Shoulder forequarter (SF)

Shoulder disarticulation (SD)
Shoulder humeral neck (SHN)

Short above-elbow (SAE)

Standard above-elbow (STAE)

Elbow disarticulation (ED)

Very short below-elbow (VSBE)

Short below-elbow (SBE)

Long below-elbow (LBE)

Wrist disarticulation (WD)
Transcarpal (TRANS)

FIG. **53-2** Levels of transverse deficiency.

Treatment Goals

I. Promote independent function.
II. Maintain integrity of distal residual limb.

Nonoperative Management

I. Therapy
   A. Assessment
      1. AROM/PROM
      2. Upper extremity manual muscle testing (observation of overall strength for infants and young children)
      3. Achievement of developmental milestones
   B. Prosthetic fitting
      1. Passive prosthesis: Once independent sitting is achieved (approximately 6 months); provides equal limb length for gross motor activity and accommodates child to wearing a socket
      2. Active body-powered prosthesis: approximately 15 months to 2 years; componentry varies by level of amputation, typically beginning with a voluntary opening terminal device; provides functional assist for bimanual activities
      3. Myoelectric prosthesis: 3 to 5 years; fitting based on individual need; in-depth discussion regarding patient/family goals is essential to determine appropriateness of myoelectric versus body-powered prosthesis
II. Nonoperative complications
   A. Skin breakdown
   B. Rejection of prosthesis

Operative Management

Surgery typically is not indicated for short below-elbow transverse deficiencies. Occasionally, a small bone spicule or rudimentary nubbins may irritate the residual limb. Excision of the bone or removal of the nubbins can alleviate this problem. The use of limb lengthening for transverse deficiencies is controversial. For individuals with below-elbow amputations, increased limb length will not eliminate the need for a prosthesis, and the expected gains do not outweigh the risks.

Postoperative Management

Therapy needs are minimal after removal of bone spicules or nubbins and may include scar management and desensitization in preparation for prosthetic fitting.

Outcomes

Children with unilateral short below-elbow deficiency function well with or without their prosthesis. This high level of function makes acceptance more difficult to achieve. Individuals with proximal deficiencies have increased reliance on their prostheses for daily function and are more apt to be consistent users.

RADIAL DEFICIENCY

Definition

Radial deficiency is a complex congenital anomaly that primarily affects the preaxial side of the limb and can be associated with systemic conditions (Table 53-1).[6-9] The reported incidence varies between 1:55,000 and 1:100,000 live births.[10] Radial deficiency is bilateral in 50% of cases and is slightly more common in males than females (3:2). The incidence of radial deficiency within the same family is small, ranging from 5% to 10% of reported cases.

Clinical Presentation

The wrist and hand are positioned in radial deviation and develop a perpendicular relationship with the forearm over time (Fig. 53-3).[11,12] This awkward position further shortens the limb and places the extrinsic flexors and extensors at a mechanical disadvantage. The articulation between the carpus and ulna is not a normal joint.[7] The fingers are often stiff and slender, with limited motion at the metacarpophalangeal (MCP) and interphalangeal (IP) joints. The preaxial index and long fingers are more affected than are the postaxial ring and small digits. Thumb anomalies affect the extrinsic and intrinsic muscles and are directly related to the degree of thumb hypoplasia.

Classification

The classification of radial deficiency is based on the degree of absence (Table 53-2).

Treatment Goals

I. Correct the radial deviation of the wrist.
II. Balance the wrist on the forearm.
III. Maintain wrist and finger motion.
IV. Promote growth of the forearm.
V. Improve the function of the extremity.

TABLE **53-1** Syndromes Associated with Radial Deficiency

Syndrome	Characteristics
Holt-Oram	Heart defects, most commonly cardiac septal defects
TAR	Thrombocytopenia absent radius syndrome. Thrombocytopenia present at birth, improves over time.
VACTERL	Vertebral abnormalities, anal atresia, cardiac abnormalities, tracheoesophageal fistula, esophageal atresia, renal defects, radial dysplasia, lower limb abnormalities
Fanconi's anemia	Aplastic anemia not present at birth, develops at about 6 years of life. Fatal without bone marrow transplantation. A chromosomal challenge test is now available for early diagnosis.

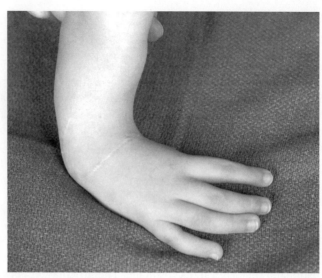

FIG. **53-3** A 3-year-old child with right radial deficiency. (Courtesy Shriners Hospital for Children, Philadelphia, Penn.)

Nonoperative Management

I. Indications
    A. Type I through type IV radial deficiency accompanied by any of the following
        1. Radial deviation positioning of wrist
        2. Potential concomitant digit, wrist, forearm, elbow, and shoulder limitations in ROM, strength, and joint stability
    B. Functional limitations may be present with increased severity of anomaly or bilateral involvement
II. Precautions
    A. Presence of concomitant systemic concerns necessitating initial medical attention

TABLE **53-2** Classification of Radial Deficiency

Type	Radiographic Findings	Clinical Features
I—Short radius	Distal radial epiphysis delayed in appearance Normal proximal radial epiphysis Mild shortening of radius without bowing	Minor radial deviation of the hand Thumb hypoplasia is the prominent clinical feature requiring treatment
II—Hypoplastic	Distal and proximal epiphyses present Abnormal growth in both epiphyses Ulna thickened, shortened, and bowed	Miniature radius Moderate radial deviation of the hand
III—Partial absence	Partial absence (distal, middle, proximal) of radius Absence of distal one-third to two-thirds of radius most common Ulna thickened, shortened, and bowed	Severe radial deviation of the hand
IV—Total absence	No radius present Ulna thickened, shortened, and bowed	Most common type Severe radial deviation of the hand

Adapted from Bayne LG, Klug MS: J Hand Surg Am 12:169-179, 1987.
Because ossification of the radius is delayed in radial deficiency, the differentiation between total and partial absence (types III and IV) cannot be established until approximately 3 years of age.
Centralization is required for types II, III, and IV.

B. Skin integrity
1. Age-related factors
2. Presence of pterygium—careful monitoring of webbed region is essential, because treatment may affect underlying abnormal blood vessels, nerves, and muscular structures
C. Joint instability
D. Extreme discomfort
III. Therapy
A. AROM/PROM
B. Splinting
1. Considerations
a. Infants and younger children: Line thermoplastic splints with moleskin or other soft padding or fabricate splints out of soft material such as neoprene
b. Increased prominence of ulnar styloid needs soft tissue protection
2. Daytime: Wrist support: Goal is to minimize radial deviation and maximize flexor posturing (Fig. 53-4).
3. Nighttime
a. Resting hand splint: Goal is to minimize IP flexion contractures and/or radial drift of digits, if present.
b. Wrist support
c. Elbow splint: Goal is to improve elbow flexion or extension contracture, if present.
4. Note: For individuals with severe Type II through Type IV deficiency, splinting often is accompanied by surgical intervention. For individuals with moderate to severe deficiency, wrist splinting typically is recommended until skeletal maturity is achieved.
C. Functional training to minimize radial deviation positioning

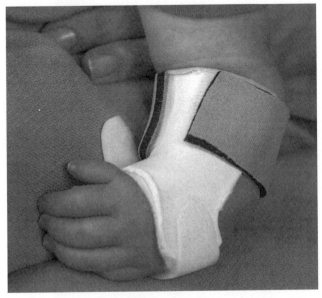

FIG. **53-4** A 6-month-old child with left radial deficiency treated with static progressive splinting. (Courtesy Shriners Hospital for Children, Philadelphia, Penn.)

IV. Nonoperative complications
   A. Skin breakdown
   B. Decreased compliance with home exercises or splint-wearing schedule
   C. Progressive functional deficits with age and growth of limb

Operative Management

Centralization is usually performed at about 1 year of age. Before central-ization, a radiograph is obtained with the wrist positioned over the distal ulna in the anteroposterior lateral projection. If the radiograph reveals reduction of the carpus onto the end of the ulna, then centralization is per-formed. If reduction is not evident, preliminary soft tissue distraction is required to stretch the taught radial structures.[13] We prefer to obtain dis-traction with the use of a pediatric Ilizarov device (Richards, Memphis, Tenn), which allows multiplanar correction (Fig. 53-5). The external fixator is applied using standard principles, with one ring positioned perpendicu-lar over the hand and wrist and one ring perpendicular to the distal forearm. The goal in soft tissue lengthening is to realign the carpus in the sagittal and coronal planes. The distal and proximal external fixator rings become more parallel as the correction progresses toward completion. After soft tissue correction has been obtained, the fixator is retained for an additional month to allow soft tissue equilibrium. Subsequently, the fixator is removed and formal centralization is performed at the same setting.

Centralization is performed with slight overcorrection of the carpus, imbrication of the ulnar capsule, dermodesis of the redundant ulnar skin, and tendon transfer to rebalance the wrist. An ulnar approach is adequate for exposure and centralization, because the radial skin and soft tissues have been elongated by stretching or application of the Ilizarov device. An ulnar bow greater than 20 to 30 degrees requires osteotomy for straightening.

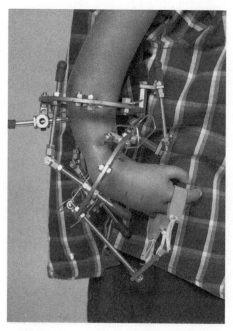

FIG. **53-5** A 4-year-old boy with right radial deficiency treated with pediatric Ilizarov fixator and finger slings. (Courtesy Shriners Hospital for Children, Philadelphia, Penn.)

Bony fixation is accomplished with longitudinal wires, which are also used to maintain the alignment of the wrist.

Postoperative Management

Centralization/Radialization

I.   Postoperative indications: types II through IV radial deficiency necessitating realignment of the distal ulna on the carpus
II. Postoperative precautions
     A. Avoid PROM wrist flexion/extension for 12 weeks after surgery or until longitudinal wires are removed.
     B. Avoid weight-bearing (e.g., crutches, cane) on upper limb extremity for 12 weeks after surgery.
III. Postoperative therapy
     A. The upper extremity is immobilized in a cast for 6 to 8 weeks; then a wrist support fabricated to maintain the postoperative position of the wrist. (The splint is worn at all times for 4 weeks, then decrease to nights only until skeletal maturity is achieved.)
     B. AROM/PROM for digits and any other affected joints until full available AROM is achieved.
     C. 12 weeks postoperatively: Initiate wrist strengthening after removal of longitudinal wires.
IV. Postoperative complications
     A. Recurrence of radial deviation deformity
     B. Loss of wrist mobility
     C. Decreased growth of forearm secondary to growth plate injury
     D. Early migration/irritation of surgically placed longitudinal wire, necessitating removal

Distraction Histiogenesis (Ilizarov)

I.   Postoperative indications (after application of external fixator): severe types II through IV radial deficiency necessitating external fixator application for soft tissue correction
II. Postoperative precautions (after application of external fixator)
     A. Avoid contact sports
     B. Showers only (no bathing)
     C. No swimming in untreated water (e.g., lake, ocean)
III. Postoperative therapy (after application of external fixator)
     A. Week 1
        1. Splints
           a. Resting hand splint to maintain digit extension for nighttime (may be fabricated intraoperatively for a younger child with limited tolerance)
           b. Finger sling attachments to distal ring of fixator for daytime use to maintain digit extension while promoting functional use of hand (see Fig. 53-5)
           c. Elbow extension or flexion splint as indicated (static progressive splinting)
        2. AROM/PROM of all uninvolved joints
        3. Edema control
        4. Instruction in pin site care

5. Physician instruction in distraction schedule
   a. Distractions may be initiated immediately postoperatively at a rate of 1 mm/day; the physician may alter the distraction rate based on the patient's ROM status and comfort level.
   b. Therapist should educate family in monitoring distractions
      (1) Provide pictorial handout of distraction instructions
      (2) Therapist may apply nail polish to distraction bars as a marker for the family to track whether distractions are progressing in the correct direction
      (3) Family may measure and record distance between rings daily
B. Patient returns to clinic every other week for reassessment
   1. Radiographs to assess limb alignment
   2. Monitor AROM/PROM of uninvolved joints (stiff digits and elbow flexion contractures are common and are exacerbated by underlying abnormal anatomy)
   3. Reassess functional status and provide adaptive techniques or devices as needed.
   4. Adjust splints, because distractions may alter fit of splint (avoid strapping or splinting close to pin sites, because this may cause irritation)
C. Once the appropriate correction is completed, the fixator is maintained for 3 to 4 weeks to allow soft tissue equilibrium.
D. After surgical removal of fixator and formal centralization, longitudinal wires may be placed to maintain positioning.
E. 10 to 12 weeks after fixator removal, wires are removed and a volar wrist support is fabricated.
   1. Splint is initially worn at all times except for exercise.
   2. Patient is instructed in AROM for wrist flexion/extension as well as continued AROM/PROM of all uninvolved joints.
   3. Continued education regarding pattern of functional use with affected arm. (Emphasize importance of decreasing active radial deviation and use of ulnar digits for function, because this may increase the potential for recurrence)
F. Patient is weaned from daytime splint wear over a period of 6 weeks.
G. Nighttime wrist splinting is recommended until skeletal maturity is achieved.
H. Patient is monitored in clinic with periodic radiographical examination.
IV. Postoperative complications
A. Recurrence of radial deviation deformity
B. Pin tract infection
C. Fracture through pin site
D. Pin loosening
E. Joint contracture

Outcomes

Centralization remains the principal procedure to realign the carpus onto the distal ulna, and it is indicated for types II, III, and IV radial deficiencies.[11,12,14,15] Numerous technical modifications have been proposed to preserve alignment over time. However, no method reliably and permanently corrects the radial deviation, balances the wrist, and allows continued growth of the forearm. Currently, maintenance of the carpus on the end of the ulna without sacrificing wrist mobility or stunting forearm growth remains a daunting task.[14,16] Some degree of recurrence is common. Factors related to recurrence include incomplete centralization, deficient motors to balance the wrist, and the natural tendency for radial deviation during eating and grooming activities.

ARTHROGRYPOSIS

Definition

Arthrogryposis, or **arthrogryposis multiplex congenital,** is a syndrome of joint contractures that are present at birth and are nonprogressive.[17] There are multiple forms of arthrogryposis that vary in presentation, severity, and number of involved joints. The joint contractures are secondary to lack of motion during fetal life. Multiple processes can lead to lack of fetal limb movement, including muscle abnormalities, nerve anomalies, a restricted intrauterine space, vascular insufficiency, and maternal illness. The precise cause often remains unknown.

There are a multitude of syndromes and genetic conditions that have features of arthrogryposis. A classic example is Freeman-Sheldon syndrome (also known as "whistling face syndrome"), an autosomal dominant condition that affects the hands and feet and includes a characteristic facial appearance.[18-20]

Classification

The degree of joint involvement may be minimal, moderate, or severe. Presentation can be divided into three groups: group I, distal hand involvement only; group II, diffuse upper extremity involvement; and group III, upper and lower extremity involvement.

Clinical Presentation

Amyoplasia (classic arthrogryposis) is the most common form; it is characterized by symmetrical positioning of the limbs.[21] Posturing of the upper extremities includes shoulder adduction and internal rotation, elbow extension, forearm pronation, wrist flexion, and hand ulnar deviation (Fig. 53-6). The digits are postured in flexion and stiff. The contracted clasped thumb is a common finding in arthrogryposis and creates functional difficulties with activities of daily living.[22,23] Additional clinical features include waxy skin devoid of skin creases, considerable muscle wasting, and a paucity of subcutaneous tissue.

Treatment Goals

I.   Individualize treatment to each child's needs.
II. Achieve independent function for self-feeding and perineal care.

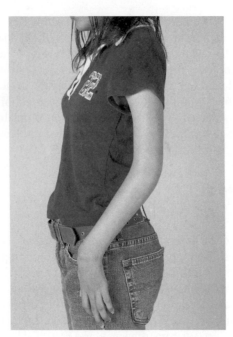

FIG. 53-6 A 12-year-old child with arthrogryposis and typical left upper extremity posturing. (Courtesy Shriners Hospital for Children, Philadelphia, Penn.)

Nonoperative Management

I.   Indications
     A. Arthrogryposis accompanied by one or more of the following
        1. Thumb limitations, ranging from narrow web space to contracted clasped thumb
        2. Potential concomitant digit, wrist, forearm, elbow, and shoulder limitations in ROM, strength, and joint stability
     B. Functional limitations may be present with increased severity of anomaly
II. Therapy
     A. AROM/PROM: Maximize PROM of all involved joints for potential future surgical interventions.
     B. Splinting
        1. To increase function (e.g., wrist support to decrease flexor positioning and increase grip strength)
        2. To promote/maintain PROM of joints
        3. Static progressive splinting and serial casting provide a low load and prolonged stretch and may be efficacious for diminishing contractures.
        4. Passive stretching, serial casting, and orthotics are most efficacious in distal arthrogryposis.[24]
        5. Joint contractures in amyoplasia are often rigid and refractory to therapy.
     C. Training in adaptive techniques

Operative Management

The timing of surgery is controversial.[23,25] Surgery is usually recommended before school age (i.e., at 4 or 5 years of age) to minimize compensatory movements and maximize mainstream school function.[23] Older children

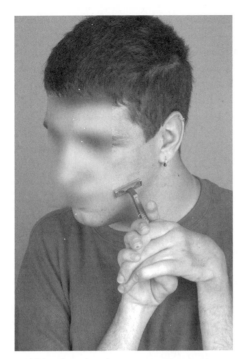

FIG. **53-7** An 18-year-old man with arthrogryposis shaving; he is using compensatory maneuvers and bimanual grasp. (Courtesy Shriners Hospital for Children, Philadelphia, Penn.)

develop adaptive maneuvers to accomplish many daily tasks (Fig. 53-7). These positions may appear awkward, but they are functional for many activities.[21] For example, tasks are often accomplished with bimanual limb use that involves scissoring of the upper limbs for grasp. Surgical recommendations must consider these adaptive maneuvers and ensure no degradation in function after surgery.

Elbow

The elbow is often the most problematic joint in children with arthrogryposis. Lack of flexion is the common impairment, and it prohibits hand-to-mouth function and many daily tasks. The first goal is restoration of passive motion. Adequate passive flexion allows the hand to be placed near the face using a tabletop or adaptive equipment. Early efforts to restore passive elbow flexion are critical and should be emphasized in therapy. Recalcitrant lack of elbow flexion requires consideration for surgical release via lengthening of the triceps and posterior capsular release.[23]

A secondary goal is restoration of active elbow flexion.[26] Potential donor muscles for elbow flexorplasty include the pectoralis major, latissimus dorsi, triceps, and flexor-pronator mass. The selection of donor is more difficult in children with arthrogryposis compared with other conditions, and the results are less predictable.[26] Detailed discussion of elbow flexorplasty and postoperative therapy is beyond the scope of this chapter.

Forearm and Wrist

Forearm pronation and wrist flexion coupled with ulnar deviation are the typical contractures (see Fig. 53-6). The wrist position is difficult to overcome via therapy because of the rigid volar structures (fascia, ligaments, tendons, skin) and the deficiency in active wrist extension. Persistent wrist flexion recalcitrant to therapy may require surgery to better position the wrist for function. Our preferred procedure is osteotomy of the midcarpus to correct both the wrist flexion and ulnar deviation. The tight forearm fascia is incised, and the wrist flexor muscles and tendons are incised or lengthened. A transverse dorsal incision and a biplanar wedge resection of the midcarpus are performed to straighten and position the wrist in slight extension. The wedge is wider at the radial and dorsal margins. The wedge of bone is removed from the midcarpus, and the osteotomy site is coapted by wrist extension. Interosseous sutures and/or percutaneous longitudinal wires are used for fixation. The extensor carpi ulnaris tendon is transferred to the radial wrist extensors.

Thumb and Fingers

The fingers are stiff, fixed in flexion, and positioned in ulnar deviation. Mild to moderate digital overlap may be present during flexion. Considerable stiffness and/or angulation creates a functional limitation. Surgical treatment to restore supple finger motion is unsuccessful.

The contracted clasped thumb may be released from the palm to enhance prehension and function (Fig. 53-8). This involves release of the taught palmar skin and adjacent structures. The skin deficit is covered by a rotation flap from the index finger. The extensor pollicis longus (EPL) is inspected for integrity and position. The EPL is often intact but malpositioned over the MCP joint. The EPL is then repositioned over the MCP joint and rerouted over the first compartment to augment thumb extension. In children with marked EPL hypoplasia, a tendon transfer (e.g., extensor indicis proprius, extensor digiti quinti) is used to increase thumb extension.

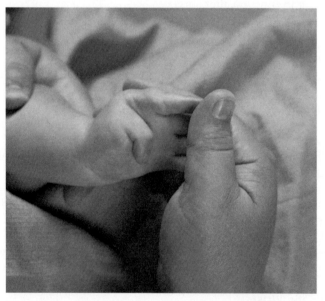

FIG. **53-8** A 9-month-old child with left contracted clasped thumb, typical of arthrogryposis. (Courtesy Shriners Hospital for Children, Philadelphia, Penn.)

Postoperative Management

Triceps Lengthening and Posterior Capsule Release

I.   Postoperative indications: persistent elbow extension contracture necessitating surgical intervention
II. Postoperative precautions
     A. Avoid PROM elbow flexion beyond maximum obtained at surgery for 6 weeks after surgery
III. Postoperative therapy
     A. Splinting
        1. The upper extremity is casted in elbow flexion of at least 90 degrees for 3 weeks.
        2. After cast removal, a posterior elbow splint is fabricated at 90 degrees flexion.
           a. Child is weaned from splint during day over period of 3 weeks.
           b. Splint is worn at night until 12 weeks after surgery.
     B. AROM/PROM
        1. Encourage use of PROM elbow flexion for functional activities (e.g., leaning forearm on table and bending trunk forward to achieve passive elbow flexion for hand-to-mouth activity)
     C. Edema control
     D. Scar management

Midcarpal Dorsal Wedge Osteotomy and Wrist Extension Tendon Transfer

I.   Postoperative indications: wrist flexion and ulnar deviation contracture necessitating bony and soft tissue correction
II. Postoperative precautions
     A. Avoid PROM wrist flexion and ulnar/radial deviation for 12 weeks after surgery.
III. Postoperative therapy
     A. Splinting
        1. The upper extremity is immobilized in a long arm cast for 6 weeks.
        2. At the time of cast removal, longitudinal wires are removed.
        3. A volar wrist support is fabricated with wrist in extension (degree of extension achieved varies after surgery, goal is to avoid tension on transfer)
           a. Child is weaned from splint during day over period of 3 weeks.
           b. Splint is worn at night until 12 weeks after surgery.
     B. AROM wrist extension tendon transfer initiated at time of cast removal
     C. AROM/PROM of all other affected joints
     D. Edema control
     E. Scar management to minimize adhesions and hypertrophy of scars
     F. Functional training

Contracted Clasped Thumb

I. Postoperative indications: contracted clasped thumb with skin deficiency and limited thumb extension necessitating surgical correction

II. Postoperative precautions
  A. Avoid PROM into thumb flexion if tendon transfer was performed for thumb extension

III. Postoperative therapy
  A. Splinting
    1. Casting for 4 to 6 weeks with longitudinal wire placed in thumb to maintain position
    2. After removal of cast and longitudinal wire, a thumb spica splint is fabricated for use at all times except during bathing, exercise, and play.
    3. Wean child from splint in day over period of 6 weeks.
    4. Continue use of night splint for 12 weeks.
  B. AROM/PROM
  C. Edema control
  D. Scar management

IV. Postoperative complications
  A. Decreased AROM/PROM of thumb

Outcomes

Early splinting and serial casting result in a rather unpredictable change in motion. Distal arthrogryposis responds better than does amyoplasia.[24] Operative intervention results in objective and subjective improvement in 75% of cases.[22] The outcome is related to the degree of contracture and the age of the patient. A tendon transfer for elbow flexion yields a variable increase in motion, depending on the quality of the donor muscle and the amount of preoperative passive motion.[26]

HYPOPLASTIC THUMB

Definition

Thumb hypoplasia occurs in varying grades and most commonly is part of radial deficiency.

Classification

The underdeveloped thumb has been classified into five types. The type of condition guides treatment recommendations (Table 53-3).[27-29]

Clinical Presentation

Severe thumb hypoplasia (types III through V) is readily apparent (Fig. 53-9). The main distinction between a thumb that can be reconstructed and a thumb that requires ablation is the presence or absence of a carpometacarpal (CMC) joint. A stable CMC joint provides a foundation for thumb reconstruction. An absent CMC joint negates the possibility of thumb reconstruction and is best treated by ablation and pollicization.

TABLE **53-3** Classification of Thumb Deficiency

Type	Findings	Treatment
I	Minor generalized hypoplasia	Augmentation
II	Absence of intrinsic thenar muscles	Opponensplasty
	First web space narrowing	First-web release
	Ulnar collateral ligament (UCL) insufficiency	UCL reconstruction
III	Similar findings as in type II plus:	IIIA: Reconstruction
	Extrinsic muscle and tendon abnormalities	IIIB: Pollicization
	Skeletal deficiency	
	Carpometacarpal joint may be stable (IIIA)	
	or unstable (IIIB)	
IV	*Pouce flottant* or floating thumb	Pollicization
V	Absence	Pollicization

The clinical differentiation between types IIIA and IIIB may be difficult.[29] The child often helps discriminate between a type IIIA and a type IIIB deficiency during the development of pinch and grasp. A stable IIIB thumb is incorporated into routine use, whereas an unstable thumb is ignored as prehension develops between the index and long digits. In addition, the stable index finger tends to reposition itself by pronation and rotation out of the palm. Mild thumb hypoplasia (types I and II) is less obvious and

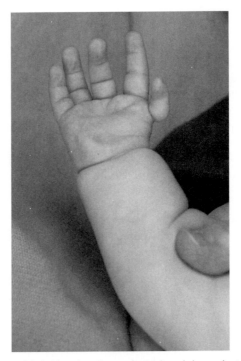

FIG. **53-9** A 1-year-old child with right grade IV thumb hypoplasia *(pouce flottant)*. (Courtesy Shriners Hospital for Children, Philadelphia, Penn.)

requires a careful examination. The first web space, MCP joint, and thenar muscles require examination for deficiencies and/or instability.

Treatment Goals

I.   Maximize function to a thumb with a stable CMC joint.
    A. Web space
    B. Joint stability
    C. Tendon transfers
II. Reconstruct a thumb via index finger pollicization in severe hypoplasia (*pouce flottant* or absence).

Nonoperative Management

I.   Indications: thumb hypoplasia types I through V that may require future surgical intervention
II. Therapy
    A. Splinting to maintain thumb web space for future surgical interventions
    B. AROM/PROM: Promote/maintain PROM of radial digit in types IIIB through V hypoplasia in preparation for future pollicization of digit
    C. Strengthening of potential donor muscles for future tendon transfer
    D. Functional training to promote use of thumb pinch versus scissor pinch (index to long digits) in types I through IIIA hypoplasia

Operative Management

Thumb Reconstruction

Thumb reconstruction in types II and IIIA requires addressing all elements of the hypoplasia. The adducted posture of the thumb is corrected with a web space deepening and reconstruction by Z-plasty or dorsal transposition flap. The MCP joint instability involves the ulnar side and is rectified by ulnar collateral ligament (UCL) reconstruction. Transfer of the abductor digiti quinti or a flexor digitorum superficialis (FDS) tendon for opposition augments the thenar hypoplasia. A type IIIA thumb may also require transfers to overcome the extrinsic musculotendinous abnormalities of the EPL and/or flexor pollicis longus tendons.

Pollicization

Pollicization is the procedure of choice for types IIIB, IV, and V hypoplasia (Fig. 53-10).[28-30] This procedure involves neurovascular transposition of the index digit to the thumb position with reconstruction of the intrinsic muscles of the thumb. The index digit must be rotated approximately 120 degrees to attain proper orientation of the new thumb. The index is shortened by removal of the diaphysis, and a metacarpal epiphysiodesis is performed to prevent excessive length of the thumb. The neurovascular bundles are carefully protected throughout the procedure. The first web space is reconstructed using skin flaps elevated from the hand and index finger. Joint and tendon reorganization is necessary for optimum pollicization (Table 53-4).

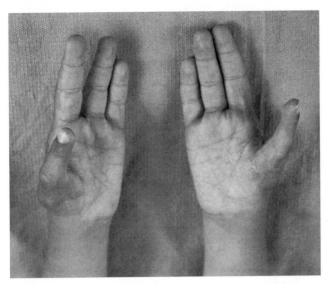

FIG. **53-10** A 5-year-old child after bilateral index finger pollicization. (Courtesy Shriners Hospital for Children, Philadelphia, Penn.)

Postoperative Management

Thumb Reconstruction

I. Postoperative indications: types I through IIIA hypoplasia necessitating surgical intervention
II. Postoperative precautions
    A. UCL repair: avoid PROM thumb palmar or radial abduction for 12 weeks after surgery
    B. Opponensplasty
        1. Avoid PROM radial abduction or thumb extension for 12 weeks after surgery
        2. Avoid resistive activities until 8 weeks after surgery
III. Postoperative therapy
    A. Z-plasty and skin flap: cast for 3 to 4 weeks, followed by whirlpool, wound care, and dressings until incisions are healed
    B. UCL repair
        1. Cast for 3 to 4 weeks, followed by splint for protection
        2. Wean from daytime splint at 6 to 8 weeks after surgery
        3. Continue splint at night until 12 weeks after surgery
        4. Initiate AROM for light play activities after cast removal

TABLE **53-4** Reconstruction during Pollicization

Index Structure	Pollicization Function
Distal interphalangeal joint	Interphalangeal joint
Proximal interphalangeal joint	Metacarpophalangeal joint
Metacarpophalangeal joint	Carpometacarpal joint
First dorsal interosseous	Abductor pollicis
First volar interosseous	Adductor pollicis
Extensor indicis proprius	Abductor pollicis longus
Extensor digitorum	Extensor pollicis longus

C. Opponensplasty
  1. Cast for 3 to 4 weeks, followed by splint for protection
  2. Wean from daytime splint at 6 to 8 weeks after surgery
  3. Continue splint at night until 12 weeks after surgery
  4. AROM of tendon transfer and place-hold exercises
      a. For FDS opponensplasty, complete isolated FDS glide with ring finger to obtain small objects (e.g., crayon, clay)
      b. Avoid use of compensatory thumb flexion during opposition exercises

IV. Postoperative complications
  A. Decreased AROM/PROM of thumb

Pollicization

I. Postoperative indications: types IIIB to V thumb hypoplasia necessitating surgical intervention
II. Postoperative precautions
  A. Avoid PROM of thumb CMC joint for 12 weeks after surgery.
  B. Avoid extreme AROM/PROM thumb extension/flexion for 12 weeks after surgery
  C. Avoid resistive activities for 12 weeks after surgery
III. Postoperative therapy
  A. Splinting
    1. Immobilize in long arm cast for 4 to 6 weeks
    2. Thumb spica splint
       a. Wean from day use at weeks 6 to 7
       b. Continue at night until 12 weeks after surgery
    3. Thumb taping: in medial direction, wrap self-adherent tape (e.g., Coban) around thumb CMC joint three times, then wrap tape around wrist three times in medial direction to position thumb into palmar abduction for enhanced tip-to-tip pinch
    4. Buddy-tape long and ring fingers to decrease scissor grasp
  B. AROM/PROM of thumb IP and MCP joints
  C. Play activities to promote thumb pinch for objects of various sizes and shapes
IV. Postoperative complications
  A. Decreased AROM/PROM of pollicized thumb
  B. Tendon adhesions

Outcomes

The results after pollicization are directly related to the status of the transposed index digit and surrounding musculature.[28,30,31] A mobile index finger transferred to the thumb position provides stability for grasp and mobility for pinch (see Fig. 53-10). In contrast, a stiff index finger provides a stable thumb for gross grasp but does not participate in pinch. For this reason, pollicization of the index finger provides good functional and cosmetic results in patients with isolated thumb hypoplasia and is less reliable in patients with radial forearm deficiencies. Early good results have been shown to persist into adulthood.[31]

SYNDACTYLY

Definition

Syndactyly is defined as an abnormal interconnection between adjacent digits and is described according to the magnitude and extent of the connection.

Clinical Presentation

Syndactyly is usually readily apparent on clinical examination. The interconnection between the digits is variable, and this guides the classification scheme. The web space between the middle and ring fingers is most frequently involved, followed by the ring/little finger interspace.[32-34] The thumb/index finger web space develops earlier than the fingers, and this is the least common pairing.

Classification

The interconnection may encompass the entire length of the adjacent digits *(complete)*, or it may be discontinued before the fingertip *(incomplete)* (Fig. 53-11). The syndactyly may involve only skin and fibrous tissue *(simple)*, or it may include bone *(complex)*. Syndactyly that occurs with other anomalies (e.g., Apert's syndrome, Poland's syndrome, macrodactyly) is referred to as *complicated* syndactyly. *Pseudosyndactyly* occurs in congenital constriction band syndrome and involves an intact web space with a distal connection between digits.[34] This is the result of intrauterine healing secondary to an insult from the amniotic bands and must be differentiated from true syndactyly.

Treatment Goals

   I.   Separate syndactyly to promote independent function of each digit.
  II.   Restore commissure using local flaps.
 III.   Reconstruct nail bed and fold using available tissue.
 IV.   Avoid separation of digits that function better as a unit than they would as individual digits with limited stability and/or motion.

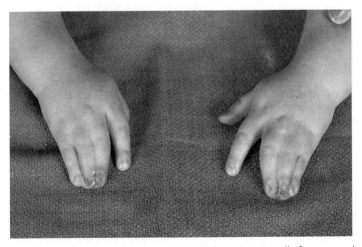

FIG. **53-11** A 1-year-old child with bilateral long/ring/small finger syndactyly. (Courtesy Shriners Hospital for Children, Philadelphia, Penn.)

Operative Management

Mild incomplete syndactyly that does not interfere with function does not require treatment. In contrast, simple syndactyly of any considerable degree warrants surgical reconstruction of the web space for improved function and appearance. The timing of release and technique of separation are both controversial, but certain guidelines should be followed[32,33] (Box 53-1).

Syndactyly release is performed with the child under general anesthesia.[34] The groin is preferred as the skin graft donor site for supplemental skin. A multitude of flap designs have been proposed for syndactyly release, and each surgeon appears to have his or her own preference.[32,33,35] A dorsal flap is favored for commissure reconstruction, because the skin is thin and easy to mobilize. On the palmar surface, the proximal transverse incision represents the level of commissure reconstruction. Subsequently, interdigitating zigzag dorsal and palmar flaps are constructed. The palmar flaps are mirror images of the dorsal flaps to optimize skin coverage after separation.

The flaps are elevated by sharp dissection, and the digits are separated from distal to proximal. The bifurcation between the common and proper neurovascular structures is identified during proximal dissection. A distal split of the digital nerves can easily be separated by microdissection. A distal arterial junction requires surgical decision-making, because ligation of a proper digital artery for acceptable commissure placement may be required. An absorbable suture is used for closure. The remaining skin defects are covered with a full-thickness skin graft.

BOX 53-1 Guidelines to Operative Release of Syndactyly

PRIORITY OF RELEASE

Border digits (thumb/index and ring/small finger web spaces) have marked differences in their respective lengths and should be separated within the first few months of life. Release prevents tethering of the longer digit, which results in a flexion contracture and rotational deformity.

In contrast, long/ring syndactyly combines digits of relatively equal lengths, and separation may be delayed until the child is older and the hand larger, facilitating surgical reconstruction. This delay is valuable, because surgery performed after 18 months of age has a lower incidence of complications and unsatisfactory results (e.g., web creep).[37]

TIMING

Surgical reconstruction should include only one side of an affected digit at a time, to avoid vascular compromise of the skin flaps or digit. Therefore, complete separation of three connected adjacent fingers requires staged surgical procedures.

COMMISSURE

A flap should be used to recreate the commissure; this avoids interdigital contracture and motion-limiting scar. Avoid skin grafting.

SKIN GRAFT

Release of a complete syndactyly results in a skin deficiency that requires grafting. The circumference of two digits separated is 22% greater than that of the same digits conjoined, and flap designs cannot mobilize additional skin.[32,33]

Proper postoperative dressings are an essential part of the operation. The dressings must apply compression across the skin graft sites and protect the separated digits. In young children, the compressive hand dressing must be reinforced by above-the-elbow plaster immobilization to prevent inadvertent removal.

Complex syndactyly often adjoins the soft tissue and bone along a portion or the entire length of the adjacent digits. This form of syndactyly is less common than simple syndactyly and is more challenging to treat, especially as the quantity of bony union increases.[34] Determination of the correct plane of cleavage, realignment of the joints, and management of the soft tissue are the difficult issues that require experience. The soft tissue coverage is more difficult and neurovascular anomalies are more frequent, complicating surgical reconstruction.

Postoperative Management

I. Postoperative indications: simple or complex syndactyly necessitating surgical intervention
II. Postoperative precautions
   A. Avoid inadvertent dressing removal.
III. Postoperative therapy
   A. Wound care: dressings are removed 2 weeks after surgery with gentle washing and application of nonadherent bandages until scabs desiccate and detach.
   B. Scar management is initiated after all areas closed; scar care products are used to prevent hypertrophic scarring.
   C. Encourage incorporation of affected hand for play activities.
IV. Postoperative complications
   A. Skin graft failure can occur as a result of hematoma, seroma, or loss of postoperative bandages. A very small amount is inconsequential and will heal by secondary intention. A substantial loss requires repeat grafting to prevent hypertrophic cicatrix formation.

Outcomes

Certain complications are predictable and should be discussed with the parent before surgery. One third of patients with isolated syndactyly and two thirds of those with complex or complicated syndactyly require additional surgery to correct web space creep or hypertrophic scar formation (Fig. 53-12).[32,34,36,37] Surgery for simple syndactyly results in a predictable outcome with adequate digital separation into individual digits with good function. In contrast, complex or complicated syndactyly cannot transform anomalous digits into normal counterparts. Underlying deficiencies in the bones, joints, and tendons prohibit such extraordinary results.

CAMPTODACTYLY

Definition

Camptodactyly is a painless flexion contracture of the proximal interphalangeal (PIP) joint that usually is gradually progressive (Fig. 53-13).[38] There is no intraarticular or periarticular swelling. The MCP and distal interphalangeal (DIP) joints are not affected, although they may develop compensatory deformities. The small finger is most commonly involved.[39,40] Other digits can be affected, although the incidence decreases toward the radial side of the hand.

Classification

Camptodactyly has been divided into three categories[39,41] (Table 53-5). A type I deformity is the most common form and becomes apparent

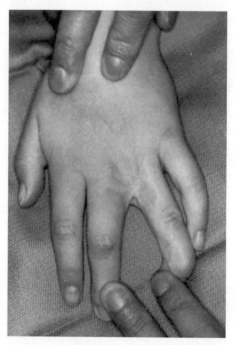

FIG. **53-12** An 8-year-old child status after syndactyly release with web creep. (Courtesy Shriners Hospital for Children, Philadelphia, Penn.)

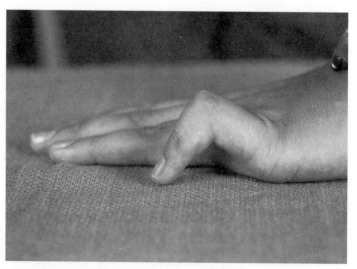

FIG. **53-13** A 15-year-old girl with left small finger camptodactyly. (Courtesy Shriners Hospital for Children, Philadelphia, Penn.)

TABLE **53-5** Types of Camptodactyly

Type	Manifestation	Description
I	Congenital	Apparent during infancy. Usually limited to the fifth finger.
II	Preadolescence	Develops between the ages of 7 and 11 years. Does not improve spontaneously and may progress to a severe flexion deformity of 90 degrees.
III	Syndromic	Multiple digits of both extremities are affected. Associated with a variety of syndromes, such as craniofacial disorders, short stature, and chromosomal abnormalities.

Adapted from Benson LS, Waters PM, Kamil NI, et al.: J Pediatr Orthop 14:814-819, 1994.

during infancy. The deformity is usually an isolated finding that is limited to the small finger. This "congenital" form affects males and females equally. A type II deformity has similar clinical features, although they are not apparent until preadolescence. This "acquired" form of camptodactyly develops between the ages of 7 and 11 years and affects females more than males. This type of camptodactyly usually does not improve spontaneously and may progress to a severe flexion deformity.[42,43] A type III deformity is often a severe deformity that usually involves multiple digits of both extremities and is associated with a variety of syndromes. This syndromic camptodactyly can occur in conjunction with craniofacial disorders, short stature, and chromosomal abnormalities.[39,43,44]

Clinical Presentation

The type I or congenital form of camptodactyly manifests with a flexion deformity noted at birth or during infancy.[41,42,45] The type II or acquired form begins with a subtle deformity that is gradually progressive. The contracture remains mild up to the age of 10 years and is rarely disabling. This small amount of flexion may go unnoticed by the patient and family, and a delay in seeking evaluation and treatment is common. During the growth spurt of adolescence, the PIP flexion deformity progresses and can advance to 90 degrees.[38,46] A gradual worsening of the PIP joint position can continue until 20 years of age.[38] The main complaint of the patient and family is the angulation of the finger and the appearance of the hand. Pain is not a common complaint and may indicate an alternative diagnosis.

Treatment Goals

I. Prevent progression of contracture.
II. Decrease PIP joint contracture.
III. Surgical correction in severe cases with functional impairment

Nonoperative Management

I. Indications
   A. Flexion contracture of one or more PIP joints
   B. A contracture of less than 30 to 40 degrees does not create a functional handicap or interfere with activities of daily living.[38,39] The individual should be instructed to accept the deformity and avoid surgical intervention.

II.   Therapy
   A. Splinting: Reports vary regarding wearing schedule.[47,48] Most
      authors recommend nighttime use to prevent progression of
      deformity. Continue splint wear until skeletal maturity is
      achieved.
      1. Static progressive splinting: more effective than dynamic
         splinting for rigid deformities.[43] Use forearm-based splint for
         infants for adequate fit and to prevent removal (Fig. 53-14).[44]
      2. Serial casting: mild prolonged stretch in extension may be
         necessary to elongate tight palmar structures followed by
         static splinting[41]
   B. PROM of affected joints

Operative Management

The natural history of camptodactyly predicts no improvement or progression of the deformity in 80% of individuals.[42] Severe involvement hinders
various occupational and sporting endeavors, such as using a computer
keyboard, playing a musical instrument, or wearing a baseball glove.[38,43]
This extreme flexion warrants treatment, although restoration of full
motion is not a realistic expectation or a reasonable goal. Secondary bony
changes about the PIP joint downgrade the outcome after surgery.[44]

   The PIP joint is usually approached via a palmar Z-plasty to lengthen
the tight skin. A graduated release of the offending agents is performed
until adequate PIP joint extension is obtained. After the skin incision, any
abnormal fascia and linear fibrous bands are released during exposure of

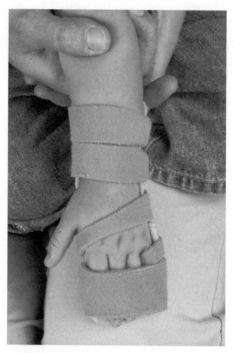

FIG. **53-14** A 1-year-old child with left small digit camptodactyly treated with static
progressive splinting. (Courtesy Shriners Hospital for Children, Philadelphia, Penn.)

the deeper structures. Additional release of the flexor tendon sheath, FDS tendon, check-rein ligaments, collateral ligaments, and palmar plate may be necessary to obtain sufficient extension.

The digit is explored for anomalous structures, with specific examination of the intrinsic muscles and FDS. Any anomalous origin or insertion of the lumbrical and/or interosseous muscle is resected.[44,46] The presence of a functioning FDS makes the tendon suitable for transfer. Transfer of the FDS tendon to the extensor apparatus lessens the PIP joint flexion force and augments PIP joint extension.[38,44] The FDS tendon is transected and withdrawn into the palm. The tendon is passed into the lumbrical canal, beneath the intermetacarpal ligament, and attached to the lateral band and central slip. The tendon is tensioned with the MCP joint positioned in 30 degrees flexion and the PIP joint held in full extension.

The extremity is immobilized with the wrist in neutral position, the MCP joints in 70 degrees flexion, and the IP joints straight. Kirschner wire fixation of the PIP joint is controversial. The choice usually is made at the time of surgery and depends on the degree of preoperative PIP joint contracture, the ease of obtaining extension, and the end-feel of the joint in extension. If K-wire fixation is chosen, the duration is limited to 3 weeks.

Postoperative Management

I. Indications: camptodactyly necessitating surgical correction
II. Precautions (if tendon transfer was included)
    A. Avoid forceful composite MCP and IP extension for 12 weeks after surgery
    B. Avoid forceful IP flexion with MCP extension for 12 weeks after surgery
    C. Avoid resistive exercises for 6 to 8 weeks after surgery
III. Therapy
    A. Splinting
       1. Cast and sutures removed 3 weeks after surgery
          a. Splint as follows
             (1) Forearm-based splint with wrist in neutral, MCP joints in 70 degrees flexion, IP joints in 0 degrees flexion
             (2) A second option is an ulnar wristlet sling maintaining the MCP joint in flexion and encouraging PIP joint extension.
          b. Goal of splint and wristlet: MCP flexion enables extrinsic extensors to extend the PIP joint until the intrinsic tendon transfer is capable and also protects FDS tendon transfer by placing slack on the tendon
          c. Splint schedule
             (1) Weeks 3 to 6: splint on at all times except for therapy, bathing, and completion of home exercise program
             (2) Weeks 6 to 8: If consistently activating transfer, discontinue splint during day except for use during strenuous activity that could cause tendon transfer to rupture; continue to wear splint at night
             (3) Week 8 to late teenage years, to prevent recurrence[47]: discontinue splint daytime, continue to wear at night
    B. Scar management

   C. AROM and place-hold exercises: to facilitate activation of tendon
      transfer (e.g., patient may be cued to attempt isolated PIP joint
      flexion of the donor digit, which should activate the FDS tendon
      and yield PIP joint extension)
   D. Functional activities: to promote PIP extension; initiated after
      consistent contraction of transferred muscle is achieved
   E. Resistive activities
      1. Week 6: Initiate light resistive strengthening.
      2. Weeks 7 to 8: Gradually increase resistive strengthening.

Outcomes

Camptodactyly is difficult to treat, and it is even more difficult to consistently achieve successful results. Conservative treatment with splinting
and passive stretching has resulted in an improvement in the amount of
PIP joint contracture.[47,48] Supervised therapy and a compliant patient are
prerequisites to the implementation of conservative management. The best
results are obtained in a well-motivated patient with a mild deformity.[49]
Prolonged diligent splinting is necessary to achieve a satisfactory outcome.

   Multiple surgical procedures have been reported for camptodactyly. The
technique is variable, and the results are scattered with respect to outcome.[38,42,49] The goal of enhancing extension without losing flexion is difficult to achieve. The outcome is less predictable in patients with severe
flexion deformities and/or secondary bony changes.

REFERENCES

General Guidelines

   1. Data System for Medical Rehabilitation: WeeFIM System Clinical Guide Version 5.1.
      State University of New York at Buffalo, Buffalo, NY, 2000
   2. Uniform Data System for Medical Rehabilitation: Guide for the Uniform Data Set for
      Medical Rehabilitation (including the FIM™ instrument), Version 5.1. State University
      of New York at Buffalo, Buffalo, NY, 1997
   3. Law M, Baptiste S, McColl MA, et al. The Canadian Occupational Performance
      Measure: an outcome measure for occupational therapy. Can J Occup Ther 57:82-87,
      1990
   4. McColl MA, Paterson M, Davies D, et al.: Validity and community utility of the
      Canadian Occupational Performance Measure. Can J Occup Ther 67:22-30, 1999
   5. Wiedrich TA: Congenital constriction band syndrome. Hand Clin 14:29-38, 1998

Radial Deficiency

   6. Kozin SH: Upper-extremity congenital anomalies: current concepts review. J Bone Joint
      Surg Am 85:1564-1575, 2003
   7. Heikel HVA: Aplasia and hypoplasia of the radius: studies on 64 cases and on epiphyseal
      transplantation in rabbits with the imitated defect. Acta Orthop Scand Suppl 39:1-155, 1959
   8. Lamb DW: Radial clubhand: a continuing study of sixty-eight patients with one hundred
      and seventeen clubhands. J Bone Joint Surg Am 59:1-13, 1977
   9. Auerbach AD, Verlander PC, Brown KE, et al.: New molecular diagnostic tests for two
      congenital forms of anemia. J Clin Lab Anal 11:17-22, 1997
  10. Lourie GM, Lins RE: Radial longitudinal deficiency: a review and update. Hand Clin
      14:85-99, 1998
  11. Bayne LG, Klug MS: Long-term review of the surgical treatment of radial deficiencies.
      J Hand Surg Am 12:169-179, 1987
  12. Bora FW Jr, Osterman AL, Kaneda RR, et al.: Radial club-hand deformity: long-term
      follow-up. J Bone Joint Surg Am 63:741-745, 1981

13. Murray JH, Fitch RD: Distraction histiogenesis: principles and indications. J Am Acad Orthop Surg 4:317-327, 1996
14. Damore E, Kozin SH, Thoder JJ, et al.: The recurrence of deformity after surgical centralization for radial clubhand. J Hand Surg Am 25:745-751, 2000
15. Watson HK, Beebe RD, Cruz NI: A centralization procedure for radial clubhand. J Hand Surg Am 9:541-547, 1984
16. McCarroll HR: Congenital anomalies: a 25-year overview. J Hand Surg Am 25:1007-1037, 2000

Arthrogryposis

17. Hall JG, Reed SD, Driscoll EP: Amyoplasia: a common, sporadic condition with congenital contractures. Part I. Am J Med Genet 15:571-590, 1983
18. Freeman EA, Sheldon JH: Cranio-carpo-tarsal dystrophy: an undescribed congenital malformation. Arch Dis Child 13:277-283, 1938
19. McCarroll HR Jr, Manske PR: The windblown hand: correction of the complex clasped thumb deformity. Hand Clin 8:147-159, 1992
20. Krakowiak PA, Bohnsack JF, Carey JC, et al.: Clinical analysis of a variant of Freeman-Sheldon syndrome (DA2B). Am J Med Genet 76:93-98, 1998
21. Sells JM, Jaffe KM, Hall JG: Amyoplasia, the most common type of arthrogryposis: the potential for good outcome. Pediatrics 97:225-231, 1996
22. Bennett JB, Hansen PE, Granberry WM, et al.: Surgical management of arthrogryposis of the upper extremity. J Pediatr Orthop 5:281-286, 1985
23. Ezaki M: Treatment of the upper limb in the child with arthrogryposis. Hand Clin 16:703-711, 2000
24. Smith DW, Drennan JC: Arthrogryposis wrist deformities: results of infantile serial casting. J Pediatr Orthop 22:44-47, 2002
25. Mennon U: Early corrective surgery of the wrist and elbow in arthrogryposis multiplex congenital. J Hand Surg Br 18:304-307, 1993
26. Van Heest A, Waters PM, Simmons BP: Surgical treatment of arthrogryposis of the elbow. J Hand Surg Am 23:1063-1070, 1998

HypoplasticThumb

27. Lister GD: Reconstruction of the hypoplastic thumb. Clin Orthop 195:52-65, 1985
28. Kozin SH, Weiss AA, Webber JB, et al.: Index finger pollicization for congenital aplasia or hypoplasia of the thumb. J Hand Surg Am 17:880-884, 1992
29. Manske PR, McCarroll HR Jr, James MA: Type III-A hypoplastic thumb. J Hand Surg Am 20;246-253, 1995
30. Buck-Gramcko D: Pollicization of the index finger: methods and results in aplasia and hypoplasia of the thumb. J Bone Joint Surg Am 53:1605-1617, 1971
31. Clark DI, Chell J, Davis TR: Pollicisation of the index finger: a 27-year follow-up study. J Bone Joint Surg Br 80:631-635, 1998

Syndactyly

32. Eaton CJ, Lister GD: Syndactyly. Hand Clin 6:555-574, 1990
33. Flatt AE: The Care of Congenital Hand Anomalies. 2nd Ed. Quality Medical Publishing, St. Louis, 1994, pp. 228-275
34. Kozin SH: Syndactyly. J Am Soc Surg Hand 1:1-13, 2001
35. Bauer TB, Tondra JM, Trusler HM: Technical modification in repair of syndactylism. Plast Reconstr Surg 17:385-392, 1956
36. Keret D, Ger E: Evaluation of a uniform operative technique to treat syndactyly. J Hand Surg Am 12:727-729, 1987
37. Richterman I, Dupree J, Kozin SH, et al.: Radiographic analysis of web height. J Hand Surg Am 23:1071-1076, 1998

Camptodactyly

38. Smith RJ, Kaplan EB: Camptodactyly and similar atraumatic flexion deformities of the proximal interphalangeal joints of the fingers. J Bone Joint Surg A, 50:1187-1203, 1968

39. Senrui H: Congenital contractures. In Buck-Gramcko D (ed): Congenital Malformations of the Hand and Forearm. London: Churchill Livingstone, 1998, pp. 295-309
40. Courtemanche AD: Campylodactyly: etiology and management. Plast Reconstr Surg 44:451-454, 1969
41. Benson LS, Waters PM, Kamil NI, et al.: Camptodactyly: classification and results of nonoperative treatment. J Pediatr Orthop 14:814-819, 1994
42. Engber WD, Flatt AE: Camptodactyly: an analysis of sixty-six patients and twenty-four operations. J Hand Surg Am 2:216-224, 1977
43. Flatt AE: Crooked fingers. In Flatt AE (ed): The Care of Congenital Hand Anomalies. 2nd Ed. Quality Medical Publishing, St. Louis, 1994, pp. 47-63
44. Kay SPJ: Camptodactyly. In Green DP, Hotchkiss RN, Pederson WC (eds): Green's Operative Hand Surgery. 4th Ed. Churchill Livingstone, Philadelphia, 1999, pp. 510-517
45. Koman LA, Toby EB, Poehling GG: Congenital flexion deformities of the proximal interphalangeal joint in children: a subgroup of camptodactyly. J Hand Surg A, 15:582-586, 1990
46. Smith PJ, Grobbelaar AO: Camptodactyly: a unifying theory and approach to surgical treatment. J Hand Surg Am 23:14-19, 1998
47. Miura T, Nakamura R, Tamura Y: Long-standing extended dynamic splintage and release of an abnormal restraining structure in camptodactyly. J Hand Surg Br 17:665-672, 1992
48. Hori M, Nakura R, Inoue G, et al.: Nonoperative treatment of camptodactyly. J Hand Surg Am 12:1061-1065, 1987
49. Siegert JJ, Cooney WP, Dobyns JH: Management of simple camptodactyly. J Hand Surg Br 15:181-189, 1990

Therapeutic Management of the Performing Artist

54

Lauren Valdata

Within the last 20 years, information about injuries in performing artists has flourished in the literature. The field of performing arts medicine now recognizes the unique nature of performance-related injuries in musicians. A survey of more than 2000 symphony orchestra musicians revealed that 76% of this population had experienced a problem that affected their performance.[1] The same survey showed that problems differed significantly depending on the instrument played (string, brass, woodwind, or percussion), the size of the instrument, and the gender of the player.[1] This chapter provides the clinician unfamiliar with injuries observed in musicians with a brief overview of common problems, evaluation guidelines, and treatment techniques.

DEFINITION AND GRADES OF INJURIES

When a musician presents with vague complaints of pain that cannot be isolated to a specific tissue or diagnosis, the injury is often categorized as an overuse syndrome. These injuries result when a biological tissue (e.g., muscle, bone, tendon, ligament) is stressed beyond its physiological limit.[2] Also included under the umbrella of overuse injuries are specific diagnoses such as lateral epicondylitis, De Quervain's syndrome or tenosynovitis, carpal tunnel syndrome, thoracic outlet syndrome (TOS), neuritis, and bursitis.

Various grading scales have been reported in the literature to help classify the irritability of the musician's symptoms. The scale proposed by Fry is broken down into five grades[3]:

Grade 1: pain at one site only and only while playing

Grade 2: pain at multiple sites

Grade 3: pain that persists well beyond the time that the musician stops playing

Grade 4: all of these, and many activities of daily living (ADLs) begin to cause pain.

Grade 5: all of these, but all ADLs that engage the affected body part cause pain

PREDISPOSING FACTORS FOR OVERUSE INJURIES IN MUSICIANS

I.   Specific factors that may predispose a musician to overuse injuries:

A. Sudden increase in practice time: This often relates to preparation for concerts, recitals, juries, and other performances. Onset of pain may coincide with attendance at special courses, where a disproportionate amount of playing occurs with respect to the musician's baseline playing time, and/or with efforts to master technically challenging phrases.[3]

B. Change in instructor: A change in an instructor usually equates with a change in pedagogy, repertoire, and/or technique. If such changes are not incorporated gradually, pain may result.

C. Multiple instruments or a change in instrument: Musicians frequently play more than one instrument. Pain that occurs when playing a primary instrument may be the result of playing a secondary instrument, or vice versa. Pain syndromes can also develop when a different instrument is purchased or substituted. Subtle differences in key positions, different bridge heights (Fig. 54-1), different string tensions, or an increase in the instrument's weight can change loading demands on muscle and connective tissue, causing less conditioned tissues to be overloaded. Injuries may also result from playing on different instruments, such as pianists encounter when on tour. (It requires greater force to produce the same musical result on a piano with stiff keys.)

D. Poorly conditioned muscles: Most athletes know that muscle strength, flexibility, and endurance play a role in preventing injuries. Some authors have compared the musician with the athlete, as both professions require agility, speed, and neuromuscular coordination.[4] Properly conditioned muscles are better able to meet the demand of strenuous rehearsals and performances. Bilateral upper quadrant and cervical flexibility and muscle endurance decrease the chances of static muscle imbalances and minimize the risk of fatigue-related injuries. Digital flexibility and endurance also prevent injuries that result from overstretching to reach keys or higher string positions, different tension levels of keys or strings, and so on.

E. Poor practice habits: Each practice session should include an actual physical warm-up of the part, warm-up on the instrument, a rest period, and a cool-down. Soft tissue can be injured during practice if the warm-up period is inadequate, absent, or overly vigorous. At least 10 minutes of rest every 50 minutes of play is mandatory. This rule of thumb is utilized even in military troop movements. The rationale is to get more function with occasional rest periods every hour, rather than lose performance levels with increased time. The onset of muscle soreness, discomfort, and/or pain may be delayed and may not appear until 24 to 48 hours after exertion. Therefore, use of discomfort, pain, or fatigue as a gauge for the need to incorporate rest periods is not recommended. A cool-down after strenuous playing is advised, using cool soaks and/or ice massage.

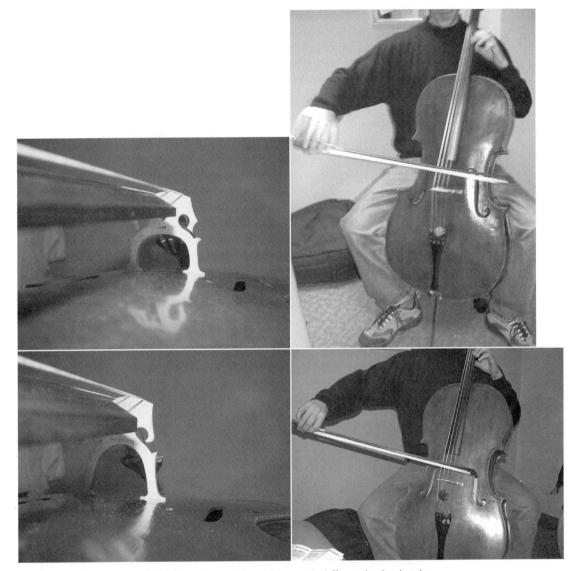

FIG. **54-1** Potential problems with different bridge heights.

F. Poor technique: Most musicians agree that their instrument has no universally accepted proper technique. In fact, developing one's own style and innovative technique may allow virtuoso playing, giving the competitive edge necessary to succeed in today's music world. If these techniques violate proper ergonomic principles and muscle balance, however, they may be detrimental in the long run.

G. Poor posture and muscle imbalances: Repetitive postural deviations (e.g., forward head) can result in muscle imbalances. The compression forces of the upper posterior cervical spine increase, and the muscles of the upper posterior cervical spine shorten while the lower posterior muscles and connective tissues lengthen.

H. Previous injury: In a survey of 468 musicians, Dawson[5] found that 51% had a traumatic injury which then caused them pain when playing their instruments. Regardless of the origin of the injury, inadequate rehabilitation of a previous injury can result in pain while playing.

I. Aggravating ADLs: The clinician needs to be aware of other activities that the instrumentalist participates in besides those related to music. Job-related activities (lifting, computer use, typing), sports (golf, tennis), or hobbies (gardening, yoga, needlework) may create, exacerbate, or perpetuate pain experienced while playing an instrument.

J. Gender: Data from various studies has suggested that there is a higher prevalence of overuse injuries in female musicians than in male musicians.[1,6,7]

K. Practice or rehearsal environment: Factors such as insufficient lighting, ambient temperature, and seating within an ensemble can contribute to painful overuse conditions. Poor lighting can cause one to tense the muscles while squinting and protracting the head to see the music. Cold and/or drafty rooms can cause muscles to tighten. The seating arrangement in an ensemble can lead to muscle asymmetries as the musician rotates to see the conductor or to avoid contact with other instrumentalists on crowded stages or in small orchestra pits.

EVALUATION OF THE MUSICIAN

I. Subjective Evaluation

The goals of the subjective evaluation should be to obtain an understanding of the musician's practice and playing habits, the location and nature of his or her pain, the irritability of the pain symptoms, previous medical interventions, and the patient's general fitness and health. The subjective examination is only as revealing as the clinician's understanding of the significance of the musician's responses to the questions posed. A knowledge of the factors that predispose to injury can assist the clinician in gaining pertinent information.

Typically, musicians are good historians. They often recall the circumstances when they first noted symptoms. A chronological history of a musician's symptoms may provide clues to the cause of the injury. A self-administered questionnaire can be a time-effective and helpful way to obtain this information (Appendix 54-1).

II. Physical Examination without the Instrument

This examination resembles other musculoskeletal examinations. The musician's posture should be observed in sitting and standing, and from the front, back, and side, looking at muscle contour for signs of atrophy or hypertrophy (Fig. 54-2). The clinician should observe whether there are static muscle imbalances such as forward head, rounded shoulders, reversed curvature of the cervical spine, or an excessive unilateral elevation of the shoulder girdle. Stretch weakness, caused by poor sitting posture, is often found in scapula adductors with compensatory shortening of the pectoral muscles.[2]

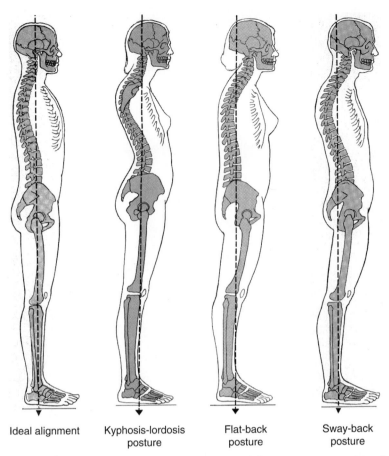

| Ideal alignment | Kyphosis-lordosis posture | Flat-back posture | Sway-back posture |

FIG. **54-2** Types of postural alignment. (From Kendall FP, McCreary EK: Muscles: Testing and Function. 4th Ed. Lippincott Williams & Wilkins, Philadelphia, 1993.)

It is also important to look for dynamic muscle imbalances and substitution patterns during movement.[8] Some examples are unequal scapular abduction with shoulder flexion, winging of the scapula with shoulder motion, shoulder external rotation with supination of the forearm, and shoulder internal rotation with pronation of the forearm.

Special tests for the cervical spine should be performed to rule out nerve root compression. Tests such as the foraminal compression test, cervical distraction test, vertebral artery test, and cervical quadrant test are all indicated.[9] If peripheral, spinal, or nerve root compression symptoms are present, sensory testing may be indicated.

The examination should include active range of motion (AROM) and passive range of motion (PROM) of the cervical spine, upper extremities, and trunk. The clinician should look for limitations or excessive amounts of joint motion, noting any pain with AROM, PROM, or overpressure. Joint laxity, or benign hypermobility, may enhance technical performance, but it is more often the reason a musician develops pain in the upper quadrant.[10-12]

Manual muscle testing to detect strength deficits in the upper quadrant should be performed only if it does not exacerbate the pain. Muscles to be included in this examination are the trunk muscles, abdominals, cervical spinal muscles, shoulder girdle, and intrinsic muscles of the hand. Special

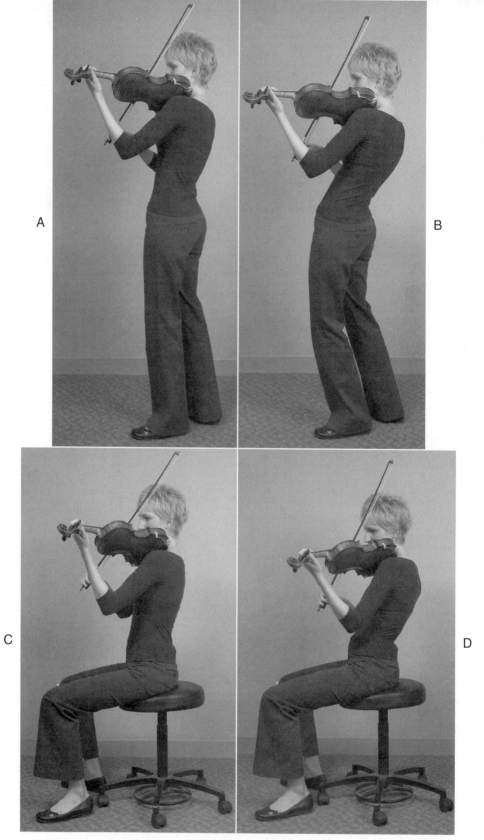

FIG. **54-3** Proper and improper standing and sitting posture. **A,** Proper standing; **B,** improper standing; **C,** proper sitting; **D,** improper sitting.

tests to detect shortened muscles, especially for the pectoralis major and minor, latissimus dorsi, hip flexors, scalene muscles, and hand intrinsics, are important to perform.

Musicians may present with specific diagnoses, such as De Quervain's syndrome or tenosynovitis, lateral epicondylitis, medial epicondylitis, TOS, carpal tunnel syndrome, or cubital tunnel syndrome, which are addressed in other chapters of this book. Please refer to the appropriate chapters for evaluation and treatment guidelines for these conditions.

III. Physical Examination with the Instrument

When evaluating the musician with his or her instrument, the clinician must keep in mind the basic principles of ergonomics and biomechanics. Whether the musician is seated or standing, the clinician should assess the musician's posture to ensure an appropriate base of support, pelvic positioning, and proper vertebral alignment (Fig. 54-3, A to D).

It is important to note whether joints are in positions that increase pressure on peripheral nerves (e.g., excessive wrist flexion or extension, consistent elbow flexion beyond 90 degrees). The proximal stabilizers (abdominals, paraspinals, rhomboids, latissimus dorsi, serratus anterior, and trapezius) should be balanced to allow the arms to move with grace and ease.[13] Additionally, the clinician should observe whether there is excessive tension in muscle groups, which can lead to premature muscle fatigue.

Musicians who play larger instruments, such as the tuba, cello, or string bass, should be evaluated on their technique of transporting the instrument. Heavy cases carried by a handle or by a shoulder strap can cause traction on the arm, which can aggravate or initiate TOS and other peripheral nerve irritations. Luggage carts or wheeled cases can be used to minimize loading on the upper extremity.

It is important to assess the practice or rehearsal setup. Playing in an ensemble often requires some spinal rotation to see both the music and the conductor. The clinician should note whether the musician's head position is excessively forward or tilted to one side, as is often the case with the "chin instruments" (violin, viola) and with the flute. These postures cause asymmetrical loading of the paraspinal and cervical muscles, which can become painful over time.

The instrument should appear to be an extension of the player; the player should not have to contort himself or herself to fit the instrument.

INSTRUMENT-SPECIFIC PROBLEMS

The literature on performing arts medicine reveals that injuries to musicians can be related to the type of instrument played. The prevalence of pain syndromes is significantly higher among string and keyboard players, compared with woodwind, brass, or percussion players.[1,14] It is helpful for the clinician unfamiliar with injuries in instrumentalists to be aware of instrument-specific problems.

A. String Instruments

Shoulder problems are common among string players. Three potential injuries are impingement syndrome, subacromial/subdeltoid bursitis, and bicipital tendinitis.[15] Cellists, violinists, violists, and bass players are at risk for development of bicipital tendinitis in the right arm because of the repetitive elbow and shoulder action required for bowing.

Classical guitar players are prone to problems in the right shoulder because of the upper extremity posture needed to clear the edge of the guitar. This posture, combined with the picking and strumming action of the fingers, can lead to a shoulder injury. Guitar players often position the left wrist in extreme flexion. This position, combined with repetitive digital flexion, makes the left hand susceptible to carpal tunnel syndrome. Repositioning of the instrument to minimize extremes of wrist flexion may help alleviate symptoms. Guitar supports are available that stabilize the guitar on the thigh at an angle that enables proper finger positioning in the left hand with minimal wrist flexion. In addition, tendinitis of the flexor and/or extensor muscles of the forearm is common even when excessive positions do not cause problems. The predisposing factors typically effect these muscle groups.

Violinists, violists, and cellists may develop cubital tunnel syndrome in either arm. The left arm is more frequently involved because of the sustained position of elbow flexion necessary to reach the fingering board.[15,16] These musicians are also prone to myofascial pain and pain secondary to muscle imbalance. The head and neck are flexed, laterally bent, and rotated, with the shoulder elevated to support the instrument. Sustaining this posture (potentially for hours) can lead to muscle pain from active, latent, or chronic trigger points in the shoulder girdle and/or neck musculature.

Harpists usually play with their arms abducted and wrists extended. This position can be taxing to the rotator cuff muscles and can increase pressure in the carpal tunnel. Additionally, this instrument requires an enormous amount of tuning. If a small tuning device is used, greater muscle forces are required. Larger, ergonomic tuners can reduce stresses to the hand and should be recommended.

B. Keyboard Instruments

Keyboard players are prone to a wide variety of pain syndromes. These include muscle imbalances, myofascial pain, and all the specific diagnoses listed under the umbrella of overuse. For example, De Quervain's syndrome may result from the crossing of the thumb under the other digits to reach a desired key. Lateral and/or medial epicondylitis may be attributed to techniques that use excessive wrist motion. Trigger points are often located in the upper trapezius muscles and levator scapulae as a result of tension and "hunching" of the shoulders while playing. Pain from poor body mechanics and/or posture may result from a piano bench that is of the improper height or incorrectly positioned. A keyboard player with relatively small hands or limited interdigital web space may experience pain from straining to achieve an octave or more with one hand.

Focal dystonia (often referred to as occupational cramp) is most frequently reported among pianists.[17] It is characterized by impairment or loss of motor control. The condition is often task specific, manifesting as involuntary flexion or extension of the fingers that occurs only while playing the instrument. The etiology and pathology of focal dystonia remains an enigma, and the disorder continues to be frustrating for clinician and musician. Despite a plethora of proposed treatments, none have been consistently effective.

C. Wind Instruments

Flutists are prone to upper quadrant myofascial pain and shoulder problems because of the way in which the instrument is designed to be held. One option for positioning the flute is with the head and neck laterally flexed to the right and the right shoulder relaxed, but this positioning can lead to cervical problems. The flutist may elect to keep the head vertical, but this requires static shoulder abduction, which can lead to tendinitis, impingement syndromes, or pain from chronic trigger points. Flutists are also susceptible to radial digital nerve compression at the base of the left index finger, because this area serves as a counterbalance to support the instrument. Piccolo players are subject to cubital tunnel syndrome in either arm because the small size of the instrument requires both elbows to be held in extreme flexion.

Clarinet, oboe, and English horn players may suffer metacarpal joint pain in the right thumb, because a large portion of the instrument's weight is supported by the thumb, distal to the interphalangeal joint. Double reed instrumentalists, such as bassoonists and oboists, may develop lateral epicondylitis, sometimes referred to as a *reed-maker's elbow*, from making reeds. Finishing a reed requires holding the reed firmly on a mandrel in one hand, while carefully shaving excess cane from the reed with a knife in the other. The repetitive ulnar deviation and extension of the wrist can lead to tendinitis.

D. Percussion Instruments

When percussion instruments are played, rapid deceleration of the forearm muscles occurs on impact with the drumhead, which then causes absorption of vibration forces by the muscles and tendons of the forearm. With repetition, inflammation of the connective tissue may result. Percussionists are prone to develop tendinitis of the wrist flexors and extensors, tendinitis of the first dorsal interossei, medial or lateral epicondylitis, and rotator cuff injuries.[18-20] Drummers in rock bands may have pathology of the cervical spine if head thrashing is part of their style, and jazz drummers may develop De Quervain's syndrome due to technique variances in play.

E. Brass Instruments

The majority of problems experienced by brass players relate to the embouchure or the temporomandibular joint. They may also have problems caused by the way in which the instrument is held, such as trombone, French horn, and trumpet mutes when using overt wrist extension.

TREATMENT

I. Goals

Treatment of injuries in musicians must be individualized based on the clinical findings of the evaluation. A primary goal of treatment is to identify and reduce unnecessary muscle tension used when playing the instrument. Some examples include pressing more firmly on the keys or strings when playing *forte* (loud), "tensing up" on difficult or technically challenging passages, and holding the instrument more tightly than necessary.

It is also necessary to identify and correct unnecessary tension used in ADLs, such as carrying objects, driving, writing, and computer use.

Musicians often use coping mechanisms such as refingerings, changes in technique, or changes in repertoire to avoid pain. It is the role of the clinician to identify coping mechanisms used by the musician to avoid pain, to uncover the underlying cause of the pain, and to educate and assist the musician in rectifying the source of the problem.

II. Absolute and Relative Rest

Most experts agree that rest is the initial treatment of choice.[16,17,21-23] The decision as to whether a period of relative rest, meaning a decrease in practice/performance time and elimination of certain aggravating ADLs, or a period of absolute rest is indicated is based on the grade of the injury. Those classified with grade IV and V injuries may initially require absolute rest and immobilization. Musicians advised of relative rest should understand that the aggravating activity should be ceased with the first sign of pain or paresthesia. It is also important to emphasize that other hand-intensive ADLs, such as gardening, computer work, or needle crafts, should be moderately decreased or avoided during the resting phase of treatment. *Overuse pain is not something that should be "worked through." The "no pain, no gain" philosophy has no role in the rehabilitation of injured musicians.*

III. Exercise Programs

Exercise programs should be specific and structured. The clinician must take the time to properly instruct the patient as to what to feel and expect with light stretching and strengthening exercises. One joint stretching exercise should provide a gentle stretch, no discomfort, nor any pain. Any discomfort that occurs after an exercise program should last no more than 15 to 20 minutes. Pain lasting longer than this is a sign that the exercise was too aggressive. Musicians tend to be very motivated and may be overzealous with exercises. Without strict guidelines, an exercise program may do more harm than good, especially if it is approached like a large-muscle-group sports program.

As discussed earlier, the role of proper posture, with and without the instrument, should be addressed. Repositioning of a music stand or seat may be needed to encourage a balanced, neutral posture. If a balanced position cannot be obtained, the musician should be instructed to stretch away from this static posture every 15 minutes while playing and frequently during the day. Some examples of instrument-specific stretches are left lateral bending of the cervical spine for flutists, right lateral bending of the cervical spine for players of chin instruments, and pectoralis major stretch for cello, oboe, and clarinet players. Muscle imbalances as a result of poor posture can be addressed with range of motion exercises, if needed, in addition to postural reeducation (Fig. 54-4), light conditioning exercises, progressing towards light strengthening exercises with a gradual increase in endurance conditioning. Swimming, Pilates, and aerobic exercises for full-body conditioning should also be tailored for the musician's full-body treatment program. Another concept is to actually hold isometrically the exact opposite position of the instrument play position (with or without

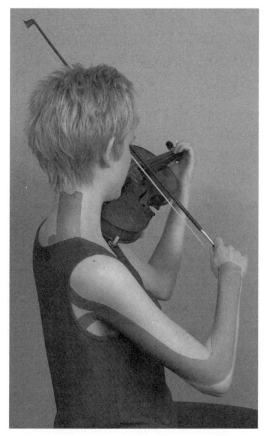

FIG. **54-4** Postural reeducation using tape.

instrument). The opposite or "un" position can assist in lengthening shortened muscles and place the overstreched muscles in a shortened position,
hence the "un" cello position, to confuse the cell memory resulting from
many years of holding the muscles in their musical positions.

IV. Role of Modalities

As in other cases of acute and chronic tendinitis, bursitis, and nerve compression, modalities such as ice, heat, phonophoresis, and iontophoresis,
as well as high-voltage galvanic stimulation (HVGS), transcutaneous electrical nerve stimulation (TENS), and other electrical stimulation modalities, may be indicated for pain reduction.

Biofeedback can be used to help the musician decrease muscle tension
with specific tasks and while at rest. When the resting state has improved,
the musician should be asked to play, keeping the feedback signal as quiet
as possible.

Video analysis can provide visual feedback to the performer. The clinician and musician together can use slow motion videography to look for
areas of tension, poor posture, and questionable technique. Sequential
videos provide a source of documentation and comparison. In the absence
of expensive equipment, mirrors may be an alternative for visual cueing
and also for simulating the "un" instrument position.

Proper alignment of the body relieves tension and results in more efficient patterns of movement. The Alexander technique and Feldenkrais are designed to show individuals how their bodies are misused and how to correct detrimental postural and movement patterns. A description of these techniques is beyond the scope of physical and occupational therapy practice; they are best learned from a certified instructor.

V. Patient Education

Education of the musician regarding good practice habits and physical fitness can minimize the chance of recurrent injury. A regular warm-up program, both away from the instrument and on the instrument, should be implemented to slowly stretch and warm the muscles before playing. A 10-minute break is necessary for every 50 minutes of play. This 10/50 ratio should be progressed to only if the musician is able to perform without complaints. This is a must during individual practice time. During ensemble breaks, the musician should put the instrument down, get up, walk around, stretch, and relax. This should be a break from upper extremity use, not time to whittle on a reed or practice a missed passage. If rehearsals do not have scheduled breaks, dangling the arms for a few seconds, resting the instrument in the lap or against the body, and doing gentle finger stretches during measures of rest can help improve circulation to the muscles and alleviate tension.

The musician should be encouraged to have practice time away from the instrument. Individual practice sessions can be taped and reviewed for self-critiquing. Listening to recordings, studying the scores or piano parts, and mentally hearing the way a piece should sound are all methods of enhancing the end performance without touching the instrument. Mental play without holding the instrument and mental play holding the instrument in the "un" position or in proper position can be initiated gradually during the return to play as well as when playing. Structured practice sessions with specific goals can maximize the benefits of the session while minimizing the playing time. By preparing well in advance for juries, auditions, rehearsals, and performances, the musician can avoid the physical dangers of "cramming."

After an injury, return to play should be implemented in a scheduled, graduated, and progressive manner. The musician should be advised to start with short practice periods and long rest periods. The specific times vary; the patient may actually begin playing for only 3 to 5 minutes initially, with a 20- to 50-minute break for rest and cool-down. Dr. Richard N. Norris has produced a very specific return-to-play chart[23] (Table 54-1). Close communication between patient and therapist assists return to the full pattern of 50 minutes play and 10 minutes rest that can be continued throughout the day. Keeping to a controlled practice schedule allows both the musician and the clinician to know the irritability and tolerance levels of the involved tissues. The pieces selected should be relatively slow and simple. Warm-up and cool-down exercises must be incorporated. Cooling for 5 to 15 minutes after practicing can lessen the effects of mild inflammatory responses. With any signs of discomfort or pain, the duration of play should be decreased and adjusted.

One of the most important tools for instrumentalists is knowing what to do if their symptoms should return. Most important, they should

TABLE **54-1** Returning to Work or Play

Levels (3-7 Days at Each)	Work Play	Rest	Work Play	Rest	Work Play	Rest	Work Play	Rest	Work Play
1	5	60	5						
2	10	50	10						
3	15	40	15	60	5				
4	20	30	20	50	10				
5	30	20	25	40	15	45	5		
6	35	15	35	30	20	35	10		
7	40	10	40	20	25	25	15	50	10
8	50	10	45	15	30	15	25	40	15
9	50	10	50	10	40	10	35	30	20
10	50	10	50	10	50	10	45	20	30

Etc.

- Start with slow and easy activity or pieces. Gradually progress to faster, more difficult tasks or pieces.
- In general, perform a maximum of 50 minutes continuous work or play with a minimum of 10 minutes rest.
- *Warm up* before working or playing!
- If pain occurs at any level, drop back to level of comfort until able to progress without pain.

From Norris RN: Musician's survival manual. ICSOM, St. Louis, 1991.

NEVER ignore pain. The instrumentalist should be instructed to immediately stop playing, try cooling the area to decrease the inflammatory response, rest, and discuss with the therapist why the problem might have returned.

VI. Role of Splints

Two categories of splints are used in the treatment of injuries in musicians. The first category includes splints that are used to support the instrument and alleviate pain caused by excessive strain on a joint or soft tissue. Examples include a modified carpometacarpal splint on the right hand of a clarinet, oboe, or English horn player; custom-formed chin rests for violin and viola players; and, for the flutist, use of an orthotic device to evenly distribute the pressure on the base of the left index finger. Various commercially available neck straps and posts can be used to support woodwind instruments.

Limitations of these devices include cost, appearance, and acceptance by both the musician and his or her colleagues. For aesthetic and/or personal reasons, the instrumentalists may be resistant to using these devices during performances; however, even if they are used only during practice, they may be helpful in controlling symptoms.

The second category of splints are those commonly used to treat tendinitis, nerve compression, and other inflammatory conditions. Splints in this category include wrist splints, thumb spica splints, and long arm splints. These splints should be used judiciously, and primarily during the acute, and perhaps the subacute, stage of injury. The longer the splints are used, the greater the risk of developing joint stiffness and muscle weakness as a result of disuse. As pain symptoms decrease, splint wear should be gradually weaned, with simultaneous incorporation of a progressive strengthening and flexibility program and use of soft supports (as opposed to a hard splint).

VII. Ergonomics of Instruments

Instruments were not designed with upper extremity ergonomics in mind. One of the best methods to reduce the risk of overuse injury for a musician is to fit the instrument to the hands and body by modifying the instrument. Instrument manufacturers can be contacted for instrument modification. Examples of ergonomic alterations include extending specific keys on the flute, clarinet, saxophone, or oboe; angling the head joint of a flute 30 degrees, beveling the top right portion of the classical guitar; and reshaping the right edge of the viola or violin. Limitations of these alterations include cost, appearance, and acceptance by both the musician and his or her colleagues. It is only with time and a universal knowledge of disease prevention, decreased symptoms, and the lack of any negative effects on the instrument's sound that such ergonomic changes may be used by the musician population.

OUTCOMES

The field of performing arts medicine (PAM) has been in existence for less than 25 years, but many articles have been published. During the full years from 1997 to 2001, a total of 1366 references were found. Over the last 200 years, 5550 references were found, with approximately 82% written in English.[24]

Problems and studies typically looked at age-specific, instrument-specific, technique-specific, and body type problems. In Dawson's study[25] of 167 performers reviewed retrospectively, the age range was 9 to 83 years, and 41.9% of the patients were men. Almost 90% were professional performers, teachers, collegiate music students, or dedicated amateurs. More than 75% played string or keyboard instruments. Among pianists, 54.7% had strains, 17.4% had inflammatory conditions, and 12.8% had nerve problems. Violinists/violists had strains (64.4%) and inflammatory problems (6.7%).

Only pianists showed a statistically significant difference in occurrence according to age: strain diagnoses were more common in the under-30 age group, and inflammatory problems in the above-30 group. Repetition and/or forceful upper extremity movements were related to the specific diagnoses. Muscle-tendon strain complaints were most common among pianists, guitarists, upper string instrumentalists, and reed instrumentalists. Inflammation of joints and tendons was seen most frequently in flutists, whereas percussionists and orchestral conductors showed a more equal distribution between the two problems.[25]

The prevalence of playing-related musculoskeletal disorders (PRMDs) in performing artists continues to be studied by many authors, and many references can be cited. Treatment outcomes appear to be needed, so as to determine the prevention and/or resolution of pain and symptoms from the different variables causing the problems. Davies and Mangion[26] studied the predictors of pain/symptoms involving three outcome indices: "frequency of pain/symptoms over the playing lifetime, frequency of pain/symptoms during the previous 12 months, and pain/symptom severity." Their results showed "a degree of cohesion between the important factors for all three outcomes."[26] Of interest, playing-related stress was significant for the previous year and the playing lifetime. Lack of warm-up and rest versus break with high stress effected more severe symptoms. Poor health, lack of fitness, and exhaustion may also have been triggers when present in conjunction with high playing loads.[26]

Prevention through instrument and postural education, general fitness, and stress release appears to be most important for musicians to continue effectively for the life of their performance years.

REFERENCES

1. Middlestadt SE, Fishbein M: The prevalence of severe musculoskeletal problems among male and female symphony orchestra string players. Med Probl Perform Art 41:41, 1989
2. Norris R: The Musician's Survival Manual: A Guide to Preventing and Treating Injuries in Instrumentalists. International Conference of Symphony and Opera Musicians, 1993
3. Fry HJH: The treatment of overuse injury syndrome. MD Med J 42:277, 1993
4. Quarrier NF: Performing art medicine: the musical athlete. J Orthop Sports Phys Ther 17:90, 1993
5. Dawson WJ: Hand and upper extremity injuries in instrumentalists: epidemiology and outcome. Med Probl Perform Art 3:19, 1988
6. Sakai N: Hand pain attributed to overuse among professional pianists: a study of 200 cases. Med Probl Perform Art 17:178, 2002
7. Roamaryn LM: Upper extremity disorders in performing artists. Maryland Med J 42:255, 1993
8. Kendall FP, McCreary EK, Provance P: Muscles: Testing and Function. 4th Ed. Williams & Wilkins, Baltimore, 1993
9. Magee DJ: Cervical spine. In Magee DJ: Orthopedic Physical Assessment. WB Saunders, Philadelphia, 1987, p. 21
10. Brandfonbrener AG: Joint laxity in instrumental musicians. Med Probl Perform Art 5:117, 1990
11. Brandfonbrener AG: Joint laxity: help or hindrance? [editorial]. Med Probl Perform Art 9:1, 1994
12. Brandfonbrener AG: Joint laxity and arm pain in musicians. Med Probl Perform Art 15:72, 2000
13. Tubiana R, Champagne P, Brockman R: Fundamental positions for instrumental musicians. Med Probl Perform Arts 4:73, 1989
14. Newmark J, Hochberg FH: "Doctor, it hurts when I play": painful disorders among instrumental musicians. Med Probl Perform Arts 2:93, 1987
15. Hoppman RA, Patrone NA: Musculoskeletal problems in instrumental musicians. In Sataloff RT, Brandfonbrener AG, Lederman RJ (eds): Textbook of Performing Arts Medicine. Raven Press, New York, 1991, p. 71
16. Amadio PC, Russotti GM: Evaluation and treatment of hand and wrist disorders in musicians. Hand Clin 6:405, 1990
17. Tubiana R: Prolonged neuromuscular rehabilitation for musician's focal dystonia. Med Probl Perform Art 18:166, 2003
18. Judkins J: The impact of impact: the percussionist's shoulder. Med Probl Perform Art 6:69, 1991
19. Judkins J: A performance application for rehabilitating the rotator cuff in the percussionist. Med Probl Perform Art 7:83, 1992
20. Chong J, Lynden M, Harvey D, et al: Occupational health problems of musicians. Can Fam Physician 35:2341, 1989
21. Winspur I, Wynn Parry CB: The Musician's Hand: A Clinical Guide. 1st Ed. Martin Dunitz Ltd, London, 1998
22. Fry JH: The treatment of overuse injury syndrome. Md Med J 42:277, 1993
23. Norris RN: The upper extremity difficulties of instrumental musicians. Mackin EJ, Callahan AD, Skirven TM, et al. (eds): Hunter-Mackin-Callahan Rehabilitation of the Hand and Upper Extremity. 5th Ed. Mosby, St. Louis, 2002, pp. 2044, 2050
24. Dawson WJ: The bibliography of performing arts medicine: a five-year retrospective review. Med Probl Perform Art 18:27-32, 2003
25. Dawson WJ: Upper extremity problems caused by playing specific instruments. Med Probl Perform Art 17:135-140, 2002
26. Davies J, Mangion S: Predictors of pain and other musculoskeletal symptoms among professional instrumental musicians. Med Probl Perform Art 17:155-168, 2002

APPENDIX **54-1**

Evaluation of Performing Artists

Name: _____

Sex: _____ **Age:** _____ **School level (if applicable):** _____

1. Do you have a previous history of trauma to your arms, neck, or back?
2a. Do you have any other significant health problems?
2b. Have you had any special tests performed? (MRI, EMG, NCV, bone scan, radiographs)
3. What instrument(s) do you play?
4. How many years have you been playing each instrument?
5. How long do you play your instrument daily? (Specify for each instrument)
6. How many hours are personal practice, rehearsals, and performance?
7. Have you had a change in your practice, playing, or performance time recently?
8. Do you have a warm-up routine?
9. If yes, how long is this routine? Is it with your instrument, without your instrument, or both?
10. How often do you rest when practicing?
11. Have you changed teachers recently? Have you changed your playing technique recently?
12. Have you consulted other musicians concerning your condition or possible technique changes to decrease your symptoms?
13. In your own words, describe your problem and what you believe to be the cause.
14. How long has your problem been going on?
15. When do you have pain? How long can you play pain free?
16. What do you do to decrease or alleviate your pain?
17. Do your symptoms increase with arpeggios, scales, trills, or other patterns?
18. How do you practice technical passages (slowly, in small segments in short time intervals, from beginning to end or reverse, from the middle)?
19. Do you tend to practice the same passage over and over until you get it right, no matter how long it takes?
20. What are you working toward musically at this time? What are your goals over the next 2 to 4 years?
21. Do you exercise regularly? (Running, swimming, aerobics, martial arts, weight lifting, etc.)

PLEASE CHECK ALL OF THE FOLLOWING THAT APPLY TO YOU:

I have been diagnosed with:

1)___ Muscle pain and tenderness
2)___ Tendinitis
3)___ Overuse syndrome
4)___ Fibromyalgia
5)___ Carpal tunnel syndrome

6)___ Ulnar nerve compression
7)___ Thoracic outlet syndrome
8)___ Neck (cervical) problems
9)___ No diagnoses have been made
10)___ Other

I have had prior therapy including:

___ Nonsteroidal antiinflammatory medications (NSAIDs)
___ Steroids: oral or injection
___ Strengthening/stretching
___ Splinting
___ Moist heat
___ Ice
___ Massage
___ Electrical stimulation

___ TENS
___ Ultrasound
___ Phonophoresis
___ Iontophoresis
___ Kinesiotaping
___ Light therapy
___ Homeopathic
___ Acupuncture
___ Chiropractic

___ Alexander technique
___ Feldenkrais
___ Biofeedback
___ Ergonomic assessment
___ Other

PLEASE CHECK ANY OF THE FOLLOWING SYMPTOMS THAT YOU EXPERIENCE:

Pain Scale from 0-10, with 0 = no pain and 10 = in Emergency Room pain

___ Discomfort
___ Pain
___ Fatigue
___ Swelling
___ Redness
___ Stiffness

___ Pins and needles
___ Weakness
___ Cramping
___ Loss of muscle control

___ Curling of fingers uncontrollably
___ Numbness
___ Other: please explain

PLEASE CIRCLE THE SENTENCE THAT MOST ACCURATELY DESCRIBES YOUR PRESENT CONDITION:

1. I have pain in one site while playing. The location and presence of the pain are relatively consistent, but the pain stops very soon after I stop playing.
2. I have pain in multiple sites while playing. The locations of these pains are consistent. The pain stops shortly after I stop playing, and I can perform other activities without pain.
3. I have pain in multiple sites while playing that persists after playing. It now interferes with *some* of my other daily activities.
4. I have pain in multiple sites while playing that persists after playing. It now interferes with *all* of my other daily activities.
5. My hand or arm is now so painful that I cannot use it for anything.

Special Considerations and Common Injuries of Athletes

55

Tracy Videon

This chapter provides a broad overview of the special considerations for rehabilitating the athlete's upper extremity. Although there are no "cookbook" rehabilitation protocols, the rehabilitation of the athlete needs special considerations.

Each athlete is unique and may have different functional demands even within the same sport. A baseball pitcher needs to throw 60 to 100 high-velocity pitches per game, whereas a baseball outfielder may throw the ball a longer distance but only once a game.

Athletes are taught and expected to endure pain. Therefore, during rehabilitation pain cannot be the only guide, nor can it be ignored. If an athlete wants to participate in a pivotal game, time may be of the essence. Sports medicine professionals also have to make the critical decision of allowing the athlete to return to play. This decision must be made with the athlete's safety, including the risk of reinjury, in mind. The expectations of coaches, fans, media, and the athletes themselves add pressure to these return-to-play decisions.

THE SPORTS MEDICINE TEAM

I. Team physician
   A. Most often an orthopedic surgeon
   B. Sets the rehabilitation guidelines
   C. Checks the stages of healing
   D. Along with selected specialists, influences the return-to-play decision
   E. Orthopedists are usually team physicians for the collegiate and professional teams. In lower-level athletics, the team physician may be an internist or primary care physician.
II. Primary care physician or pediatrician
   A. Already has an established relationship with the athlete
   B. May be the first physician consulted after an athletic injury

C. If insurance dictates, may need to be consulted for diagnostic testing and/or follow-up care with the specialist
III. Certified Athletic Trainer (ATC)
    A. Educated in the prevention, care, recognition, and rehabilitation of athletic injuries
    B. Ideally, on hand at all athletic events to provide pregame taping or splinting and immediate care after an injury to decrease any inflammatory response
    C. May not be able to provide sufficient rehabilitative services because of lack of space and time and availability of equipment
    D. May be able to serve as a liaison to school officials
IV. Rehabilitation specialist
    A. May be either a physical or an occupational therapist
    B. Many high-level teams have a strength and conditioning coach.
V. Coach
    A. Supports the athlete both on and off the field
    B. Can encourage the athlete throughout the rehabilitative process
    C. Needs to understand when and under what circumstances the athlete will return to play
    D. May be used as a resource with information on demands placed on the athlete
VI. School nurse
    A. Can dispense medications or provide ice throughout the school day
    B. Can also serve as a liaison to school officials
VII. Parents
    A. If the athlete is younger than 18 years of age, must be informed regarding all levels of care
    B. May be the main enforcer of home therapies

REHABILITATION PROCESS

I. Differences in athletes compared with the general population
    A. In prime physical condition
    B. Must maintain cardiovascular conditioning
    C. Must maintain strength in noninjured extremities and core
    D. Make sure all muscle groups of injured area are in balance
    E. Must understand the limits of the injury and the consequences of breaking those limits
    F. Psychological changes
    G. Special considerations for the young athlete
        1. Skeletal immaturity
            a. Can have growth plate or physeal fracture
            b. Greenstick (or incomplete) fracture
        2. Soft tissue growth versus bone growth
            a. Flexibility may be compromised, leading to overuse injuries
            b. Avulsion fracture may be more likely than a soft tissue injury
II. Inflammation
    A. Phase I
        1. Acute inflammatory process occurs during first 12 to 48 hours after injury

2. Therapeutic goal is to decrease the amount of tissue damage.
   a. Aggressive use of rest, ice, compression, and elevation (RICE) to injured area to stop further tissue damage
   b. Medical management
3. If the inflammation can be controlled, rehabilitation can be accelerated
B. Phase II (repair and regeneration)
   1. Occurs from 3 days to 6 weeks or more after injury
   2. Goals
      a. Therapy goals should be performance-based, not time-based, unless directed otherwise by the physician
      b. Goals should be to decrease the formation of scar tissue, control inflammation, and return to functional activities
      c. Short-term goals should be set constantly, achieved, and set again[1]
         (1) Allows the athlete to understand the progression
             (a) Ensures that progress is going as planned
             (b) Allows athlete to see how much progress is being made and stay motivated
             (c) Allows the athlete to understand limitations
         (2) Allows the therapist to see how quickly or slowly an athlete is progressing
         (3) Should include daily, weekly, and monthly goals
   3. Exercise regimens
      a. Pain-free range of motion (ROM) can start immediately, including active (AROM), active-assisted (AAROM), and passive (PROM)
      b. Isometric strengthening should start as soon as possible
      c. As allowed, isotonic and isokinetic strengthening should start
         (1) Concentric contractions
         (2) Eccentric contractions
      d. Sport-specific activity
         (1) Goal is to dynamically stabilize the joint
         (2) Break down functional activities into many sequences
         (3) Progress rehabilitation of each sequence separately
             (a) Mimic motions with Theraband (e.g., throwing)
             (b) Simulate equipment (e.g., weighted stick for bat)
             (c) Perform less rigorous version of activity (e.g., throwing 20 ft instead of 60 ft)
   4. Modalities
      a. Goal is to decrease the inflammatory response
         (1) Ultrasound: consider any contraindications (e.g., over a growth plate)
         (2) Intermittent compression devices
         (3) Edema massage
         (4) Paraffin bath
         (5) Direct current stimulation
      b. Goal is to decrease pain
         (1) Interferential electrical stimulation
         (2) Massage
         (3) Whirlpool bath

(4) Fluidotherapy
(5) Joint mobilization
C. Phase III (remodeling)
1. Occurs at approximately 3 weeks after injury and may last up to 1 year
2. Important that the athlete be aware of this phase and continue with a maintenance rehabilitation program

PSYCHOLOGICAL CONSIDERATIONS

I.   Initial reaction
A. Anxiety
B. Fear
C. Guilt about letting down team, coach, and parents
D. Past experiences may cause pessimism
II. Loss of an athlete's normal routine
A. Grieving process
1. Denial
2. Anger
3. Bargaining
4. Depression (loss of self-esteem or self-worth, loss of control of situation)
5. Acceptance
III. Allow the athlete to participate in goal setting[2]
A. Therapist must be firm, but understanding, in helping set the goals.
IV. Allow other members of the sports medicine team to encourage the athlete
A. Help stop destructive behaviors
B. Help support positive behaviors
V.   Stay connected with team (maintain support system)
A. Attend strategy sessions
B. Conditioning sessions

COMMON INJURIES

One of the most challenging areas of athletic medicine and rehabilitation is the case of the overhead or throwing athlete. This includes baseball pitchers, softball pitchers, volleyball hitters, swimmers, tennis players, and track and field throwing athletes. The mechanics of throwing play a large role in any upper extremity injury, whether it is in the shoulder, elbow, or hand. With any of these athletes, it is important to communicate with other members of the sports medicine team to check the player's mechanics. This may prevent aggravation of the current injury as well as injury in the future. Mild modifications to body mechanics may make a large difference in safe participation.

I.   Shoulder injuries
A. Rotator cuff tendonitis, including impingement
1. Caused by repetitive motions, most often in throwing athletes
2. Can be traumatic from direct forces, such as in men's lacrosse or football

      3. May be able to participate in the sport with restriction
        a. Number of pitches thrown
        b. Stop when pain reaches a certain level
        c. Limit playing or practice time
        d. Alter mechanics of techniques (e.g., throwing)
        e. Continue therapy outside sports participation
    B. Rotator cuff tear
      1. Usually from a traumatic event
      2. May be barred from participation for a significant period
    C. Biceps tendonitis
      1. Usually a result of overuse
      2. Can be a throwing athlete
        a. Check the mechanics of throwing
      3. Possible anatomical predisposition
    D. Shoulder separation
      1. Caused by a direct fall on arm
        a. On outstretched arm
        b. On elbow
        c. On shoulder
    E. Shoulder dislocation
      1. Posterior dislocation is usually from direct force, such as being hit in football, ice hockey, rugby, or men's lacrosse
      2. Anterior dislocation is usually from external rotation/abduction force on humerus, such as throwing that is impeded
        a. Quarterback hit in throwing motion
        b. Lacrosse player being stick-checked during the throwing motion

II.   Elbow injuries
    A. Lateral epicondylitis (popularly known as "tennis elbow")
      1. Also found in golf, racquetball, and baseball
      2. Repetitive forces from holding implement
      3. Check the weight, size, and other characteristics of implement to make sure it matches the athlete's capabilities[3]
    B. Medial epicondylitis
      1. More common in baseball pitchers and javelin throwers
      2. Check mechanics of throw
    C. Medial and lateral collateral strains/tears
      1. Usually from traumatic forces (e.g., gymnasts, baseball pitchers, elbow being caught around another player)
      2. One of most feared injuries of the thrower is the ulnar collateral ligament rupture.
      3. Participate with protective equipment such as a brace
    D. Dislocation
      1. Traumatic
        a. Fall on extended elbow
        b. Sudden, violent unidirectional blow to elbow
      2. May also have fracture or neurovascular disruption
III.   Hand injuries
    A. Mechanism
      1. Fall on outstretched hand
      2. Direct blow

3. Weight-bearing
4. Rotational force (gymnastics)
B. Ligamentous injuries[4]
1. Collateral ligament
a. "Jammed finger"
b. Either a hyperextension force or varus or valgus force to the joint
c. May be able to buddy-tape the finger or splint it
2. Volar plate
a. Caused by a severe hyperextension force
C. Tendon injuries[4]
1. Mallet finger: distal interphalangeal (DIP) joint
a. Caused by a blow to the tip of finger (usually from a ball)
b. Splint into extension for 6 to 8 weeks
c. Consult with physician about participation
2. Boutonniere deformity: proximal interphalangeal (PIP) joint
a. Caused by trauma to the top of the finger
b. Splinting required
c. Consult with physician about participation
3. Jersey finger: flexor digitorum profundus (FDP) tendon rupture
a. Finger gets caught in jersey of another player
D. Fracture[4]
1. Crush (usually to tip)
2. Bend or twist (usually midshaft)
3. Spiral (finger gets twisted)

RETURN TO PLAY

I. Host (athlete)
A. Mentally ready
1. Ready to return to where injury took place
2. Playing style is similar to preinjury level
B. Ready to return physically
1. Player may not need full ROM
2. Basic movements are relatively pain free
3. Able to perform basic movements with adequate strength
4. Must be able to complete an effective sequence without further damaging the injury
5. Change of role on team
a. Soccer player not making throw-in from sideline
b. Baseball player becoming designated hitter instead of pitcher
II. Environment (game play or practice)
A. Protective equipment
1. Braces with restraining devices
a. Must be comfortable
b. Should restrict intended motion but not other needed movements
c. Check to make sure device is legal
2. Padding to help disperse force
a. Hard shell
(1) May need padding to cover

           (2) Must not be too bulky

           (3) Should not restrict motions

        b. Foam doughnuts

           (1) May surround injured area

           (2) Must be secured each time an athlete participates

           (3) Does not interfere with athletic function

     3. Finger splints

        a. Be able to hold implement

        b. Perform function without functional use of that finger

III.   Agency (force)

    A. Most difficult to control

    B. Evaluate kinds of forces the athlete encounters

       1. No contact with other players

       2. Contact with other players (football)

       3. Contact with other objects (e.g., balls, sticks)

    C. Indirect forces (e.g., ball striking a racquet)

RETURN TO PLAY CHECKLIST

    I.   Can the athlete perform functional activities?

       A. Can the athlete play with certain limitations?

       B. Does everyone (coach, athlete, parents, teammates) understand those limitations?

       C. Can the athlete's role on the team be modified?

       D. Does the athlete have the cardiovascular conditioning necessary?

       E. Is the core (trunk) in proper condition?

       F. Is the entire shoulder-elbow-wrist complex in balance?

   II.   Is the athlete mentally ready to play?

  III.   Can the athlete decrease the risk of reinjury with the use of protective equipment?

       A. Is the protective equipment legal?

       B. Is it comfortable to wear?

       C. Does it allow the athlete to function?

  IV.   Can the athlete withstand the forces that will be expected in the field of play?

   V.   Once the game or practice is completed, what should the athlete do?

       A. Ice

       B. Rehabilitative exercises

       C. Continue with formal therapy

REFERENCES

1. Kahanov L, Fairchild PC: Discrepancies in perceptions held by injured athletes and athletic trainers during the initial injury evaluation. J Athletic Training 29:70-75, 1994
2. Wagman D, Khelifa M: Psychological issues in sport injury rehabilitation: current knowledge and practice. J Athletic Training 31:257-261, 1996
3. Manners JA: Equipment in Golf and Tennis [oral presentation]. Salisbury University Sports Medicine Symposium, Salisbury, MD, January 18, 2003
4. Combs JA: It's Not "Just a Finger." J Athletic Training 35:168-178, 2000

Management of Upper Extremity Amputations 56

Lorie Theisen

Complete or partial loss of an upper extremity is devastating, whether the loss is due to trauma or advanced disease. A comprehensive treatment program is necessary for the patient with a complete or partial amputation of the hand or limb. Each patient with an amputation has a unique set of circumstances that includes, but is not limited to, the level of amputation, the condition of the residual limb, the condition of the contralateral limb, and the stage of adjustment to the loss.

DEFINITION

The initial phase of rehabilitation begins during the initial hospitalization. Later phases of rehabilitation usually occur in an outpatient setting. As a result of the typically shorter inpatient stay, many initial phase treatment goals are addressed on an outpatient basis.

Fitting a patient within 1 month after trauma with an upper extremity prosthesis (even a temporary device) increases acceptance of the prosthesis.[1-3] Prosthetic training also has been shown to have a positive effect on function.[4]

SURGICAL PURPOSE

To remove useless or nonviable extremity parts that have been severely damaged by disease or trauma. Amputations are commonly performed for life-threatening infections, irreversible vascular compromise, tissue damage beyond hope of repair, and advanced loss of function so that the extremity becomes a biological parasite for the patient (Fig. 56-1). Rarely, chronic pain is a reason for amputation. The level of amputation is important and must be determined by the surgeon. The more length that can be safely preserved, the better the prognosis is for efficient and compliant prosthetic wear and use.

TREATMENT PURPOSE

I. Promote early mobilization.
II. Promote proper shaping of the residual stump.

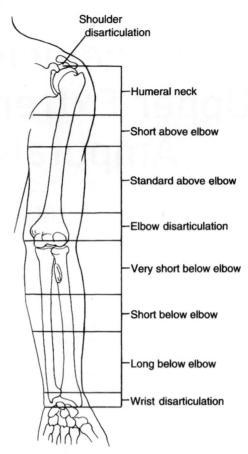

Shoulder disarticulation

—Humeral neck

—Short above elbow

—Standard above elbow

—Elbow disarticulation

—Very short below elbow

—Short below elbow

—Long below elbow

—Wrist disarticulation

FIG. **56-1** Upper extremity amputations are performed for useless or nonviable parts severely damaged by disease or trauma.

III.   Maximize independence in activities of daily living (ADLs).
IV.   Provide orientation to the next rehabilitation phase (i.e., initial phase rehabilitation should orient the patient to follow-up with outpatient treatment).
V.   Introduce options with regard to upper extremity prosthesis, if indicated.

TREATMENT GOALS

I.   Promote wound healing.
II.   Reduce edema of residual stump.
III.   Control or reduce incisional and phantom pain.
IV.   Maintain or increase active range of motion (AROM) and passive range of motion (PROM) of residual upper extremity joints.
V.   Promote ADL independence.
VI.   Explore patient's and family's feelings about loss of limb.
VII.   Explore resources for continuation of preprosthetic training, prosthetic training, and other necessary services.

POSTOPERATIVE INDICATIONS/PRECAUTIONS FOR THERAPY

I.   Indications: any patient with an amputation, complete or partial, who is otherwise medically stable and able to participate in ADLs and exercise programs.

II. Precautions
     A. Unstable medical status
     B. Others as noted by physician

POSTOPERATIVE THERAPY

I.   Evaluation
     A. Database should include age, sex, hand dominance, occupation, avocations, date of injury, date of surgery, level of amputation, mechanism of injury, current medical status, past medical history.
     B. Note skin condition at site of amputation. Note other structures (e.g., tendon, bone) that may have suffered trauma in both upper extremities.
     C. Presence of edema, girth measurements bilaterally to compare involved and uninvolved extremity.
     D. ROM of residual joints and of sound upper extremity: ROM of the uninvolved extremity is necessary for comparison with the residual joints. Pay special attention to shoulder girdle and radioulnar joints. In a below-elbow amputation, maximizing supination and pronation is an important goal.
     E. Muscle strength of residual musculature and of sound upper extremity: Adhere to precautions with respect to orthopedic condition and other soft tissue injuries.
     F. Presence and quality or description of pain.
     G. Sensibility and hypersensitivity at stump.
     H. ADL status.
     I. Posture and balance.
     J. Note need for additional support from a social worker or psychologist.

II. Treatment plan
     A. Wound care as prescribed by physician: Adhere to special precautions (e.g., skin graft).
     B. Edema control: Consider use of compression pump, elevation, and stump wrapping as condition of vascular system and soft tissues allows.
     C. Splinting as necessary for protecting any repaired structures or for decreasing limitations in ROM
     D. AROM, active-assisted range of motion (AAROM), or PROM exercise program as indicated, paying special attention to shoulder girdle and radioulnar joints
     E. Consider transcutaneous electric nerve stimulation (TENS) for pain control.
     F. Desensitization program as condition of wounds allows; include deep pressure when tolerated
     G. ADL training should include compensatory techniques and adaptive equipment. Consider use of temporary pylon to aid in ADL independence.

H. Postural exercises, if indicated
I. Initiate appropriate intervention from a social worker, psychologist, or psychiatrist.
III.   Discharge planning evaluation from inpatient unit
   A. Identify initial problems and current status and any additional problems.
   B. Note progress or lack of progress; include explanation for lack of progress (e.g., complications).
   C. Potential for additional rehabilitation
   D. Follow-up plan
      1. Location and date of initial visit for further outpatient rehabilitation
      2. Follow-up with primary surgeon
      3. Social work, psychologist, or psychiatrist follow-up as indicated
      4. Follow-up via amputee clinic or physician for prosthetic prescription and other necessary services

POSTOPERATIVE COMPLICATIONS

I.   Infection
II.   Delayed healing
III.   Decreased ROM due to immobilization period
IV.   Neuroma and other scar adherence problems

EVALUATION TIMELINE

I.   Initial assessment when medically stable
II.   Reevaluation every week thereafter during initial phase of rehabilitation
III.   In late phases of rehabilitation, reevaluate at least monthly.

PROSTHETIC TRAINING

Treatment Goals

I. Educate patient and family regarding prosthetic fabrication, fitting, and training.
II. Identify specific goals of prosthesis for ADLs, work tasks, and avocational interests.
III. Collaborate with prosthetist, physician, patient, and family to determine the type of prosthesis.
IV. After completion and delivery of the prosthesis, evaluate patient and family about the prosthetic parts, care of the prosthesis, and the wearing schedule.
V. Independence in doffing and donning the prosthesis
VI. Success in basic control of the prosthesis for positioning and opening and closing the terminal device[5] (Fig. 56-2)
VII. Functional use training via application of learned control for ADL activities.
VIII. Progress to functional training for avocational and vocational activities

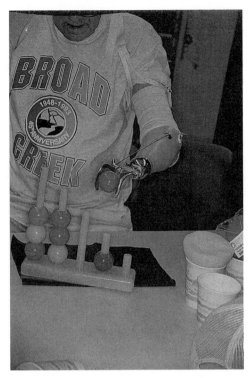

F I G . **56-2**   Maintaining pressure on objects while reaching.

Treatment Plan

I.   Provide verbal and written education to patient as to terminology, treatment specifics, and resources available regarding upper extremity prosthesis.
II.   Orientation to and practice of donning and doffing process
III. Training in opening, closing, and prepositioning terminal device
IV.   Manipulation of various graded activities
V.   Application of skills learned in control training to functional tasks (e.g., cutting food, dressing). Practice challenging activities such as inserting paper into an envelope, wrapping a package, and picking up a Styrofoam cup without crushing the cup with terminal device pressure.
VI.   Identify specific terminal devices or characteristics of the prosthesis needed for the patient's specific goals, such as work or sports terminal devices.[5]

OUTCOMES

Outcomes research in patients with upper extremity amputation is elusive. Few articles have been written about the outcomes after amputation and fitting of upper extremity prosthetics. Experts cite the uniqueness of each case, the limited measurements available to assess function, and the relatively small population of patients.[6] Factors such as level of amputation, hand dominance, psychosocial issues, type of prosthesis, and training in the use of the prosthesis all have a major effect on the outcome in patients with loss of limb.

Some of the research available investigates the ability of health care providers to return the patient to his or her prior level of function. Patients may discover methods to perform particular activities that may or may not involve the use of a prosthesis. Datta and colleagues[7] reported that 73.2% of patients returned to work, yet 33.75% rejected their prosthesis. Gaine and associates[8] described the satisfaction rate of prosthetic use in patients suffering a traumatic upper extremity amputation and in those with congenital deformities. They reported that early prosthetic fitting, rehabilitation, and posttraumatic counseling lead to the optimum functional state of the patient. Overall satisfaction of upper limb amputees with their prosthesis was also investigated by Davidson.[9] She looked at prosthetic use, current needs, and preferences of upper extremity amputees in Australia and concluded that a multitude of factors influence outcomes, including the patient's comfort when wearing the prosthesis, the type of activity to be performed (home, work, and leisure tasks), the patient's personality and psychological status, and the support system. Successful rehabilitation programs address all of these areas.

REFERENCES

1. Malone J, Fleming L, Roberson J, et al.: Immediate, early and late postsurgical management of upper-limb amputation. J Rehabil Res Dev 21:33, 1984
2. Fletchall S, Hickerson W: Early upper extremity prosthetic fit in patients with burns. J Burn Care Rehabil 12:234, 1991
3. Pinzur MS, Angelats J, Light TR, et al.: Functional outcome following upper limb amputation and prosthetic fitting. J Hand Surg Am 19:836-839, 1994
4. Lake C: Effects of prosthetic training on upper extremity prosthesis use. J Prosthet Orthot 9:3, 1997
5. Michael JW, Gailey RS, Bowker JH: New developments in recreational prostheses and adaptive devices for the amputee. Clin Orthop (256):64-75, 1990
6. Otto J: Outcomes measurements in upper-limb prosthetics: why so elusive? The O&P Edge, January 2003. Available at: http://www.oandp.com (accessed April 6, 2005)
7. Datta D, Selvarajah K, Davey N: Functional outcome of patients with proximal upper limb deficiency—acquired and congenital. Clin Rehabil 18:172-177, 2004
8. Gaine WJ, Smart C, Bransby-Zachary M: Upper limb traumatic amputees: review of prosthetic use. J Hand Surg Br 22:73-76, 1997
9. Davidson J: A survey of the satisfaction of upper limb amputees with their prosthesis, their lifestyles, and their abilities. J Hand Ther 15:62-70, 2002

SUGGESTED READINGS

Atkins D, Meir R III: Comprehensive Management of the Upper Extremity Amputee. Springer-Verlag, New York, 1989
Helpa M: The Union Memorial Hospital Lower Extremity Amputee Program. Union Memorial Hospital, Baltimore, MD, 1990
Nico D, Daprati E, Rigal F, et al.: Left and right hand recognition in upper limb amputees. Brain 127:120-132, 2004
Olivett B: Adult amputee management and conventional prosthetic training. In Hunter J, Schneider L, Mackin E, et al. (eds): Rehabilitation of the Hand: Surgery and Therapy. 3rd Ed. Mosby, St. Louis, 1990, p. 1057
Pinzur MS, Angelats J, Light TR, et al.: Functional outcome following traumatic upper limb amputation and prosthetic limb fitting. J Hand Surg Am 19:836, 1994
Upper Limb Prosthetics. 2nd Rev. New York University Post-Graduate Medical School, New York, 1986

Social Work Services   57

Ann Leman-Domenici

The clinical skills and services of a social worker can be an integral part of the interdisciplinary treatment offered to patients with injuries to the hand or upper extremity.

The social work role in this ambulatory, rehabilitative setting is a consultative one to staff, physicians, patients, and families. The primary focus is to explore the patient's and family's emotional reaction to the hand or upper extremity injury; what the injury means to them in terms of loss and change in their lives, and how they have typically coped with change in the past. It is important to be supportive and to challenge the patient and family to use some of those beneficial skills in the present situation. Also, the social worker asks the patient and family to clarify their understanding and expectations of treatment. According to Richard K. Johnson[1]:

> The assessment also might involve exploration of how the injured person is handling grief. The person's sense of grief flows from the experience of loss; a loss of the use of one's hand, [even] if only temporary, is significant. The loss triggers not only apprehensions over the future functioning of the hand but also the loss of employment, income and self-image as a productive, contributing person in a company or a family, if only a short while. The stages of grief involving denial, depression and anger are important aspects to be assessed.

Many psychosocial factors can be triggered as a result of a trauma or injury, including issues of body image, sexuality, and self-identity; changes in physical activity and preinjury recreational or leisure activities; changes in fulfilling social and familial roles; and issues of responsibility and employment.

The stated message in a psychosocial assessment is that the treatment team wants to learn the best way of treating the whole injured worker so that there will be a successful recovery and rehabilitation. The patient with a hand or upper extremity injury requires understanding, empathy, support, and education in establishing realistic goals.

Psychosocial support for these patients should begin as soon as possible after the injury. To accomplish this, in our facility, both Clinical Social Work services and Behavioural Medicine consultations are available to hospitalized patients. Social Work services are available to patients and families in the outpatient, ambulatory setting during clinic visits, therapy, and work hardening programs, both at the hospital and at the satellite sites off campus.

It is vitally important for the patient and the family to be able to tell their story, the facts of the injury, and their feelings associated with those facts to someone on the team.

DEFINITION

Referrals for social work services are typically received from physicians, hand therapists, work rehabilitation therapists, rehabilitation nurses, and family members through direct referrals.

TREATMENT INDICATIONS

Important indicators for referral include the following:
- I. Adjustment to injury issues
- II. Alcohol/drug abuse and/or recovery issues
- III. Anxiety
- IV. Depression
- V. Specific diagnoses
  - A. Complex regional pain syndrome (CRPS)
  - B. Traumatic upper extremity amputation
  - C. Chronic pain
  - D. Posttraumatic stress disorder (PTSD)
- VI. Conversion reactions
- VII. Factitious disorder
- VIII. Family problems
- IX. Financial issues
- X. High stressors
- XI. Lack of social supports
- XII. Marital problems
- XIII. Previous psychiatric treatment
- XIV. Pharmacy assistance/prescriptions
- XV. Transportation to treatment issues

ASSESSMENT

The social worker completes a comprehensive written psychosocial assessment, including the following information:
1. The presenting problem as perceived by the patient
2. Insurance coverage (Workers Compensation claim, Medicare, medical assistance, self-pay, commercial insurance), financial and legal status
3. Understanding of diagnosis, cause of symptoms, and expectations of treatment
4. Patient's support network, family composition, family/marital status
5. Education and/or level of literacy, work history, current job, length of employment, job satisfaction
6. Current affective and cognitive functioning

7. Stressors and emotional state; symptoms of depression
8. Current medications
9. Alcohol/drug usage
10. Activities of daily living (ADLs): What is a typical day like?
11. Prior mental health treatment
12. Preexisting/concurrent medical problems
13. Difficulty with the law

After the assessment is complete, the social worker collaborates with the patient, the therapist, the physician, and the rehabilitation specialist to initiate a treatment plan for the patient that includes action steps and appropriate referrals. This is not a passive process in which the patient is the receiver of the social worker's treatment; rather, it is an active process of communication and negotiation to achieve mutual treatment goals.

Additionally, the patient's spouse or significant other is invited to participate in the sessions. At times, a telephone interview is the best alternative to obtain information and enlist support toward the recommended plan of treatment. Especially if the recommendation is for a psychiatric evaluation, the spouse or significant other may need assistance also, or couples counseling may be recommended.

TREATMENT GOALS

Treatment goals vary depending on the identified and agreed-upon problem. Diagnostic indicators for specific problems are presented here, based on the treatment indications listed earlier.

I. Adjustment to injury issues: The treatment goal is to provide information, referral, and emotional support and to advocate on behalf of the patient. Examples include the following:
   A. Basic information on the Workers Compensation system is provided. Patients are directed to their representing attorney for specific concerns.
   B. Overall orientation to the institution's purpose and philosophy, with clarification of the roles and responsibilities of patient and institution. Patients are encouraged to take ownership of their care.
   C. Information and referral to community resources as appropriate
      1. Adult literacy and/or General Educational Development (GED) program to improve skills and to provide a productive, structured activity
      2. Encourage volunteer employment to reduce boredom, increase activity level, and promote self-esteem
      3. Referral to the State Division of Rehabilitation Services
      4. Recommend participation in a senior center for social support and to reduce isolation and symptoms of depression for senior citizens
      5. Referral to support groups
      6. Referral to shelters and/or group homes
      7. Referral to church-sponsored programs
II. Alcohol, drug abuse, and addictions (e.g., eating, smoking, gambling): The treatment goal is to identify the problem, educate the patient about the treatment options available, and make a recommendation for treatment to the patient and physician.

In addition, the social worker reinforces and supports the program of recovery being used.

    A. Documented use (e.g., emergency room) of alcohol/drugs when the injury occurred

    B. Use of alcohol to self-medicate for pain management

    C. Use of prescription narcotics for more than 2 to 3 months after the injury or surgery

    D. Patient arrives for hand treatment under the influence

    E. Self-identified recovering alcoholic or addict who is working a 12-step program. The stress of the injury and rehabilitation can place such an individual at high risk for relapse.

    F. Cigarette addiction that is compromising the physical outcome of the injury.

    G. Gambling behavior that is interfering with financial resources to engage or follow through with treatment.

III. Anxiety: The treatment goal is to identify the symptoms and provide education and treatment recommendations. Anxiety disorders are treated by a combination of cognitive behavior therapy and medication and usually require a psychiatric evaluation.

    A. Phobic disorder: The essential feature is fear of an activity, situation, or object that results in a desire to avoid the same. If the avoidance behavior or fear is a significant source of distress and interferes with social or role functioning, treatment is indicated.

    B. Panic disorder: The essential feature is a sudden onset of intense apprehension, fear, or terror, associated with feelings of impending doom. Symptoms include dyspnea, palpitations, chest pain, dizziness or unsteady feelings, sweating, faintness, trembling or shaking, or hot/cold flashes.

IV. Depression: The treatment goal is to identify the symptoms, educate the patient about available treatments, and make a recommendation for treatment to the patient and physician. Typical treatment involves medication and psychotherapy. Symptoms include the following:

    A. Loss of interest or pleasure in all or almost all usual activities; withdrawal from family and friends

    B. Appetite disturbance, at either extreme (increased appetite and weight gain or loss of appetite and weight loss)

    C. Sleep disturbance

    D. Concentration difficulties; increased forgetfulness

    E. Suicidal ideation

V. Specific diagnoses

    A. CRPS or chronic pain: The treatment goal is to identify symptoms of depression and educate the patient about the benefits of antidepressants in pain management and the symptoms of depression. Also, the patient may be referred to a CRPS support group.

    B. Traumatic upper extremity amputation: The treatment goal is to identify symptoms of loss, anger, and depression and to provide counseling for adjustment to the injury. Referral to the Amputee Association of America is a standard procedure. Psychiatric evaluation is often indicated.

C. PTSD: recognition that the hand patient experienced an event outside the range of usual human experience. The four major characteristics of PTSD are as follows:
   1. Persistent re-experiencing of the traumatic event
   2. Recurrent distressing dreams of the event
   3. Sudden acting or feeling as if the traumatic event were recurring (flashback episodes)
   4. Persistent avoidance of stimuli associated with the traumatic event

VI. Conversion reactions: The treatment goal is to identify symptoms and related issues and refer the patient for psychiatric evaluation. The main symptom is a loss or change in physical functioning that suggests a physical disorder but is an expression of a psychological conflict or need. The disturbance is not under the voluntary control of the patient.

VII. Factitious disorder with physical symptoms: The treatment goal is to identify symptoms and refer the patient for psychiatric evaluation. The essential feature is the presentation of physical symptoms that are not real. An example is self-inflicted tourniqueting of the upper extremity.

VIII. Family problems: The treatment goal is to identify and educate the patient about available resources.
   A. History of physical, sexual, and/or emotional abuse or domestic violence
   B. Bereavement issues when there is loss of a family member
   C. Child's reaction to a parent's injury

IX. Financial issues: The treatment goal is to identify the problem and the potential resources and make the necessary referrals.
   A. Referral to the Department of Social Services for medical assistance, general public assistance, food stamps, Transitional Emergency Medical Housing Assistance (TEMHA).
   B. Referral to the internal mechanisms of the hospital for financial assistance.

X. Stressors are high: The treatment goal is to identify the stressors and educate the patient in stress management techniques using a cognitive behavioral approach.
   A. Progressive muscle relaxation exercises and self-hypnosis
   B. Encourage self-nurturing activities
   C. Affirming positive gains

XI. Lack of social supports: The treatment goal is to engage the patient in recognizing the problem and brainstorming solutions.
   A. Encourage and direct the patient to volunteer in some capacity
   B. Encourage the patient to participate in church-related activities
   C. Encourage participation in a support group

XII. Marital problems: The treatment goal is to identify couples issues as the problem and to refer couples for counseling.

XIII. Previous and/or current psychiatric treatment: The treatment goal is to obtain from the patient the name and telephone number of the previous or current treating mental health professional. If behavioral changes are observed during the course of treatment of the injury, contact can be initiated with this resource person.

XIV. Transportation to treatment: The treatment goal is to facilitate the patient's treatment. It may be appropriate to contact the insurance carrier, explain the problem, and negotiate a solution.
   A. Bus tokens
   B. Cab vouchers

SUMMARY

Patients with hand or upper extremity injuries are just like anyone else. They may worry about the past, present, and future; their jobs; their families; the direction and fabric of their lives; and their health and capabilities.

I have experienced the continuum of responses—patients who were initially angry at their physicians for referring them to a social worker and patients who were eternally grateful for the referral. It has always been a privilege for me when another human being willingly or even reluctantly shares thoughts and feelings, fears, frustrations, and sense of loss, in an effort to process individual experience. Social work services assist the patient and family in this endeavor.

REFERENCE

1. Johnson RK: Psychological evaluation of patients with industrial hand injuries. Occup Injuries 3:567, 1986

SUGGESTED READINGS

Cone J, Hueston JT: Psychological aspects of hand injury. Med J Aust 1:104, 1974
Chan J, Spencer J: Adaptation to hand injury: an evolving experience. Am J Occup Ther 58:128-139, 2004
Grunert BK, Devine CA, Matloub HS, et al.: Sexual dysfunction following traumatic hand injury. Ann Plast Surg 1:46, 1988
Grunert BK, Devine CA, McCallum-Burke S, et al.: On-site work evaluation: desensitizing for avoidance reactions following hand trauma. J Hand Surg Br 14:239, 1989
Grunert BK, Matloub HS, Sanger JR, et al.: Treatment of posttraumatic stress disorder after work related hand trauma. J Hand Surg Am 15:511, 1990
Grunert BK, Smith CJ, Devine CA, et al.: Early psychological aspects of traumatic hand injury. J Hand Surg Br 13:177, 1988
Inaba K, Goecke M, Sharkey P, et al.: Long-term outcomes after injury in the elderly. J Trauma 54:486-491, 2003
Lai CH: Motivation in hand-injured patients with and without work-related injury. J Hand Ther 17:6-17, 2004
Mendelson R, Burech J, Polack EP, et al.: The psychological impact of traumatic amputations—a team approach: physicians, therapists and psychologist. Occup Injuries 3:577, 1986
Meyer TM: Psychological aspects of mutilating hand injuries. Hand Clin 19:41-49, 2003
Michael AJ, Michaels CE, Moon CH, et al.: Psychosocial factors limit outcomes after trauma. J Trauma 44:644-648, 1998
Pascarelli EF, Hsu YP: Understanding work-related upper extremity disorders: clinical findings in 485 computer users, musicians and others. J Occup Rehabil 11:1-21, 2001
Pransky GS, Benjamin KL, Savageau JA, et al.: Outcomes in work related injuries: a comparison of older and younger workers. Am J Ind Med 47:104-112, 2005
Zatzick DF, Jurkovich GJ, Gentilello L, et al.: Post traumatic stress, problem drinking and functional outcome after injury. Arch Surg 137:200-205, 2002

Industrial Rehabilitation Services

58

Donna M. Keegan and Robert C. Kahlert

Hand or upper extremity injuries, including those suffered on the job, can affect a patient's ability to return to work, even at the conclusion of traditional medical treatment and rehabilitation. With this in mind, industrial rehabilitation services were developed in the 1970s. During the next decade, focus on these services shifted from dealing with work injuries from a psychosocial or behavioral model only, termed **work adjustment**, to assessment of an injured worker's physical abilities and limitations in the work setting, or what has become known as **industrial rehabilitation**.

As occupational and physical therapists became involved in this field, which previously was addressed primarily by vocational evaluators, they assisted in defining functional capacity evaluation and work hardening services, which are ideally provided by a team of professionals with experience in the vocational, medical, and psychological arenas. By 1989, the Commission on Accreditation of Rehabilitation Facilities (CARF) had established specific standards for the practice of work hardening programs. The 2003 CARF standards classify these services as Occupational Rehabilitation Programs.

Current industrial rehabilitation programs may include functional capacity evaluations, work conditioning, work hardening, on-site therapy, post-offer job screenings, job analysis, injury prevention education classes, and ergonomic evaluations. This chapter primarily focuses on protocols for functional capacity evaluations, work hardening, and ergonomics for upper extremity injuries.

DEFINITIONS AND TIMELINES

Functional Capacity Evaluations

"The Functional Capacity Evaluation Process consists of evaluation procedures, questionnaires, and observations, which document the patient's ability to perform work from a physical, medical, behavioral, and ergonomic perspective… This process will help to determine if that worker can return to work safely."[1]

Ideally, the functional capacity evaluation should take place over two client visits, to accurately evaluate the client's response to testing and to reduce the cumulative effects of fatigue or pain. Both sessions should be scheduled so that the evaluation can be completed within 1 week, to more closely simulate work demands. Finally, the process should conclude with a team meeting to formulate appropriate goals and recommendations. The functional capacity evaluation may stand on its own to provide a clear picture of the individual's work capabilities for job placement, or it may be followed by a work hardening program.

Work Hardening

"A Comprehensive Occupational Rehabilitation Program is an interdisciplinary, outcomes-focused, individualized program. Through the comprehensive assessment and treatment provided by occupational rehabilitation specialists, the program addresses the medical, psychological, behavioral, physical, functional and vocational components of employability and return to work. The simulated/real work used in the program addresses the complexities of the persons served and their work environments."[2]

Generally, work hardening is a daily program of either half-day or full-day sessions (up to 8 hours) of work simulation, conditioning, and education. The program lasts for an average of 4 weeks, with adjustment as necessary to meet the client's specific goals.

Ergonomics

Ergonomics is a science that utilizes information pertaining to human anatomy, physiology, and anthropometry to design or adapt functional activities. Its practitioners assess an individual's endurance, effectiveness, health, and safety while performing work, sports, and leisure activities, as well as activities of daily living (ADLs). The application of ergonomic principles is intended to provide preventive strategies for **cumulative trauma injuries** and **work-related musculoskeletal disorders (WMSDs)**. WMSDs are musculoskeletal disorders that occur or are exacerbated by an individual's interaction with tools, equipment, or environment.

Symptoms of cumulative trauma injuries and WMSDs may begin with fatigue, numbness, tingling, burning, discomfort, or pain. If the activities contributing to these symptoms are not modified, they may eventually result in difficulty performing job duties, ADLs, and leisure activities. A comprehensive activity analysis or job analysis is essential when attempting to prevent or reduce cumulative trauma injuries or WMSDs with ergonomics. Data are gathered for activity analysis or job analysis from interviews, observations, and physical data collections. Ergonomic risk factors can be identified after completion of a comprehensive activity analysis. Recommendations are made to eliminate or reduce the severity of the ergonomic risk factors.

Ergonomics is most effective when it is implemented in tandem with medical management. Cumulative trauma injuries and WMSDs are cured most quickly when symptoms are identified early and interventions to alleviate symptoms are initiated immediately. WMSDs are most preventable when ergonomics is an integral component of a health and safety program. Optimal results from an ergonomics program can be obtained only if the program is a continuous process, because the individual's daily activities and environment are in constant change.

PURPOSES/GOALS

I. Functional capacity evaluation
   A. Assess the injured worker's abilities and limitations related to work or job demands.
   B. Clarify job demands and vocational status.
   C. Compare current performance of work simulations to required job demands.
   D. Evaluate consistency of effort and pain behaviors as they affect work performance.
   E. Assess work-related behaviors.
   F. Determine whether further services are needed (including work hardening) and provide a thorough baseline for subsequent treatment.
II. Work hardening
   A. Facilitate gradual, progressive improvement in physical skills and work tolerances.
   B. Physical conditioning and endurance training.
   C. Provide psychosocial preparation for return to work, and identify any related barriers to work performance.
   D. Ensure safety in the workplace, and provide education in topics such as proper body mechanics and injury prevention.
III. Ergonomics
   A. Prevent cumulative trauma injuries and WMSDs.
   B. Improve health and safety.
   C. Increase efficiency in performing activity or job duty.
   D. Reduce discomfort in performing activity or job task.
   E. Decrease fatigue while performing activity or job duty.
   F. Increase employee morale and job satisfaction.
   G. Decrease employer's Workers' Compensation claims and cost of work injuries.
   H. Maintain or increase worker productivity.
   I. Increase employer profitability.

ADMISSION CRITERIA

In general, patients eligible for industrial rehabilitation services should meet the following admission criteria: (1) have one or more physical limitations that may affect job performance or work potential, (2) be medically stable, (3) have a primary diagnosis or symptoms of musculoskeletal injury, and (4) have written referral or clearance from a physician. To participate in work hardening, the patient should also meet the following criteria: (1) have completed a baseline evaluation or functional capacity evaluation that documents the probable benefit from a work hardening program, and (2) have a vocational goal or job target. Functional capacity evaluations and work hardening programs are typically initiated after the client has reached maximum benefit from more traditional types of occupational and/or physical therapy. Functional capacity evaluations and work hardening programs usually are covered through Workers' Compensation insurance carriers, rather than general health insurance companies. Ergonomic assessments are recommended when a client experiences musculoskeletal symptoms from interaction with an activity. Ergonomic programs may be covered by Workers' Compensation carriers or by employers.

EVALUATION AND TREATMENT GUIDELINES

I. Functional capacity evaluation
    A. Vocational specialist
        1. Interview injured worker/client.
            a. Work history
            b. Educational background
            c. Current employer information
            d. Current source of income
            e. Behavioral and attitudinal status
            f. Cognitive status
            g. Detailed information about job demands and requirements
            h. Social status
        2. Contact client's employer.
            a. Confirm job demands.
            b. Clarify employment status and/or schedule a job site analysis.
            c. Resolve any return-to-work issues.
        3. Obtain and review job description with client.
            a. O*Net Dictionary of Occupational Titles[3] and computerized occupational information systems
            b. Client report
            c. Employer's verbal and/or written job descriptions
            d. Communicate job information to therapist.
    B. Rehabilitation technician
        1. Assess client's current cardiovascular status.
        2. Determine current fitness level.
        3. Communicate any contraindications for return to work or further participation in evaluation or work hardening program (e.g., hypertension).
    C. Occupational/physical therapist
        1. Interview injured worker/client.
            a. History of current injury
            b. Past medical history
            c. Client report of functional abilities/limitations
            d. All current subjective information from client as it relates to injury
        2. Evaluate client's functional abilities/limitations.
            a. Volumetric or circumferential measurement (edema)
            b. Musculoskeletal evaluation, as applicable to client's injury and function
                (1) Range of motion
                (2) Manual muscle testing

TABLE **58-1**   Standard Physical Demands of Work (Materials Handling, lb)

Frequency	Sedentary	Light	Medium	Heavy	Very Heavy
Occasionally (1%-33% of day)	10	20	21-50	50-100	>100
Frequently (34%-66% of day)	<10	10	10-25	25-50	>50
Constantly (67%-100% of day)	<10	<10	10	20	>25

      (3) Sensation
      (4) Gross and fine coordination
      (5) Grip/pinch strength
      (6) Posture, gait, flexibility, balance
  c. Determine maximum voluntary effort in lifting, carrying, pushing, and pulling.
  d. Determine physical demand level and endurance for materials handling (Table 58-1).
  e. Consistency of effort using several measures
  f. Tolerance to working positions
  g. Work simulations related to specific job demands (Fig. 58-1)

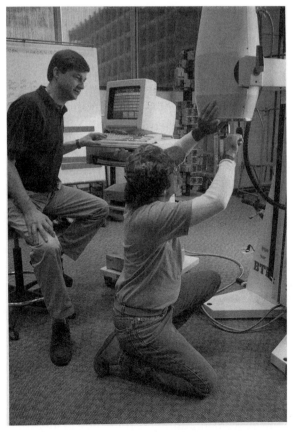

FIG. **58-1** Work simulation utilizing Baltimore Therapeutic Equipment (BTE) Work Simulator. (Courtesy Curtis Work Rehabilitation Services, Baltimore, MD.)

       3. Arrange and facilitate team meeting.
       4. Communicate results and recommendations.
       5. Compose report, using all data collected as well as information from team members.
    D. Interdisciplinary team
       1. Attend team meeting to communicate results and develop recommendations.
       2. Foster client communication and determine need for treatment.
II. Work hardening
    A. Vocational specialist
       1. Prepare list of job demands specific to job targeted; this becomes part of the individual program plan.
       2. Conduct educational lectures regarding return-to-work issues.
       3. Act as liaison between employer and team.
    B. Occupational/physical therapist
       1. Act as case manager for work hardening team.
          a. Design an individualized treatment plan, including work simulation activities.
          b. Orient client to work hardening activities.
          c. Promote client participation in program.
          d. Set short-term and long-term goals.
          e. Consider/implement recommendations of other team members regarding service provision.
          f. Consistently reevaluate client progress.
          g. Complete weekly progress reports.
          h. Communicate with physician, referral source, and all relevant external and internal team members.
          i. Arrange and facilitate team meetings.
          j. Facilitate discharge planning.
          k. Modify treatment plan as needed.
             (1) Ensure that work simulations are appropriate and progressive during entirety of program.
             (2) Ensure that conditioning/strengthening activities are appropriate.
       2. Teach and reinforce proper body mechanics.
       3. Conduct group and/or individual education on pertinent topics.
       4. Make recommendations for job or tool modifications or any adaptive equipment.
       5. May perform job site analysis or ergonomic consultation.
    C. Psychologist
       1. Review client questionnaires related to injury adjustment.
       2. Determine need for psychological services.
       3. Perform initial assessment if warranted.
       4. Conduct weekly coping and/or educational sessions.
       5. Counsel clients individually if necessary.
    D. Rehabilitation technician
       1. Supervise clients during performance of job simulation, strengthening, and conditioning exercises
       2. Alert therapists to any issues of concern.

E. Interdisciplinary team
  1. Participate in weekly client updates and provide input as needed throughout the program to ensure comprehensive client care.
  2. Foster client participation in the program and client self-advocacy skills.
  3. Attend biweekly team meetings with the client to assist in discharge planning.
  4. Determine appropriate discharge goals and final client disposition and recommendations.
  5. Participate in program evaluation and continuous operation improvement activities.
III. Ergonomics
  A. Analysis of activity or job
    1. Determine essential tasks or job duties to accomplish the activity or achieve the goals of the job.
    2. Identify sequence of tasks and procedures required to perform the activity. Determine the amount of time spent performing each individual task or function.
    3. Assess the level of skill, technical knowledge, or experience required to perform the activity or job.
    4. Identify the number of people available to perform the activity.
    5. Examine relationships with supervisors, coworkers, and customers. Determine what relationships are required to effectively perform the job.
    6. Assess the consequences of the task's being eliminated or achieved through automation.
    7. Determine the physical demand level of the activity. Determine whether the job is in the Sedentary, Light, Medium, Heavy, or Very Heavy category.
    8. Identify physical movements and working positions required to perform the task. Working positions may include sitting, standing, walking, climbing, balancing, stooping, kneeling, crawling, reaching, handling, fingering, and feeling.
    9. Assess forces and pressures that must be exerted to perform essential tasks.
    10. Determine range of motion or body movements required to perform the activity.
    11. Identify tools, materials, and equipment used to perform the activity. Evaluate weights and dimensions of objects involved in the activity. Measure size of handles and knobs to operate tools and machinery.
    12. Assess environmental conditions and working conditions, including temperature, moisture, vibration, confined spaces, noises, lighting, and exposure to hazardous materials.
  B. Evaluation of risk factors for cumulative trauma or WMSDs
    1. Awkward postures
      a. Postures that do not incorporate the natural curves of the spine
      b. Positions with spine rotation
      c. Forward shoulders and elevated scapulas
      d. Joint angles deviating from a resting position or neutral position

        e. Joint positions or movements outside the midrange of motion
- (1) Flexion, extension, or abduction of the shoulder
- (2) Internal or external rotation of the shoulder
- (3) Flexion or extension of elbow
- (4) Supination or pronation of forearm
- (5) Flexion, extension, ulnar deviation, or radial deviation of wrist

        f. Pinching with hand

2. Static postures
- a. Maintaining positions against gravity
- b. Holding objects for extended periods
- c. Remaining in one position for extended period without opportunity to change position

3. Force
- a. Muscle force required to perform activity
- b. Quick motions against external resistance
- c. Gripping and pinching

4. Repetition
- a. Frequent movements or exertions
- b. Inadequate pauses or breaks

5. Compression
- a. Tool handle pressure over carpal tunnel
- b. Elbows resting on hard surface
- c. Body part compressed against equipment, machinery, or workstation

6. Vibration
- a. Power tools
- b. Operating equipment or machinery resulting in whole-body vibration

7. Temperature
- a. Cold
- b. Heat

8. Poor physical conditioning

C. Ergonomic hazard prevention and controls

1. Engineering controls
- a. Workstation (Box 58-1; Fig. 58-2) should be designed to accomplish the following:
  - (1) Fit the size of the individual performing the activity.
  - (2) Be adjustable if more than one person uses the same workstation.
  - (3) Promote good posture.
  - (4) Enable job activity to be performed with joints in neutral position.
  - (5) Enable change of positions while maintaining safe postures.
  - (6) Allow for either dominance preference.
- b. Tool and equipment use
  - (1) Design tool handles to accommodate a forceful grip when forceful exertions are required.
  - (2) Use power tools to limit repetition of joint movements.
  - (3) Select power tools with the least vibration.

BOX 58-1   Ergonomic Checklist for a Computer Workstation

Chair should have a padded seat and provide good thigh support without contacting back of lower legs.

Chair back should provide good lumbar support and promote sitting with a neutral spine.

Hips should be at back of chair and level or slightly higher than knees.

Feet should rest firmly on floor or footrest.

Shoulders should be relaxed with upper arms resting comfortably at side.

Armrests should be padded and provide support when shoulders are relaxed. Armrests should not interfere with workstation or ability to reach with upper extremities.

Forearms should be parallel to the floor when working on the keyboard or mouse. Height of chair or height of keyboard can be adjusted to properly position forearms.

An adjustable-height keyboard tray can be used to properly position the keyboard and mouse.

Wrists should be in a neutral position when fingertips are resting on the keys.

A padded wrist rest should be used to rest wrists when taking a break from typing.

Monitor should be positioned directly in front of operator.

Height of monitor should place top row of characters at eye level when sitting with good posture.

Monitor should be positioned 18 to 30 inches away from operator. Monitor should be approximately an arm's distance away when operator is using the keyboard.

Document holder should be used when viewing monitor and document. Document holder should be located directly next to monitor.

Workstation accessories should be located within easy reach (e.g., stapler, telephone, tape dispenser, note pad)

Telephone headsets should be used when frequently communicating on the telephone or when the telephone is used while performing other tasks.

Workstation should have sufficient space to allow unrestricted movement of extremities.

Computer operator should be provided the opportunity to frequently change positions throughout the day. Micro stretch breaks should be taken every 20 to 30 minutes with intensive typing.

---

   (4) Design tools that minimize contact stress in the hand.

   (5) Use tools that have good balance in the hand.

   (6) Adapt tool handles to promote a firm grip.

   (7) Consider tools with a long lever arm if forceful exertions are required to perform a task.

   (8) Design or adapt the angle of the tool handle to minimize awkward postures of wrist when using the tool.

   (9) Use vices or clamps to stabilize work piece.

(10) Consider mechanical devices for frequent material handling and for heavy lifting or carrying. Mechanical devices may include hoists, carts, hand trucks, or conveyor systems.

(11) Use stools or ladders to prevent reaching overhead.

(12) Select appropriately fitting gloves to enhance gripping or for protection from the cold.

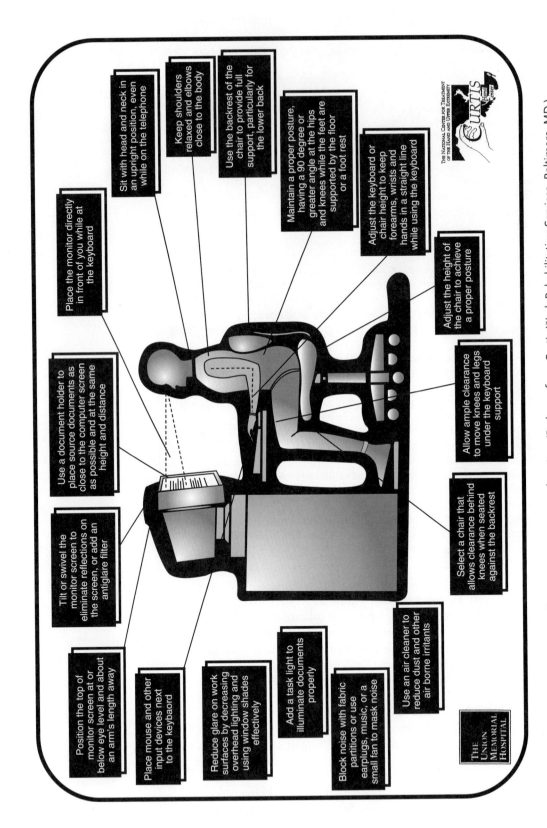

FIG. **58-2**   Ergonomically correct computer workstation. (Redrawn from Curtis Work Rehabilitation Services, Baltimore, MD.)

2. Administrative controls
   a. Enlarge jobs to limit repetition of a specific job duty.
   b. Use job rotation to rotate workers to jobs that do not require the same motions or muscle exertions.
   c. Alternate job duties throughout the day.
   d. Provide appropriate breaks to prevent muscle fatigue or to allow muscles adequate time to recover.
   e. Keep equipment maintained and tools sharpened to minimize risk factors.
   f. Consider alternative methods for performing the activity.
   g. Provide workers time to perform warm-up exercises.
   h. Encourage early reporting of symptoms of WMSDs.
   i. Establish a return-to-work program.
3. Education and training
   a. Educate employer and workers regarding risk factors for cumulative trauma disorders or WMSDs.
   b. Provide information to workers regarding signs and symptoms of cumulative trauma disorders or WMSDs.
   c. Teach proper stretching and strengthening exercises to minimize risk of musculoskeletal disorders.
   d. Instruct workers to report signs and symptoms of WMSDs early.
   e. Educate individuals on proper body mechanics and posture while performing tasks. Emphasize working in a neutral position.
   f. Provide education on proper use of tools and equipment.
   g. Instruct worker on proper maintenance of tools.
   h. Instruct individuals to use their largest joints and muscles to perform an activity.
   i. Emphasize the use of two hands to perform a task whenever possible.
   j. Train client to perform activity or job duty without jerking, tugging, or using quick, forceful exertions. Train client to use smooth, controlled motions to perform the activity.
   k. Train client to limit use of force when the task can be completed with a reduction in force.
   l. Instruct clients to use ergonomic principles for work, ADLs, and leisure activities.

REFERENCES

1. Blankenship K: Industrial Rehabilitation I. American Therapeutics, Inc., Macon, GA, 1990
2. Medical Rehabilitation Standards Manual. Commission on Accreditation of Rehabilitation Facilities, Tucson, AZ, 2003
3. O*Net Dictionary of Occupational Titles, 1998-1999 Edition. JIST Works, Inc., Indianapolis, IN, 1998

SUGGESTED READINGS

Armstrong TJ, Franzblau A, Haig A, et al.: Developing ergonomic solutions for prevention of musculoskeletal disorder disability. Assist Technol 13(2):78-87, 2001
Bernard BP: Musculoskeletal disorders and workplace factors. NIOSH publication 97-141. Cincinnati, OH: U.S. Department of Health and Human Services, National Institute for Occupational Safety and Health, Cincinnati, OH, 1997

Conrad KM, et al.: Initiating an ergonomic analysis: a process for jobs with highly variable tasks. AAOHN J 48: 423-429, 2000

Demers L: Work Hardening: A Practical Guide. Andover Medical Publishers, Boston, 1992

Good Practice Manual for the Rehabilitation of the Injured Worker. Maryland Injured Workers Task Force, Baltimore, Revised 1993

Isernhagen S: The Comprehensive Guide to Work Injury Management. Aspen Publishers, Gaithersburg, MD, 1995

King PM, et al.: A critical review of functional capacity evaluations. Phys Ther 78:852-866, 1998

Kuhn M, Kneidel T: Is work hardening effective. Indus Rehabil Q 3:1, 1990

Larson BA, Ellexson MT: Blueprint for ergonomics. Work 15:107-112, 2000

National Safety Council, Accredited Standards Committee Z365: Control of Cumulative Trauma Disorders. National Safety Council, Itasca, IL, 1998

Revised Handbook for Analyzing Jobs. U.S. Department of Labor, Washington, DC, 1991

U.S. Department of Health and Human Services: NIOSH Publications on Video Display Terminals. 3rd Ed. USDHHS, National Institute of Occupational Safety and Health, Cincinnati, OH, 1999

U.S. Department of Labor, Occupational Safety and Health Administration: Effective Ergonomics: Strategy for Success. February 3, 2004. Available at: http://www.osha.gov/SLTC/ergonomics/index.html (accessed April 6, 2005).

U.S. Department of Labor, Office of Disability Employment Policy: Job Analysis: An Important Employment Tool. October 1994. Available at: http://www.dol.gov/odep/pubs/fact/analysis.htm (accessed April 6, 2005).

Warren N: Work stress and musculoskeletal disorder etiology: the relative roles of psychosocial and physical risk factors. Work 17:221-234, 2001

Wilkens PM: Preventing work-related musculoskeletal disorders in VDT users: a comprehensive health promotion program. Work 20:171-178, 2003

Evidence-Based Practice in Hand and Upper Extremity Therapy

59

Heather DeLaney

As our field becomes increasingly complex with improved surgical and non-surgical treatments for a variety of problems involving the upper extremity, it is imperative that every hand therapist engage in evidence-based practice to ensure the future of our profession. David Sackett, a leader in evidence-based medicine, defines it as "the conscientious, explicit and judicious use of current best evidence in making decisions about the care of the individual patient. It means integrating individual clinical expertise with the best available external clinical evidence from systematic research."[1]

"The economic challenges confronting healthcare today have forced practitioners to justify clinical decisions according to an identified body of knowledge and to challenge the theory base that forms the foundation of their profession."[2] Every clinician has had to justify his or her services to insurance companies in order to be compensated. Clinicians have a daily need for valid information about diagnosis, prognosis, therapy, and prevention, despite limitations of time and resources.[3]

The purpose of evidence-based medicine is to replace the traditional medical paradigm, which is based on authority. Evidence-based medicine relies on the use of randomized controlled trials, systematic reviews, and other sources. It is important that the therapist be able to determine what is clinically relevant, critically evaluate the literature, and incorporate the information into practice.

THE PRACTICE OF EVIDENCE-BASED MEDICINE

The following steps outline a method of incorporating evidence-based medicine into daily practice[4]: (1) convert the need for information into an answerable question; (2) track down the best evidence to answer the question; (3) perform critical appraisal of the evidence for its validity, impact, and applicability; (4) integrate the information into clinical practice; and (5) evaluate effectiveness and efficiency. Details of these steps are presented next.

I. Convert the need for information into an answerable question. Construct a well-built search strategy.[5]
   A. Patient: Describe the clinical problem in terms of the patient's disease or general health condition.
   B. Intervention: The intervention may be any of the following:
      1. Clinical examination
      2. Prevention
      3. Prognosis
      4. Etiology
      5. Differential diagnosis
      6. Diagnostic test results
      7. Self-improvement
   C. Expected outcome: Ask the following questions:
      1. What can I hope to accomplish?
      2. Have all clinically relevant options been considered?
      3. What could the intervention really affect?
II. Track down the best evidence by following these steps[6]:
   A. Translate the clinical question into a usable search strategy.
   B. Select an appropriate database resource.[7]
      1. MEDLINE (http://www.medlineplus.gov): the National Library of Medicine's premier computerized bibliographic database; covers the fields of medicine, nursing, and health and rehabilitation sciences from the 1950s to the present.
         a. Provides only the abstract.
         b. Obtain full text article from a local medical/health library or the National Network of Libraries of Medicine's Loansome Doc program.
         c. MEDLINE is accessible via the American Physical Therapy Association web site
      2. CINAHL (http://www.cinahl.com): Cumulative Index of Nursing and Allied Health Literature; includes citations from 1228 journals dated 1982 to the present.
         a. Search CINAHL web site (requires a fee).
         b. Use local college or health professional library to access (usually free)
      3. The Cochrane Library (http://www.thecochranelibrary.com)
         a. Covers all areas of health care.
         b. Is made up of several databases to provide systematic reviews of literature that help summarize the results from a number of studies.
         c. The Cochrane Library can be accessed via their web site for a fee.
III. Critical appraisal of the evidence. It is imperative that a clinician understand the processes, definitions, and analytic procedures of research in order to structure an investigation.
   A. Levels of evidence[8]
      1. Systematic reviews: summarize and combine the results of several studies.
         a. Are said to have the highest level of evidence, because they minimize bias and random error
         b. "Only as strong as the design of the studies they summarize"[8]

      c. Caution must be taken, because judgments and choices are made by the researchers, which may introduce bias.
  2. Randomized controlled trials
    a. Bias is addressed through the following precautions:
      (1) Randomization: Experimental and control groups are essentially equal.
      (2) Blinding: Subjects and researchers are unaware of group assignment.
      (3) Other methods
    b. A strong causal relationship can be established because the treatment effect is isolated and manipulated.
    c. Bias may still exist, especially if volunteers were used.
    d. Careful consideration of the inclusion criteria is required to apply the results of the study to an individual patient.
  3. Cohort study: a prospective or longitudinal study
    a. This type of study monitors subjects over a period of time, usually for the purpose of describing developmental changes in a particular group.[2]
    b. These studies do not use blinding or randomization.
    c. Unknown confounding variables may play a role in the outcomes.
  4. Case-control study
    a. Cross-sectional or retrospective study to look at rare outcomes
    b. The retrospective nature of this study makes it susceptible to confounding factors.
  5. Case series reports
    a. Reports describe the process of patient/client management and the outcomes for a single patient or group of patients.
    b. Because these are strictly descriptive reports, no causal relationships can be established.
  6. Expert opinion
    a. The lowest level of evidence
    b. Unsystematic in nature and of unknown quality
B. Validity[2]
  1. Subjects
    a. Should not have sampling bias
    b. Should define the target population
    c. Sampling methods: random versus convenience[2]
      (1) Random sample: method of selecting subjects in which each subject has an equal chance of being chosen
      (2) Convenience sample: selection of the most available subjects for a study
    d. The number of subjects should be adequate to demonstrate a statistically significant difference if one exists
  2. Design
    a. Experimental versus nonexperimental
    b. Is the design appropriate for the question at hand?
    c. Are the subjects randomly assigned to groups?
  3. Instrumentation
    a. Specific devices should be described.
    b. Reliability of the instrument should be discussed, including intrarater or interrater reliability.

    4. Procedures
      a. The sequence of events should be listed in chronological order.
      b. Independent and dependent variables should be operationally defined to allow reproduction of study and application to clinical situations.
    5. Data analysis
      a. Descriptive and inferential statistics should be provided.
        (1) Descriptive statistics: statistics used to describe and summarize sample characteristics and their relationships
        (2) Inferential statistics: statistics concerned with testing a hypothesis and using sample data to determine relationships and make generalizations
      b. Are the statistical procedures used appropriate?
    6. Results
      a. No subjective comment should be interjected.
      b. All subjects should be accounted for.
    7. Discussion/conclusion
      a. Major conclusions regarding results and hypothesis should be stated.
      b. Should answer questions presented
  C. Applicability: "Can the results be applied to my patient?"[9]
    1. Similar demographics
    2. Severity
    3. Comorbidities
    4. Other prognostic factors
    5. Are there any compelling reasons why the results should not be applied?
    6. Are the benefits worth the harms and/or costs?
IV. Integrate the evidence with clinical expertise, patient preferences, and the unique biology of the patient in question, and apply it to practice.[10]
V. Evaluate your effectiveness and efficiency in executing all of the steps, seeking ways to improve them both for the next time.

CONCLUSION

The practice of evidence-based medicine is a process of career-long, self-directed, problem-based learning. Developing clinical questions that are specific to one's own patient population and then searching current databases may be the most productive way to keep current with literature.[1] "Ultimately, we as clinicians are expected by payers, patients, and the clinical community to use tests and interventions that have an acceptable level of research support."[8]

REFERENCES

1. University of North Carolina Health Sciences Library: What Is EBM? Available at: http://www.hsl.unc.edu/services/tutorials/ebm/welcom.htm (accessed April 14, 2005)
2. Portney LG, Watkins MP: Foundations of Clinical Research: Applications to Practice. Appleton and Lange, Norwalk, CT, 1993
3. Centre for Evidence-Based Medicine: Why the sudden interest in EBM? Available at: http://www.cebm.utoronto.ca/intro/interest.htm (accessed April 6, 2005)

4. Centre for Evidence-Based Medicine: Formulating Answerable Clinical Questions. Available at: http://www.cebm.utoronto.ca (accessed April 14, 2005)
5. University of North Carolina Health Sciences Library: Literature Search. Available at: http://www.hsl.unc.edu/services/tutorials/ebm/welcom.htm (accessed April 14, 2005)
6. University of Massachusetts Medical School: Components of EBM. Available at: http://www.library.umassmed.edu/EBM (accessed April 14, 2005)
7. American Physical Therapy Association: How to Find Information in the Physical Therapy Literature. Available at: http://www.APTA.org/research/factsheet_tips/howtofindresearch_related (accessed April 6, 2005)
8. Glaros S: All evidence is not created equal: a discussion of levels of evidence. PTMagazine 11(10):42-52, 2003
9. University of Alberta: Systematic Review. Available at: http://www.med.ualberta.ca/ebm/ebm.htm (accessed April 14, 2005)
10. University of North Carolina Health Sciences Library: Evaluating Evidence. Available at: http://www.hsl.unc.edu/services/tutorials/ebm/welcom.htm (accessed April 14, 2005)

Index

A

Acetic acid solution, in wound cleansing, 10
Acromioplasty, anterior, definition of, 346
Active motion dysfunction, in brachial plexus injury,
        202-203, 203f
Activity modification, for shoulder tendonitis, 332
Acute burn stage
    postoperative therapy for, 32-34
    treatment goals for, 31
Addictions, identification of, 723-724
Adverse mechanical tension (AMT), 198
Agee force-couple, for intraarticular middle phalanx
        fracture, 571, 572f
Alcohol abuse, identification of, 723-724
Allodynia, definition of, 151
American Society for Surgery of the Hand (ASSH),
        and International Federation of Hand
        Surgeons (IFSSH)
    impairment determination principles of, 77-78
    motor function impairment evaluation of, 79-80
Amputation
    congenital, 660
    digital, 597-603
        evaluation timeline for, 602
        nonoperative therapy for, 599-600
        outcomes of, 602-603
        partial, definition of, 597
        postoperative therapy for, 600-602
        surgical purpose of, 598-599
        treatment goals for, 599
    management of, 715-720
        evaluation timeline for, 718
        outcomes of, 719-720
        postoperative therapy in, 717-718
        prosthetic training in, 718-719, 719f
        surgical purpose in, 715, 716f
        treatment goals in, 716
        treatment purpose in, 715-716
    preservation of amputated part after, 581

AMT (adverse mechanical tension), 198
Angiofibroblastic tendinosis, 399
Anterior acromioplasty, definition of, 346
Anterior interosseous nerve
    compression of, 87
        postoperative therapy for, 92
    muscles innervated by, 90t
Anterior transposition, for ulnar nerve compression,
        101-102
Antibiotics, topical, in wound cleansing, 10
Antihistamines, in scar management, 42
Area localization of touch, sensibility testing for, 67-68
Arm, replantation of, postoperative therapy for, 591-592
Arthritis
    conservative management of, 649-658
        evaluation in, 650-651
        nonoperative indications/precautions for, 650
        splinting in, 651-652, 652f-654f
        treatment goals for, 649
        treatment purpose of, 650
    definition of, 649
    of elbow, 431f
    of metacarpophalangeal joint, arthroplasty for, 625.
            See also Metacarpophalangeal (MCP) joint,
            arthroplasty of.
    of thumb carpometacarpal joint, 617, 618f
    of wrist, arthroplasty for, 524, 524f
Arthrodesis
    intercarpal, definition of, 530, 531f
    small joint, of hand, 641-646. See also Small joint
            arthrodesis, of hand.
    wrist, 529-535. See also Wrist, arthrodesis of.
Arthrogryposis, 669-674, 670f, 671f, 672f
    classification of, 669
    clinical presentation of, 669, 670f
    definition of, 669
    nonoperative management of, 670
    operative management of, 670-672
    outcomes of, 674

Page numbers followed by f indicate figures, t, tables; b, boxes.

Arthrogryposis *(Continued)*
  postoperative management of, 673-674
  treatment goals in, 669
Arthropathy, cuff tear, definition of, 347
Arthroplasty
  basal joint, 617-623. *See also* Carpometacarpal (CMC)
      joint, thumb, arthroplasty of.
  distal interphalangeal, 633-640. *See also* Distal
      interphalangeal (DIP) arthroplasty.
  elbow, 431-437. *See also* Elbow, arthroplasty of.
  metacarpophalangeal joint, 625-631. *See also*
      Metacarpophalangeal (MCP) joint, arthroplasty of.
  proximal interphalangeal, 633-640. *See also* Proximal
      interphalangeal (PIP) joint(s), arthoplasty of.
  shoulder, 389-395. *See also* Shoulder, arthroplasty of.
  thumb carpometacarpal joint, 617-623. *See also*
      Carpometacarpal (CMC) joint, thumb,
      arthroplasty of.
  wrist, 523-527. *See also* Wrist, arthroplasty of.
Arthroscopy
  definition of, 453
  elbow, 423-430. *See also* Elbow, arthroscopy of.
  wrist, 453-459. *See also* Wrist, arthroscopy of.
Artist, performing. *See also* Musician.
  therapeutic management of, 689-705
Athlete
  injuries in, 707-713
    elbow, 711
    hand, 711-712
    psychological considerations for, 710
    rehabilitation process for, 708-710
    return to play after, 712-713
    shoulder, 710-711
  sports medicine team for, 707-708
Atraumatic multidirectional glenohumeral instability,
      362-364
Avulsion fractures, nondisplaced
  of fingers, nonoperative therapy for, 552-553
  of thumb, nonoperative therapy for, 551-552
Axial flap, definition of, 22
Axial pattern flap, 19f
Axillary interval, brachial plexus neuropathy and, 195, 196

B

Bankart lesion, 360
Bankart procedure, for traumatic glenohumeral
      instability, 360
Basal joint arthroplasty, 617-623. *See also* Carpometacarpal
      (CMC) joint, thumb, arthroplasty of.
Baseball finger, 293-297. *See also* Mallet finger.
Behavior modification, in brachial plexus injury
      management, 206-207, 206f
Berger's test, positive, in carpal tunnel syndrome, 87
Biceps tendonitis, in athletes, 711
Biofeedback, in injury management in musician, 699
Bony avulsions, nondisplaced, definition of, 548
Boutonniere deformity, 302-308
  in athlete, 712
  causes of, 302
  definition of, 302, 303f
  evaluation timeline for, 308
  nonoperative therapy of, 304-305, 305f, 306f, 307f
    indications/precautions for, 304

Boutonniere deformity *(Continued)*
    operative indications/precautions for, 305-307
    postoperative therapy for, 307-308, 635-636, 637f
      complications of, 308
      indications/precautions for, 307
    treatment and surgical purpose for, 303-304
    treatment goals for, 304
BPN (brachial plexus neuropathy), 195
Brachial plexus gliding exercises, 131
Brachial plexus injuries, 195-214
  definition of, 198-199
  evaluation timeline for, 212
  nonoperative therapy for, 200-211
    complications of, 211
    evaluation in, 200-205
    indications/precautions for, 200
    treatment in, 205-211
      general considerations for, 205-206
      rehabilitative phase of, 209-211
      restoration phase of, 208-209, 210f
      symptom control phase of, 206-207, 206f, 208b
  outcomes of, 212
  postoperative therapy for, 211-212
    complications of, 212
    indications/precautions for, 211
  surgical indications for, 211
  traction (BPTI), 198
    thoracic outlet syndrome compared with, 198t
  treatment goals in, 200
  treatment purpose in, 199
Brachial plexus neuropathy (BPN), 195
  compressive, 198
Bracing, for humeral shaft fractures
  with collar and cuff, 379-380, 380f
  functional, 378, 380, 381f
Brass instruments, injuries specific to, 697
Burns, 29-37
  definition of, 30
  evaluation timeline for, 36
  fourth-degree, definition of, 30f, 31
  full-thickness, definition of, 30f, 31
  functional outcomes of, 36
  partial-thickness, definition of, 30, 30f
  postoperative complications of, 35-36
  recovery from, stages of, 31
  severity of, 29
  surgery for, indications for, 32
  therapy for, postoperative
    in acute burn stage, 32-34
    indications/precautions for, 32
    reconstruction stage of, 35
    in rehabilitation stage, 34-35
  treatment goals for, 31-32
Buttonhole deformity, 302-308. *See also* Boutonniere
      deformity.

C

Calcium alginate, as wound dressing, 11, 13t
Calcium channel blocker injection, in scar management, 42
Camptodactyly, 681-686, 682f, 683t, 684f
  classification of, 682-683, 683t
  clinical presentation of, 683
  definition of, 681-682, 682f

Camptodactyly *(Continued)*
  nonoperative management of, 683-684, 684f
  operative management of, 684-685
  outcomes of, 686
  postoperative management of, 685-686
  treatment goals for, 683
Capitate fractures, 463
Capsular release of elbow, therapy after, 419-420
Capsulectomy
  metacarpophalangeal, 605-615
    anatomy of joint and, 607f
    definition of, 606
    evaluation timeline for, 611-615
    outcomes of, 615
    postoperative complications of, 611
    postoperative therapy for, 608-609, 610f
    surgical purpose of, 606
    treatment goals for, 607
  proximal interphalangeal, 605-615
    anatomy of joint and, 607f
    definition of, 606
    evaluation timeline for, 611-615
    outcomes of, 615
    postoperative therapy for, 608-609, 611,
      612f-614f
    surgical purpose of, 606
    treatment goals for, 607
Carpal bones
  fractures of, 461-474
    definition of, 462-463
    evaluation timeline for, 472-473
    nonoperative therapy for, 465-466, 467f
      complications of, 470
      indications/precautions for, 465
    outcomes of, 473
    postoperative therapy for, 470
      indications/precautions for, 470
    surgical purpose in, 464-465
    treatment goals for, 465
  proximal row of, removal of, 517-521. *See also*
      Proximal row carpectomy (PRC).
Carpal instability, 461-474
  definition of, 463-464
  evaluation timeline for, 472-473
  nonoperative therapy for, 466-468, 469f
    complications of, 470
    indications/precautions for, 465
  outcomes of, 473
  postoperative therapy for, 470-472
    indications/precautions for, 470
  surgical purpose in, 464-465
  treatment goals for, 465
Carpal instability combined (CIC), 464
Carpal instability dissociative (CID), 463-464
Carpal instability nondissociative (CIND), 464
Carpal tunnel
  anatomy of, 88f
  median nerve impingement in, 87
Carpal tunnel syndrome
  release for, postoperative therapy for, 92
  wrist splint for, 91f
Carpectomy, proximal row, 517-521. *See also* Proximal row
      carpectomy (PRC).

Carpometacarpal (CMC) joint, thumb
  arthritis of, 617, 618f
  arthroplasty of, 617-623
    definition of, 618, 619f
    evaluation timeline for, 621
    outcomes of, 621-622
    postoperative therapy for, 619-621, 620f
    surgical options in, 617-618
    surgical purpose of, 619
    treatment goals for, 619
  reconstruction of, 618, 619f
Centralization, in radial deficiency, 666-667
Cervical extensor strengthening exercise, 134
Chondral defects, arthroscopy for, postoperative
      therapy for, 456
Cleansing, wound, 10
Collagen, synthesis of, in wound healing, 39, 40f
Collagen maturation process, in wound healing,
      influencing, 12-13
Complex extensor reconstruction, 319-326
  definition of, 320
  evaluation timeline for, 322
  outcomes of, 322-325, 323t, 324f, 324t, 325f
  postoperative therapy for, 320-321, 322f
    complications of, 322
    indications/precautions for, 320, 321f
  surgical purpose of, 320
  treatment goals for, 320
Complex regional pain syndrome (CRPS), 215-223
  definition of, 215-216
  evaluation timeline for, 222
  International Association for the Study of Pain
      criteria for, 215b
  nonoperative treatment of, 218-221, 219f, 220f, 221f
    complications of, 221
    indications/precautions for, 216-218, 217f
  outcomes in, 222
  postoperative complications in, 222
  postoperative therapy for, 221
  treatment goals in, 216
  treatment purpose for, 216
Compression, nerve
  median, 87-95. *See also* Median nerve compression.
  radial, 109-120. *See also* Radial nerve palsy.
  ulnar, 97-107. *See also* Ulnar nerve compression.
Compression neuropathy, thoracic outlet syndrome from, 121
Compressive garments
  in burn rehabilitation, 34, 35f
  in scar management, 42, 45, 45f
Congenital hand differences, 659-688
  arthrogryposis as, 669-674, 670f, 671f, 672f. *See also*
      Arthrogryposis.
  camptodactyly as, 681-686, 682f, 683t, 684f. *See also*
      Camptodactyly.
  hypoplastic thumb as, 674-678. *See also* Thumb, hypoplastic.
  radial deficiency as, 663-669. *See also* Radial deficiency.
  syndactyly as, 679-681, 679f, 680b, 682f
  therapy evaluation of, guidelines for, 659-660
  transverse deficiency as, 660-662, 660f, 661f
Conservative treatment program with wrist gauntlet, for
      triangular fibrocartilage complex injuries, 478
Coronoid, fracture of, with posterior elbow dislocation,
      411, 411f

Corticosteroid, interlesional injection of, in scar management, 42
Costoclavicular interval, brachial plexus neuropathy and, 195, 196
Creams, topical, in scar management, 46
Crescent-shaped tears, definition of, 347
CRPS. *See* Complex regional pain syndrome (CRPS).
Cryosurgery, in scar management, 42
Cubital tunnel, anatomy of, 97, 98f
Cubital tunnel syndrome
  definition of, 98
  nonoperative treatment of, 100-101, 101f
  postoperative therapy for, 102-103
Cuff tear arthropathy, definition of, 347
Cumulative trauma injuries, 728
Cutaneous flap, definition of, 22

D
Dakin solution, in wound cleansing, 10
Dargan's classification, of extensor tendon repair results, 288t
Darrach procedure, for ulnar head resection, 507, 508f
  therapy after, 511-512
DD. *See* Dupuytren's disease (DD).
De Quervain's tenosynovitis, 441
  nonoperative therapy for, 445-446, 446f
    indications/precautions for, 444
  postoperative therapy for, 449
    complications of, 450
Debridement, wound, 10-11
Debridement treatment program, for triangular fibrocartilage complex injuries, 477, 478-479
Decompression, for ulnar nerve compression, 101
Deep partial-thickness burns
  definition of, 30, 30f
  postoperative therapy for, in acute stage, 33
Desensitization
  definition of, 151
  evaluation timeline for, 161
  outcomes of, 161-162
  postinjury indications/precautions for, 152-153
  postoperative complications of, 160-161
  postoperative program for, 153-155, 154f
  purpose of, 152
  three-phase, record form and protocol for, 164
  treatment goals for, 152
Diaphragmatic breathing, in brachial plexus injury management, 207
Diaphragmatic breathing exercise, 134
Digit Widget, in scar management, 42
Digital nerve, repair of, studies of, 146t
DIP joint. *See* Distal interphalangeal (DIP) joint.
Discrimination, texture, definition of, 54
Dislocation(s)
  dorsal, definition of, 572
  elbow, 409-422. *See also* Elbow, fractures and dislocations of.
    in athlete, 711
  shoulder, in athlete, 711
  volar, definition of, 572
Distal interphalangeal (DIP) joint, arthroplasty of, 633-640
  definition of, 633
  evaluation timeline for, 638

Distal interphalangeal (DIP) joint, arthroplasty of (*Continued*)
  outcomes of, 638-639
  postoperative therapy for, 636-637, 638f
  surgical purpose of, 633-634
  treatment goals for, 634
Distal radioulnar joint (DRUJ), instability of, ulnar head resection for, 507-515. *See also* Ulna, head of, resection of.
Distraction histiogenesis, in radial deficiency management, 667-668
Dorsal dislocation, definition of, 572
Dorsal ganglion excision, arthroscopy for, postoperative therapy for, 456
Drainage, in wound evaluation, 7
Dressings, wound, 11
Drop finger, 293-297. *See also* Mallet finger.
Drug abuse, identification of, 723-724
DRUJ (distal radioulnar joint), instability of, ulnar head resection for, 507-515. *See also* Ulna, head of, resection of.
Duchenne's sign, in ulnar nerve palsy, 175, 176f
Dupuytren's disease (DD), 539-545
  definition of, 540, 540f, 541f
  evaluation timeline for, 544
  genetic origin of, 539
  nonoperative indications/precautions for therapy of, 541
  outcomes of, 544
  postoperative therapy for, 541-543, 542f, 543f
    complications of, 543
    indications/precautions for, 541
  surgical purpose in, 540
  treatment goals in, 541
Dupuytren's fasciectomy, wound in, 7, 8f
Dynamic extensor outrigger, for radial nerve palsy, 111, 111f
Dysesthesia, definition of, 151

E
Early Active Short Arc Motion (SAM) protocol, after extensor tendon repair, 276-278, 277f
Early passive motion method, of postoperative therapy, after extensor tendon repair, 282-284, 283f
  in thumb zones TIII through TV, 286, 286f
ECRL. *See* Extensor carpi radialis longus (ECRL).
ECU (extensor carpi ulnaris) tendonitis, 442
Edema, management of, in complex regional pain syndrome, 218, 219f
EDM (extensor digiti minimi) tendonitis, 442
Elbow, 397-437
  arthritis of, 431f
  in arthrogryposis, operative management of, 671
  arthroplasty of, 431-437
    definition of, 431
    evaluation timeline for, 436
    operative indications for, 434
    outcomes of, 436
    postoperative therapy for, 435
      complications of, 436
      indications/precautions for, 434-435
    surgical purpose of, 433
    treatment goals of, 434

Elbow *(Continued)*
  arthroscopy of, 423-430
    advantages of, 423
    in capsular release for contractures of elbow, 425-426, 426f
    in diagnostic evaluation, 423-424
    evaluation timeline for, 428-429
    for lateral release, 426
    operative indications/precautions for, 426-427
    in osteochondritis dissecans, 425
    outcomes of, 429
    in removal of loose bodies, 424
    surgical purpose of, 426
    in synovectomy, 425
    therapy after, 427-428
    treatment goals with, 426
  capsular release of, therapy after, 419-420
  epicondylitis of, 399-407. *See also* Epicondylitis.
  fractures and dislocations of, 409-422
    definition of, 409-413, 410f, 411f, 412f
    evaluation timeline for, 420
    nonoperative therapy of, 414-416
      complications of, 416
      indications/precautions for, 413
    outcomes of, 420-421
    postoperative therapy for, 416-420
      complications of, 420
      indications/precautions for, 416
    surgical purpose in, 413
    treatment goals in, 413
  golfer's. *See also* Epicondylitis.
    definition of, 400
  injuries to, in athletes, 711
  tennis. *See also* Epicondylitis.
    definition of, 399-400
Elective wound, definition of, 3
Electrical stimulation, functional, in scar management, 45
Energy conservation, in conservative management of arthritis, 656
Entrapment neuropathy, thoracic outlet syndrome from, 122
EPI (extensor indicis proprius) syndrome, 442
Epicondylitis, 399-407
  in athlete, 711
  definition of, 399
  evaluation timeline for, 405
  nonoperative therapy for, 402-404
    complications of, 404
    indications/precautions for, 401-402
  operative indications/techniques for, 404
  outcomes of, 405-406
  postoperative therapy for, 404-405
    indications for, 404
  treatment goals for, 401
  treatment purpose in, 400-401
Epicritic sensation, definition of, 53
Epineurium, 139
EPL (extensor pollicis longus) tendonitis, 441-442
Ergonomics, 728-729
  computer workstation checklist, 735b, 736f
  evaluation and treatment guidelines for, 733-735, 737
Essex-Lopresti fracture, 412

Evidence-based medicine, 739-742
  converting need for information into answerable questions in, 740
  critical appraisal of evidence in, 740-742
  evaluating effectiveness and efficiency in, 742
  integrating evidence in clinical expertise in, 742
  practice of, 739-742
  tracking down best evidence in, 740
Exercise(s)
  after extensor tendon repair, 283
    for Zones III and IV, 276-277, 279, 280f
  after flexor tenolysis, 263-267
  after rotator cuff repair, 348-355, 349f, 350f-351f, 352f, 353f, 354f
  in conservative management of arthritis, 655-656
  in digital replantation, 587-589, 587f, 588f, 589f
  in Dupuytren's disease, 543
  in humeral shaft fracture management, 380-383, 382f
  in injury management in musician, 698-699
  in metacarpophalangeal arthroplasty, 627-628
  postoperative, in distal radius fractures, 499-501
  in postoperative therapy, for total shoulder arthroplasty, 393
  in proximal humeral fracture management, 373-374
  in rehabilitation of injured athlete, 709
  for shoulder tendonitis, 333, 334f-340f
  in thumb carpometacarpal joint arthroplasty, 620
  in triangular fibrocartilage complex injuries, 480
Extensor carpi radialis brevis (ECRB), brand transfer of, to intrinsics with tendon graft, 180, 180f
Extensor carpi radialis longus (ECRL)
  brand transfer of, to intrinsics with tendon graft, 180, 180f
  transfer of, to flexor digitorum profundus, 183-184, 183f
Extensor carpi ulnaris (ECU) tendonitis, 442
Extensor digiti minimi (EDM) tendonitis, 442
Extensor indicis proprius (EPI) syndrome, 442
Extensor pollicis longus (EPL) tendonitis, 441-442
Extensor tendon(s), 271-326
  anatomy and physiology of, 271, 272f, 273f
  imbalance of, 293-309
    boutonniere deformity as, 302-308. *See also* Boutonniere deformity.
    mallet finger as, 293-297. *See also* Mallet finger.
    swan-neck deformity as, 297-302. *See also* Swan-neck deformity.
  reconstruction of, complex, 319-326. *See also* Complex extensor reconstruction.
  repair of
    definition of, 275
    evaluation timeline for, 287
    management of, 271-293
    outcomes of, 287-290, 288t
    postoperative complications of, 286
    postoperative therapy in, 276-286
      complications of, 286
      indications/precautions for, 275-276
      for thumb zones TI and TII, 284-285
      for thumb zones TIII through TV, 285-286, 286f
      for Zones I and II, 276
      for Zones III and IV, 276-280, 277f, 279f, 280f
      for Zones V, VI, and VII, 280-284, 281f, 283f
      for Zones VIII and IX, 284

Extensor tendon(s) *(Continued)*
   repair of *(Continued)*
      surgical purpose of, 275
      treatment goals for, 275
   tendinopathies of, 441-442, 442f
   trauma to, classification of, 271, 274f
Extensor tenolysis, 311-317
   definition of, 311
   evaluation timeline for, 316
   indications for, 311, 312f
   operative indications/precautions for, 312-313
   outcomes of, 317
   postoperative therapy for, 313-315, 314f, 315f, 316f
      complications of, 315-316
   treatment goals for, 311
Extrinsic tendon healing, 227

F

Fasciectomy, Dupuytren's, wound in, 7, 8f
Fasciocutaneous flap, definition of, 22
FCR tendonitis. *See* Flexor carpi radialis (FCR) tendonitis.
FCU tendonitis. *See* Flexor carpi ulnaris (FCU) tendonitis.
FDP. *See* Flexor digitorum profundus (FDP).
FDS. *See* Flexor digitorum superficialis (FDS).
Fibroplasia, in wound healing, 39
Finger(s)
   amputation of, 597-603. *See also* Amputation, digital.
   arthrodesis in, 641-646. *See also* Small joint arthrodesis, of hand.
   in arthrogryposis, operative management of, 672
   interphalangeal joint arthroplasty in, 633-640. *See also* Distal interphalangeal (DIP) joint, arthroplasty of; Proximal interphalangeal (PIP) joint(s), arthroplasty of.
   jersey, in athlete, 712
   ligament injuries of, 548, 548f
      evaluation timeline for, 557-558
      nonoperative therapy for, 552-553
      outcomes of, 558-559
      postoperative therapy for, 555-556
      treatment and surgical purpose for, 550
   mallet, 293-297. *See also* Mallet finger.
      in athlete, 712
   replantation of, postoperative therapy for, 585-589, 586f, 587f, 588f, 589f
   syndactyly and, 679-681, 679f, 680b, 682f
   trigger, 443
      anatomy of, 442f
      nonoperative therapy for, 447, 448f
         indications/precautions for, 445
      postoperative therapy for, 449-450
         complications of, 450
Fingertip-wrinkling test, 59-60
Fixation, of distal radius fractures
   external, 490-497, 491f, 492f, 493f, 494f, 495f-497f
   internal, open reduction and, 497-502, 498f, 500f-501f
Flaps, skin, 17-27. *See also* Skin flaps.
Flexor carpi radialis (FCR) tendonitis, 443
   nonoperative therapy for, 447
      indications/precautions for, 445
Flexor carpi ulnaris (FCU) tendonitis, 443
   nonoperative therapy for, 447
      indications/precautions for, 445

Flexor digitorum profundus (FDP), transfer of extensor carpi radialis longus to, 183-184, 183f
Flexor digitorum superficialis (FDS)
   of middle finger, intrinsic rebalancing of, 178-181, 179f, 180f
   of ring finger, transfer of, to adductor pollicis, 181-182, 182f
Flexor pollicis longus (FPL)
   repair of
      dynamic splint for, 238f
      outcomes of, 242-243
      static dorsal blocking splint for, 234f
      therapy protocol for
         with dynamic splint, 239b
         with static splint, 236b
   transfer of, postoperative therapy for, 169-170, 170f
Flexor tendon(s), 227-269
   injury to, zones of, 228f, 229t
   involvement of, in ulnar and median nerve repair, postoperative care in, 144-145
   reconstruction of, 245-259
      definition of, 246
      overview of, 245-246
      primary tendon grafting in. *See* Primary tendon grafting.
      staged. *See* Staged tendon reconstruction.
   repair of, 227-244
      evaluation timeline for, 239-240
      outcomes of, 241-243, 242t
      postoperative complications of, 239
      postoperative therapy in, 231-239, 232b, 233f, 234f, 235b-236b, 237f, 238b, 238f, 239b
         early active mobilization protocols for, 233-234, 234f, 237f, 238-239, 240b-241b
         early passive mobilization protocols for, 231, 233, 233f, 234f, 235b-236b, 237f-238f, 238b-239b
         immobilization protocol for, 230b, 231
         indications/precautions for, 229-230
      surgical and treatment purpose in, 227-228
      treatment goals in, 228-229
   tendinopathies of, 443
Flexor tenolysis, 261-269
   definition of, 261, 262f
   evaluation timeline for, 268
   postoperative complications in, 268
   postoperative therapy for, 263-267, 264f, 265f, 266f, 267f
      indications/precautions for, 263
   surgical and treatment purpose of, 261-263
Fluidotherapy, for desensitization, 155
Forearm, in arthrogryposis, operative management of, 671-672
FPL. *See* Flexor pollicis longus (FPL).
Fracture(s)
   in athlete, 712
   avulsion, nondisplaced
      of fingers, nonoperative therapy for, 552-553
      of thumb, nonoperative therapy for, 551-552
   capitate, 463
   carpal, 461-474. *See also* Carpal bones, fractures of.
   definition of, 561
   digital, rehabilitation of, 561-580. *See also* Phalanx fractures.
   distal radius. *See* Radius, distal, fractures of.

Fracture(s) *(Continued)*
    elbow, 409-422. *See also* Elbow, fractures and dislocations of.
    hamate, 462
    healing of
        based on fixation, 563f
        timeline for, 562f
    humeral, 369-387. *See also* Humeral fractures.
    lunate, 462-463
    phalanx, rehabilitation of, 561-580. *See also*
        Phalanx fractures.
    pisiform, 463
    scaphoid, 462
    trapezial, 462
    trapezoid, 463
    triquetrum, 462
Free flaps, 20
Free tissue transfer
    postoperative management of, 25
    vascularized, definition of, 21
Froment's sign, in ulnar nerve palsy, 175, 176f
FTSG. *See* Full-thickness skin grafts (FTSG).
Full-thickness burns
    definition of, 30f, 31
    postoperative therapy for, in acute stage, 33-34
Full-thickness skin grafts (FTSG), 18
    definition of, 21
Functional bracing, for humeral shaft fractures, 378
Functional capacity evaluations, 727-728
Functional electrical stimulation (FES), in scar
    management, 45
Fusion, joint. *See also* Arthrodesis.
    definition of, 641

G
Gauntlet splint, for radial nerve palsy, 111, 112f
Gauze, as wound dressing, 11
Glenohumeral instability, 359-367
    acquired, 359, 364-366, 366f
    atraumatic multidirectional, 359, 362-364
    traumatic unidirectional, 359-362
        clinical presentation of, 359-360
        complications of, 362
        postoperative rehabilitation in
            goals of, 360-361
            treatments in, 361-362
        surgical purpose in, 360
Glenohumeral joint
    arthritis of, 390f
    instability of, 359-367. *See also* Glenohumeral instability.
Gliding
    in brachial plexus injury management, 207, 210-211
    peripheral nerve, 196-197
    tendon
        after repair, 272-274
        exercises for, after flexor tenolysis, 266-267, 266f
Gnosis, tactile, definition of, 54
Golfer's elbow. *See also* Epicondylitis.
    definition of, 400
Graft(s)
    nerve, sensibility testing for, 56
    skin, 17-27. *See also* Skin grafts.
Graphesthesia, definition of, 54
Grasping force control, in sensory reeducation, 159

Grip force maintenance, in sensory reeducation, 159
Guyon's canal
    ulnar nerve compression in
        definition of, 99
        postoperative therapy for, 103-104
    ulnar nerve in, 97-98, 99f

H
Hamate fracture, 462
Hand, 537-646
    arthroplasties in, 617-640. *See also under* Arthroplasty.
    congenital differences in, 659-688. *See also* Congenital
        hand differences.
    digital amputation in, 597-603. *See also* Amputation,
        digital.
    digital fracture rehabilitation and, 561-580. *See also*
        Phalanx fractures.
    Dupuytren's disease of, 539-545. *See also* Dupuytren's
        disease (DD).
    injuries to, in athletes, 711-712
    ligament injuries of, 547-560. *See also*
        Ligament(s), hand.
    metacarpophalangeal capsulectomy in, 605-615. *See also*
        Capsulectomy, metacarpophalangeal.
    proximal interphalangeal capsulectomy in, 605-615.
        See also Capsulectomy, proximal interphalangeal.
    ray resection in, 597-603. *See also* Ray resection.
    replantation of, 581-595. *See also* Replantation.
        postoperative therapy for, 590-591
    small joint arthrodesis of, 641-646. *See also* Small joint
        arthrodesis, of hand.
    tendinopathies of, 441-452. *See also* Tendinopathy(ies),
        wrist and hand.
Hand Screen, 66-67
    form for, 65f, 66
    procedure for, 63
Healing
    tendon, 227
    wound
        dressing characteristics and, 13t
        phases of, 39
        physiology of, 4-6, 5f
Heat, in scar management, 45
Hemiarthroplasty, shoulder. *See also* Shoulder,
        hemiarthroplasty of.
    definition of, 390
    evaluation timeline for, 395
    operative indications/precautions for, 394
    postoperative complications of, 394
    postoperative therapy for, 394
    treatment goals for, 394
Hemiresection-interposition technique, of ulnar head
        resection, 507-508, 508f
High-voltage galvanic stimulation (HVG)
    after proximal row carpectomy, 519, 519f
    for shoulder tendonitis, 332
Hill-Sachs lesion, 360
Humeral fractures, 369-387
    distal, 409-410, 410f
        nonoperative therapy for, 414-415
        postoperative therapy for, 417-418
    proximal, 369-377
        anatomy and, 370, 370f

Humeral fractures *(Continued)*
  proximal *(Continued)*
    classification of, 370-372, 371f, 372b
    clinical union of, 370
    clinical unity of, 369-370
    definition of, 370-372
    evaluation timeline for, 376
    nonoperative therapy for, 373-374
      complications of, 374-375
      indications/precautions for, 372-373
    operative indications/precautions for, 375
    outcomes of, 376-377
    postoperative therapy for, 375, 376b
      complications/considerations for, 375-376
    surgical purpose in, 372
    treatment goals for, 372
  shaft, 377-385
    classification of, 378, 378f
    definition of, 378
    evaluation guidelines for, 384
    indications for, 379
    nonoperative therapy of, 379-383, 380f, 381f, 382f
    operative indications/precautions for, 383
    outcomes of, 385
    postoperative therapy for, 383-384
    precautions/contraindications for, 379
    treatment goals for, 379
    treatment purpose in, 379
HVG (high-voltage galvanic stimulation), for shoulder
    tendonitis, 332
Hydrocolloids, impermeable, as wound dressings, 11, 13t
Hydrogel, semipermeable, as wound dressing, 11, 13t
Hydrogen peroxide, in wound cleansing, 10
Hyperalgesia, definition of, 152
Hypersensitivity, definition of, 54, 152
Hypertrophic scar, definition of, 40
Hypoplastic thumb, 674-678. *See also* Thumb, hypoplastic.

I

IASP (International Association for the Study of Pain)
    criteria for complex regional pain
    syndrome, 215b
Ilizarov device, in radial deficiency management, 666, 666f,
    667-668
Immersion particles, for desensitization, 153, 154f, 164
Immobilization, after tendon transfer for median nerve
    palsy, early mobilization versus, 171-172, 172t
Immobilization method, of postoperative therapy, after
    extensor tendon repair
  in finger and wrist extensors, zone V, VI, and VII,
    280-282, 281f
  in thumb zones TIII through TV, 285
Impermeable hydrocolloids, as wound dressings, 11
Impingement, median nerve, 87-95. *See also* Median
    nerve compression.
Industrial rehabilitation services, 727-738
  admission criteria for, 729-730
  definitions/timelines for, 727-729
  evaluation and treatment guidelines for, 730-737
    ergonomics and, 733-737, 735b, 736f
    functional capacity evaluation and, 730-732, 731f, 731t
    work hardening and, 732-733
  purposes/goals of, 729

Infection, wound, 8, 9f
Inflammatory phase, of wound healing, 39
Innervation density, definition of, 54
Instruments, musical, injuries specific to, 695-697
Intercarpal arthrodesis
  definition of, 530, 531f
  indications for, 531
Interferential electrical stimulation, for shoulder
    tendonitis, 332
International Association for the Study of Pain (IASP) criteria
    for complex regional pain syndrome, 215b
International Federation of Hand Surgeons (IFSSH),
    and American Society for Surgery of the
    Hand (ASSH)
  impairment determination principles of, 77-78
  motor function impairment evaluation of, 79-80
Interscalene triangle, brachial plexus neuropathy and, 195
Intersection syndrome, 441
  nonoperative therapy for, 446
    indications/precautions for, 444-445
  postoperative therapy for, 449
Intrinsic tendon healing, 227
Iontoporesis, in scar management, 46
Island flap, definition of, 22

J

Jeanne's sign, in ulnar nerve palsy, 175, 176f
Jersey finger, in athlete, 712
Joint(s)
  carpometacarpal, of thumb, arthroplasty of, 617-623.
    See also Carpometacarpal (CMC) joint, thumb,
    arthroplasty of.
  distal interphalangeal. *See* Distal interphalangeal (DIP)
    joint.
  metacarpophalangeal. *See* Metacarpophalangeal (MCP)
    joint.
  protection of, in conservative management of arthritis,
    652, 654-655
  proximal interphalangeal. *See* Proximal interphalangeal
    (PIP) joint(s).
  radioulnar, distal, instability of, ulnar head resection for,
    507-515. *See also* Ulna, head of, resection of.
  trapeziometacarpal, 617. *See* Carpometacarpal (CMC)
    joint, thumb.
Joint fusion. *See also* Arthrodesis.
  definition of, 641

K

Keloid scar, definition of, 40
Keyboard instruments, injuries specific to, 696

L

Laser surgery, in scar management, 42
Lidocaine patch, in scar management, 42
Ligament(s)
  carpal, injury to, 463-464. *See also* Carpal instability.
  hand
    functions of, 547
    injuries to, 547-560
      definitions of, 548-549
      evaluation timeline for, 557-558
      nonoperative therapy for, 550-554, 551f, 552f, 553f, 554f
      operative indications/precautions for therapy in, 555

Ligament(s) *(Continued)*
  hand *(Continued)*
    injuries to *(Continued)*
      outcomes of, 558-559
      postoperative therapy for, 555-556
      treatment goals for, 550
Lunate fracture, 462-463
Lunotriquetral instability, 464
  nonoperative therapy for, 467-468
  postoperative therapy for, 472
Lunotriquetral tears, arthroscopy for, postoperative
    therapy for, 455

M

Mallet finger, 293-297
  in athlete, 712
  conservative treatment of, 293
  definition of, 294, 294f
  evaluation timeline for, 297
  nonoperative therapy for, 295, 296f
    complications of, 296
    indications/precautions for, 295
  postoperative therapy for, 297
  treatment and surgical purpose of, 294
  treatment goals for, 294-295
Marginal convergence, definition of, 347
Massage, in scar management, 45
Matched ulna resection, 508, 509f
Matsen procedure, for traumatic glenohumeral instability, 360
Mechanoreceptors, definition of, 54
Medial transposition, for ulnar nerve compression, 102
Median nerve
  injury to
    high, tendon transfer for, postoperative therapy in,
      169-170, 170f
    low, tendon transfer for, postoperative therapy in,
      167-169, 167f, 168f, 169f
  muscles innervated by, 90t
  repair of
    with flexor tendon involvement, postoperative care in,
      144-145
    studies of, 146t
    at wrist level, postoperative therapy for, 141-143,
      142f, 143f
Median nerve compression, 87-95
  complications of
    nonoperative, 91
    postoperative, 92
  definition of, 89
  evaluation timeline for, 93
  outcomes of, 93
  pathologic anatomy and staging of, 89
  sites for, 87b
  therapy for
    nonoperative, 90-91
      indications/precautions for, 90
    operative, indications/precautions for, 91
    postoperative, 92
  treatment and surgical purpose in, 89
  treatment goals in, 89
Median nerve palsy, tendon transfers for, 165-173.
    See also Tendon transfers, for median
    nerve palsy.

Metacarpophalangeal (MCP) joint
  arthroplasty of, 625-631
    definition of, 625
    evaluation timeline for, 629
    outcomes of, 629
    postoperative therapy for, 627-629
    surgical purpose of, 625-626
    treatment goals in, 626
  capsulectomy of, 605-615. *See also* Capsulectomy,
    metacarpophalangeal.
  of finger, arthrodesis of, 641-646. *See also* Small joint
    arthrodesis, of hand.
  of fingers, injuries to, postoperative therapy for, 555-556
  structures limiting motion of, 605-606
  of thumb
    arthrodesis of, 641-646. *See also* Small joint
      arthrodesis, of hand.
    injuries to, 547, 548f
      postoperative therapy for, 555
      treatment and surgical purpose for, 549-550
Midcarpal dorsal wedge osteotomy, in arthrogryposis
    management, 673
Midcarpal instability
  palmar, nonoperative therapy for, 468, 469f
  postoperative therapy for, 472
Miller's classification, of extensor tendon repair results, 287t
Mobilization protocols, for flexor tendon repair
  early active, 233-234, 234f, 237f, 238-239, 240b-241b
  early passive, 231, 233, 233f, 234f, 235b-236b, 238b-239b,
    327f-238f
Monofilament testing
  errors in, 67
  protocol for, 62-67
    hand mapping procedure in, 63
    Hand Screen in, 63, 65f, 66-67
    procedural details in, 63-66
    questions in, 62-63
  for touch-pressure detection threshold level, 61-67
Monteggia lesions, 411-412, 412f
Motor function
  effects of nerve lesions on, 148-149
  impairments of, evaluation of, ASSH and IFSSH
    guidelines for, 79-80
Motor retraining, in postoperative therapy of ulnar/median
    nerve repair, 142
Moving two-point discrimination test, 71
Muller's classification system, for humeral shaft fractures,
    378, 378f
Muscle testing, in sensibility testing, 60-61
Muscles, innervations of, 90t
Musculocutaneous flap, 19f
  definition of, 22
Musculoskeletal disorders, work-related, 728
Musician
  evaluation of, 692-695, 704-705
    physical examination in
      with instrument, 695
      without instrument, 692-695, 693f, 694f
    subjective, 692
  injuries in
    grades of, 689
    outcomes of, 702-703
    overuse, predisposing factors for, 690-692, 691f

Musician *(Continued)*
  injuries in *(Continued)*
    treatment of, 697-702
      ergonomics of instruments in, 702
      exercise programs in, 698-699
      goals of, 697-698
      modalities in, 699-700
      patient education in, 700-701
      rest in, 698
      splints in, 701
    problems in, instrument-specific, 695-697
    therapeutic management of, 689-705
Myocutaneous flap, definition of, 22
Myofascial trigger points, 199t

N

Neer's Classification System, for proximal humeral
        fractures, 370-371, 371f
Nerve(s)
  biomechanics of, 196-197
  compression of, sensibility testing for, 55-56
  injuries to, 51-223
    sensibility testing in, 53-85. *See also* Sensibility testing.
  lesions of
    desensitization after, 151-155. *See also* Desensitization.
    effects of, on motor function, 148-149
    sensory reeducation after, 151, 155-160. *See also*
        Sensory reeducation.
    median, compression of, 87-95. *See also* Median nerve
        compression.
    peripheral, structure and function of, 139
    repair of, 139-149. *See also* Nerve repair.
    ulnar, compression of, 97-107. *See also* Ulnar
        nerve compression.
Nerve conduction velocity, in sensibility testing, 60
Nerve graft
  postoperative therapy for, 144
  preoperative care for, 144
Nerve mobilization techniques, for brachial plexus injury, 207
Nerve repair
  definition of, 139, 140f
  delayed primary, preoperative care for, 144
  evaluation time line for, 145
  with flexor tendon involvement, postoperative care in,
        144-145
  operative indications and precautions for, 141
  outcomes of, 145, 146t
  postoperative complications of, 145
  postoperative therapy for, 141-144, 142f, 143f
  purpose of, 140
  sensibility testing for, 56
  treatment goals in, 140-141
Nervous system, as continuum, 197-198, 197f
Neural tissue examination, in brachial plexus injury,
        202-204, 203f, 204f-205f, 205t
Neuropathic disease, sensibility testing for, 56-57
Neuropathy
  brachial plexus, 195
  compression, thoracic outlet syndrome from, 121
  entrapment, thoracic outlet syndrome from, 122

O

Object manipulation, in sensory reeducation, 159-160
Ointments, natural, in scar management, 46

Olecranon, fractures of, 410, 410f
  nonoperative therapy for, 415
  postoperative therapy for, 418
Opponensplasty, 167-169, 167f, 168f, 169f
  postoperative therapy for, 678
Orthopedic Trauma Association Classification, of
        proximal humeral fractures, 371-372, 372b
Osteotomy, midcarpal dorsal wedge, in arthrogryposis
        management, 673

P

Pain management
  in complex regional pain syndrome, 218, 219f
  in conservative management of arthritis, 655
Palpation, in brachial plexus injury, 205
Paper tape, in scar management, 46
Partial-thickness burns
  definition of, 30, 30f
  postoperative therapy for, in acute stage, 32-33
Passive motion dysfunction, in brachial plexus injury,
        203-204, 204f-205f, 205t
Patient education
  in brachial plexus injury, 207
  in complex regional pain syndrome, 220
  in conservative management of arthritis, 652
  for musician with injuries, 700-701
Pectoral muscle stretching exercise, 132-133, 133f
Pectoralis minor stretching exercise, 133
Pedicle flaps, 19-20, 19f, 20f
  definition of, 22
Percussion instruments, injuries specific to, 697
Performing artist. *See also* Musician.
  therapeutic management of, 689-705
Peripheral nerves
  gliding of, 196-197
  structure and function of, 139
Phalanx fractures, 561-580
  distal, 562-566
    evaluation timeline for, 566t
    nonoperative therapy for, 563-564
    outcomes of, 566
    postoperative therapy for, 564-566
    treatment goals for, 563
    treatment purpose in, 563
  middle, 566-576
    evaluation timeline for, 566t
    intraarticular, 571-576
      evaluation timeline for, 566t
      nonoperative therapy for, 573-575
      outcomes of, 576
      postoperative therapy for, 575-576
      treatment purpose in, 572
    nonoperative therapy for, 568-569
    outcomes of, 570-571
    patterns of, 567, 567f
    postoperative therapy for, 569-570
    treatment goals for, 568
    treatment purpose in, 568
  proximal, 577-579
Phalen's test, 57, 58f
  positive, in carpal tunnel syndrome, 87
Pharmacological therapy, in complex regional pain
        syndrome, 221

Phonophoresis, for shoulder tendonitis, 332
PIN (posterior interosseous nerve) syndrome, 113-117.
        See also Posterior interosseous nerve (PIN)
        syndrome.
Pisiform fractures, 463
Point localization of touch, sensibility testing for, 67-68
Pollicization, for hypoplastic thumb, 676, 677f, 677t
    postoperative therapy for, 678
Posterior capsule release, in arthrogryposis
        management, 673
Posterior interosseous nerve (PIN) syndrome, 113-117
    definition of, 113
    nonoperative therapy for, 113-114
    operative indications and technique for, 115
Postural abnormalities, thoracic outlet syndrome from,
        121-122
Postural exercises, for thoracic outlet syndrome, 131-134,
        133f, 134f
Posture
    modifications of, in brachial plexus injury
        management, 207
    musician's, evaluation of, 692, 693f, 694f
Povidone-iodine solution, in wound cleansing, 10
Power pinch, restoration of, 181-182, 181f, 182f
PRC (proximal row carpectomy), 517-521. *See also*
        Proximal row carpectomy (PRC).
Prehension pattern correction, in sensory
        reeducation, 159
Pressure, maintained, for desensitization, 154
Primary tendon grafting
    definition of, 246, 247f
    evaluation timeline for, 257
    flexor tenolysis after, 261-269. *See also* Flexor tenolysis.
    outcomes of, 258
    postoperative complications of, 257
    postoperative therapy for, 253
        indications/precautions for, 252-253, 253f
    postoperative treatment goals for, 250-252
    preoperative therapy for, 248-249, 250f-252f
        goals of, 247-248
        indications for, 248
    surgical purpose of, 246-247
Progressive nerve mobilization techniques, in brachial
        plexus injury, 208-209
Pronator syndrome
    anatomy of, 88f
    postoperative therapy for, 92
Prosthesis
    after amputation, training for, 718-719
    elbow
        constrained, 431
        semiconstrained, 432, 432f, 433
        unconstrained, 432, 433f, 434f
    shoulder
        hemiarthroplasty, 390, 391f. 392f
        unconstrained, 389-390, 390f, 391f
    wrist, 523-524
Protective sensation, definition of, 54
Provocative tests
    in brachial plexus injury, 205
    definition of, 54
Proximal interphalangeal (PIP) joint(s)
    arthroplasty of, 633-640

Proximal interphalangeal (PIP) joint(s) *(Continued)*
    definition of, 633
    evaluation timeline for, 638
    outcomes of, 638-639
    postoperative therapy for, 634-636, 635f, 636f, 637f
    surgical purpose of, 633-634
    capsulectomy of, 605-615. *See also* Capsulectomy,
        proximal interphalangeal.
    injuries to, 548
        postoperative therapy for, 556
    structures limiting motion of, 605-606
Proximal row carpectomy (PRC), 517-521
    arthroscopic, postoperative therapy for, 457
    definition of, 517, 517f
    evaluation timeline for, 520
    outcomes of, 520-521
    postoperative therapy for, 518-520, 519f
        complications of, 520
        indications/precautions for, 518
    surgical purpose of, 518
    treatment goals of, 518
Pseudomonas, wound infected with, 8, 9f
Pseudosyndactyly, 679

R
Radial collateral ligament (RCL)
    injuries to, 547
    tears of, incomplete
        definition of, 548
        of fingers, nonoperative therapy for, 552-553
        of thumb, nonoperative therapy for, 551-552, 551f
Radial deficiency, 663-669
    classification of, 663, 664t
    clinical presentation of, 663, 664f
    definition of, 663
    nonoperative management of, 664-666, 665f
    operative management of, 666-667, 666f
    outcomes of, 668-669
    postoperative management of, 667-668
    syndromes associated with, 663t
    treatment goals of, 663
Radial nerve
    compression of, 109-120. *See also* Radial nerve
        compression.
    course and distribution of, 109, 110f
    repair of, 143-144
    studies of, 146t
Radial nerve compression
    posterior interosseous nerve syndrome as, 113-117.
        See also Posterior interosseous nerve (PIN)
        syndrome.
    radial nerve palsy as, 110-113
    radial tunnel syndrome as, 113-117. *See also*
        Radial tunnel syndrome.
    Wartenberg syndrome as, 117-119
Radial nerve palsy, 110-113
    definition of, 110
    evaluation and treatment guidelines for, 111-112
    in humeral shaft fracture, splinting for, 380, 381f
    nonoperative therapy for, 111
    operative indications for, 112-113
    tendon transfers for, 187-194. *See also* Tendon transfers,
        for radial nerve palsy.

Radial sensor nerve compression, provocative test for, 59, 59f
Radial styloidecotmy, arthroscopic, postoperative therapy for, 457
Radial tunnel syndrome
  definition of, 113
  nonoperative therapy for, 114-115
  operative indications and technique for, 115
  postoperative complications of, 117
  postoperative management for, 115-117
Radialization, in radial deficiency management, 667
Radiation, in scar management, 42
Radioulnar joint, distal, instability of, ulnar head resection for, 507-515. *See also* Ulna, head of, resection of.
Radius
  dislocations of, 411
    nonoperative therapy for, 415-416
    postoperative therapy for, 419
  distal, fractures of
    external fixation of, 490-497, 491f, 492f, 493f, 494f, 495f-497f
      definition of, 490-492, 491f, 492f, 493f
      evaluation timeline for, 495, 497
      postoperative complications of, 494-495
      postoperative therapy in, 493-494, 494f, 495f, 496f-497f
      treatment goals for, 492-493
    history/overview of, 489-490
    intraarticular, arthroscopy for, postoperative therapy for, 455-456
    open reduction and internal fixation of, 497-502, 498f, 500f-501f
      definition of, 497-498, 498f
      evaluation timeline for, 502
      outcomes of, 502-503
      postoperative complications of, 501-502
      postoperative therapy in, 499-501, 500f-501f
      treatment goals of, 498-499
    treatment and surgical purpose of, 490
    unstable, fixation of, 489-505
  proximal, fractures of, 410-411, 410f
    nonoperative therapy for, 415
    postoperative therapy for, 418-419
Random flap, 19f
  definition of, 22
Range of motion (ROM)
  after complex extensor reconstruction, 321, 322f
  after Darrach procedure for ulnar head resection, 511-512
  after elbow arthroscopy, 427-428
  after extensor tendon repairs, 280-282
    timing of, 274-275
  after extensor tenolysis, 314, 314f
  after proximal row carpectomy, 519
  after tendon transfers for radial nerve palsy, 189, 191
  after ulnar wafer resection, 513
  in conservative management of arthritis, 655-656
  in digital amputation, 601
  in digital replantation, 586
  in Dupuytren's disease, 543
  in elbow fracture/dislocation rehabilitation, 416-420
  in epicondylitis, 402
  in extensor tendon repair, 272

Range of motion (ROM) *(Continued)*
  in flexor tendon reconstruction
    postoperative, 253, 255
    preoperative, 249
  in humeral shaft fracture management, 380-381, 382, 383
  in metacarpophalangeal capsulectomy, 609
  in physical examination of musician, 693
  in postoperative therapy
    of radial nerve repair, 144
    of total shoulder arthroplasty, 393
    of ulnar/median nerve repair, 141-142
  in proximal humeral fracture management, 373-374
  in proximal interphalangeal capsulectomy, 611, 613f
  in radial deficiency management, 665
  in ray resection, 601
  in scar management, 45
  tendon excursions created by, 274
  in thumb carpometacarpal joint arthroplasty, 620
  in triangular fibrocartilage complex injuries, 480
Ray resection
  definition of, 597-598, 598f, 599f
  evaluation timeline for, 602
  outcomes of, 602-603
  postoperative therapy for, 600-602
  surgical purpose of, 598-599
  treatment goals for, 599
RCL. *See* Radial collateral ligament (RCL).
Reconstruction stage of burn
  postoperative therapy for, 35
  treatment goals for, 32
Reconstruction treatment program, for triangular fibrocartilage complex injuries, 477, 479
Reeducation
  definition of, 54
  sensory, 151, 155-160. *See also* Sensory reeducation.
Referred touch, definition of, 54
Regional anesthesia, in complex regional pain syndrome, 220-221, 221f
Rehabilitation stage of burn
  postoperative therapy for, 34-35
  treatment goals for, 31
Replantation, 581-595
  arm, postoperative therapy for, 591-592
  definition of, 581, 582, 583f
  digital, postoperative therapy for, 585-589, 586f, 587f, 588f, 589f
  evaluation timeline for, 592-593
  hand, postoperative therapy for, 590-591
  immediate postoperative complications in, 584
  operative indications/precautions for, 583-584
  outcomes of, 593
  postoperative therapy for, 585-592
    complications of, 592
    indications/precautions for, 584
  surgical purpose of, 582
  thumb, postoperative therapy for, 589-590
  treatment goals for, 582-583
Revascularization, definition of, 582
Rheumatoid wrist synovectomy, arthroscopic, postoperative therapy for, 456-457
ROM. *See* Range of motion (ROM).

Rotator cuff
 functions of, 345
 injuries to
  in athletes, 710-711
  causes of, 345-346
Rotator cuff repair, 345-358
 arthroscopic-assisted open, definition of, 347
 arthroscopic evaluation for, 346
 complete arthroscopic, definition of, 347
 definition of, 346
 evaluation timeline for, 355
 mini-open, definition of, 347
 outcomes of, 356
 postoperative therapy in, 348-355, 349f, 350f-351f,
    352f, 353f, 354f
  complications of, 355
  for incomplete or small tears, 348-351, 349f,
    350f-351f, 352f
  indications/precautions for, 348
  for major tears, 351-354, 353f, 354f
  for massive tears, 355
 surgical purpose of, 347
 treatment goals in, 347-348

S

Sagittal band (SB)
 injuries to
  nonoperative therapy for, 553-554
  postoperative therapy for, 556
  treatment and surgical purpose for, 550
 purpose of, 548
 tears of, definitions of, 549
Saline, in wound cleansing, 10
Saturday night palsy, definition of, 110
Sauve-Kapandji procedure, for ulnar head resection, 509, 509f
 therapy after, 512-513, 512f
SB. See Sagittal band (SB).
Scalene muscle stretching exercise, 132, 132f
Scaphoid fractures, 462
 arthroscopy for, postoperative therapy for, 456
Scapholunate instability, 464
 nonoperative therapy for, 467-468
 postoperative therapy for, 471-472
Scapular adductor strengthening exercise, 133, 133f
Scapulothoracic stabilization techniques, in brachial
    plexus injury, 209
Scar(s)
 evaluation of, 41-42
 formation of, 39
 hypertrophic, definition of, 40
 keloid, definition of, 40
 management of
  definition of, 40
  medical interventions in, 42
  therapeutic interventions in, 42, 44f-45f, 45-46
 maturation of, 39
 nonoperative complications of, 46
 nonoperative outcomes of, 46
 revision surgery for, 46-48
 surgical, self-rating scale for, 42, 43f
 therapy of
  goals of, 40

Scar(s) (Continued)
 therapy of (Continued)
  nonoperative, 41-46, 43f-45f
   indications/precautions for, 41
  purpose of, 40
Schenck dynamic traction splint, for intraarticular
    middle phalanx fracture, 571, 573f
Semipermeable films, as wound dressings, 11, 12f, 13t
Semipermeable foams, as wound dressings, 11, 13t
Semmes-Weinstein Monofilament Test, 61, 61f
 interpretation of, and relationship to function, 81-82
Sensation
 definition of, 54
 epicritic, definition of, 53
 protective, definition of, 54
Sensibility, definition of, 54
Sensibility testing, 53-85
 computerized, 72
 definitions for, 53-54
 goals of, 55
 indications and precautions for, 55-57
 muscle testing in, 60-61
 nerve conduction velocity in, 60
 outcomes of, 72-73
 point or area localization of touch in, 67-68
 precautions for, 57
 provocative tests in, 57-59, 58f-59f
 purpose of, 55
 for sympathetic nerve status, 59-60
 two-point discrimination test in
  for innervation density, 68-71
  moving, 71
 vibration detection in, 71-72
Sensory function, impairments of, determination of,
    ASSH and IFSSH principles for, 77-78
Sensory management, in complex regional pain syndrome,
    218, 219f
Sensory reeducation
 definition of, 152
 evaluation timeline for, 161
 outcomes of, 161-162
 postinjury indications/precautions for, 153
 postoperative complications of, 161
 postoperative program for, 155-160
  design of, 155-156, 156f
  early-phase, 156-157, 157f
  five-stage, 158-160
  late-phase, 157-158, 158f
 purpose of, 152
 treatment goals for, 152
Sensory testing
 quantitative, 83-84
 relative guideline for, 85
Shoulder, 327-396
 arthroplasty of, 389-395
  total, 389-309
   evaluation timeline for, 395
   operative indications/precautions for, 392
   postoperative therapy for, 393
   surgical purpose of, 391-392
   treatment goals for, 392
 dislocation of, in athlete, 711

Shoulder *(Continued)*
  glenohumeral instability in, 359-367. *See also*
      Glenohumeral instability.
  humeral fractures and, 369-387. *See also* Humeral fractures.
  injuries to, in athletes, 710-711
  rotator cuff repairs in, 345-358. *See also* Rotator cuff repairs.
  tendonitis of, 329-344
    anatomy associated with, 331f
    evaluation timeline for, 341-342
    nonoperative therapy for, 332-333, 334f-340f
      complications of, 341
      indications/precautions for, 332
    outcomes in, 342
    postoperative therapy for, 341
    treatment goals for, 331-332
    treatment purpose in, 331
Shoulder girdle motion exercise, 132
Silicone gel sheets, in scar management, 42, 44f
Skin, functions of, 29
Skin creases, 228f
Skin flaps, 17-27
  characteristics of, 17t
  definition of, 21
  evaluation timeline for, 26
  free, 20
  functional outcomes of, 26
  indications for, 18-19, 22
  location of, 22
  pedicle, 19-20, 19f, 20f
  postoperative complications of, 25-26
  postoperative evaluation of, 23
  postoperative management of, 24-25
  precautions for, 23
  short-term goals for, 17
  surgical purpose of, 22
  therapy with, 23-25
  treatment goals for, 22
Skin grafts, 17-27
  characteristics of, 17t
  definition of, 21
  evaluation timeline for, 26
  full-thickness (FTSG), 18
    definition of, 21
  functional outcomes of, 26
  indications for, 17-18, 22
  location of, 22
  postoperative complications of, 25-26
  postoperative evaluation of, 23
  postoperative management of, 24
  precautions for, 23
  short-term goals for, 17
  split-thickness (STSG), 17-18
    definition of, 21
  surgical purpose of, 22
  "take" of, 18
  therapy with, 23-25
  treatment goals for, 22
SLAP (superior labrum anterior-posterior) lesion, 364-366
Small joint arthrodesis, of hand, 641-646
  evaluation timeline for, 645
  fixation methods for, 642f
  outcomes of, 645-646, 645t

Small joint arthrodesis, of hand *(Continued)*
  postoperative therapy for, 644-645, 644f
  treatment and surgical purpose of, 643
  treatment goals for, 643
Smith-Hastings procedure, 181-182, 181f, 182f
Social work services, 721-726
  definition of, 722
  indications for, 722
  psychosocial assessment as, 721, 722-723
  psychosocial support as, 721-722
  treatment goals for, 723-726
    adjustment to injury issues in, 723
    alcohol/drug abuse/addictions and, 723-724
    anxiety and, 724
    in chronic pain, 724
    in complex regional pain syndrome, 724
    conversion reactions and, 725
    depression and, 724
    factitious disorder with physical symptoms and, 725
    family problems and, 725
    financial issues and, 725
    lack of social supports and, 725
    marital problems and, 725
    in posttraumatic stress disorder, 725
    previous/current psychiatric treatment and, 725
    stressors and, 725
    transportation problems and, 726
    in traumatic upper extremity amputation, 724
Sodium hypochlorite, in wound cleansing, 10
Soft tissue mobilization, in brachial plexus injury, 208
Somatic block, in complex regional pain syndrome, 221
Splinting
  after Darrach procedure for ulnar head resection, 511
  after partial wrist arthrodesis, 532, 532f
  after Sauve-Kapandji procedure for ulnar head resection,
      512-513, 512f
  after total wrist arthrodesis, 532-533
  after ulnar wafer resection, 513
  in boutonniere deformity, 305, 305f, 306f, 307, 308
  in camptodactyly, 684, 684f
    postoperative, 685
  in carpal fractures, 465-466, 467f
  in carpal tunnel syndrome, 90, 91f
  in complex extensor reconstruction, 320-321, 321f
  in cubital tunnel syndrome, 100-101, 101f
  in digital amputation, 600-601
  in digital replantation, 585, 586f
  in DIP arthroplasty, 636-637, 638f
  in distal radius fracture, 492, 493, 493f, 494f, 499-500,
      500f-501f
  in dorsal hand burns, 33, 33f
  in Dupuytren's disease, 542, 542f
  in epicondylitis, 402, 403f
  in extensor tendon repair
    with early passive motion method of postoperative
        therapy, 282, 283f, 284
    with immobilization method of postoperative
        therapy
      for Zones III and IV, 276, 277f, 278-280, 279f
      for Zones V, VI, and VII, 280, 281f,
          281-283, 283f
  in extensor tenolysis, 314-315, 315f, 316f

Splinting *(Continued)*
  in flexor tendon reconstruction
    postoperative, 253-255, 254f, 255f, 256
    preoperative, 249, 250f-252f
  in flexor tendon repair, 233, 233f, 234f, 235b-236b,
      237f-238f, 238b-239b, 240b, 241b
  in flexor tenolysis, 263, 264f, 265, 265f, 266
  in full-thickness burns, 33, 34
  in injuries in musicians, 701
  in intraarticular middle phalanx fracture, 571-572,
      572f, 573f
  in ligament injuries
    of fingers, 552-553, 552f
    of thumb, 551-552, 551f
  in mallet finger, 295, 296f
  in median nerve repair, 141, 142-143, 142f
  in metacarpophalangeal arthroplasty, 627-628, 628f
  in metacarpophalangeal capsulectomy, 605-609, 610f
  in middle phalanx fractures, 568, 568f
  in palmar midcarpal instability, 468, 469f
  in PIP arthroplasty, 634-636, 635f, 636f, 637f
  in pollicization for hypoplastic thumb, 678
  in proximal interphalangeal joint capsulectomy, 605-609,
      611, 612f-613f
  in radial deficiency, 665, 665f
  in radial nerve palsy, 111, 111f-112f
  in ray resection, 600-601
  in sagittal band injuries, 554, 554f
  in small joint arthrodesis of hand, 644-645, 644f
  in tendon transfers for radial nerve palsy, 189, 190f-191f,
      191-192, 192f
  in thumb carpometacarpal joint arthroplasty, 620, 620f
  in triangular fibrocartilage complex injuries, 479-480,
      479f, 480f
  in trigger digits, 447, 448f
  in ulnar nerve repair, 141, 142-143, 142f, 143f
Split-thickness skin grafts (STSG), 17-18
  definition of, 21
Sports medicine, 707-713. *See also* Athlete.
Staged tendon reconstruction
  definition of, 246, 248f, 249f
  evaluation timeline for, 257
  flexor tenolysis after, 261-269. *See also* Flexor tenolysis.
  outcomes of, 258
  postoperative complications of, 257
  postoperative therapy for, 253-256, 254f, 255f
    indications/precautions for, 252-253, 253f
  postoperative treatment goals for, 249-252
  preoperative therapy for, 248-249, 250f-252f
    goals of, 248
    indications for, 248
  surgical purpose of, 247
Stener lesions, 547-548, 548f
  definition of, 549
Stener-like lesions, definition of, 549
Stereognosis, definition of, 54
Stiles-Bunnel procedure, modified, 180-181
Stress, application of, in scar management, 45
String instruments, injuries specific to, 695-696
STSG. *See* Split-thickness skin grafts (STSG).
Subacromial impingement, 329-330. *See also* Shoulder,
    tendonitis of.

Superficial partial-thickness burns
  definition of, 30, 30f
  postoperative therapy for, in acute stage, 32
Superior labrum anterior-posterior (SLAP) lesion, 364-366
Surgery
  for burns, indications for, 32
  laser, in scar management, 42
  scar revision, 46-48
Surgical wound, definition of, 3
Swan-neck deformity, 297-302
  anatomy in, 298f
  causes of, 297-298
  classification of, 298
  definition of, 298, 299f
  evaluation timeline for, 302
  nonoperative therapy for, 300
    complications of, 300
    indications/precautions for, 299-300
  operative complications of, 301-302
  postoperative therapy for, 301, 636
    indications/precautions for, 300-301
  treatment and surgical purpose of, 298-299
  treatment goals in, 299
Sympathetic block, in complex regional pain syndrome,
    220, 221f
Sympathetic nerve, status of, sensibility testing for, 59-60
Syndactyly, 679-681, 679f, 680b, 682f
Synovectomy, rheumatoid wrist, arthroscopic,
    postoperative therapy for, 456-457

T
Tactile gnosis, definition of, 54
Tendinopathy(ies)
  definition of, 441
  wrist and hand, 441-452
    definition of, 441-443
    evaluation timeline for, 450-451
    nonoperative therapy for, 445-447, 446f
      complications of, 447
      indications/precautions for, 444-445, 444f
    outcomes of, 451
    postoperative therapy for, 449-450
      complications of, 450
      indications/precautions for, 447, 449
    treatment goals for, 444
    treatment purpose for, 443-444
Tendinosis, elbow
  lateral, definition of, 399-400
  medial, definition of, 400
Tendon(s)
  extensor, 271-326. *See also* Extensor tendon(s).
  flexor, 227-269. *See also* Flexor tendon(s).
  healing of, 227
  inflammation of. *See* Tendonitis.
  injuries to, 225-326
  transfers of, 165-194. *See also* Tendon transfers.
  wrist
    anatomy of, 443f
    extension, transfer of, in arthrogryposis management, 673
Tendon gliding
  after repair, 272-274
  exercises for, after flexor tenolysis, 266-267, 266f

Tendon grafting, primary, definition of, 246
Tendon transfers
    definition of, 166, 177, 187
    for median nerve palsy, 165-173
        evaluation timeline for, 170-171
        for high median nerve injury, postoperative therapy in,
            169-170, 170f
        for low median nerve injury, postoperative
            therapy in, 167-169, 167f, 168f, 169f
        outcomes of, 171-172, 171t, 172t
        postoperative complications of, 170
        postoperative indications/precautions for, 167
        postoperative therapy for, 167-170
        treatment goals for, 166-167
    purpose of, 165, 166
    for radial nerve palsy, 187-194
        evaluation timeline for, 193
        nonoperative complications of, 189
        outcomes of, 193
        postoperative complications of, 193
        postoperative indications/precautions for therapy in, 189
        postoperative therapy in, 189
        precautions for, 188
        preoperative therapy for, 188-189, 190f-191f
        purpose of, 187, 188
        treatment goals for, 188
    for ulnar nerve palsy, 175-185
        evaluation timeline in, 184
        for low ulnar nerve injury, postoperative therapy for,
            178-182, 179f, 180f, 181f, 182f
        postoperative complications of, 184
        postoperative indications/precautions for, 178
        purpose of, 177
        treatment goals for, 177-178
Tendonitis, 399
    biceps, in athletes, 711
    extensor carpi ulnaris, 442
    extensor digiti minimi, 442
    extensor pollicis longus, 441-442
    rotator cuff, in athletes, 710-711
    shoulder, 329-344
Tennis elbow. See also Epicondylitis.
    definition of, 399-400
Tenosynovitis, De Quervain's. See De Quervain's
        tenosynovitis.
TENS (transcutaneous electrical nerve stimulation)
    for desensitization, 154-155
    for shoulder tendonitis, 332
Terminal median nerve, muscles innervated by, 90t
Texture discrimination, definition of, 54
Texture(s), graded, for desensitization, 153, 164
TFCC. See Triangular fibrocartilage complex (TFCC).
Thoracic outlet syndrome (TOS), 121-137, 198
    brachial plexus traction injury compared with, 198t
    causes of, 121-122
    definition of, 123-124
    diagnosis of, 122-123
    evaluation timeline for, 135
    nonoperative therapy for, 125-134
        accessory joint movement therapy in, 131
        brachial plexus gliding exercises in, 131
        conservative management in, 128-134

Thoracic outlet syndrome (TOS) (Continued)
    nonoperative therapy for (Continued)
        driving position in, 130, 130f
        general precautions in, 130-131
        history in, 125
        indications/precautions for, 124-125
        muscle spasm/tension management in, 131
        pain management in, 131
        patient education in, 128-131
        physical examination in, 125-127
        postural exercises in, 131-134, 133f, 134f
        posture in, 128-129, 128f
        pretreatment evaluation in, 125-127
        ROM exercises in, 134
        sleep positions in, 129, 129f
        treatment in, 127-134
        working in, 129-130
    operative management of
        indications/precautions for, 134
        techniques for, 134
        therapy and complications after, 135
    outcomes of, 135
    sites of compression in, 121, 122f
    treatment purpose and goals for, 124
Thumb
    arthrodesis in, 641-646. See also Small joint arthrodesis,
        of hand.
    in arthrogryposis, operative management of, 672, 672f
    carpometacarpal joint of, arthroplasty of, 617-623. See also
        Carpometacarpal (CMC) joint, thumb.
    contracted clasped, in arthrogryposis management, 674
    hypoplastic, 674-678
        classification of, 674, 675t
        clinical presentation of, 674-676, 675f
        definition of, 674
        nonoperative management of, 676
        operative management of, 676, 677f, 677t
        outcomes of, 678
        postoperative management of, 677-678
        reconstruction of, 676
        treatment goals for, 676
    ligament injuries of, 547-548, 548f
        evaluation timeline for, 557
        nonoperative therapy for, 551-552
        outcomes of, 558
        postoperative therapy for, 555
        treatment and surgical purpose for, 549-550
    reconstruction of, postoperative management of,
        677-678
    replantation of, postoperative therapy for, 589-590
Tinel's sign, in brachial plexus injury, 202
Tissue expanders, 20
    postoperative management of, 25
Tissue transfer, free
    postoperative management of, 25
    vascularized, definition of, 21
TOS. See Thoracic outlet syndrome (TOS).
Total shoulder arthroplasty (TSA). See also Shoulder,
        arthroplasty of, total.
    definition of, 389-390
Total wrist arthrodesis
    definition of, 530, 530f

Total wrist arthrodesis *(Continued)*
    indications for, 531-532
    postoperative therapy for, 532-533
Touch
    point or area localization of, sensibility testing for, 67-68
    referred, definition of, 54
Touch-pressure threshold detection level, definition of, 54
Transcutaneous electrical nerve stimulation (TENS)
    for desensitization, 154-155
    for shoulder tendonitis, 332
Transposition
    anterior, for ulnar nerve compression, 101-102
    medial, for ulnar nerve compression, 102
Transverse deficiency, 660-662, 660f, 661f
Trapezial fracture, 462
Trapeziometacarpal joint, 617. *See also* Carpometacarpal
            (CMC) joint, thumb.
Trapezoid fractures, 463
Trauma, glenohumeral instability from, 359-362. *See also*
            Glenohumeral instability, traumatic unidirectional.
Traumatic open wound, definition of, 3
Triangular fibrocartilage complex (TFCC)
    anatomy of, 475, 476f
    debridement of
        evaluation and treatment timeline for, 481-483
        postoperative complications of, 484
    definition of, 475
    injuries to, 475-487
        degenerative, 475-476, 476, 478f
            treatment indicaitons/technique for, 478-479
        nonoperative management of, 479
            timeline for, 479-481
        operative indications for, 481
        traumatic, 475, 476, 477f
            treatment indications/technique for, 477-478
        treatment indications/technique for, 477-479
    peripheral tear of, primary tear of, 484-486
Triceps lengthening, in arthrogryposis management, 673
Trigger digits, 443
    nonoperative therapy for, 447, 448f
        indications/precautions for, 445
    postoperative therapy for, 449-450
        complications of, 450
Trigger finger, anatomy of, 442f
Trigger points, myofascial, 199t
Triquetrum, fracture of, 462
TSA (total shoulder arthroplasty). *See* Shoulder,
            arthroplasty of, total.
    definition of, 389-390
Tuning forks, in vibration testing, 71-72
Two-point discrimination test
    computerized, 72
    for innervation density, 68-71
    moving, 71

U

U-shaped tears, definition of, 347
UCL. *See* Ulnar collateral ligament (UCL).
Ulna
    dislocations of, 411, 411f
        nonoperative therapy for, 415-416
        postoperative therapy for, 419

Ulna *(Continued)*
    head of, resection of, 507-515
        Darrach procedure for, 507, 508f
        evaluation timeline for, 513-514
        hemiresection-interposition technique of,
            507-508, 508f
        matched procedure for, 508, 509f
        operative indications/precautions for, 510
        outcomes of, 514
        postoperative therapy for, 511-513, 512f
            complications of, 513
            indications/precautions for, 511
        Sauve-Kapandji procedure for, 509, 509f
        surgical purpose of, 510
        treatment goals for, 510
        ulnar wafer resection in, 509-510, 510f
    proximal, fractures of, 410
        nonoperative therapy for, 415
        postoperative therapy for, 418
Ulnar collateral ligament (UCL)
    injuries to, 547
    tears of, incomplete
        definition of, 548
        of fingers, nonoperative therapy for, 552-553
        of thumb, nonoperative therapy for,
            551-552, 551f
Ulnar nerve
    injury to
        high, tendon transfer for, postoperative therapy in,
            183-184, 183f
        low, tendon transfer for, postoperative therapy in,
            178-182, 179f, 180f, 181f, 182f
    provocative test for, 57, 58f
    repair of
        with flexor tendon involvement, postoperative
            care in, 144-145
        studies of, 146t
        at wrist level, postoperative therapy for, 141-143,
            142f, 143f
Ulnar nerve compression, 97-107
    in cubital tunnel, 97, 98f
    definitions of, 98-99
    evaluation timeline for, 104-105
    in Guyon's canal, 97-98, 99f
        definition of, 99
    nonoperative treatment of
        complications of, 101
        indications/precautions for, 100
        for mild compression, 100-101
    outcomes for, 105
    surgical purpose in, 99
    surgical treatment of, 101-102
        complications after, 104
        indications/precautions after, 102
        therapy after, 102-104
    treatment goals in, 99
Ulnar nerve palsy
    signs of, 175
    tendon transfers for, 175-185. *See also* Tendon transfers,
            for ulnar nerve palsy.
Ulnar wafer resection, 509-510, 510f
    therapy after, 513

Ultrasound
   for desensitization, 155
   for shoulder tendonitis, 332
Upper limb tension testing (ULTT), in brachial plexus
      injury, 203-204, 204f-205f, 205t

V

Vasomotor management, in complex regional pain
      syndrome, 218, 219f, 220f
Verapamil injection, in scar management, 42
Vibration, graded, for desensitization, 153-154,
      154f, 164
Vibration testing, 71-72
   computerized, 72
Video analysis, in injury management in
      musician, 699
Volar dislocation, definition of, 572
Volar ganglion excision, arthroscopy for, postoperative
      therapy for, 456

W

Wartenberg syndrome, 117-119
Wartenburg's sign, in ulnar nerve palsy, 175, 176f
Whirlpool therapy, in Dupuytren's disease, 542
Wind instruments, injuries specific to, 697
Work adjustment, 727
Work hardening, 728
   roles of industrial rehabilitation team members in,
      732-733
Work-related musculoskeletal disorders (WMSDs), 728
Wound
   burn, 29-37. See also Burns.
   care of, 3-15
      surgical purpose of, 4
      treatment goal in, 4
   cleansing of, 10
   complications of, 13
   debridement of, 10-11
   definition of, 3
   dressings for, 11
      characteristics of, healing and, 13t
   environment of, protecting, 10-11
   evaluation of, 6-8, 8f, 9f
   healing of
      dressing characteristics and, 13t
      phases of, 39
      physiology of, 4-6, 5f
   infected, 8, 9f
   management of, 1-50
   physiology of, 4-6, 5f
   scar management in, 39-50. See also Scar(s).
   skin grafts and flaps for, 17-27. See also Skin flaps;
      Skin grafts.

Wound (Continued)
   therapy for, 4-13
      indications/precautions for, 4
      influencing collagen maturation process in, 12-13
      minimizing mechanical influence in, 12
      protecting environment in, 10-11
Wrist, 439-536
   arthrodesis of, 529-535
      definition of, 530
      evaluation timeline for, 533-534
      operative indications/precautions for therapy in, 531-532
      outcomes of, 534
      postoperative complications in, 533
      postoperative therapy for, 532-533, 532f
      surgical purpose of, 530
      treatment goals of, 531
   in arthrogryposis, operative management of, 671-672
   arthroplasty of, 523-527
      definition of, 523-524
      evaluation timeline for, 526
      outcomes of, 526-527
      postoperative therapy for, 525-526, 526f
         complications of, 526
         considerations/precautions for, 524-525
      surgical purpose of, 524
      treatment goals of, 524
   arthroscopy of, 453-459
      operative indications/precautions for, 454-455
      outcomes of, 458
      portals for, 453, 454f
      postoperative therapy for, 455-457
         complications of, 457
         indications/precautions for, 455
      surgical purpose of, 453
      timeline for, 457-458
      treatment goals for, 453-454
   carpal fractures and instabilities and, 461-474. See also
         Carpal bones.
   joints of, 461
   proximal row carpectomy and, 517-521. See also
         Proximal row carpectomy (PRC).
   tendinopathies of, 441-452. See also Tendinopathy(ies),
         wrist and hand.
   triangular fibrocartilage complex injuries and, 475-487.
         See also Triangular fibrocartilage complex (TFCC).
   unstable distal radius fractures and, 489-505. See also
         Radius, distal, fractures of, unstable.
Wrist extension tendon transfer, in arthrogryposis
      management, 673
Wrist tenodesis, in extensor tendon repair, 283

Z

Zancolli lasso procedure, 178-180, 179f